REHABILITATION OF THE HEAD INJURED ADULT

REHABILITATION OF THE HEAD INJURED ADULT

MITCHELL ROSENTHAL, Ph.D
ASSISTANT PROFESSOR OF REHABILITATION MEDICINE
TUFTS UNIVERSITY SCHOOL OF MEDICINE
DIRECTOR OF REHABILITATION PSYCHOLOGY
NEW ENGLAND MEDICAL CENTER
DIRECTOR OF TRAINING
TUFTS-NEW ENGLAND MEDICAL CENTER
  MEDICAL REHABILITATION RESEARCH AND TRAINING CENTER
BOSTON, MASSACHUSETTS

ERNEST R. GRIFFITH, M.D.
MEDICAL DIRECTOR
INSTITUTE OF REHABILITATION MEDICINE
GOOD SAMARITAN HOSPITAL
PHOENIX, ARIZONA

MICHAEL R. BOND, M.D., Ph.D., FRCS, MRC Psych., MRCP, DPM
PROFESSOR AND CHAIRMAN
DEPARTMENT OF PSYCHOLOGICAL MEDICINE
UNIVERSITY OF GLASGOW
GLASGOW, SCOTLAND, UNITED KINGDOM

J. DOUGLAS MILLER, M.D., Ph.D., FRCS Ed., FRCS Glas., FACS
PROFESSOR AND CHAIRMAN
DEPARTMENT OF SURGICAL NEUROLOGY
THE ROYAL INFIRMARY
UNIVERSITY OF EDINBURGH
EDINBURGH, SCOTLAND, UNITED KINGDOM

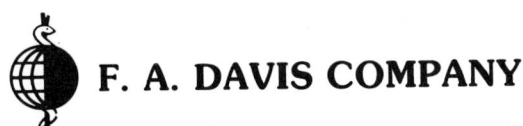

F. A. DAVIS COMPANY   Philadelphia

Copyright © 1983 by F.A. Davis Company
Second printing 1984

All rights reserved. This book is protected by copyright. No part of it may be reproduced, stored in a retrieval system, or transmitted in any form or by any means, electronic, mechanical, photocopying, recording, or otherwise, without written permission from the publisher.

Printed in the United States of America

Library of Congress Cataloging in Publication Data
Main entry under title:

Rehabilitation of the head-injured adult.

   Includes bibliographical references and index.
   1. Head—Wounds and injuries—Complications and sequelae. 2. Brain damage—Patients—Rehabilitation. I. Rosenthal, Mitchell, 1949– . [DNLM: 1. Head injuries—Rehabilitation. WE 706 R345]
RD521.R45   1983   617'.51044   82-23504
ISBN 0-8036-7625-5

THIS BOOK IS DEDICATED TO THE FAMILIES OF HEAD-INJURED PERSONS.

FOREWORD

Although head injury is 10 times more frequent than spinal injuries, there is much less chance that the victim of head injury will be fortunate enough to find a coherent and expertly conceived rehabilitation program. The problems of paraplegia are fairly stereotyped and well understood, with solutions available for most of them. By comparison, the disabilities after head injury are complex and varied and are seldom fully recognized; even when they are, their management is often difficult. The main reason for this is that mental deficits dominate—and these interfere both with the patient's ability to cope and with the capacity for cooperation with those trying to help the patient. No wonder that therapists not sensitive to the subtleties of brain damage often tend to reject head-injured patients; even families and friends find them a trial. The aggressive muscular approach that so often pays off with paraplegic patients is doomed to failure with most head injuries. Yet many patients make a good recovery, whereas others can be taught to cope with their altered selves and to make a new life by capitalizing on their remaining assets. In this regard, head-injured patients present a challenge, responding to which can prove most rewarding for those therapists who are prepared to make the effort.

There is a welcome awakening in the therapeutic community on both sides of the Atlantic to the needs of the head-injured patient. Courses on this topic have been consistently oversubscribed, and by a broad spectrum of disciplines—physicians, nurses, and social workers, as well as those more conventionally associated with rehabilitation.

This book is for all of the health-care community interested in rehabilitating head-injured patients. It endeavors to explain the many facets of head injury in the acute and late stages, with a view to improving understanding of how to plan not only rehabilitation but also studies in rehabilitation. The latter are needed not only in order to devise and test new techniques, but also so that methods already in use can be re-examined with a view to discarding those found not to be effective. In the call for more rehabilitation, however, there is need to resist the temptation to indulge in action for its own sake, or to accept as self-evident that more rehabilitation must always mean more benefit for patients. Rehabilitation depends on the intensive use of the scarcest of all resources—skilled personnel. We should therefore seek to deploy such skills in an appropriate manner—that is to say, in circumstances in which they are both necessary and effective. Only in that way will patients and society benefit most from our efforts.

Bryan Jennett, M.D.
University of Glasgow
Glasgow, Scotland

PREFACE

For the victim, family member, and health-care professional, head injury has always been something of a "puzzle." The event creating the injury occurs suddenly without warning. From that instant, the course of medical and rehabilitative management proceeds, but ultimately may not resolve the nagging questions posed by family members: "Will he ever be the same person again?" "What kind of life can he have now that he is brain-damaged?" Head injury often strikes persons within the prime of their lives—aged 16 to 35 years. Often, these victims are, at the time of injury, in the midst of carving out social, vocational, and economic patterns that typically last a lifetime. Yet, in the case of severe head injury, all of this is changed—often permanently. Within the past few decades, the advances in neurosurgical diagnostic and management techniques have enabled many persons to survive the immediate consequences of the injury. However, this newly head-injured person and the family are then faced with the difficulties inherent in continued survival and the challenge of regaining a measure of productivity and happiness.

Those professionals concerned with rehabilitation have only recently truly awakened to the plight of head-injured persons. That is not to say that head-injured persons have not received rehabilitative services for the past 30 years. Instead, I would suggest that the impression of "irreversibility of damage to brain tissue" has led many to behave as if rehabilitation efforts were rarely successful in restoring the person to a meaningful, productive existence. The public has also been frightened by head injury, perhaps because of its close association with the concept of brain damage, which has often incorrectly been equated with "mentally retarded," "emotionally disturbed," "physically crippled," and the like. Though the process of neural reconstitution and recovery from head injury is still not fully understood, those practicing within the medical and allied health community appear to be more hopeful about the future prospects of head-injured patients.

The "puzzle" of head injury is partly attributable to the extraordinary array of physical and mental sequelae of the injury, and the lack of adequate, scientifically based methods of treating these deficits in a systematic, effective manner. The fact that no two head injuries result in the exact same sequelae precludes broad generalizations for rehabilitation management and necessitates individualized treatment programs. In the not-so-distant past, many well-meaning practitioners equated head injury with stroke and dealt with these two populations in a similar manner. However, the research and clinical experiences gained in the past decade have highlighted the important differences in the initial neurologic insult and eventual residual deficits. One such finding—namely, that head injury usually results in diffuse brain damage, while stroke often is focal and unilateral in its locus—has helped to explain the greater variety of physical and mental deficits following head injury. For example, a stroke patient with a right brain insult may experience motor paralysis on the left side, spatial disorientation, dysarthria, and emotional lability. In contrast, a closed head injury impacting on the right hemisphere may cause a "contre-coup" effect, which may result in diffuse damage. The manifestations of this injury could include bilateral motor weakness, subtle language deficits, post-traumatic amnesia, motor slowing, impaired perception, emotional blunting, altered sensation, and so forth. In addition, the head-injured victim often sustains associated injuries, which may include leg fractures, spinal cord injury, and facial lacerations.

The sum total of head injury may often be the temporary or permanent displacement of the victim and family. The victim may struggle for many years to accept and understand what has really happened. Life can become a series of frustrations and obstacles that often lead to exasperating failures. Head-injured persons return to the community to find that previous friendships and rewarding activities have been greatly restricted. After the euphoria accompanying discharge from the hospital subsides, relationships with spouse, family members, and significant others become strained. Economic hardship becomes a new reality. Some head-injured persons describe their houses as "feeling like a prison." A fight for emotional, social, and economic independence is likely to be a long, painful one.

The initial impetus for the writing of this text comes from our collective involvement in the Annual Post-Graduate Course on the Rehabilitation of the Brain Injured Adult, sponsored by the Medical College of Virginia. When initiated in 1977, no other annual course on head injury was ongoing in the United States. The first program was planned with the hope that 50 to 100 rehabilitation professionals would attend. More than 250 applications were received for that course. By 1981, at least 10 major hospitals had initiated annual courses in head injury, involving more than 2000 health-care professionals per year. Clearly, the compelling nature of the topic has been established. No fewer than 30 hospitals and rehabilitation centers have opened specialized head-injury units within the past 5 years.

A second motivating force for producing this book has been the dearth of previous texts or articles directed toward educating the rehabilitation professional about head injury. The last book of this type was published in 1969. Drs. Walker and Caveness edited a book entitled *The Late Effects of Head Injury*, which was a compilation of papers from a symposium. At each meeting about head injury, rehabilitation professionals posed the question, "Why doesn't someone publish a book about rehabilitation and head injury?" Finally, we decided to answer this question by compiling the current volume.

Since this book is the first text on head-injury rehabilitation in many years, we have attempted to be as comprehensive as possible. The attempt to adequately cover such a broad topic is fraught with perils. By presenting a comprehensive overview of the subject, we have not been able to provide as much depth on some topics as we would like. Thus, the physician may be disappointed at the relatively few chapters devoted exclusively to medical assessment and management. Yet other texts may fulfill this need, such as the recently published book by Bryan Jennett and Graham Teasdale, *Management of Head Injuries* (F. A. Davis, 1981). Certain rehabilitation professionals may feel that their specialty area, such as nursing or physical therapy, has not been given adequate space. Regrettably, the field of head injury encompasses so many disciplines that the volume would have exceeded 1000 pages if material was presented for every group of professionals involved with brain injury—for example, nutrition, law, recreational therapy, education, psychiatry, and orthopedic surgery. Nonetheless, we are of the opinion that the content of the book will be valuable for all those concerned with head injury, regardless of their specific area.

Another difficulty in writing this book was to strike a balance between an academic and a clinical point of view. Predictably, the point of view varies depending on each chapter's author. We have designed the book not only to highlight important research advances of the

PREFACE

past decade but to allow clinicians to find it useful as a guide to clinical practice. It is our sincere hope that each reader will find something of value that will generalize to his or her clinical practice.

This book owes its existence to a great many people. First and foremost, we are indebted to our contributors, whose long and hard labors have resulted in this text. I am personally grateful to the indefatigable efforts of my co-editors, Drs. Griffith, Bond, and Miller. Without their assistance, the book would likely still be in the planning stages. The support and editorial assistance provided by Mr. Bob Martone has been exceedingly valuable. I would like to express my deep appreciation to my colleagues who had a major role in planning and running the series of head-injury courses that led to the volume, especially Richard and Christi Eisenberg, Linda Diehl, Rita Riani, Robin McNeny, Jean Cerny, and others at the Medical College of Virginia. I also appreciate the support and encouragement provided by my colleagues at the Department of Rehabilitation Medicine, Tufts-New England Medical Center—especially my chairman, Dr. Bruce Gans. My thanks are also extended to Dr. Roberta Trieschmann, Dr. Cynthia Dember, and Dr. Paul Karoly, all of whom were important influences in my early career as a graduate student. The assistance of Mrs. Sarah McGillowey in typing the final manuscript is gratefully acknowledged. Finally, I express my heartfelt appreciation to my wife Peggy, daughter Michelle, and parents Morris and Edythe for their love, support, and encouragement.

Mitchell Rosenthal

CONTRIBUTORS

YEHUDA BEN-YISHAY, Ph.D.
Associate Professor of Clinical Rehabilitation Medicine, Co-Director, Head Trauma Program, New York University Medical Center, New York, New York; Visiting Associate Professor of Clinical Rehabilitation Medicine, University of Tel Aviv School of Medicine, Tel Aviv, Israel

SHELDON BERROL, M.D.
Clinical Assistant Professor of Rehabilitation Medicine, Stanford University; Senior Consultant, Santa Clara Valley Medical Center, San Jose, California; Assistant Clinical Professor of Physical Medicine and Rehabilitation, University of California, San Francisco, Oakland, California

JOHN P. BOLGER, M.S.
Rehabilitation Psychologist, Head Trauma Program, Woodrow Wilson Rehabilitation Center, Fishersville, Virginia

MICHAEL R. BOND, M.D., Ph.D., FRCS, MRC Psych., MRCP, DPM
Professor and Chairman, Department of Psychological Medicine, University of Glasgow, Glasgow, Scotland, United Kingdom

D. NEIL BROOKS, Ph.D.
Senior Lecturer in Clinical Psychology, Department of Psychological Medicine, University of Glasgow; Clinical Psychologist, Greater Glasgow Health Board, Glasgow, Scotland, United Kingdom

JOHN J. CARONNA, M.D.
Professor and Vice-Chairman, Department of Neurology, The New York Hospital-Cornell Medical Center, New York, New York

JEAN CERNY, O.T.R.
Supervisor, Department of Occupational Therapy, Medical College of Virginia Hospital, Richmond, Virginia

LINDA NIELSON DIEHL, R.N., M.S.
Director of Nursing, Sheltering Arms Hospital, Virginia Rehabilitation Center for Adults; Assistant Professor of Rehabilitation Medicine, Medical College of Virginia, Virginia Commonwealth University, Richmond, Virginia

LEONARD DILLER, Ph.D.
Chief, Behavioral Sciences, Professor of Clinical Rehabilitation Medicine, Co-Director, Cognitive Remediation Program, New York University Medical Center, New York, New York

RICHARD P. GREENBERG, M.D., Ph.D.
Assistant Professor of Neurosurgery, Medical College of Virginia, Virginia Commonwealth University, Richmond, Virginia

ERNEST R. GRIFFITH, M.D.
Medical Director, Institute of Rehabilitation Medicine, Good Samaritan Hospital, Phoenix, Arizona

MICHAEL GROHER, Ph.D.
Assistant Chief, Audiology and Speech Pathology, Veterans Administration Medical Center, New York, New York

EMILY HACKLER, R.N., M.A.
Clinical Associate Department of Physical Medicine and Rehabilitation, University of California-Irvine College of Medicine, Orange, California

WILLIAM J. HAFFEY, Ph.D.
Staff Neuropsychologist, Casa Colina Hospital for Rehabilitative Medicine, Pomona, California

JOHN A. JANE, M.D., Ph.D.
Professor and Chairman, Department of Neurosurgery, University of Virginia Medical Center, Charlottesville, Virginia

BRYAN JENNETT, M.D., FRCS
Dean, Faculty of Medicine; Professor of Neurosurgery, University of Glasgow, Southern General Hospital, Glasgow, Scotland, United Kingdom

WILLIAM J. LYNCH, Ph.D.
Director, Brain Injury Rehabilitation Program, Palo Alto Veterans Administration Medical Center, Menlo Park, California

DIANE KARAICA, A.A.
Occupational Therapy Assistant, Brain Injury Program, Casa Colina Hospital for Rehabilitative Medicine, Pomona, California

ROBIN McNENY, O.T.R.
Senior Staff Therapist, Department of Occupational Therapy, Medical College of Virginia Hospital, Richmond, Virginia

J. DOUGLAS MILLER, M.D., Ph.D., FRCS Ed., FRCS Glas., FACS
Professor and Chairman, Department of Surgical Neurology, The Royal Infirmary, University of Edinburgh, Scotland, United Kingdom

CRAIG A. MUIR, Ph.D.
Director of Neuropsychology Service, Casa Colina Hospital for Rehabilitative Medicine, Pomona, California

CONTRIBUTORS

JANE H. MUIR, R.P.T.
Program Manager, Brain Injury Program, Casa Colina Hospital for Rehabilitative Medicine, Pomona, California

ARTHUR J. NELSON, Ph.D., R.P.T.
Professor and Chairman, School of Physical Therapy, New York University Medical Center, New York, New York

PAULINE G. NEWLON, M.S.
Research Assistant, Department of Neurosurgery, Medical College of Virginia, Virginia Commonwealth University, Richmond, Virginia

KATHRYN J. OTT, B.S.N.
Staff Nurse, Brain Injury Program, Casa Colina Hospital for Rehabilitative Medicine, Pomona, California

REBECCA W. RIMEL, R.N., N.P.
Director, Clinical Head Injury Research Unit, Assistant Professor of Neurosurgery, University of Virginia Medical Center, Charlottesville, Virginia

MITCHELL ROSENTHAL, Ph.D.
Assistant Professor of Rehabilitation Medicine, Tufts University School of Medicine; Director of Rehabilitation Psychology, New England Medical Center; Director of Training, Tufts-New England Medical Center Medical Rehabilitation Research and Training Center, Boston, Massachusetts

ROBERT M. SMITH, M.Ed.
Chief, Speech Pathology and Audiology, Veterans Administration Medical Center, Lebanon, Pennsylvania

MARGARET SUTKO, Ph.D.
Staff Psychologist, Brain Injury Program, Casa Colina Hospital for Rehabilitative Medicine, Pomona, California

JEROME S. TOBIS, M.D.
Professor and Chairman, Department of Physical Medicine and Rehabilitation, University of California-Irvine College of Medicine, Orange, California

PAULA E. WAHLSTROM, O.T.R.
Senior Staff Therapist, Department of Occupational Therapy, Rancho Los Amigos Hospital, Downey, California

CONTENTS

SECTION 1 NATURE OF THE PROBLEM 1

Chapter 1 SCALE AND SCOPE OF THE PROBLEM 3
Bryan Jennett, M.D.

   SEVERITY OF INJURY 4
   NATURE OF THE DISABILITY 5
   RECOVERY AFTER HEAD INJURY 6
   REFERENCES 8

Chapter 2 CHARACTERISTICS OF THE HEAD-INJURED PATIENT 9
Rebecca W. Rimel, R.N., N.P.
John A. Jane, M.D., Ph.D.

   PATIENT CHARACTERISTICS 11
      Age and Sex 11
      Socioeconomic Status 12
      Medical History 13
      Cause of Injury 13
      Location of Injury 14
      Time of Injury 14
   SEVERITY OF INJURY 14
      Glasgow Coma Scale 15
      Clinical Course 16
      Length of Hospital Stay 18
   OUTCOME 18
      Outcome at Discharge 19
      Outcome at Three Months 19
   SUMMARY 20

REFERENCES 21
BIBLIOGRAPHY 21

Chapter 3 TYPES OF DISABILITY 23
Ernest R. Griffith, M.D.

PHYSICAL IMPAIRMENTS AND RESULTING DISABILITIES 24
- Motor Impairments 24
- Sensory Impairments and Aberrations 24
- Disabilities of Physical Function Resulting From Motor and Sensory Impairments 25
- Pre-Existing Physical Impairments 26
- Disabilities Resulting From Associated Injuries 26
- Disabilities Resulting From Medical Complications 26

COMMUNICATION DISABILITIES 27
PSYCHOLOGIC DISABILITIES 27
SOCIAL DISABILITIES 30
EDUCATIONAL AND VOCATIONAL DISABILITIES 30
"MINOR BRAIN TRAUMA" 31
SUMMARY 31
REFERENCES 31

CONCLUSION 33
Michael R. Bond, M.D., Ph.D., FRCS, MRC Psych., MRCP, DPM

SECTION 2 EARLY METHODS OF ASSESSMENT AND TREATMENT 35

Chapter 4 EARLY EVALUATION AND MANAGEMENT 37
J. Douglas Miller, M.D., Ph.D., FRCS Ed., FRCS Glas., FACS

PATHOPHYSIOLOGY OF HEAD INJURY 37
- Premorbid Status of the Brain 37
- Primary Impact Damage to the Brain 38
- Primary Impact Damage to the Scalp, Skull, Dura, and Other Structures 39
- The Concept of Concussion 40

SECONDARY INSULTS TO THE INJURED BRAIN 41
- Arterial Hypoxemia 41
- Arterial Hypotension 42
- Anemia 42
- Hyponatremia 42
- Post-Traumatic Intracranial Hematoma 43
- Brain Swelling 43
- Raised Intracranial Pressure 43

CONTENTS

      Intracranial Infection   44
      Hydrocephalus   44
      Post-Traumatic Epilepsy   45
   SECONDARY DAMAGE TO THE INJURED BRAIN   45
      Brain Distortion, Shift, and Herniation   45
      Hypoxic/Ischemic Brain Damage   46
   DIAGNOSIS IN HEAD INJURY   46
      Determinants of Head Injury   46
      Triage of Head-Injured Patients   47
      Evaluation of the Comatose Head-Injured Patient   48
   MANAGEMENT OF SEVERE HEAD INJURY   51
      Early Measures at the Scene of the Accident and in Transit   51
      Management in the Emergency Room   51
      Operative Management of Head Injury   52
      Management in the Intensive-Care Unit   52
      Treatment of Raised Intracranial Pressure   53
   PROCESS OF RECOVERY FROM HEAD INJURY   53
   FACTORS THAT HAVE A MAJOR INFLUENCE ON OUTCOME FROM SEVERE HEAD INJURY   55
   REFERENCES   56
   BIBLIOGRAPHY   58

Chapter 5   **THE NEUROLOGIC EVALUATION**   59
      John J. Caronna, M.D.

   THE ACUTE PHASE   59
      Regulation of Consciousness   60
      Pathophysiology of Coma   61
   IMMEDIATE MANAGEMENT OF THE COMATOSE PATIENT   63
      Maintenance of Respiration   63
      Blood Chemistries and Dextrose Administration   63
      Nasogastric Intubation   64
      Blood Pressure   64
      Pulse   64
      Traumatic Injuries   64
      Hypothermia   64
      Fever   65
      Neurologic Examination   65
      Neurologic Assessment in the Recovery Stage   68
   PREDICTION OF OUTCOME IN COMA   68
      Head Injury   69
      Medical Coma   69
   ASSESSMENT OF OUTCOME   70
      When to Assess Outcome   70
      Outcome After Head Injury   71
      The Vegetative State After Head Injury   71
      Conclusion   71
   REFERENCES   71

Chapter 6 ASSESSMENT OF BRAIN FUNCTION WITH MULTIMODALITY EVOKED POTENTIALS 75
Pauline G. Newlon, M.S.
Richard P. Greenberg, M.D., Ph.D.

MULTIMODALITY EVOKED POTENTIALS 77
  Multimodality Evoked Potentials in Comatose Patients 77
  Analysis of Data 78
  Detecting Brain Dysfunction With Sensory Evoked Potentials 82
MULTIMODALITY EVOKED POTENTIAL AND PROGNOSIS 87
  Severity of Dysfunction 87
  Extent of Dysfunction 88
  Secondary Insults 88
  Serial Evaluation: Dynamics of Recovery 91
  Early Multimodality Evoked Potentials and Clinical Recovery 91
SUMMARY 95
REFERENCES 95
BIBLIOGRAPHY 96

Chapter 7 STANDARDIZED METHODS OF ASSESSING AND PREDICTING OUTCOME 97
Michael R. Bond, M.D., Ph.D., FRCS, MRC Psych., MRCP, DPM

WHY MEASURE OUTCOME? 97
THE PROCESS OF MEASUREMENT 97
AIMS OF MEASUREMENT 100
MEASURES OF OUTCOME 100
ASSESSMENT OF SEVERITY OF INJURY 100
  Assessment of Post-Traumatic Amnesia 100
  Measurement of Coma Duration 101
NEUROLOGIC ASSESSMENT OF OUTCOME 103
ASSESSMENT OF MENTAL OUTCOME 105
  Cognitive and Perceptual Functions 105
  Assessment of Personality and Behavior 107
ASSESSMENT OF OVERALL OUTCOME 108
ASSESSMENT OF SOCIAL ADJUSTMENT 111
CONCLUSION 112
REFERENCES 112

CONCLUSION 115
J. Douglas Miller, M.D., Ph.D., FRCS Ed., FRCS Glas., FACS

SECTION 3 SPECIFIC PROBLEMS RELATED TO HEAD INJURY 117

Chapter 8 POST-TRAUMATIC EPILEPSY 119
Bryan Jennett, M.D.

CONTENTS

FEATURES OF EARLY (FIRST WEEK) EPILEPSY 119
FEATURES OF LATE EPILEPSY 120
PREDICTING LATE EPILEPSY 120
PREVENTION OF LATE EPILEPSY 122
EPILEPSY AND DRIVING 123
REFERENCES 124

Chapter 9 SPASTICITY 125
Ernest R. Griffith, M.D.

ETIOLOGY AND PATHOPHYSIOLOGY OF SPASTICITY 126
CLINICAL PICTURE 129
EVALUATION OF SPASTICITY 130
MANAGEMENT 132
SUMMARY 139
REFERENCES 139

Chapter 10 DEFICITS IN ACTIVITIES OF DAILY LIVING 143
Robin McNeny, O.T.R.

BASIC ACTIVITIES OF DAILY LIVING 143
  Feeding 143
  Dressing 146
  Hygiene Skills 147
ADVANCED LIVING SKILLS 148
  Communication Skills 148
  Home Living Skills 149
  Family Relationships 149
  Time Management 150
  Financial Management 151
  Social Roles 151
  Driving 151
  Other Issues 152
CONCLUSION 153
REFERENCES 153

Chapter 11 COMMUNICATION DISORDERS 155
Michael Groher, Ph.D.

OPEN VERSUS CLOSED HEAD TRAUMA 156
DURATION OF UNCONSCIOUSNESS 157
EFFECTS OF FOCAL AND DIFFUSE DAMAGE ON COMMUNICATION 157
APHASIA SECONDARY TO TRAUMATIC AND VASCULAR ORIGINS 158
SPECIFIC SPEECH AND LANGUAGE DEFICITS 159
THE PROBLEM OF DYSARTHRIA 160
RECOVERY OF COMMUNICATION 161
SUMMARY 163
REFERENCES 164

Chapter 12 COGNITIVE DEFICITS 167
Yehuda Ben-Yishay, Ph.D.
Leonard Diller, Ph.D.

DIFFERENT APPROACHES TO DEFINING COGNITIVE DEFICITS 167
Psychometric Tradition 168
Clinical Neurologic Approach 168
Learning Theory Approach 169
Rehabilitation Approach 170
Use of Norms 170

PROBLEMS IN ESTABLISHING THE LONG-TERM MENTAL SEQUELAE OF TRAUMATIC HEAD INJURY 171

PROBLEMS IN THE ASSESSMENT OF FUNCTIONAL LIMITATIONS DUE TO MENTAL SEQUELAE OF HEAD INJURY 172

IRM APPROACH TO ASSESSMENT OF COGNITIVE DEFICITS IN HEAD TRAUMA 176
Barriers to Functional Normalcy 176
Baseline Measures 178
Process and Outcome Measures 181

SUMMARY 181
REFERENCES 182

Chapter 13 DISORDERS OF MEMORY 185
D. Neil Brooks, Ph.D.

WHAT KINDS OF MEMORY DEFICIT WILL A PATIENT SUFFER? 185
Deficits Found Early After Injury 185
More Delayed Deficits 186

WHAT IS THE REASON UNDERLYING DEFICITS IN MEMORY? 186
Long- and Short-Term Memory 187
Storage or Retrieval? 187
Memory Sensitivity 187

CAN THE DEFICITS BE PREDICTED? 188
Disturbance of Consciousness Level 188
Signs of Focal Brain Damage 189

HOW RAPIDLY DOES MEMORY RECOVER, AND TO WHAT LEVEL? 190

DOES MEMORY TEST PERFORMANCE RELATE TO "EVERYDAY" MEMORY? 192

HOW MAY MEMORY FUNCTIONS BE IMPROVED? 192
SUMMARY AND CONCLUSIONS 194
REFERENCES 194

Chapter 14 BEHAVIORAL SEQUELAE 197
Mitchell Rosenthal, Ph.D.

FACTORS THAT CONTRIBUTE TO BEHAVIORAL DYSFUNCTION 197
Premorbid Factors 198

Site of Lesion 198
Environmental Factors 200
COURSE OF RECOVERY 201
OUTCOME STUDIES 202
SECONDARY BEHAVIORAL DISTURBANCES 203
Denial 203
Depression 204
Dependence Upon Others 205
MINOR HEAD INJURY 205
CONCLUSION 206
REFERENCES 207

Chapter 15 EFFECTS ON THE FAMILY SYSTEM 209
Michael R. Bond, M.D., Ph.D., FRCS, MRC Psych., MRCP, DPM

THE HEAD-INJURED PATIENT AND THE FAMILY 209
PHYSICAL AND MENTAL CONSEQUENCES OF INJURY 210
PSYCHOSOCIAL CONSEQUENCES OF THE SYMPTOMS OF SEVERE HEAD INJURY FOR FAMILIES OF INJURED PERSONS 213
CONCLUSION 216
REFERENCES 216

Chapter 16 EDUCATIONAL AND VOCATIONAL DEFICITS 219
John P. Bolger, M.S.

BRAIN FUNCTION 219
PRE-INJURY STRENGTHS AND WEAKNESSES 220
EFFECTS OF UNIVERSAL DEFICITS 220
EFFECTS OF SPECIFIC DEFICITS 221
REMEDIATION 222
CONCLUSION 223
REFERENCES 224

CONCLUSION 227
Mitchell Rosenthal, Ph.D.

SECTION 4 SPECIALIZED METHODS OF ASSESSMENT 229

Chapter 17 MEDICAL ASSESSMENT 231
Sheldon Berrol, M.D.

CRITERIA FOR REHABILITATION 232
Evidence of Neurologic Improvement 232
Medical Stability 232
Post-Traumatic Amnesia 233
Cranial Nerve Deficits 233

Late Effects of Facial Bone Fractures 234
Epilepsy 235
Infections 235
Post-Traumatic Hydrocephalus 235
Cranioplasty 236
Oral-Feeding Status 236
Heterotopic Ossification 236
Airway Obstruction 237
Skeletal Trauma 237
Hypothalamic Functions 237
CONCLUSION 238
REFERENCES 238

Chapter 18 MOTOR ASSESSMENT 241
Arthur J. Nelson, Ph.D., R.P.T.

MOTOR PROBLEMS OF THE HEAD-INJURED ADULT 242
OBSERVATIONAL PHASE OF ASSESSMENT 242
Motor Examination 242
MUSCLE TONUS AND MYOTATIC REFLEXES 244
HEAD-DROPPING TEST 245
ASSESSMENT OF SENSORY RESPONSIVENESS 245
Stereognosis 246
Two-Point Discrimination 246
Bilateral Simultaneous Stimulation 246
Body Schema 247
Visual Function 248
TONIC REFLEXES 248
Tonic Labyrinthine Reflex 248
TRIGGERED RESPONSES 248
EQUILIBRIUM REACTION 249
Seated Position 249
The Arm-Dropping Test 249
Pronation and Supination of Forearms 249
Sitting Balance When Disturbed 250
Sitting to Standing 251
The Standing Position 252
AUTOMATIC BEHAVIORS 253
Locomotion (Forward) 253
Functional Ambulation Score 253
ASSESSMENT OF HAND FUNCTION 253
RECORDING OF MOTOR BEHAVIOR 255
DYNAMOMETRY 255
Validity and Reliability of the Dynamometer 259
SUMMARY AND CONCLUSIONS 259
REFERENCES 260
APPENDIX 1. MOTOR BEHAVIOR INVENTORY 261
Instructions for Assessment and Rating of Motor Behavior 261

APPENDIX 2. SENSORY INVENTORY   266
   Instructions for Sensory Inventory   266

Chapter 19 OCCUPATIONAL THERAPY EVALUATION   271
Paula E. Wahlstrom, O.T.R.

REVIEW OF MEDICAL HISTORY   271
GENERAL EVALUATION PROCEDURES   272
MOTOR CONTROL   273
   Range of Motion   273
   Muscle Tone   273
   Muscle Strength   273
SENSATION   274
PERCEPTUAL-MOTOR   274
   Visual Awareness   274
   Somatosensory Functions   275
   Form and Space   275
   Motor Planning   276
ACTIVITIES OF DAILY LIVING (ADL)   276
   Self-Care Skills   276
   Home Skills   276
   Community Skills   277
GOAL SETTING   277
SUMMARY   277
REFERENCES   278

Chapter 20 SPEECH AND LANGUAGE ASSESSMENT   279
Robert M. Smith, M.Ed.

ASSESSMENT OF LANGUAGE AND COGNITIVE FUNCTION   279
   Cognitive Evaluation   279
   Language Evaluation   281
ASSESSMENT OF THE NEUROMUSCULAR SPEECH SYSTEM   283
   Dysarthria   283
   Apraxia of Speech   283
   Motor Speech Evaluation   283
NATURAL RECOVERY PROCESS   285
   Brain Trauma Recovery Levels   286
CONCLUSION   287
REFERENCES   287
BIBLIOGRAPHY   289

Chapter 21 NEUROPSYCHOLOGIC ASSESSMENT   291
William J. Lynch, Ph.D.

DEFINITION AND BACKGROUND   291
DESCRIPTION OF THE PROMINENT TEST BATTERIES   292
   Halstead-Reitan Battery   292

Luria's Neuropsychological Investigation   293
Luria-Nebraska Neuropsychological Battery   293
ADDITIONAL TECHNIQUES   297
  Language Functions   297
  Memory Functions   298
NEUROPSYCHOLOGIC ASSESSMENT IN REHABILITATION SETTINGS   299
  Baseline Determinations   299
  Identification of Strengths and Weakness   299
  Prescriptions for Treatment   300
  Prediction and Determination of Outcome   300
  Organization and Presentation of Neuropsychologic Data   302
SUMMARY   305
REFERENCES   307

CONCLUSION   309
Ernest R. Griffith, M.D.

SECTION 5   TREATMENT APPROACHES   311

Chapter 22   STRATEGIES FOR IMPROVING MOTOR CONTROL   313
Arthur J. Nelson, Ph.D., R.P.T.

MECHANISMS OF RECOVERY FROM CENTRAL NERVOUS SYSTEM LESIONS   313
  Diaschisis or Cerebral Shock   313
  Equipotentiality   313
  Vicarious Function   314
  Behavioral Substitution   314
  Functional Reorganization   314
  Supersensitivity of Denervation   314
  Collateral Sprouting   315
  Regeneration   315
PRINCIPLES OF IMPROVING MOTOR CONTROL   315
  Management During the Acute Phase   315
  Subacute Phase (Postcomatose Patient)   317
  Supplemental Treatment   329
CONCLUSION   333
REFERENCES   333

Chapter 23   REMEDIATION OF PERCEPTUAL DYSFUNCTION   335
Paula E. Wahlstrom, O.T.R.

TREATMENT APPROACHES   336
POSITIONING TECHNIQUES   338

CASE STUDIES 342
FUNCTIONAL SKILLS 343
GOAL SETTING 343
CONCLUSION 343
REFERENCES 344

Chapter 24 REALITY ORIENTATION THERAPY 345
Jean Cerny, O.T.R.
Robin McNeny, O.T.R.

GOALS OF THE REALITY ORIENTATION PROGRAM 345
COMPONENTS OF REALITY ORIENTATION PROGRAM: ENVIRONMENTAL PROGRAM 346
  Positive Staff Attitude 346
  Consistent Approach 346
  Environmental Stimulation 346
COMPONENTS OF THE REALITY ORIENTATION PROGRAM: STRUCTURED GROUP SESSIONS 348
THE OCCUPATIONAL HISTORY 351
THE TREATMENT PROGRAM 351
CONCLUSION 353
REFERENCES 353

Chapter 25 TREATMENT OF COMMUNICATION DISORDERS 355
Robert M. Smith, M.Ed.

ROLE OF THE SPEECH AND LANGUAGE PATHOLOGIST 355
  Evaluation Team 355
  Coma-Arousal Task Force 356
  Task Force for Swallowing Dysfunction 356
  Cognitive Retraining Task Force 356
  Provider of Speech Pathology Therapeutic Service 357
TREATMENT APPROACHES FOR COMMUNICATION DISORDERS 357
  Communication Problems Owing to Cognitive Dysfunction 357
  Aphasia Therapeutic Program 359
  Treatment of Dysarthria 361
ALTERNATE FORMS OF COMMUNICATION 363
  Manual Communication 363
  Communication Aids 364
SUMMARY 365
REFERENCES 365

Chapter 26 COGNITIVE REMEDIATION 367
Yehuda Ben-Yishay, Ph.D.
Leonard Diller, Ph.D.

DEFINING THE OBJECTIVES OF COGNITIVE REMEDIATION 368
   Considerations of Context 368
   Consideration of Scope 369
SUMMARY 378
REFERENCES 378

Chapter 27 TREATMENT OF BEHAVIORAL DEFICITS 381
Craig A. Muir, Ph.D.
William J. Haffey, Ph.D.
Kathryn J. Ott, B.S.N.
Diane Karaica, A.A.
Jane H. Muir, R.P.T.
Margaret Sutko, Ph.D.

REHABILITATION AS A BEHAVIORAL PROCESS 381
DEFINITIONS OF BEHAVIORAL PRINCIPLES 382
PUBLISHED APPLICATIONS 384
   Chemotherapeutic Approaches 385
CURRENT TREATMENT APPLICATIONS 386
   Inpatient Settings 386
   Transitional Living Programs 388
   Day Treatment Programs 389
SUMMARY 390
REFERENCES 391

Chapter 28 PATIENT-FAMILY EDUCATION 395
Linda Nielson Diehl, R.N., M.S.

FACTORS IN PLANNING AN EDUCATIONAL INTERVENTION 397
TYPES OF INTERVENTIONS 397
   Reality Orientation 397
   Home Visits 397
   Educational Group Approaches 398
   Family Conferences 399
   Self-Help Groups 399
METHODOLOGIC CONSIDERATIONS 400
CONCLUSION 400
REFERENCES 401
APPENDIX. HOME VISIT EVALUATION FORM 403

Chapter 29 METHODS OF FAMILY INTERVENTION 407
Mitchell Rosenthal, Ph.D.
Craig A. Muir, Ph.D.

THEORETICAL FRAMEWORK FOR FAMILY INTERVENTION 408
   Effects of Psychosocial Deficits on the Family System 409
ESTABLISHING THE NEED FOR INTERVENTION 410
   Analysis of Premorbid History 411

Identifying the Nature, Severity, and Duration of Deficits 411
Understanding "Signals" From the Family 412
HIGH-RISK FAMILIES 412
FACTORS TO CONSIDER BEFORE INITIATING AN INTERVENTION 412
TYPES OF FAMILY INTERVENTION TECHNIQUES 413
Patient-Family Education 413
Family Counseling 414
Family Therapy 415
NONPROFESSIONAL INTERVENTION 416
CONCLUSION 417
REFERENCES 418

Chapter 30 REINTEGRATION INTO THE COMMUNITY 421
Emily Hackler, R.N., M.A.
Jerome S. Tobis, M.D.

BACKGROUND OF THE PROBLEM 421
ABOUT LONG-TERM SURVIVORS 422
Anosognosia 424
Fact or Fiction 426
The Police and Head-Injured Individuals 427
LOCKED IN GRIEF SYNDROME 428
THE COMMUNITY 429
IMMEDIATE ENVIRONMENT 430
BEHAVIORAL CONTROLS 431
OTHER CONSIDERATIONS 431
OPTIMAL CARE FOR HEAD-INJURED PERSONS 432
CONCLUSION 433
REFERENCES 434

CONCLUSION 435
Mitchell Rosenthal, Ph.D.

INDEX 437

Section 1

NATURE OF THE PROBLEM

Chapter 1

SCALE AND SCOPE OF THE PROBLEM

Bryan Jennett, M.D.

Head injuries are very common. Just how common is difficult to discover because many are not serious enough to warrant admission to the hospital, and statistics about emergency room attenders are unreliable and incomplete. Deaths, however, are readily detected and provide a guide to the relative frequency of injuries in different places. In different parts of the United States, there are 22 to 25 fatal head injuries per 100,000, more than twice as many as in Britain, Sweden, or Japan.[1] About 7 million head injuries are estimated to occur annually in the United States,[2] with about 500,000 persons admitted to the hospital.

Many patients admitted are injured only mildly, in that they stay in the hospital for only a few days; in Britain, more than two thirds are discharged in 2 days or less. Yet each of these numerous patients, passing rapidly through the hospital emergency room and wards, may suffer for several weeks from symptoms of impaired functioning, both mentally and socially; whereas a few will develop a serious accident neurosis that can last for months or even years. At the other end of the scale are patients who remain in coma for several days, even weeks. During that period, they require assiduous assistance from physiotherapists if they are not to develop pulmonary complications that may be fatal, or limb contractures that may cause lasting disability. Most of these seriously injured patients will have major disabilities for some months, and many of them will never be quite the same people again; some will have a major disability, mental or physical, for the rest of their lives. Since their average age is under 30 years, this means many years of disability, which will persist long after the patient loses contact with the hospital system. Although the number of these severe injuries is relatively small, the population of disabled survivors of head injury in the community is much greater than would be expected from statistics based on the annual occurrence of new cases. Exactly how many patients this amounts to at any one time (the prevalence of disability due to head injury) is difficult to calculate without some kind of census in a defined community. One estimate in Britain arrived at a figure of 150 markedly disabled persons per 100,000, and head injury is much less common in the United Kingdom than in many parts of the world.

A word of warning is needed about the epidemiology of head injury—about counting the numbers of head injuries that occur, the nature of the victims, and the causes of the injury. The basis of the calculation should be the community—not a single hospital, or a single service. This is because all kinds of selection processes operate to determine where patients go after injury. Many of these processes are unrecognized, and some are difficult to determine even if they are looked for. The distribution of causes, for example, will be quite different in the emergency room than in the intensive-care unit or the autopsy room; this is because the cause is related to the severity of the injury. Hence, road accidents are the major cause of serious head injuries, whereas minor head injuries are mostly due to other factors,[3] such as falls and fights.

SEVERITY OF INJURY

The problems of management, both in the acute stage and for later rehabilitation, are so different for injuries of different severity that it is vital to understand how to assess severity. It is obviously brain damage that matters, not scalp lacerations or skull fractures. The brain damage may be primary, sustained at the moment of impact; or it may be secondary, the result of subsequent pathologic processes. These processes include brain swelling, intracranial hematoma, and the effects on the brain of extracranial events such as blood loss, arterial hypotension, and pulmonary complications. The commonest combined effect of these various secondary processes is production of widespread ischemic brain damage, and this can occur within hours after injury. In some cases, it is obvious that secondary brain damage is dominant, in that the patient was clearly not adversely affected soon after injury; for example, the patient may have talked before lapsing into coma. In other cases, it is a matter of conjecture how much of the brain damage has resulted from primary or from secondary factors, but in either event the therapist has to deal with the net effect of these two kinds of damage.

Of most importance for rehabilitation are the nature and location of the brain damage. It has already been explained that secondary ischemic damage is widespread throughout the brain; in most cases, the impact damage also affects many parts of the brain. Thus, wherever the blow on the head or the location of the skull fracture, there are usually contusions of the cortex in both frontal and temporal lobes; and there is commonly disruption or stretching of nerve fibers in the white matter of the cerebral hemispheres and the brain stem.[3,4] Even when there is a clear focal lesion, such as an intracranial hematoma causing hemiplegia, this is seldom the only site of brain damage. This is one reason for the difference in the disability produced by head injury, as compared with that produced by cerebrovascular accident. The latter is usually a strictly focal lesion, and the main rehabilitation issue is the focal neurophysical deficit. By contrast, the widespread nature of the brain damage after head injury is probably responsible for the dysfunction that affects so many aspects of mental activity.

The most consistent effect of diffuse brain damage, even when it is mild, is impairment of consciousness. The best guide to the severity of this damage is the degree and duration of altered consciousness. In the emergency room, it is useful to classify patients into those who are already talking when they arrive, and those who are not. The talkers can be divided into those who have a period of amnesia following their injury, and those who can remember everything clearly. In those who are unconscious on arrival, the depth and duration of coma provide the best guide to the severity of the diffuse damage, and this is readily recorded in terms of the Glasgow Coma Scale (see Chapter 2 for further discussion). It should be noted that a severe compound depressed fracture with brain issuing from the wound is compatible with there having been no loss of consciousness and no amnesia whatever because the brain damage was focal.

After the patient has recovered, the best guide to the severity of the diffuse damage is the duration of the post-traumatic amnesia (PTA). An advantage of this indicator is that it can be assessed in conversation with the patient months after injury and without reference to records relating to the early management of the patient. This makes it of particular value to the rehabilitation team that inherits the patient some time after injury, often from another institution. Patients are asked how long it was before they "came to," in that they themselves were aware of their surroundings; patients must not report what their relatives have told them about this, because relatives usually equate this with when patients first began to talk, and that is long before the beginning of continuous memory for day-to-day events. There is no need to seek a very accurate figure for PTA; what matters is whether it lasted minutes, hours, days, or weeks, as indicated in Table 1-1. There is now abundant evidence that the duration of PTA correlates well with late outcome, as well as with the interval before patients return to work, and also with the occurrence of late traumatic epilepsy (see Chapter 8).

NATURE OF THE DISABILITY

After both mild and severe injuries, it is useful to distinguish between the mental and physical components of disability, while acknowledging that what matters is the net effect of these on the overall social functioning of the individual. It is also important to distinguish persisting complaints or deficits that reflect incomplete recovery from those that develop anew. The latter include traumatic epilepsy, as well as secondary psychosocial problems resulting from reactions of the patient and family to the accident and its consequences. Although there is a certain amount of overlap between the disabilities suffered after mild and severe injuries, the differences are more striking than the similarities.

The symptoms that predominate after mild injury (often dubbed the postconcussional syndrome) are seldom suffered after severe injury—when patients will usually deny ever having had headaches, dizziness, or even anxiety. That is not to imply that the symptoms complained of after mild injury are imaginary or psychologically induced, as was once believed. Indeed, there is now ample evidence that these symptoms have their basis in physiologic disorders, albeit short-lived. Better means of testing the ability of these patients to process information, and of measuring mild vestibular abnormalities and other physiologic functions, now make it clear that the complaints of these patients can be explained on an organic basis. There is also pathologic evidence that even mild concussion causes visible structural damage in the brain; evidence of stretching and rupture of nerve fibers can be found in the white matter of the brains of patients who die from other causes after having recovered from mild head injury. If the symptoms of these mildly injured patients are ignored or are unsympathetically dealt with, there is a real risk of secondary anxiety and depression, leading to neurosis.

After severe injury, the characteristic of the disability is the combination of mental and physical deficits, which often leads to a greater degree of social disability than would be expected from the separate deficits. In most cases, the mental dysfunction predominates in contributing to the social handicap, and it also impedes the rehabilitation of the physical deficits, because motivation is reduced and patients often reject the efforts of those trying to help them. The physical deficits comprise those related to cerebral hemisphere function (sensorimotor hemiplegia, dysphasia, and epilepsy) and those caused by damage to the brain stem and cranial nerves. Mental deficits include memory disorder on a day-to-day or even an

TABLE 1-1. Duration of Post-traumatic Amnesia (PTA) and Severity of Injury

PTA Duration	Severity
Less than 5 min	Very mild
5 to 60 min	Mild
1 to 24 hr	Moderate
1 to 7 days	Severe
1 to 4 weeks	Very severe
More than 4 weeks	Extremely severe

hour-to-hour basis, cognitive impairments that can be measured by psychometric tests, and personality disorders. The latter are both the most common and often the most disabling; they frequently occur in patients who have little or no physical deficit and whose performance on formal psychologic tests is not greatly impaired.[5] Yet personality change may not be immediately evident, unless care is taken to invite family and friends to compare the patient's present overall behavior with that before the injury. Personality change is also the least tractable of the disabilities for therapeutic intervention.

A further factor that contributes to the overall disability of the head-injured patient in many cases is the patient's pretraumatic psychosocial status. The victims of head injury are not a random sample of their age group; they include an undue proportion of people with some kind of social deviancy. They are risk takers in cars and on motorcycles, and they are drinkers and declared alcoholics. And although the young brain may have more potential for recovery than an older one, youth is often not helpful in the social sense. Some of the younger patients are still facing the turmoil of adolescence and greatly resent the enforced dependence on their parents that brain damage inevitably produces. Others are on the threshold of their careers and cannot accept any special arrangements to be made, unlike the man with 30 years of good service in the same job behind him. Those who are married have seldom been so for long, and these marriages frequently break down under the stress of brain damage; by contrast, the man who has been married for 30 years, and was perhaps expected to retire soon anyway, may be more readily accepted by his wife when he is left with hemiplegia after a cerebrovascular accident.

RECOVERY AFTER HEAD INJURY

Little is understood about the process of recovery after head injury, by any standards a remarkable phenomenon. The patient lying unconscious, temporarily apneic and pulseless, may get up and walk away only minutes later. Or the patient may be in coma for several days, and it may be weeks before the patient is restored to full consciousness. And some such patients never do get back to their own selves, or anything like them. Rehabilitation aims to influence this process favorably, either to hasten the restoration of function or to ensure that recovery is eventually more complete than it would have been without therapy. This treatment can be rationally based only if it is founded on some hypothesis of the process of recovery.

It seems probable that different biologic activities operate at different stages of the injury. Recovery of consciousness after a stunning blow takes only minutes, whereas there are severely injured patients who report continuing improvement in some neurologic functions a year or more after the injury. Changes in the first minutes after injury presumably indicate the resolution of transitory dysfunction that may not have any structural component. Recovery after several days is more likely due to the resolution of temporary structural abnormalities such as edema and vascular permeability. The mechanism that underlies recovery over months or years is much less easily explained. The extent to which alternative, perhaps normally redundant, pathways are brought into action as a substitute for structures that have been rendered permanently functionless is uncertain. Whether recovery is due to restoration of activity in recovering structures or diversion to others, it seems likely that the restoration of function is essentially a learning process. The poorer prospects for recovery in older patients may have several explanations: a reduced capacity to learn, a less resilient vascular system, and a more limited neuronal reserve by way of alternative pathways.

As there are different biologic processes taking place at different times after injury, so the objectives and techniques of rehabilitation also differ as the time since injury increases and the patient's condition changes. In the first month after severe injury, the aim is to prevent complications—those in the chest that may threaten life, and those in the limbs that may cause permanent crippling.

It is in the next 3 to 6 months that therapeutic rehabilitation interventions are likely to have their greatest impact. As the degree of recovery against time is recorded, one must decide when to abandon efforts to restore old skills to damaged parts, in favor of teaching how to substitute new skills using unaffected parts. It may be that the success of rehabilitation for permanent paraplegics is the certainty that walking will never be possible, so that no time is lost before turning attention to what can be done without walking. There is a need to be readier to recognize when such a point has been reached with hemiplegia or dysphasia, and to seek substitution rather than flogging a functionally dead horse. This is certainly the theme of rehabilitation after 6 months or more—when the need is to analyze not only the patient's disability but also the patient's capability. Only then is it clear how to encourage the patient to adapt physically and mentally to the changed status so that the patient and family may adjust socially in an appropriate way. This is no easy matter when it is the mental and emotional sphere that is most drastically changed; but unless that effort is made, there is little to look forward to.

In all this there is another responsibility for the therapists: to influence the attitudes of the family, to prepare them for the difficult months ahead, to support and counsel them during these months, and to help them to understand their brain-damaged family member. If this is accepted as a part of rehabilitation from the outset, it should be possible to anticipate, and so to minimize, the most harmful of secondary psychologic reactions (and interactions) of the patient and family, reactions that can be a serious impediment to optimal recovery. An important element in this counseling is the setting of realistic goals based on properly calculated predictions, not on false hopes. To hold out promises of dramatic further functional recovery once the likelihood of this has passed is not only unkind but can be a positive hindrance to a sensible attitude of rehabilitation.

An aspect of rehabilitation that is too often neglected is research—into how effective present methods are, and into new approaches. The obvious emotional need to respond to disability by action can lead to unquestioning acceptance of the doctrine that more therapy means better recovery. This is a costly assumption, considering that rehabilitation is a labor-intensive activity that depends on skilled personnel, a resource that money cannot always buy. The effectiveness of therapy, whether an organized system or a single technique, can be judged only if there are reliable means of comparing either the rate of recovery or the state of recovery at a given (fixed) time after injury. That is why there are chapters on the assessment of outcome later in this book. There is need also to be able to quantify the treatment given—its type, its dose, and its timing. Also, it is necessary to distinguish between skill-specific therapy and the general benefits of enthusiastic amateurs, whether these be other health professionals or members of the family. Only if these factors are recognized is it possible to plan a rehabilitation program that is realistic and economic, rather than pretentious and expensive.

If rehabilitation is to be taken seriously, like a potent drug or an effective surgical procedure, then it deserves to be assessed by the same standards. That entails seeking answers to the same kinds of questions. What is the best method and what is the most effective dose? When should treatment start, and when should it finish? Are there adverse effects of some forms of rehabilitation, and can some patients become addicted?

One of the most important goals is to provide continuity of care for a program that will be intensive for a few months but may last for the rest of life. Family members are the only persons able to provide this. They should be recruited as members of the therapeutic team as early as possible after the patient emerges from coma. They should be taught what to do and encouraged to do it; as time passes, they should be told what they may need to do differently. This is not just economically sensible; it is the only way to ensure that the patient can adapt to the community.

REFERENCES

1. Jennett, B and MacMillan, R: *Epidemiology of head injury.* Br Med J 282:101, 1981.
2. Caveness, WF: *Incidence of craniocerebral trauma in the United States in 1976 with trend from 1970 to 1975.* Adv Neurol 22:1, 1979.
3. Jennett, B and Teasdale, G: *Management of Head Injuries.* Contemporary Neurology Series, Vol 20, Plum, F (ed). FA Davis, Philadelphia, 1981.
4. Adams, JH, et al: *Brain damage in fatal non-missile head injury.* J Clin Pathol 33:1132, 1980.
5. Jennett, B, et al: *Disability after severe head injury: Observations on the use of the Glasgow Outcome Scale.* J Neurol Neurosurg Psychiatry 44:285, April 1981.

Chapter 2

CHARACTERISTICS OF THE HEAD-INJURED PATIENT

Rebecca W. Rimel, R.N., N.P.
John A. Jane, M.D., Ph.D.

Over the years, there has been a steady increase in the number of persons sustaining head injury. More persons die on American highways each year in automobile accidents than were lost in the entire Vietnam conflict, and central nervous system (CNS) trauma is the single most common cause of death in these accidents. The head is injured in more than two thirds of all automobile accidents, and head injury is the cause of death in about 70 percent of fatal cases.[1] Trauma is currently the third most common cause of death in the United States and is the primary cause of death in persons under age 38.[2] Because of its potentially devastating physical, psychologic, and social consequences, head injury is one of the most critical problems facing the health-care system.

The medical problems of patients who survive head injury are enormous, and the socioeconomic impact on our society is staggering. Even though head injury is recognized as one of the major health problems in our society, the epidemiology is not well described because of problems in patient identification and definition of the severity of injury. In recent years, the epidemiology of head injury has received much attention, and as a result of such studies, a wide range of incidence figures has resulted.[3,4] Studies that are confined to small geographic localities are felt to be more reliable; this is due in part to fewer methodologic problems. It is difficult, therefore, to give valid incidence rates for CNS trauma. The variation in estimates of head injuries in the United States is demonstrated in Table 2-1. A recent survey conducted by the National Institute of Neurological and Communicative Disorders and Stroke, the most recent and largest survey of its kind in the United States, provides data on the occurrence of new cases of head injury, type and cause of injury, admission and duration of hospital stay, and frequency of existing cases of injury.[5] Comparisons of these findings and data collected at the University of Virginia are discussed in this chapter.

The goal of this chapter is to provide an overview of the characteristics of head-injured patients. Each person, whether practicing in an acute-care or a rehabilitation setting, will be involved not only with the patients sustaining head trauma but with their families as well. Therefore, a better knowledge of the characteristics of these patients, the mechanism of injury, and implications for management is useful for providing improved patient care as well as education and counseling directed at the patient, the family, and the public.

In September 1977, the Department of Neurosurgery at the University of Virginia began a prospective data bank of patients with CNS injuries in central Virginia. The major emphasis of this project was the identification and study of all patients who sustained injury in a well-

TABLE 2-1. Incidence of Head Injury

Source	Description	Incidence/100,000	Total USA
National Surveys and Estimates			
National Center for Health Statistics	All head injuries except deaths	3,900	8,111,000
Caveness	Excluding lacerations of scalp and face	915	1,900,000
Health Interview Survey	Household interview survey	600	1,275,000
Research Triangle for NINCDS	Hospitalized patients	185	422,000
Hospital Discharge Survey	Hospitalized patients	170	353,000
Annegers and Kurland	Traumatic unconsciousness or post-traumatic amnesia or skull fracture	↑ 300 est	
England and Wales	Hospitalized patients	430	
San Diego County	Death or hospitalization	295	

defined geographic area. The University of Virginia, located in central Virginia, provides the only neurologic coverage for a 13-county area. All head injuries requiring neurosurgical care are treated at one center, thus providing an opportunity for population-based studies where the bias of selection factors is minimized. During the 20-month period from October 1, 1977, to May 30, 1979, this prospective study resulted in a data bank of 1248 patients from which the data presented here are derived.

PATIENT CHARACTERISTICS

AGE AND SEX

All studies have reported that head trauma is two or three times more common in males than in females. In our series, occurrence of CNS trauma in males was approximately two times greater than that in females for most age categories. Even though the male predominance exists over most categories, the differences in sex are greatest between ages 15 and 24.

For the age distribution of CNS injuries, three age groups were found to exceed the overall incidence of 24 per 10,000 population in our study. This was demonstrated first in age groups 15 through 29 years, with the highest age group, 15 through 19 years, showing an incidence of 42 per 10,000. Another high-risk age group was ages 75 and over, where the incidence was 30 per 10,000 population. Lowest incidence of injury occurred in the 5-through-9 age group. The overall age distribution for head injuries can be seen in Figure 2-1. In this series and others, there was no important difference in the occurrence of head injuries between the white and nonwhite population based on local census data.

The aim in assessing demographic and epidemiologic data in such a study is that certain significant characteristics will become evident that will help in the identification of a population at risk. Such is the case when looking at age distribution. If one looks at the frequency of the

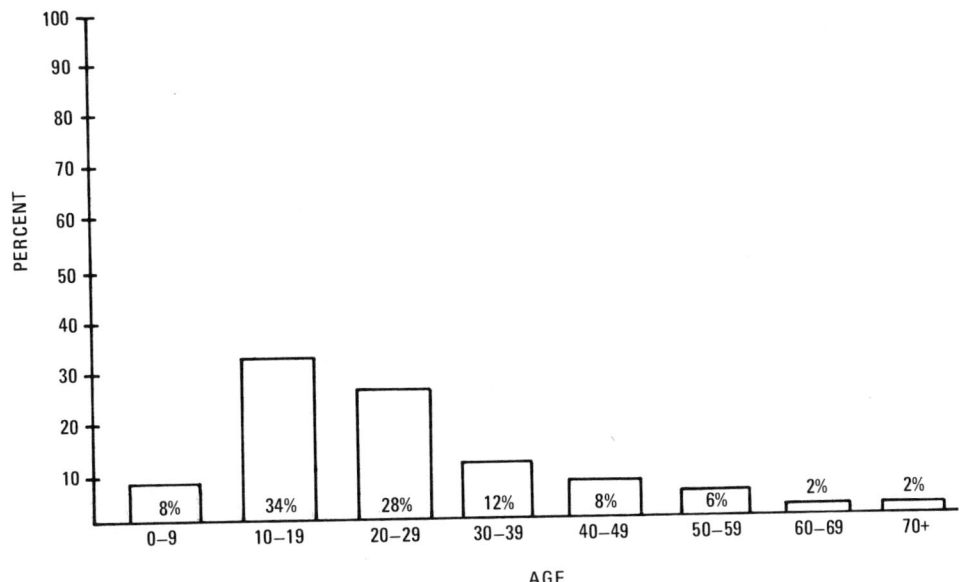

FIGURE 2-1. Age distribution for CNS trauma due to head injury.

age distribution, it can be quite deceiving. As expected, the greatest number of patients is between ages 10 and 19 (34 percent). The elderly population comprises a very small percentage, with fewer than 4 percent of the patients over age 65. However, calculation of the incidence figures based on the population for the central Virginia catchment area shows that two age groups are at risk for head injury: the 10-to-30-year-olds as expected, but also the elderly population.

SOCIOECONOMIC STATUS

Other significant descriptive characteristics were evaluated, including marital status, type of employment, and overall socioeconomic status. Of those injured, 59 percent were single, which is 20 percent higher than the population base as a whole. Twenty-nine percent of the patients were married, and the remainder were either widowed or divorced. In this series, the majority of patients (75 percent) earned less than $10,000 a year. Differences in salaries within specific geographic areas must be considered, however; therefore, the employment status provides a more objective overview of the group's socioeconomic status. Figure 2-2 shows the distribution of CNS trauma patients by employment status. The largest category is that of "student," which comprises 24 percent of the population. The existence of a large university in Charlottesville results in a greater proportion of students in the patient population. The "unemployed" patients are particularly noteworthy since their incidence of CNS trauma is almost three times that of their proportion in the total population.

Data on the education completed by the patient population reveal that approximately 25 percent of the patients had fewer than 8 years of education, 50 percent had 8 to 12 years, and 25 percent had 12 years or more of education. In our series, the patients who sustained head trauma were predominantly from a lower socioeconomic class. In a national study conducted from July 1965 through June 1976, the occurrence of head injury was related to income. Differences such as these can be due in part to the type of interview procedures used

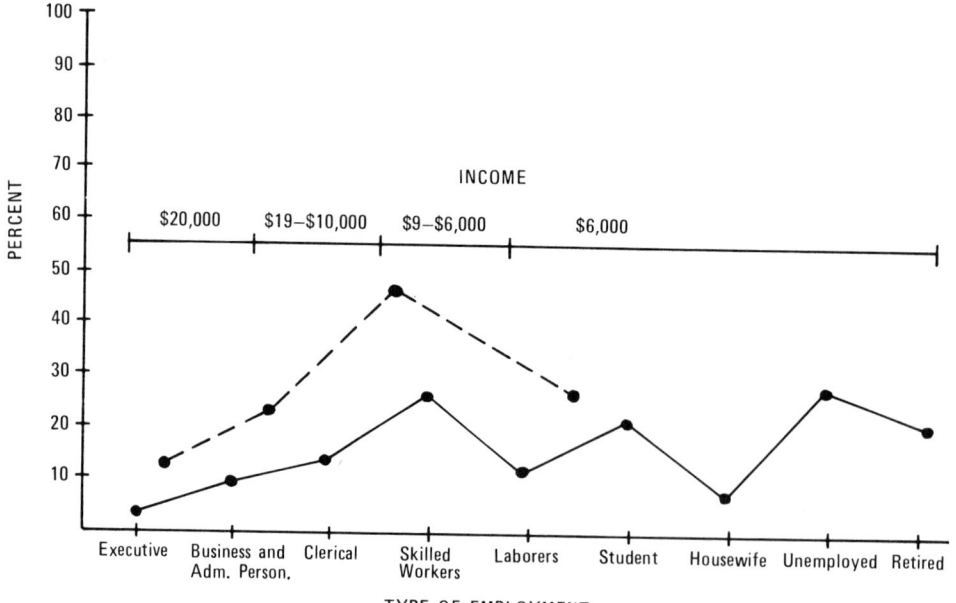

FIGURE 2-2. Type of employment and income.

in a given study. Selecki and coworkers[6] found that among neurosurgical admissions in South Wales and Australia, laborers and craftsmen were disproportionately represented. Persons in the lower socioeconomic class had considerably more head injuries caused by assaults and household accidents. Traffic accidents were not related to socioeconomic class.

MEDICAL HISTORY

Another interesting factor that also identifies potential patients at risk for head trauma is those admitted for a previous head injury prior to the current insult. In this series, 31 percent of all patients studied were previously hospitalized for a head injury. The question that presents itself is whether people who have already had a head injury are at high risk for a second injury. The literature seems to differ on this question. Partington[1] found no increased risk for a second head injury in children who had previous insult. However, in a study conducted in Minnesota, the incidence of a subsequent head injury in adults was about three times that of a first head injury in a general population. Among those who had more than one head injury, the incidence of a subsequent head injury was eight times that of the general population. Therefore, based on these data and our experience, it seems that adult patients who sustain a single head injury are indeed at high risk of another insult.

In evaluating other aspects of the medical history, 25 percent of the patients interviewed stated that they had received some type of professional treatment for alcohol abuse. A significant number (20 percent) had also been treated for heart disease or high blood pressure or both. These and other disorders requiring treatment, such as psychiatric illness (11 percent), seizures (4 percent), and drug abuse (4 percent), are all identifying characteristics of the population at risk for head trauma. With such information available, we can direct preventive educational programs at this patient group during hospitalization and rehabilitation in the hope of decreasing the rate of readmission for successive injuries.

CAUSE OF INJURY

Another means of identifying high-risk groups for head trauma deals with the cause and mechanisms of injury. A review of the literature shows that the major causes of injury are similar in Australia, Wales, England, Canada, and the United States. In the majority of series, more than half of the patients are involved in traffic accidents, with falls being the next major cause of injury.[7] The rate of occurrence from the Head and Spinal Cord Injury Survey[5] does not show geographic differences in the cause of injury. Some interesting data are available demonstrating how the cause of injury differs with the age of the patient. In our series, when age-specific incidence rates were evaluated based on the cause of injury, there was an overwhelming predominance of motor vehicle accidents, and most cases of head injury occurred in the age group between 15 and 24 years. The difference between this series and ours, however, is related to falls. Most cases of head injury from falls in the National Institutes of Health (NIH) series were seen in the group under age 15. In our study, falls were the second most frequent cause of injury, with a definite rise in incidence in those aged 70 and over.

Causality data are valuable in proposing programs designed to reduce traffic accidents and minimize their consequences. One strategy would be to encourage the use of safety measures such as seat belts and protective head gear. In patients admitted to our medical center, fewer than 14 percent reported that they were wearing seat belts at the time of injury. Of the patients involved in motorcycle accidents, only 58 percent were wearing helmets even though Virginia has a requirement for such equipment. One might argue that those who are involved in the care of the head-injured patient must become actively involved in designing preventive programs and supporting legislation for mandatory and improved safety measures. In automotive accidents, it was the driver (71 percent) who most frequently sustained a head injury, and this injury was often the result of a single-car accident (58 percent). More than half of the patients who were injured reported that the vehicle was traveling in excess of the 55-mile-per-hour speed limit. Most frequently, the victim was riding in the front seat (87 percent) of a full-sized (calculated from the wheel-base size) car (75 percent). Only 12 percent of patients were injured as a result of interpersonal violence. Approximately 80 percent of all assaults—including gunshot wounds, beatings, and knifings—were either self-inflicted or a result of domestic problems. This picture differs significantly from that in larger urban areas where more assaults are the result of violent crimes.

The most significant contributing factor to all accidents was alcohol use. Blood alcohol levels were obtained on 86 percent of all patients studied, and 72 percent of these patients had a positive blood alcohol level on admission; 52 percent were considered legally intoxicated, with a blood alcohol level of 0.10 percent or higher.

LOCATION OF INJURY

As expected from the large number of traffic accidents, more than half (58 percent) of the head injuries occurred on the highway. Most accidents occurred on small two-lane roads and secondary highways; only 5 percent occurred on the major interstate highways or freeways. In part, this is because there are fewer major highways in the localities studied and also because safety conditions on secondary roads are often poor. Twenty-six percent of the injuries occurred at home or school, and an additional 8 percent took place at work. These injuries, in some cases, could have been prevented with educational safety programs directed at hazards found in the home and at industrial sites. Health-care professionals should take an active role in community-oriented programs directed toward preventive measures for the population at risk for head injury. These include legislative changes and an increase in public awareness of the risks of driving while intoxicated, which contributes substantially to the increasing number of patients sustaining head trauma each year.

TIME OF INJURY

Most studies show an increase in head trauma during the summer. In the study conducted in Minnesota, the occurrence of head trauma was highest in the summer and fall. Bicycle and motorcycle accidents were highest in the summer, whereas falls were slightly more common in the winter than in other seasons. In our series, the incidence of head injury was highest in September, owing in part to the large number of students returning to school, followed closely by the three summer months. December, January, and February were the three months with the lowest occurrence of injury.

As may be expected, nearly half of all CNS injuries occurred during the weekend. Peak periods were Saturday (25 percent) and Sunday (20 percent). Similar data on time of occurrence can be very useful for health-care planning and staffing for emergency departments and trauma wards. The daily occurrence of CNS injury shows a definite pattern, with the hour between 5 and 6 AM demonstrating the lowest point of occurrence. The peak times for CNS trauma in our series occur between 3 and 7 PM (26 percent). After 7 PM, the occurrence rate progressively declines until 5 AM.

SEVERITY OF INJURY

As mentioned previously, the University of Virginia is in a rural locality with a large geographic catchment area. Four community hospitals strategically located throughout this area refer all head injuries to our medical center. There is approximately a 100-mile radius surrounding the University of Virginia that is devoid of hospitals or emergency medical care. Because of the referral patterns, long periods of time between injury and treatment by either rescue squad personnel or community hospitals often occur. In our series, 65 percent of the patients waited 30 minutes or longer for treatment, and 20 percent did not receive emergency care for 3 hours or longer. More than 30 percent traveled distances greater than 30 miles to the hospital from the site of injury. Often, what happens during the first hour postinjury can decide the eventual outcome for the patient. Long transport times often occur in rural areas; this differs from the rapid emergency medical services found in the urban setting. Transfer of the head-injured patient in the community is most important since there is a long period of time when the patient is open to additional insult to the nervous system. At the University of Virginia, we assist the local hospital in arranging transfer through collaboration with the neurosurgical service by telephone. These protocols, as in any phase of management, are of no value unless there is a high degree of compliance. Through implementation of these programs with early prehospital intervention, the morbidity and mortality of head-injured patients presumably can be greatly reduced. If advances are to be made in decreasing the morbidity and mortality of the head-injured patient, persons knowledgeable in the management of head trauma must take an active role in training programs, seminars, and clinical practice for personnel working in the prehospital and acute-care areas as well as in rehabilitation.

In contrast to the situation in the larger metropolitan areas, all emergency vehicles and ambulances in central Virginia are staffed totally by volunteers and contain only equipment bought with contributions from the community. The training of these volunteer personnel in the care of the head-injured patient at the site of injury has been undertaken by the Department of Neurosurgery. The long transport times to the medical center mean that often the Emergency Medical Technician (EMT) is responsible for the care of patients during this most critical time. The major emphasis of the training programs has been placed on maintenance of airway, ventilation, and adequate circulation. Other aspects include history and physical assessments and various transport methods. The importance of aggressive early management of the head-injured patient cannot be overemphasized. Less than an hour's attention to the principles of basic life and brain support acutely may reduce the cost of subsequent hospitalization and rehabilitation by hundreds of days, thousands of man-hours, and tens of thousands of dollars. More importantly, appropriate critical care at the right time can conserve human faculties that would otherwise be lost forever to the victim, the family, and the community. (See Chapter 4 for further discussion of acute management.)

GLASGOW COMA SCALE

The study of the epidemiology, treatment, and outcome of head injuries has been impaired because of difficulty defining the type and severity of injury. Only after development of a method of grading the severity of injury can accurate figures on the incidence and outcome from head trauma be given. In addition to description of the problem of head injury and its impact on society, a major clinical question to be answered in such research is the effect of different treatment modalities on outcome. In order to accomplish this goal and compare data between centers, the use of an injury severity scale has been implemented. Changes in the level of consciousness constitute the earliest sign of neurologic deterioration after head injury. Unfortunately, meaningful evaluation of the parameters of neurologic function has been hampered by the use of unstandardized and purely descriptive terminology. In order to quantitatively designate the severity of head injury and predict outcome, Teasdale and Jennett[8] developed the Glasgow Coma Scale (Table 2-2). This scale relates "consciousness" to motor response, verbal response, and eye opening (see Chapter 5 for further discussion of the Glasgow Coma Scale).

In the patient population studied at the University of Virginia, 25 percent were comatose at admission, with a Glasgow Coma Scale score of 8 or less according to the Jennett criteria.[8] The remaining patients had altered levels of consciousness, with 49 percent sustaining "minor head injuries" with a Glasgow Coma Scale score of 12 or better. Much investigation has been directed toward severe head injuries, or a Glasgow Coma Scale score of 8 or less. However, our preliminary findings demonstrate that patients sustaining minor head trauma are left with significant morbidity 3 months after discharge.

In addition to the Glasgow Coma Scale scores, data were collected on loss of consciousness at the time of injury. Of all patients studied, 93 percent were unconscious following their injury. However, only 42 percent of these patients were still unconscious upon arrival in the emergency department. The majority of patients (54 percent) remained unconscious for 30 minutes or less. Caution should be taken when such data are reviewed since the length of unconsciousness was recorded in some cases through self-report. When possible, such data were collected from a family member or close friend who witnessed the event. The duration of unconsciousness in many cases was also influenced by the alcohol intake of the patients.

Another measure of the degree of trauma to the head was the presence of a skull fracture. Data on the type and location of fracture are presented in Table 2-3.

CLINICAL COURSE

As is often the case in a busy emergency department, head-injured patients usually remained in diagnostic or holding units for long periods of time. In this study, 40 percent of the head-injured patients remained in the emergency department for 4 hours or longer. The reasons for long delays in the emergency department are varied. Usually, however, the head-injured patient presents a difficult diagnostic and management problem. The majority of patients studied received a skull roentgenogram (94 percent) while in the emergency department, and 34 percent underwent CT scanning.

The medical management and diagnosis of head trauma are often complicated by extracranial injury. Obviously, the patient with multiple-system involvement requires more di-

TABLE 2-2. Glasgow Coma Scale

	Examiner's Test	Patient's Response	Assigned Score
Eye Opening	Spontaneous	Opens eyes on own	4
	Speech	Opens eyes when asked to in a loud voice	3
	Pain	Opens eyes when pinched	2
	Pain	Does not open eyes	1
Best Motor Response	Commands	Follows simple commands	6
	Pain	Pulls examiner's hand away when pinched	5
	Pain	Pulls a part of body away when examiner pinches patient	4
	Pain	Flexes body inappropriately to pain (decorticate posturing)	3
	Pain	Body becomes rigid in an extended position when examiner pinches victim (decerebrate posturing)	2
	Pain	Has no motor response to pinch	1
Verbal Response (Talking)	Speech	Carries on a conversation correctly and tells examiner where he is, who he is, and the month and year	5
	Speech	Seems confused or disoriented	4
	Speech	Talks so examiner can understand victim but makes no sense	3
	Speech	Makes sounds that examiner can't understand	2
	Speech	Makes no noise	1

TABLE 2-3. Skull Fractures

24% of all patients admitted for CNS trauma sustained a skull fracture.
38% of the fractures were open.
10% of the fractures were depressed (≤ 3 mm).

Location of Fracture	
Frontal	39%
Basilar	21%
Parietal	19%
Occipital	14%
Temporal	7%

agnostic and surgical procedures, and often experiences a more difficult clinical course and requires additional rehabilitation. Other than lacerations, orthopedic injuries occurred most frequently in this population (Table 2-4). Owing to multiple trauma, surgical procedures other than neurosurgical intervention were required in a large number of patients. Twelve percent required chest drainage, and 11 percent needed laparotomy. Eight percent of the population sustained a concomitant cervical fracture and required skeletal traction. Patients requiring intracranial procedures had burr holes (14 percent), craniotomy (19 percent), and then intracranial pressure (ICP) monitoring (20 percent). In those patients monitored, 62 percent had elevation of the initial ICP readings, with an ICP of greater than 15 mm Hg. The initial management of the severely head-injured patient was directed toward controlling the ICP and providing basic life support.

By noting some of the more common injuries sustained by the head-injured patient and their initial treatment, persons involved in rehabilitation can better plan for the future needs of the patient after discharge from the acute-care hospital. In addition, staff-education programs for persons involved in acute management can be directed toward assuring that a well-prepared team will be available for the initial care of the patient. Through anticipation of the care required by the critically ill patient and adequate preparation, valuable time can be saved, which may result in a decrease in morbidity and mortality for the head-injured patient.

Even with the best-prepared and best-educated staff, certain patients cannot be saved. Two percent of those admitted to the study died in the emergency department before ad-

TABLE 2-4. Extracranial Injuries

82% of all patients admitted had one or more extracranial injuries	
Facial fractures	13%
Chest	
Hemothorax/pneumothorax	9%
Rib fracture/lung contusion	10%
Abdomen	
Spleen injury	4%
Liver or bowel injury	11%
Genitourinary injury	3%
Orthopedic	
Upper extremity fracture	14%
Lower extremity fracture	19%
Pelvic fracture	4%
Hip fracture	2%
Laceration	
Laceration of head	61%
Laceration, other	20%

mission. Of those admitted, 22 percent required observation in an intensive-care unit. During hospitalization, 39 percent underwent additional surgical procedures, and 52 percent of the patients required consultation by a clinical service other than neurosurgery. Most frequently, orthopedic surgery was involved in the care of these patients because of the high incidence of fractures and concomitant spinal injuries. Many patients require a multidisciplinary approach to varied problems; this often involves designing a program to maximize the patient's abilities and at the same time developing plans that are feasible for the staff. In the patients studied, 31 percent required physical therapy during their hospitalization in addition to that provided by the nursing staff, 17 percent needed occupational therapy, and 8 percent required speech therapy. These programs should be initiated during the acute management of the head-injured patient in order to ensure the patient the opportunity for maximal recovery. Through anticipation of the needs of the head-injured patient, a comprehensive plan of care can be instituted that will result in a decrease in secondary problems often requiring prolonged hospitalization and rehabilitation.

LENGTH OF HOSPITAL STAY

The majority of patients (51 percent) were hospitalized for 7 days or less; however, 17 percent of the patients studied were hospitalized for more than 15 days. In the National Head and Spinal Cord Injury Survey, patients under age 15 had the shortest hospital stay, probably because patients in this group usually sustained their injuries as a result of falls. Patients in the 15- to 24-year age group had the longest hospital stay, again probably owing to the cause of injury, that is, automobile accidents. In the older population, medical complications often resulted in the prolonged hospitalization. In the study at the University of Virginia as well as that reported by the NIH survey, men remained hospitalized longer than women. These data suggest that not only are men more frequently the victim of head injuries, but their injuries tend to be more severe.

OUTCOME

The most important goal in the care of the head-injured patient who survives is to maximize the chance for a good recovery, and every therapeutic intervention should be directed toward achieving a good outcome. This demands a detailed knowledge of patterns of morbidity. Unfortunately, studies have not adequately addressed the problem of morbidity after head trauma, although there have been numerous reports on the overall mortality; however, their results vary greatly. With the head-injured patient, however, the degree of morbidity is often quite difficult to assess. The prognosis is of particular importance after head injury, because the outcome can vary so widely and so dramatically. New methods of treatment are often expensive or hazardous or both, and are justified only in relation to outcome without intervention.

In the majority of outcome studies, mortality is based on patients sustaining nonpenetrating injuries to the head, which excludes gunshot wounds. In evaluating mortality at the University of Virginia in patients admitted with a Glasgow Coma Scale score of 8 or less, the overall mortality was 70 percent. However, when gunshot wounds were excluded from the analysis, the mortality in the same group was reduced to 48 percent. In a further analysis of patients with nonpenetrating injuries, the mortality drops dramatically with increasing Glasgow Coma Scale scores. In patients admitted with a coma score between 9 and 11, mortality was 6 percent; in patients with scores of 12 and 13, mortality was 1 percent; and no mortality was observed at scores of 14 and 15. Our data and those presented by others demonstrate the value of the Glasgow Coma Scale as a prognostic indicator of mortality after head injury.

OUTCOME AT DISCHARGE

Attempts have been made at many centers to categorize late outcome after head trauma. One measure used widely in the literature is the Glasgow Outcome Scale, developed by Jennett and Bond to assess the outcome of patients sustaining CNS trauma.[7] This scale served as a baseline method for assessing the degree of recovery achieved by the head-injured patients in our study. According to the scale, survivors are placed in one of four levels depending on the degree of functioning and independence that they maintained. The scale presents broad categories of morbidity but does not evaluate the often subtle cognitive impairment of the patient. The Glasgow Outcome Scale at discharge for the patients studied is summarized in Table 2-5.

Seventy-two percent of the patients returned home after discharge from acute-care centers, and 7 percent required additional hospitalization at another facility. During this time, 14 percent of the entire head-injured population were not considered self-sufficient in activities of daily living. Of these patients, 50 percent required institutional care, and 50 percent were cared for by a family member. These figures demonstrate clearly that many patients who were having significant problems with activities of daily living were in fact sent home without the benefit of a rehabilitation program. This was due in part to a shortage of appropriate facilities to accommodate the large number of injuries occurring each year.

How soon outcome becomes stable has yet to be established, and studies are proceeding. It seems that outcome in most survivors of head injury becomes fixed at approximately 6 months; although improvement may continue after this time, it seldom is sufficient for a survivor to move into a better category on the Glasgow Outcome Scale.[7] Unfortunately, a limited amount of research on head-trauma recovery has been published to date. Yet, considering that in many studies patients are followed for 3 to 5 years, and that the Glasgow Coma Scale and Glasgow Outcome Scale have only recently been implemented, a greater amount of consistent information on the outcome of head injury can be expected.

OUTCOME AT THREE MONTHS

In order to better assess the impact of head trauma on the patient and family and to gain some knowledge about the recovery over time, all patients were seen in a follow-up clinic 3 months postinjury. During the clinic, the patient's physical and psychologic status was assessed. Data were collected on various outcome measures such as the Glasgow Outcome Scale, employment status, and physical complaints expressed by the patients. Outcome data were available on 79 percent of the population. The Glasgow Outcome Scale was used as a baseline assessment of a recovery at 3 months (Table 2-6).

TABLE 2-5. Glasgow Outcome Scale (at Discharge)

Dead	7%
Vegetative	4%
Severely disabled	8%
Moderately disabled	12%
Good recovery	69%

TABLE 2-6. Glasgow Outcome Scale (3 Months Postinjury)

Vegetative	4%
Severely disabled	8%
Moderately disabled	22%
Good recovery	66%

TABLE 2-7. Length of Unemployment After Injury

0–7 days	32%
8–14 days	11%
15–30 days	14%
31–60 days	8%
61–89 days	2%
90 days and more	33%

TABLE 2-8. Frequency of Problems After Head Injury

Problem	% of Patients
Physical complaints (headaches, blurred or double vision, vertigo)	81
Seizures	1
Memory difficulties	42
Change in marital status	4

Other factors noted in the assessment of outcome were changes in employment and financial status owing to the injury. Thirty-three percent of the patients interviewed 3 months after discharge were unemployed because of their injury, and an additional 4 percent had changed their employment. Sixty-two percent of the total patients contacted at follow-up had some change in their financial status owing to their injury. The length of unemployment noted in the patients is shown in Table 2-7. In patients with multiple-system involvement, it was difficult to determine the extent to which associated injuries affected the length of unemployment.

Data outlining the frequency of subjective problems encountered at 3 months are presented in Table 2-8.

SUMMARY

The aim of evaluating descriptive data is that certain significant characteristics might become evident that will help in the identification of a population at risk for head trauma. Such information can be of value to those involved in rehabilitating these patients, in patient education, and in development of care plans, and may also promote an increasing awareness of potential problems for the patient, family, and community after discharge.

The large number of problems exhibited in patients at follow-up and the extended length of unemployment reflect the high incidence of morbidity after trauma. Outcome measures are still in the early stages of development, and further research in the area of recovery may reveal useful information that can be used to direct different treatment methods and rehabilitation programs with the hope of decreasing the morbidity from head injury.

REFERENCES

1. PARTINGTON, MW: *The importance of accident-proneness in the aetiology of head injuries in children.* Arch Dis Child 35:215, 1960.
2. *It's an emergency.* Newsweek, Nov 21, 1977:105.
3. JAGGAR, J, ET AL: *Epidemiology of central nervous system trauma: Preliminary findings presented at 107th APHA Meeting,* November 1979.
4. JENNETT, B AND MACMILLAN, R: *Epidemiology of head injury.* Br Med J 282:101, 1981.
5. KARLSBERK, WD, ET AL: *The National Head and Spinal Cord Injury Survey: Major findings.* J Neurosurg 53:519, 1980.
6. SELECKI, BR, ET AL: *A retrospective study of neuro-traumatic admission to a reaching hospital: Part 1. General aspects.* Med J Aust 2:113, July–Dec 1967.
7. BOND, MR: *Assessment of outcome after severe brain damage.* Lancet 1:489, 1975.
8. TEASDALE, G AND JENNETT, B: *Assessment of coma and impaired consciousness: A practical scale.* Lancet 2:81, 1974.

BIBLIOGRAPHY

BRUCE, DA, ET AL: *Outcome following severe head injuries in children.* J Neurosurg 48:679, 1978.

DUCKER, TB, BLAYLOCK, RL, and PEROT, PL: *Emergency care of patients with cerebral injuries.* Postgrad Med 55(1):102, 1974.

JENNETT, B: *Some aspects of prognosis after severe head injury.* Scand J Rehabil Med 4:16, 1972.

RIMEL, RW, EDLICH, RF, AND JANE, JA: *An injury severity scale for comprehensive management of central nervous system trauma.* Journal of the American College of Emergency Physicians 8(2):97, 1979.

TEASDALE, G AND JENNETT, B: *Assessment and prognosis of coma after head injury.* Acta Neurochir (Wien) 34:45, 1976.

Chapter 3

TYPES OF DISABILITY

Ernest R. Griffith, M.D.

Residual effects of head injury are often pervasive, involving multiple life functions. The combination of physical and mental impairments may create a total life disability that is greater than the sum of its parts.[1] Although the severity, extent, and duration of residual disabilities are functions of the severity and extent of head injury, so-called "minor" head injury may produce significant and lasting sequelae.[2,3]

To avoid confusion in terminology, several definitions are offered:

An *impairment* is the alteration in the function of an anatomic part due to disease, injury, or birth defect.

A *disability* is a state of less than normal function due to impairment. The terms disability and dysfunction are used interchangeably.

A *handicap* is the difference between normal function and the deficient function (disability) created by the impairment.

This chapter will be concerned with the identification of categories of disabilities, briefly noting the major and most frequently encountered disabilities under each category. It is convenient to categorize life functions as physical, communicative, psychologic, social, educational, and vocational. Each of these spheres of function may be altered after head trauma. Physical disabilities are frequently less severe and have less impact on other life functions than do psychologic disabilities.[4] Furthermore, major physical disabilities are often accompanied by mental disabilities, whereas mental dysfunctions not infrequently occur without physical disabilities.

The multiplicity of dysfunctions resulting from head injury requires a systematic method of identification and quantification of each disability. In clinical rehabilitation settings adaptations of the Problem-Oriented Medical Record have been widely used for purposes of identification.[5-7] Baseline and follow-up comparative measurements of the severity of disabilities (the handicaps) present a greater challenge owing to difficulties in quantifying degrees of nonphysical dysfunctions. However, a number of systems—some specific to head injury—have been described for this purpose.[8-13]

PHYSICAL IMPAIRMENTS AND RESULTING DISABILITIES

MOTOR IMPAIRMENTS

Disorders of movement and posture are listed in Table 3-1. Of these, spasticity, bradykinesia, ataxia, hemiparesis, and tremors are the commonest lingering disorders that compromise function. Bradykinesia is a frequent component of other movement disorders that may profoundly affect mobility and other activities of daily living. Ataxia, or discoordinate, dyssynergic movement and faulty balance, may be related to lesions of the cerebellum and its tracts or other areas of the brain. Apraxia refers to the inability to produce a skilled movement upon request despite the capability of producing the movement spontaneously. Rigidity states include decerebrate and decorticate posturing, and the less commonly occurring Parkinson-like cogwheel or lead-pipe rigidity. In our experience, rigidity states associated with posturing usually evolve into other forms of motor dysfunction, such as spasticity, or disappear. Various limb pareses (weakness) or plegias (paralyses) are encountered, at times coexistent with neuropathic bowel and bladder dysfunction. Hemiparesis is the most common of this group of disorders. Most often when one side is primarily involved, more subtle motor deficits exist on the "normal side." Dyskinesias encompass dystonia, choreiform and athetoid movements, and ballism. Muscle tone is greatest and movement least in the posturings of dystonia. Choreiform movements are continuous, rapid, unpredictable, bizarre, seemingly purposeful, involuntary, and proximal in distribution. Athetoid movements are continuous, slow, writhing, variform, involuntary, and distal in distribution. Ballisms are hyperkinetic involuntary flailings of extremities. The dyskinesias, other than athetosis, are rarely seen in head-injured patients. When present, dyskinesias, like parkinsonian signs, are usually the consequence of tranquilizing drug effects. Tremors are predictable, timed, involuntary movements that may occur at rest or with movement or both. They are frequent concomitants of other movement disorders, particularly ataxia and spastic states. Many of these motor impairments and associated swallowing difficulties may be initiated or intensified by drugs such as antispasmodics, antiepileptics, tranquilizers, and sedatives.

SENSORY IMPAIRMENTS AND ABERRATIONS

All modalities of sensitivity may be altered by head trauma. Loss, diminution, or perversion of sense of pain, temperature, position, touch, and pressure may occur in various patterns, usually in a hemisensory distribution. Cortical sensory deficits may occur singly or in combinations. These modalities include graphesthesia, stereognosis, two-point discrimination, simultaneous tactile stimulation, and deep pain. Special sensory deficits often involve vision, hearing, smell, and taste.[3] The most frequent and disabling of these special sensory

TABLE 3-1. Disorders of Movement-Posture

1. Spasticity
2. Bradykinesia
3. Ataxia
4. Apraxia
5. Rigidity states
6. Hemiparesis-hemiplegia
7. Quadriparesis-quadriplegia
8. Triparesis-triplegia
9. Monoparesis-monoplegia
10. Dyskinesias
11. Tremors

TABLE 3-2. Types of Visual Impairment

1. Neurologic impairments
    a. Field cuts due to optic chiasm, tract, radiation injuries
    b. Visual perceptual deficits
    c. Diplopia due to extraocular muscle palsies
    d. Gaze palsies
    e. Nystagmus
    f. Other tracking disorders
    g. Decreased acuity or blindness due to optic nerve atrophy
    h. Cortical blindness
    i. Impairment of global stereopsis
    j. Defects in color vision
2. Impairments due to ophthalmologic injuries
    a. Decreased acuity, blindness, scotomata due to
        i. Retinal injuries
        ii. Globe injuries
        iii. Intraocular hemorrhage
        iv. Glaucoma
    b. Diplopia due to extraocular muscle or orbit injuries

deficits involve the visual and auditory systems. A variety of visual deficits is listed in Table 3-2. Although common, extraocular palsies are often reversible. Field cuts are somewhat less frequent and less likely to disappear. Of greatest long-term consequence are the perceptual deficits, tracking disorders, and peripheral and central types of blindness.

Hearing disorders, including tinnitus and partial or complete deafness, may be peripherally or centrally induced. Trauma of the tympanic membrane and ossicular dislocation are examples of the former. Lesions of the auditory nerve or temporal lobe are representative of the latter. Such central injuries are more likely to cause permanent hearing deficits. Damage to the olfactory bulbs producing anosmia or parosmia is often unrecognized until long after the initial injury.[3] Vestibular deficits or instability may produce vertigo, nystagmus, and associated autonomic symptoms.

Persisting pain syndromes may produce physical as well as psychologic disabilities. A listing of common pain entities is presented in Table 3-3. In these syndromes, the thalamic and other hyperpathic states are the rarest but most disabling and difficult to treat. Any of these states can produce chronic pain behaviors that greatly interfere with life functions, but most of the musculoskeletal conditions are fairly self-limited.

DISABILITIES OF PHYSICAL FUNCTION RESULTING FROM MOTOR AND SENSORY IMPAIRMENTS

The functional equivalents of motor and sensory deficits are primarily *physical disabilities*. These disabilities involve an array of activities of daily living (ADL) as depicted in Table 3-4.

TABLE 3-3. Pain Syndromes

1. Shoulder-hand syndrome
2. Other painful shoulder syndromes
3. Causalgic syndromes related to fractures, peripheral nerve injuries, other associated injuries
4. Heterotopic bone formation
5. Painful muscle spasms, rigidity
6. Thalamic syndrome
7. Other hyperpathic states of CNS damage
8. Chronic neck or back pain associated with spinal injury, movement or postural disorders

TABLE 3-4. Activities of Daily Living

1. Mobility spectrum
   a. Bed mobility
   b. Transfers
   c. Wheelchair mobility
   d. Ambulation
   e. Driving
   f. Public transportation
2. Self-care skills
   a. Dressing
   b. Bathing, grooming
   c. Toileting, hygiene
   d. Feeding, swallowing
3. Homemaking and home activities
4. Outside activities (errands, shopping, etc.)

Physical disabilities often are eventually resolved as mild handicaps. Thus the great majority of head-injured individuals become nearly or fully independent in activities of daily life.[14] Public transportation and driving are the mobility functions most likely to require continuing assistance. Usually, motor deficits constitute the basis for difficulties in public transportation, whereas mental dysfunction is the major cause of inability to drive. The other ADL areas in which independence may not be attainable are homemaking, home activities, and outside activities.

Motor and sensory impairments may profoundly affect *communicative functions,* which will be further categorized and described in the following section of this chapter. Their effect on *psychologic, social, vocational,* and *educational functions* will be indicated in those sections of the chapter.

PRE-EXISTING PHYSICAL IMPAIRMENTS

Medical disorders of the cardiovascular, respiratory, renal, gastrointestinal, neurologic, or other body systems may have limited life functions significantly before the injury, and enhance the effects of impairments created by the injury. Therefore, assessment of life functions must take into account pre-existing levels of function.

DISABILITIES RESULTING FROM ASSOCIATED INJURIES

Vehicular accidents often produce trauma in multiple sites in addition to the brain. Thoracic, abdominal, spinal, craniofacial, and bony trauma are among the most common associated injuries.[3] Although potentially life-threatening, these injuries seldom result in long-term functional deficits. Notable exceptions are the problems of cosmetic defects and chewing-swallowing difficulties imposed by craniofacial trauma.

DISABILITIES RESULTING FROM MEDICAL COMPLICATIONS

Neurologic complications pose a threat to life as well as the potential for magnifying the severity of residual brain dysfunction. The principal nervous system complications are listed in Table 3-5. Seizures and hydrocephalus are the two conditions in this group that have the greatest potential impact on long-term function. Both of these disorders may occur after a long latency period.

Added insult of these complications may have the same pervasive effects on life functions as the original trauma.

TABLE 3-5. Neurologic Complications

1. Infection
   a. Brain abscess
   b. Meningitis—often after rhinorrhea or otorrhea
   c. Wound infection
   d. Osteomyelitis of skull
2. Recurrent hemorrhage
3. Hydrocephalus
4. Elevated intracranial pressure
5. Decreased intracranial pressure
6. Seizures
7. Vascular injuries—thrombus, aneurysm
8. Pneumocele
9. Leptomeningeal cysts

Adapted from Rosner, M: *Neurological Complications of Head Injuries.* Presented at Conference on Rehabilitation of the Traumatic Brain-Injured Adult, Williamsburg, Va, June 1979

General medical complications may threaten life and enhance morbidity, but are much less likely than neurologic complications to cause residual disabilities. A representative listing of these disorders is provided in Table 3-6. Of this group, the disorders that most often have the greatest potential to produce persisting disabilities are unrecognized drug toxicities, respiratory obstruction, overeating, heterotopic bone formation, contractures, decubitus ulcers, and upper urinary tract infections.

Prompt recognition and intervention will generally obviate permanent disabilities stemming from these complications.

COMMUNICATION DISABILITIES

Physical impairments such as ataxia, dyskinesias, and spasticity can produce dysarthrias, aphonia, pseudodyslexia (due to ocular instability), prosody defects, and dysgraphia (Table 3-7). Cortical lesions of critical sites produce apraxias, aphasias, dyslexias, and dysgraphias. Confused language may be the result of memory and perceptual deficits, or behavioral abnormalities. Severe mental deficits will produce nonspecific poverty of language. Of the communication dysfunctions, aphasias are often the most disabling and resistive to treatment, although they probably are not as common as articulation deficits. These disabilities are considered in further detail elsewhere in this book.

PSYCHOLOGIC DISABILITIES

Almost invariably, the deficits impinging most severely on other life functions are the psychologic disabilities. All areas of brain function are subject to disablement since head trauma is so often a diffuse process. Inasmuch as the many varieties of dysfunction are treated in detail throughout this book, a brief identification and categorization of the chief problems will be provided in tabular form (Table 3-8). The most persistent of these disabilities include memory deficits, decreased abstraction and learning abilities, poor judgment and quality control, poor initiative, difficulty in generalization, short attention span, distractability, reduced motor speed, reduced eye-hand coordination, poor depth perception, spatial disorientation, impulsivity, irritability, depression, poor self-image, denial of consequences of the disability, childlike behavior, and dependency.

TABLE 3-6. General Medical Complications

1. Infection
   a. Pulmonary
   b. Genitourinary
   c. Infections of monitoring devices
   d. Septicemia
2. Drug toxicities
   a. Allergic reactions
   b. CNS depression
   c. Movement disorders
   d. Renal failure, other organ system toxicities
3. Gastrointestinal hemorrhage
4. Upper respiratory trauma, infection, obstruction from intubation
5. Embolic—pulmonary, systemic
   a. Thrombophlebitis
   b. Fat emboli
6. Endocrine-metabolic disorders
   a. Electrolyte-fluid imbalances
   b. Malnutrition
   c. Overeating-obesity
   d. Pituitary failure
   e. Inappropriate antidiuretic hormone secretion
   f. Cushing syndrome due to steroid administration
7. Musculoskeletal disorders
   a. Heterotopic bone formation
   b. Osteoporosis
   c. Disuse muscle atrophy
   d. Contractures
   e. Secondary injuries: falls, etc.
8. Peripheral neuropathies
   a. Drug induced
   b. Compression neuropathies
9. Hematologic disorders
   a. Anemias
   b. Bleeding diatheses
10. Dermatologic disorders
    a. Acne, drug induced
    b. Decubitus ulcers
    c. Dependent edema
    d. Injuries: self-induced, restraints, etc.
11. Autonomic disturbances
    a. Hypertension
    b. Sweating disorders
    c. Hyperventilation
12. Urinary tract disorders
    a. Infection
    b. Calculi
    c. Postcatheter urethral stricture
    d. Neuropathic bladder dysfunction

TABLE 3-7. Communication Disabilities

1. Aphonia
2. Dysarthrias and other articulation deficits
3. Prosody abnormalities
4. Aphasias: mixed, receptive, and expressive; paraphasias
5. Apraxias
6. Dyslexias, pseudodyslexias
7. Dysgraphias
8. "Confused" language

TABLE 3-8. Psychologic Disabilities

A. Cognitive-intellectual
  1. Disorders of consciousness
  2. Disorientation
  3. Memory deficits
  4. Decreased abstraction
  5. Decreased learning abilities
  6. Language-communication deficits
  7. General intellectual deficits
  8. Deficits in processing-sequencing information
  9. Illogical thoughts
  10. Poor judgment
  11. Poor quality control
  12. Inability to make decisions
  13. Poor initiative
  14. Verbal, motor perseveration
  15. Confabulation
  16. Difficulty in generalization
  17. Short attention span
  18. Distractability
  19. Fatigability
  20. Perplexity
  21. Dyscalculia
B. Perceptual-perceptual motor
  1. Reduced motor speed
  2. Reduced eye-hand coordination
  3. Poor depth perception
  4. Spatial disorientation
  5. Poor figure-ground perception
  6. Auditory perceptual deficits
  7. Anosognosia
  8. Autotopagnosia
  9. Tactile, auditory, visual neglect
  10. Apraxias
C. Emotional
  1. Apathy
  2. Impulsivity
  3. Irritability
  4. Aggressiveness
  5. Anxiety
  6. Depression
  7. Emotional lability
  8. Silliness
D. Behavioral-personality
  1. Lack of goal-directed behavior
  2. Lack of initiation
  3. Poor self-image, reduced self-worth
  4. Denial of disability or its consequences
  5. Aggressive behavior
  6. Childlike behavior
  7. Bizarre, psychotic ideation and behavior
  8. Loss of sensitivity and concern for others: selfishness
  9. Dependency, passivity
  10. Indecision
  11. Indifference
  12. Slovenliness
  13. Sexual disturbances
  14. Drug, alcohol abuse

Adapted from Rosenthal, M: *Psychological Deficits in the Brain-Injured Adult and Family.* Presented at Conference on Rehabilitation of the Traumatic Brain-Injured Adult, Williamsburg, Va, June 1979.

SOCIAL DISABILITIES

Most social dysfunctions relate directly to the psychologic disabilities enumerated in Table 3-8. Physical impairments, particularly those involving cosmesis, profoundly affect self-image and self-worth. The net effects of such psychologic and physical impairments are outlined in Table 3-9. Of these disorders, social withdrawal, marital stress, loss of leisure skills, need for structure, dependence, legal-business problems, and employment-financial difficulties occur with highest frequency.

Tobis and colleagues[15] have brought attention to the role of pre-injury psychologic factors on postinjury outcomes. They reported that a large percentage of their patients were beset by pre-injury problems, including marital discord, family strife, dependent behavior, educational difficulties and early dropout, frequent job changes and unemployment, and drug and alcohol abuse. Obviously, levels of postinjury psychologic functions will not ordinarily exceed those of pre-injury function. Indeed, these pre-existing circumstances may have precipitated the injury, and thus render the individual susceptible to recurrent injury.

Psychologic disabilities are not confined to the victim of head trauma. They occur in family members, friends, school and work associates, and society at large.[16] Consider the reaction of the family: disbelief, grief, mourning, depression, false hope, overestimation and underestimation of capabilities, guilt, disinterest, rejection, and so forth. The consequences of these reactions may include restriction to a custodial role, alienation, infidelity, divorce, sibling regression and rivalry, reversal of child-parent role, and behavioral-emotional problems in children. Society may react in ignorance, misunderstanding, or apathy to the "crazy" behaviors of both victim and family. Thus, society itself becomes "disabled": impaired in its attempts toward restoration of family and victim. Moreover, society's overreactions to aggressive or inappropriate behaviors may provoke additional problems that might well have been avoided.

EDUCATIONAL AND VOCATIONAL DISABILITIES

Mental disabilities pose the greatest obstruction to vocational and educational pursuits. Specific learning disorders, general mental deficits, communication problems, behavioral and emotional aberrations, and disorders of consciousness are among the many elements that conspire to reduce or prohibit competitive employment or education. Even in instances where individuals return to their former occupational or educational status, interpersonal relationships may be strained to the point of repetitive altercations. Tardiness, absenteeism, and deficient

TABLE 3-9. Social Disabilities

1. Social withdrawal
2. Lack of acceptance by family, associates
3. Family role identity problems
4. Marital stress
5. Sexual dysfunction
6. Inappropriate social behaviors
7. Loss of leisure skills and interests
8. Need for structure
9. Legal infractions
10. Dependence in legal-business affairs
11. Unemployment-financial difficulties
12. Inability to profit from experience

Adapted from Rosenthal, M: *Psychological Deficits in the Brain-Injured Adult and Family.* Presented at Conference on Rehabilitation of the Traumatic Brain-Injured Adult, Williamsburg, Va, June 1979.

work production and quality may be poorly tolerated by superiors and peers. The educational or vocational milieu must be painstakingly structured to the needs of the client. Physical disabilities may present architectural or transportational barriers. Slow, clumsy motor performance with or without sensory deficits may severely impede work production. Medicolegal aspects of compensations frequently act as an inhibitory influence on gainful employment.

"MINOR BRAIN TRAUMA"

The functional consequences of seemingly minor brain injury may have been grossly underestimated. The postconcussion syndrome is a constellation of dizziness-vertigo, impaired concentration, fatigability, depression, alcohol intolerance, irritability-restlessness, headache, insomnia, and defective memory.[3] However, evidence mounts as to lingering effects on psychologic, vocational, and educational functions.[17] The types of disabilities in these categories are similar to those already described, although they may diminish over many months.

SUMMARY

An attempt has been made to categorize the multiple disabilities accruing from head injury according to the functions that have been disturbed. The disabilities may incorporate all life functions, including those in the physical, psychologic, social, vocational, and educational spheres. Although the severity of these disabilities is related to the severity of brain injury, seemingly minor trauma can produce residual dysfunctions that significantly affect the lives of the victims, their families, and society at large.

Disabilities, particularly psychosocial dysfunctions, are often permanent. However, they may be amenable, even long after maximal neurologic recovery, to significant improvements as the result of rehabilitation. Therefore, it is essential that trained rehabilitation professionals anticipate, recognize, and develop management strategies for these functional problems.

REFERENCES

1. JENNETT, WB AND BOND, MR: *Assessment of outcome after severe brain damage.* Lancet March 1975:480.
2. SYMONDS, CP: *Concussion and its sequelae.* Lancet 1:1, 1962.
3. BUKAY, L AND GLASAUER, F: *Head Injury.* Little, Brown & Co, Boston, 1980.
4. BOND, MR: *Assessment of the psychological outcome after severe head injury.* Acta Neurochir (Wien) 34:57, 1976.
5. MILHOUS, RL: *Problem oriented medical record in rehabilitation management and training.* Arch Phys Med Rehabil 53:488, 1970.
6. GRANGER, CV AND DELABARRE, EM, JR: *Programmed examination formats: Use in rehabilitation medicine.* Arch Phys Med Rehabil 55:235, 1974.
7. DINSDALE, S, ET AL: *Problem oriented medical records: Their impact on staff communication.* Arch Phys Med Rehabil 56:269, 1975.
8. MOSKOWITZ, E AND MCCANN, C: *Classification of disability in the chronically ill and aging.* J Chronic Dis 5:343, 1957.
9. SARNO, JR, SARNO, M, AND LEVITA, E: *The functional life scale.* Arch Phys Med Rehabil 54:214, 1973.
10. REINSTEIN, L, STAAS, W, AND MARQUETTE, C: *A rehabilitation evaluation system which compliments the problem oriented medical record.* Arch Phys Med Rehabil 56:396, 1975.

11. Evans, CD, et al: *Rehabilitation of the brain-damaged survivor.* Injury 8:80, 1976.
12. Grosswasser, Z, et al: *Re-evaluation of prognostic factors in rehabilitation after severe head injury.* Scand J Rehabil Med 9:141, 1977.
13. Lezak, MD, Cosgrove, JM, and Wooster, N: *Portland Adaptability Inventory.* VA Hospital, Portland, Ore, 1980.
14. Lewin, W: *Rehabilitation needs of the brain injured patient.* Proc R Soc Med 63:8, 1970.
15. Tobis, J, Pure, K, and Sheridan, J: *Rehabilitation of the Severely Brain Injured Patients.* Presented at the American Congress of Rehabilitation Medicine, San Diego, Calif, November 1976.
16. Lezak, MD: *Living with the characterologically altered brain injured patient.* Journal of Clinical Psychiatry 30:592, 1978.
17. Rimel, R: *An Assessment of Recovery Following Head Trauma.* Presented at the Conference on Rehabilitation of the Traumatic Brain-Injured Adult, Williamsburg, Va, June 1979.

CONCLUSION

Michael R. Bond, M.D., Ph.D., FRCS, MRC Psych., MRCP, DPM

    The needs of head-injured persons are ill-served in most communities, and only within recent years has a strong movement toward providing for them started to develop. If those involved are to provide, as Jennett stated in Chaper 1, the most appropriate resources for rehabilitation (the type of resources, their amount, and the time of their delivery in terms of the recovery process), then they must have several types of information. They must be able to identify the population at risk, and must know its age range and sex structure, social characteristics, and the type of personal and environmental resources available for injured persons and their families. Good epidemiologic studies are rare, but the work presented in Chapter 2 by Rimel and Jane gives a very good account of the characteristics of a particular population in the United States; recently, Jennett and MacMillan have produced similar information for western Scotland. Both groups support and greatly amplify the information available from previous studies scattered through the literature and set a scene in which we see victims of severe injuries as, most often, being younger men from lower socioeconomic groups with a higher incidence of previous head injuries than noninjured people, and frequently with evidence of pretraumatic social maladjustment. About half are married, and most are on the threshold of adult life. Thus, they are personally and socially a vulnerable group, often lacking means to influence policy makers in our society. By the very nature of their injuries, many are prevented from voicing their thoughts and feelings in a coherent and positive way, leaving the greater part of their burdens to be shouldered by their relatives. Fortunately, organized help from groups of relatives is developing rapidly, and the National Head Injury Foundation Inc. in the United States and Headway in Britain seem likely to do for head-injured persons what societies for other groups of handicapped people (spastic, mentally handicapped, paraplegic, and multiple sclerosis patients, to name but a few) have been doing successfully for many years.

    Apart from knowing our patients or clients and their families, we must be fully conversant with the types of deficits they may have before we can apportion resources. In Chapter 3, Griffith outlines the full range of possibilities, indicating the most frequent physical and mental problems occurring after injury. This overview acts as an introduction to later chapters in which details of mental, social, and physical problems are explored together with their natural history. Knowledge of this kind is fundamental to the development of critical evaluative studies of methods of rehabilitation.

Section 2

EARLY METHODS OF ASSESSMENT AND TREATMENT

Chapter 4

EARLY EVALUATION AND MANAGEMENT*

J. Douglas Miller, M.D., Ph.D., FRCS Ed., FRCS Glas., FACS

The final outcome in any patient who suffers a head injury is determined by three sets of factors: the pre-injury status of the brain, the total amount of immediate damage done to the brain by the impact of the head injury, and the cumulative effects of secondary insults and pathologic damage to the already injured brain that are produced by systemic and intracranial mechanisms that come into play at various times after the accident that produced the head injury. Ideal management of patients with head injuries is aimed at minimizing the primary-impact damage and preventing or treating secondary insults so as to provide the best possible recovery consistent with the premorbid status of the brain.

In this chapter, the pathophysiology of head injury—the ways in which primary and secondary brain damage are produced—will be described. A system of clinical and laboratory assessment and diagnosis is presented that provides for rapid triage of cases so as to render urgent treatment to those patients who most require it. The principles and practice of managing head-injured patients are described, starting at the scene of the accident and following the patient in transit, through the emergency room to the intensive-care unit and the ward. Indications for surgical treatment are defined, and surgical procedures are described briefly. Finally, the relationship between various physiologic, neurologic, and diagnostic factors and the outcome from injury is presented. Emphasis will be given to those factors that carry a high probability that the patient will suffer severe disability from the head injury, for it is in such patients that early intensive rehabilitation measures should be directed. This is not a simple problem, however. Most current studies of outcome from head injury place the greatest emphasis on predicting a fatal outcome. Such an outcome is, of course, of no interest to the rehabilitationist. But, as Bricolo and coworkers[1] have recently pointed out, predicting severe morbidity is much more difficult than predicting death. Many of the factors that are instrumental in predicting a fatal outcome are of little or no value in predicting severe disability.

PATHOPHYSIOLOGY OF HEAD INJURY

PREMORBID STATUS OF THE BRAIN

Although head injuries occur most commonly in young men, they can and do affect all sectors of the community, including persons who have for one reason or another already sustained brain damage. In virtually all forms of head injury, both mild and severe, variable numbers of cerebral neurons and axons are irreversibly injured. When a head injury happens

---

*Supported by USPHS grant NS12587

to a person who has already lost a sizable population of neurons because of a previous brain injury but has made a good recovery, the result is usually much worse.

> A 54-year-old man slipped while cleaning a chicken coop, striking his head on a concrete floor. The patient was unconscious for 15 minutes but thereafter recovered consciousness fully. He was admitted to the hospital for observation because he had been unconscious and because skull x-ray films revealed a linear skull fracture. When a full history was obtained, it transpired that 1 year previously the same patient had been involved in an automobile accident and had sustained a closed head injury that had rendered him unconscious for 5 days. The patient had made a good recovery from this injury and had returned after 2 months to his occupation of farming, functioning apparently as well as he did prior to injury. Following this second, evidently less severe injury, however, the patient never fully recovered. His personality changed completely; he was unable to manage any of his own affairs, never ventured out of the house unless accompanied by someone else, was incapable of making even the simplest decisions, lost interest in all social and sexual activities, and was described by his wife as having become a completely different person.

For similar reasons, in patients who have already suffered a cerebrovascular accident, hydrocephalus, or encephalitis, a relatively minor head injury can be crippling. In addition, it is a truism that the older the patient who sustains a head injury, the less satisfactory is the recovery.

When assessing the potential of any head-injured patient for recovery, it is extremely important to obtain the best possible assessment of the pre-injury status of the patient. This can be obtained from school or college tests, previous medical examinations, results of job interviews, or interviews with members of the family. This status defines the upper limit for recovery for that patient, and in some head-injured patients it may fall far short of "normal."

PRIMARY IMPACT DAMAGE TO THE BRAIN

Depending on the nature, direction, and magnitude of the forces applied to the skull and brain at impact, primary damage to the brain can be any of one, two, or all of the following three types.[2]

Local Brain Damage

Local brain damage refers to brain injury that is localized to the site of impact on the skull. The damage may take the form of contusion and/or laceration. It may be superficial or may extend deeply into the brain. It may be mild, consisting of slight subpial hemorrhage, or it may be severe, with extensive brain necrosis and a surrounding area of local brain edema. Because of this edema, such damaged areas can swell and act as an intracranial space-occupying lesion. When the local injury has been of sufficient severity to interrupt the pial surface and cause laceration of the brain, then secondary bleeding can produce a subdural or intracerebral hematoma.

In the early stages, the propensity of such local lesions to be associated with telltale neurologic signs depends entirely on the location of injury. When, for example, the local injury is over the motor cortex, then contralateral weakness of the face and arm is to be expected. When, on the other hand, the brain lesion is in the frontal area, there may be little or no neurologic dysfunction to accompany quite severe local brain injury.

When swelling progresses to the point where brain shift and herniation are occurring, then a new set of neurologic signs will emerge, so-called "false-localizing signs." These include oculomotor or abducent nerve palsies and unilateral weakness of the arm or leg.

Polar Brain Damage

When the head is subjected to acceleration or deceleration, the brain can move to a limited extent within the skull and dural envelope. When this motion is suddenly arrested because the frontal and temporal poles impact against the walls of the anterior and middle cranial fossae, damage is done to the tips of the temporal and frontal lobes and to the orbital surface of the frontal lobe. This damage is in the form of contusion and/or laceration to the brain. Damage to the occipital pole can occur but is much less common. Just as with focal brain injury, these polar lesions can swell and be subject to intracranial hemorrhage, leading to the formation of sizable intracranial mass lesions. Because of their anterior location, such lesions are often not associated with abnormal neurologic signs until the swelling has reached the point of producing brain distortion and shift. This process may take 2 or 3 days. These polar lesions are one reason for delayed deterioration after head injury or for the existence of a lucid interval in which the patient who has been briefly comatose recovers consciousness but then deteriorates into coma once more.

> A 45-year-old man fell in the street after a drinking bout, was briefly unconscious, and was admitted to the hospital in a lethargic state, able to speak but confused and disoriented. No focal neurologic signs were detected. There was a linear skull fracture in the right temporal bone. On the second day after injury, the patient was recognized to have expressive dysphasia, right homonymous hemianopsia, and mild weakness of the right face and arm. Angiography revealed a large right temporal mass that proved at operation to be a combination of contused brain and subdural and intracerebral hematoma.

Diffuse Brain Injury

As a further consequence of the swirling movements that the brain may make inside the cranial cavity during a head injury, widely scattered shearing of axons within their myelin sheaths may occur. This damage to the white matter is intense in no single location, but its cumulative effect is nevertheless dramatic. In patients who have suffered this type of brain injury in relative isolation from focal and polar damage, the neurologic picture is fairly typical. The patient is observed to be deeply comatose from the start, often with abnormal motor function consisting most frequently of extensor posturing of the upper and lower limbs occurring spontaneously or in response to painful stimulation. The patient remains in this state for many weeks, during which time spontaneous eye opening returns. The patient does not, however, give clear evidence of any organized response to the environment, and recovery is into a vegetative state. If the patient dies, usually because of an intercurrent infection or other medical problem, autopsy reveals a brain that looks externally normal but in which there is a moderate degree of ventricular enlargement, scattered axonal retraction balls, and microglial stars and demyelination in areas where the scattered axons converge into tracts such as the cerebral peduncles. A common accompaniment of this type of injury is tearing of the corpus callosum.

When this type of diffuse brain injury is particularly severe, the areas of damage may be larger and extend more deeply to form distinct petechial hemorrhages in the white matter. With increasing severity of injury, the lesions tend more and more to extend into the brain stem. The lesions of the corpus callosum and some hemorrhagic, dorsally placed midbrain lesions are due to the impingement of the relatively mobile brain against the free edges of the falx cerebri and tentorium cerebelli, respectively, during the phase of maximum acceleration or deceleration of the head.

PRIMARY IMPACT DAMAGE TO THE SCALP, SKULL, DURA, AND OTHER STRUCTURES

In head injury, the brain is seldom, if ever, injured in isolation. Injuries to the structures that surround the brain are of significance for two reasons. They may provide a clue as to the site and nature of the impact. They may in themselves be responsible for complications that will play a major role in affecting the outcome from injury; examples of this would be epidural hemorrhage complicating linear skull fracture and producing severe brain compression, and meningitis complicating basal skull fracture associated with tearing of the dura mater and the mucosal lining of the paranasal sinuses.

The significance of a fracture of the skull is frequently a hotly debated medicolegal issue. To the layman, the presence of skull fracture signifies that a great deal of force has been exerted against the skull, and this must be synonymous with a considerable degree of brain damage and, therefore, a severe head injury. In many cases, this is true, but there are important exceptions to this rule. When no motion is imparted to the head but the skull is crushed, extensive linear fractures can result with little or no associated brain damage. Conversely, and not uncommonly in children, the capacity of the skull to bend in relation to a force can permit considerable brain injury to occur in the absence of a skull fracture. Where a moderate force is exerted against a very limited area of the skull—for example, under a hammer blow to the frontal region—a considerable amount of rather dramatic bony damage can result, with small, splintered bone fragments driven into the brain with severe but localized underlying brain damage; yet there may be no loss of consciousness, prolonged coma, or even any abnormal neurologic signs. This is because the rest of the brain has remained intact.[3]

The principal significance of damage to the structures that surround the brain is first that it may be associated with bleeding that, if inside the cranial cavity, soon becomes an urgent problem because of the limited space available for the expansion of the hematoma, and secondly that the introduction of infection into the intracranial cavity is facilitated. In this respect, the integrity of the dural envelope is of considerable importance. Once this is breached, infection is a strong possibility. If the dura remains intact, intracranial infection is rare.

> A 4-year-old boy was admitted from an infectious disease hospital to the neurosurgical unit with meningitis and a small puncture wound in the forehead that oozed watery fluid. Five days previously, he had fallen in the home and impaled himself on the axle of a toy truck. This had been pulled out by the mother. When the child became ill 3 days later with headache, vomiting, and fever, the injury was not mentioned to the family doctor, and the patient was referred to the infectious disease hospital as a case of meningitis. The puncture wound in the forehead extended through the skull and dura mater into the frontal lobe. The meningitis was clearly related to this injury.

THE CONCEPT OF CONCUSSION

One of the continuing puzzles in the pathology of head injury is the pathologic basis for the phenomenon of concussion, in which a person becomes briefly unconscious after a blow to the head, recovers consciousness, and goes on to make an apparently perfect recovery. Loss of consciousness implies major interference with the function of the reticular activating system in the brain stem. Features of concussion that also suggest brain stem dysfunction are changes in blood pressure, pulse rate, and respiration. Although most patients make an apparently full recovery, as many as one third of patients who have sustained a so-called minor injury have post-traumatic symptoms that may last many weeks or even months, in the form of persistent headaches, dizziness, and incoordination sufficient to prevent return to work.[4] Whereas some such patients have a pre-injury background of neurotic problems and no detectable postinjury neurologic deficit, just as many patients have persistent signs of mild neurologic dysfunction if these are searched for assiduously. Examples are finger and hand incoordination or vestibular dysfunction shown on nystagmography.[5]

Because these are minor injuries and do not result in death, there is virtually no supportive pathologic evidence to indicate the loci of brain damage that are associated with the syndrome of concussion. Indeed, it is possible that the entire phenomenon may be based on dysfunction rather than observable pathologic damage. Its rapidly reversible state suggests transient physiologic or biochemical dysfunction, possibly of neurotransmitter mechanisms, but in the absence of real proof, all of this is speculative.

Another approach to this problem has been to study animal models of concussive head injury. There are major drawbacks in comparing function and dysfunction in animal and human nervous systems. Differences in the relative proportions of fore and hind brain and in the relationships between brain and the surrounding skull greatly hamper the analogy between "concussive" injury in an animal and the same phenomenon in the human. It is, however, possible to define a fairly stereotyped physiologic response to concussive injury in all experimental animals that have been studied so far, ranging from the mouse to the primate.[6] This response consists of rapid but transient elevation of arterial blood pressure; irregular respiration or apnea, the duration of which is related to the severity of injury; and a decrease in electroencephalographic activity, the duration of which is also a function of the severity of injury. Intracranial pressure is transiently elevated, the height and duration of the increase in pressure again being loosely related to the severity of injury. Following these immediate changes, there is dysfunction of the cerebrovascular system such that the normal responses to changes in arterial carbon dioxide tension and blood pressure are impaired or abolished. In the midline structures in the brain stem, there is temporary impairment of blood-brain barrier function. Whether this same sequence of events occurs in the human is not known for certain, but it is at least likely.[7]

In ranking the severity of concussional head injuries in the human and in trying to assess how much long-term dysfunction and damage are to be expected, one of the most useful yardsticks at the present time is the duration of post-traumatic amnesia (PTA), measurement of which is unavailable in the experimental animal. Post-traumatic amnesia is the length of time from the point of injury until continuous memory returns. Its duration is usually at least three times that of the period of observed loss of consciousness. An injury that is followed by a PTA of less than 1 hour's duration is considered mild. Early return to work with no sequelae is anticipated. When PTA is between 1 and 24 hours, the injury should be considered moderate in severity. Post-traumatic problems of headache, dizziness, incoordination, and some persisting abnormal neurologic signs are more frequent. When the PTA is between 1 day and 1 week, the injury should be considered severe and the family warned that post-traumatic sequelae of the injury with some degree of subtle permanent disability are to be anticipated. When PTA lasts more than 7 days, the injury is considered very severe, and a full return of neurologic function after such an injury would be the exception rather than the rule.[8]

SECONDARY INSULTS TO THE INJURED BRAIN

The energy requirements of the brain are surprisingly high. There is no capacity for storage of energy-rich substrates. The supply of oxygen and glucose to the brain must therefore be plentiful and continuous. Interruption in that supply is followed within seconds by neurologic dysfunction and within a few minutes by neuronal damage that is soon irreversible. It is unfortunate that following severe head injury, several conditions occur frequently, all of which conspire in one way or another to decrease the energy supply to the injured brain. These insults may be of systemic or of intracranial origin.[9]

ARTERIAL HYPOXEMIA

The most common of the systemic insults is arterial hypoxemia, which is present in more than one third of severely head-injured patients on arrival at a major hospital from the scene of the accident. When arterial Po_2 falls below 60 mm Hg, desaturation of arterial blood begins to occur, with consequent fall in the volume of oxygen that is carried per unit volume of blood. Under normal circumstances, this is compensated for by a brisk cerebral vasodilatation. It appears, however, that in the damaged brain, this compensatory boost in blood flow is also interfered with, and the net result is a reduction in carriage of oxygen to the most severely injured parts of the brain.

Causes of arterial hypoxemia range from obstruction of the airway by blood or foreign bodies to transporting the patient flat on the back with no airway so that the tongue can fall back and obstruct the airway. More complex causes include arteriovenous shunting of blood in the lung and development of respiratory distress syndrome, the cause of which is unclear at present. Hypoxemia is truly a complication of head injury, being equally common in patients with head injury alone and in those with multiple injuries. We have encountered hypoxemia in 36 percent of 225 comatose patients with head injury, and found it to be associated with a significant increase in mortality.[10]

ARTERIAL HYPOTENSION

When arterial blood pressure is reduced, there is normally a compensatory cerebral vasodilatation that preserves cerebral blood flow despite the fall in perfusion pressure. In the injured brain, this capacity is diminished. The severely head-injured patient is, therefore, extremely vulnerable to the effects of a reduction of blood pressure, because any fall in blood pressure can lead to a reduction in cerebral blood flow.

Arterial hypotension is seldom, if ever, produced by head injury alone. This is not to say, however, that it does not occur in patients with head injury. It was recorded in 16 percent of 225 head-injured patients presenting to the Medical College of Virginia Hospitals in coma.[10] In all of these cases, the patients had suffered additional major systemic injuries, including fractures of the pelvis, injuries to the abdominal and thoracic viscera, and major long bone fractures. Severe multiple injuries are, however, present in approximately half of comatose head-injured patients. Arterial hypotension is, therefore, not uncommon and must always be looked for. When systolic arterial pressure is less than 95 mm Hg in a head-injured patient, an assiduous search should be made for further injury. This search should, if necessary, include intraperitoneal lavage to detect occult intra-abdominal bleeding.[11]

ANEMIA

Although traditional teaching is that hemorrhage is followed only sometime later by significant hemodilution, low hematocrits are not uncommon on admission to the hospital in patients with severe head injury who have also sustained other significant systemic injuries. This problem was present in 10 percent of a series of 225 severely head-injured patients.[10] The recording of a hematocrit of less than 30 percent should carry the same significance as arterial hypotension in prompting a careful search for other injuries.

HYPONATREMIA

Following severe head injury, blood electrolytes must be carefully monitored. Of particular significance is the serum sodium level, which must not be allowed to fall below 120 mEq per liter. The danger of hyponatremia lies in the accompanying reduction of serum osmolality and the tendency of damaged brain to imbibe water osmotically from the blood stream. This results in widespread and severe brain swelling with elevated intracranial pressure.

POST-TRAUMATIC INTRACRANIAL HEMATOMA

No matter the severity of the head injury, ranging from the mildest bump with no loss of consciousness to the most severe injury associated with instant and prolonged unconsciousness, there is always the risk that intracranial bleeding may complicate the injury and become a life-threatening problem in its own right. The hemorrhage most commonly begins at the time of injury and by the time of admission to hospital, on average 3 hours later, a 40 percent incidence of intracranial hematomas was recorded in 225 comatose head-injured patients.[10,12] The classic clinical picture of the intracranial hematoma is of a short period of unconsciousness followed by regaining of consciousness, then secondary loss of consciousness due this time to compression of the brain by the hematoma. This lucid interval occurs in only a proportion of head-injured patients. Many more patients with intracranial hematomas are unconscious from the outset. But if the hematoma remains undetected and untreated, such patients will show progressive deterioration of neurologic function, then respiratory and cardiovascular function, leading to death.

The acute subdural hematoma is also formed of solid clotted blood. It forms between the inner surface of the dura and the brain, covered by arachnoid and pia mater. Subdural hemorrhage may originate from torn veins linking the brain surface with the dura. This tearing is caused by the motion of the brain relative to the inside of the skull that occurs with sudden acceleration or deceleration. It is more likely to occur when the brain is atrophic, as seen in the elderly or in persons who are suffering from diffuse brain atrophy due, for example, to chronic alcoholism. Another source of subdural hemorrhage is bleeding from a small sclerotic artery on the surface of the brain. The most common source of acute subdural hemorrhage, however, is bleeding from the edges of a cerebral laceration. In such cases, there is usually a combination of subdural and intracerebral blood clot. This happens not infrequently at the frontal or at the temporal pole and is then characterized by the term "burst temporal lobe."

Intracerebral hematomas may form as described in conjunction with acute subdural hematoma or in isolation deeper within the brain. These latter hemorrhagic lesions are of uncertain etiology. Many clinicians believe that they represent hemorrhage into areas of ischemic necrosis rather than true traumatic lesions. With the advent of computerized tomography, such deep intracerebral lesions have been more frequently recognized, particularly those that develop after a delay of several days from the time of injury, lending credence to the view that they represent secondary hemorrhage into an already necrotic area of brain.[13]

BRAIN SWELLING

That the injured brain has a propensity to swell is not in doubt. Dispute still exists, however, as to the precise cause of this swelling. In the area of brain that surrounds contusion or laceration, brain swelling appears to be mainly due to the formation of cerebral edema, an accumulation of water in the intracellular and/or interstitial space. Diffuse post-traumatic swelling of the brain, however, appears to be a different phenomenon, and is more likely caused by engorgement or congestion of cerebral blood vessels. The volume that is therefore increased in this circumstance is cerebral blood volume, not brain water content.[14]

RAISED INTRACRANIAL PRESSURE

Since intracranial hemorrhage and brain swelling occur in what is virtually a rigidly enclosed space, it is not surprising that intracranial pressure (ICP) should frequently be elevated in patients with head injury. In a large series of comatose patients with severe head injury (now more than 350 cases), abnormal elevations of intracranial pressure have been recorded at some time in more than 50 percent of patients.[10,15]

In the normal adult, pressure in the cerebrospinal fluid or epidural space should remain in the range of 0 to 10 mm Hg in the recumbent position. Pressures over 20 mm Hg mean are definitely abnormal; and when ICP reaches 40 mm Hg mean, there is invariably neurologic dysfunction and impairment of the electric activity of the brain in all head-injured patients. This is because at pressures over 40 mm Hg the ICP becomes a limiting factor in the determination of cerebral blood flow.[16] The perfusion pressure of the brain is equivalent to the difference between arterial and intracranial pressure, and a minimum perfusion pressure of 50 mm Hg is necessary in the normal subject. In the patient with head injury, the minimum required perfusion pressure may be much higher. While severe elevations of ICP (>40 mm Hg) are strongly associated with severe morbidity and a high mortality, even the milder elevations of ICP (20 to 40 mm Hg) are associated with increased morbidity.[15]

INTRACRANIAL INFECTION

Complication of a head injury by intracranial infection is always a tragedy. It is not only that such an occurrence should always be preventable, but also that meningitis, suppurative encephalitis, or brain abscess adds rapidly and insidiously to morbidity and mortality. The development of meningitis in a comatose head-injured patient is extremely hard to spot. Nuchal rigidity and mild elevations of body temperature (to 101°F) are common sequelae of traumatic subarachnoid hemorrhage. The only factor which signals that these signs are due to meningitis and not subarchnoid blood is unexplained deterioration in the neurologic status of the patient. If the patient is already deeply comatose, this deterioration may take the patient to the point of death before the meningitis can be detected.

Intracranial infection can arise because of compound injuries of the head in which a scalp puncture or laceration, skull fracture, and dural tearing are all in continuity. Basal skull fractures may be compound if the fracture extends into one of the paranasal air sinuses and there is associated tearing of the dura mater and the mucosal lining of the sinus. Sharp objects can easily penetrate the floor of the anterior cranial fossa via the cheek, the roof of the orbit, or the nose. Postoperative intracranial infection may occur because of inadequate debridement of a contaminated wound or as a complication of a surgical operation. Introduction of intraventricular or subdural catheters for measurement of intracranial pressure is another potential source of intracranial infection. The dura mater is an extremely effective barrier to the development of intracranial infection. When it is breached either traumatically or surgically, the possibility of meningitis or abscess formation must always be considered.

HYDROCEPHALUS

The normal pathways by which cerebrospinal fluid (CSF) passes from the fourth ventricle over the surface of the brain to be absorbed into the cerebral venous sinus system can be obstructed as a result of particularly copious subarachnoid hemorrhage caused by head injury or during the resolution of basal meningitis. When the CSF pathways have been obstructed in this way, the ventricular system expands at the expense of the cerebral white matter. The process of recovery in the head-injured patient ceases and is followed by further slow deterioration in mentation, gait, and urinary control. This is a relatively rare occurrence after severe head injury, but it is important to detect because a relatively simple CSF shunting operation can often reverse the neurologic deterioration and set the patient back on the road to recovery.

Unfortunately, the most common cause of increase in size of the ventricular system is so-called hydrocephalus ex vacuo in which the ventricles are enlarging secondary to post-traumatic loss of white matter. In this circumstance, the enlarged ventricles are merely a telltale sign of the presence of severe brain damage. Cerebrospinal fluid shunting procedures have no influence whatsoever on the outcome of these cases.

POST-TRAUMATIC EPILEPSY

Epileptic seizures always pose a threat to the brain. At a time when the increased neuronal activity in the brain is making demands for more blood and oxygen, the patient is likely to become hypoxemic because of respiratory difficulties during the seizure. The ensuing hypoxic insult to the brain may destroy any chances for a useful recovery from severe head injury.

Epileptic seizures can occur at any time after head injury, from a few minutes after impact to several years after the original injury. Early epileptic seizures are particularly common in young children. Seizures that develop later than 1 week from the time of injury are defined as late-onset epilepsy. These later-developing seizures are much more likely to recur and persist. Factors that are associated with an increased propensity for the development of seizures include missile wounds of the head, any type of intracranial hematoma, and intracranial infection.[17] More detailed information on the causes, significance, and management of post-traumatic epilepsy are found in a later chapter (see Chapter 8).

SECONDARY DAMAGE TO THE INJURED BRAIN

BRAIN DISTORTION, SHIFT, AND HERNIATION

When an intracranial mass lesion such as a hematoma develops, brain in the immediate vicinity exhibits viscoelastic properties, becomes distorted, and tends to flow away from the distorting mass. The cortex under an epidural hematoma will show concave indentation, which remains for several minutes or hours after the hematoma has been evacuated. Neurologic dysfunction appropriate to the indented area is probably due to vascular compression on the surface of the brain. Thus, a temporoparietal epidural hematoma situated over the motor strip is frequently associated with contralateral facial and brachial weakness.

During the initial compensatory phase of the development of an intracranial mass lesion, the distorted brain fills up spaces normally occupied by CSF, the subarachnoid space becomes obliterated, and the lateral ventricles become smaller. As the process continues, brain herniates from one intracranial compartment to the others. The cingulate gyrus on the side of the mass lesion herniates under the free edge of the falx. This callosal herniation may occlude one or both anterior cerebral arteries.

The medial portion of the temporal lobe herniates through the gap between the midbrain and the free edge of the tentorium cerebelli. This process compresses and distorts the cerebral peduncle, causing a progressive motor dysfunction. First there is contralateral hemiparesis; then, due to cut-off of the normal rostral modulating influences, abnormal motor activity appears in the form of decorticate and decerebrate rigidity. Impairment of the rostral inflow to the reticular activating system of the brain stem also produces loss of consciousness. As herniation progresses, the oculomotor nerve becomes compressed between the posterior cerebral and superior cerebellar arteries, causing an ipsilateral third nerve palsy. This is manifest by dilatation of the ipsilateral pupil with loss of the pupillary response in that eye to light shone into either eye. Ptosis and lateral deviation of the eye may also become evident, the latter due to unopposed action of the lateral rectus muscle.

At the same time that the medial temporal structures are herniating through the tentorial hiatus, there is a general downward axial displacement of the brain stem toward the foramen magnum. This process is associated with vegetative disturbances in the form of impaired respiration leading to apnea; and changes in the blood pressure, which rises, and the pulse rate, which slows. This medullary impairment may be made worse by the development of tonsillar herniation in which the cerebellar tonsils prolapse through the foramen magnum and compress the medulla.

In addition to the obvious functional disturbances in the integrity of the reticular formation, oculomotor nerves, and vasopressor and respiratory centers, visible secondary brain damage can often be seen in fatal cases in the form of hemorrhages usually located centrally in the midbrain and lower brain stem. These secondary hemorrhagic lesions are thought to result from downward traction on the central perforating branches of the basilar artery, producing either direct rupture of the vessels or ischemic necrosis with secondary hemorrhage into the necrotic zones.[18]

HYPOXIC/ISCHEMIC BRAIN DAMAGE

In addition to brain damage that is a direct result of trauma or is secondary to the compressing effect of an intracranial mass lesion, a third type of post-traumatic brain damage has received much attention in recent years. This damage is indistinguishable from that which results from the imposition of severe hypoxic or ischemic insult to the brain. It is exceedingly common. Graham and colleagues[19] recorded ischemic brain damage in 91 percent of 151 patients who had died from severe head injuries. Ischemic damage is widespread; it occurs most commonly in the hippocampus (81 percent), basal ganglia (79 percent), scattered in the cerebral cortex, both in the arterial distribution zones and in the water shed between them (46 percent), and in the cerebellum, most commonly in the water shed zone between the distributions of the superior and posterior inferior cerebellar arteries (44 percent).

The distribution of these pathologic changes suggests multiple etiologies. These include arterial hypotension and hypoxemia, both of which are known to be relatively common in patients with severe head injuries, particularly when complicated by multiple systemic injuries. Other contributory causes are raised intracranial pressure, cerebral vasospasm, brain edema, and the combination of these physiologic insults with disordered cerebral vascular autoregulation. Dysregulation of cerebral blood flow is a known accompaniment of cerebral trauma.[20] It results in a situation where any reduction in cerebral perfusion pressure caused by either a fall in blood pressure or a rise in intracranial pressure is no longer accompanied by a compensatory vasodilatation to preserve cerebral blood flow. Relatively small reductions in perfusion pressure may therefore cause cerebral blood flow to fall rapidly to ischemic levels. The cerebral vasodilator response to hypoxemia is also impaired by trauma. Thus, the head-injured patient is in the particularly dangerous situation of both suffering frequently from hypoxemia and lacking the necessary defense mechanisms that would normally protect the brain against it. Cerebral vasospasm and brain edema, both of which have also been recorded in patients with severe head injury, act not only to reduce resting cerebral blood flow but also to impair the compensatory vasodilator mechanisms, thus placing the brain in double jeopardy.

DIAGNOSIS IN HEAD INJURY

DETERMINANTS OF HEAD INJURY

The diagnosis that a patient has sustained a head injury is not usually in doubt. Nevertheless, occasions arise in which a patient is found lying comatose at home or in the street and it is uncertain whether or not a significant head injury has been sustained. Doubt is often increased when alcohol or drugs are invoked as the possible cause of the patient's coma. In such circumstances, it cannot be stressed too strongly that the correct procedure when in doubt is to treat the patient as if he or she had sustained a serious head injury. The management that is provided will be appropriate for the patient who is suffering from drug-induced coma, but the converse does not hold true. Galbraith and colleagues[21] found that the majority of male patients with head injury seen at a major city hospital had some degree of alcohol intoxication. Extremely high blood alcohol levels were encountered in some of this group of patients without having produced coma. Several comatose patients with high blood alcohol levels were harboring large intracranial hematomas. It was concluded that in any comatose patient in whom head injury is suspected, the assumption that the coma is due to alcohol rather than brain injury or compression is more often wrong than right.

Epilepsy is another common source of confusion in patients who have sustained a head injury. The sudden onset of coma due to the rapid enlargement of an intracranial hematoma may be wrongly attributed to epilepsy in which the clonic phase of the seizure is assumed to have occurred unobserved. Valuable time may then be wasted awaiting return of consciousness in a patient who is in fact continuing to deteriorate rapidly because of progressive brain compression.

In summary, the correct way to manage lethargic or comatose patients in whom no clear history of head injury has occurred, but in whom it is suspected, is to proceed as if the patient had sustained a head injury and apply the appropriate diagnostic measures. The urgency with which this process is carried out depends upon the consciousness level of the patient when first seen at the hospital and during subsequent evaluation. What is required is a practical method of diagnostic triage of patients who are known or suspected to have suffered a head injury.

TRIAGE OF HEAD-INJURED PATIENTS

A simple method of triage of head-injured patients has been used at the Medical College of Virginia.[12] Patients can easily be allotted into one of three clearly definable grades.

A grade I category is assigned when the patient is alert and oriented to time, place, and person on examination at the hospital. Such a patient may have been rendered briefly unconscious by the injury but by the time he or she is seen in the hospital emergency room is now fully alert. The decision to admit such patients to the hospital is based on the history of loss of consciousness or the discovery of features, such as skull fracture, that warrant observation for 24 or 48 hours lest the patient's condition subsequently deteriorate due to intracranial hemorrhage or brain swelling.

The grade II category is assigned when the patient is lethargic or drowsy yet able to speak and answer simple questions and/or obey simple commands such as "show me two fingers," "put out your tongue," or "open and close your eyes." If the neurologic examination reveals a patient to be suffering from weakness of the face, arm, or leg or if the patient complains of severe headache and is vomiting intermittently, such patients are also assigned a grade II category.

These patients must all be admitted to the hospital for observation, and before discharge computed tomography (CT) of the cranial contents should be carried out to ensure that intracranial hematoma is not present. It is our practice in such patients to carry out CT within 24 hours after admission. Because of the relatively high consciousness level of certain patients, a certain leeway is available in which neurologic evaluation gives adequate warning of the patient's deterioration. When the patient is already in coma, however, the situation becomes quite different.

When patients are unable to obey simple commands, they are placed in a grade III category, which signifies coma. Such patients are usually unable to utter formed words, and most will not open their eyes to command or even to painful stimulation. Neither of these conditions, however, is a prerequisite for the allocation of grade III status. Patients in this status are considered to be at considerable risk from further neurologic deterioration due to brain compression or post-traumatic swelling. Definitive diagnostic and management measures must be undertaken immediately. It is our practice to have CT carried out in such patients as soon as it is possible to move the patient safely from the emergency room. In the subsequent section, the way in which the evaluation and management of such patients is carried out is described in more detail.

EVALUATION OF THE COMATOSE HEAD-INJURED PATIENT

It is impossible to make a valid assessment of neurologic function in a patient who is hypoxemic or shocked. The very first step is therefore to ensure that the patient has an adequate airway, is adequately oxygenated, and has satisfactory arterial blood pressure and peripheral circulation.

The patient must be examined from head to toe for injuries. Patients who have sustained their head injury in automobile accidents will have other major systemic injuries in at least half the cases. Signs of head injury include swelling of the scalp that may indicate an underlying fracture and bleeding from the nose or ear, particularly if this is mixed with CSF. Cerebrospinal fluid can be detected by allowing the blood-stained fluid to drip onto filter paper or a piece of gauze. A pale halo appearing around the blood drop indicates that CSF is also present. This is proof not only that the patient has sustained a basal skull fracture but also that the dura and arachnoid surrounding the brain are torn. Telltale bruising in the periorbital areas and behind the ears appears only after several hours and usually is not present on this first assessment in the emergency room.

In examining the rest of the body, particular care must be taken to detect spinal injury and soft tissue injuries around the major joints and always to remember the possibility of occult intra-abdominal hemorrhage. At the Medical College of Virginia, peritoneal lavage is performed on most comatose head-injured patients because of the frequent detection of intra-abdominal hemorrhage even in patients whose blood pressure is still normal.

The neurologic evaluation of the comatose patient in the emergency room must be brief and objective. Fortunately, the intense study of this problem in the last 20 years has made this a relatively simple matter. Most necessary information to indicate the neurologic status of the patient can be obtained rapidly by a relatively simple examination. The first determination is the conscious level. This is best defined by placing the patient on the appropriate point on the Glasgow Coma Scale.[22] This scale consists of three elements: the eye opening, motor, and verbal responses to standard stimuli. The scale is shown in Table 4-1. The preferred pain stimulus consists of the application of heavy pressure on the nail bed of the little finger. To compare the response on both sides it may also be necessary to apply pain to the sternal area. In addition, it is important to include a painful stimulus above the neck, in the supraorbital area. This will select the patient who is quadriplegic from concomitant neck injury, unresponsive to painful stimuli applied to the limbs, yet conscious and responsive to pain applied above the neck.

TABLE 4-1. Glasgow Coma Scale

Eye Opening	Best Motor Response	Verbal Commands
4 Spontaneous	6 Obeys commands	5 Oriented
3 To command	5 Localizes pain (purposeful)	4 Disoriented
2 To pain	4 Flexor withdrawal (semipurposeful)	3 Words
1 Nil to pain	3 Abnormal flexor (decorticate)	2 Sounds
	2 Extensor (decerebrate)	1 Nil to pain
	1 Nil (flaccid)	

EARLY EVALUATION AND MANAGEMENT

Other important elements of the initial neurologic examination are the pupil response to light and the eye movement reflexes. In assessing the pupil response to light, distinction must be drawn between abnormalities caused by damage to the optic or oculomotor nerves and abnormalities caused by central dysfunction in the brain stem. Pupil abnormalities confined to one eye are usually peripheral. Comparison of the direct and consensual light responses will permit distinction between second and third cranial nerve lesions. Bilateral abnormalities of the pupil light response, in contrast, are almost always due to central dysfunction.

The eye movement reflexes may be tested by eliciting the oculocephalic, or "doll's eye," reflex. In this test, the head is moved rapidly to the side, and the tendency for the eyes to revert to vertical gaze is examined. The test should be done only when it is certain that the patient's cervical spine is intact. In the comatose patient, a normal response is the tendency for the eyes to look vertically toward the ceiling no matter what the position of the head. Abnormal responses in such patients may consist of skew deviation of the eyes or no response at all. Bilateral abnormalities again imply brain stem dysfunction. Unilateral impairment of the "doll's eye" response may be a result of oculomotor nerve dysfunction.

A more powerful test of reflex eye movement is the oculovestibular response, which is elicited by syringing 20 ml of ice-cold water into the ear. This test can be done only when the tympanic membrane is known to be intact and is contraindicated in patients who have blood and/or CSF coming from the ear. A "normal" response in the comatose patient is tonic deviation of both eyes toward the irrigated ear. Bilateral abnormalities are virtually always due to brain stem dysfunction, and complete failure of the oculovestibular response with no movement of the eyes whatsoever indicates severe brain stem dysfunction and/or damage.

The next stage in the patient's assessment that should be carried out in the emergency room is to obtain plain x-ray films of both the skull and the cervical spine. Skull x-ray films are useful not only to detect fractures but also to detect intracranial foreign bodies or intracranial air. The latter is always an abnormal finding and indicates the presence of dural tearing and communication between the outside and the subarchnoid space, commonly via paranasal air sinuses. The x-ray films of the cervical spine should be scrutinized not only for fractures or dislocations of the cervical spine but also for swelling of the prevertebral soft tissue shadow. This is often the only clue that the patient has a previously dislocated and unstable cervical spine that happens to have reduced while the patient is in the recumbent position.

When these assessments have been carried out and the patient's condition is stable with good airway, adequate oxygenation, and adequate circulation with a normal blood pressure, it is judged safe for the patient to be moved to the radiology department for CT. This atraumatic study has been a major advance in head-injury care. It is possible to detect intracranial hematomas compressing the brain, both those lying outside the brain in the epidural and subdural space and intracerebral hematomas that lie within the substance of the brain (Fig. 4-1).[23] A hematoma may sometimes be of the same density as brain and therefore not distinguishable from brain substance on CT. Nevertheless, the mass effect is detectable by distortion of the ventricular system and shift of identifiable structures such as the choroid plexus and pineal gland. Computed tomography will also identify hemorrhagic or lucent areas within the brain suggesting infarct or edema, intracranial foreign bodies, intracranial air, and fractures of the skull.

If CT is unavailable, intracranial hematomas can be detected by arteriography or air ventriculography. Both of these diagnostic measures yield less information than CT does. Under ideal circumstances, all of the above diagnostic assessment can be accomplished within 1 hour after the patient's arrival at the hospital. At this stage, it is possible to make definitive plans for specific management of the head-injured patient depending on the neurologic and CT findings. Based on a series of nearly 400 comatose head-injured patients, a constant ratio of 40 percent of patients have intracranial hematomas associated with significant brain shift and herniation. These patients require immediate surgical treatment.

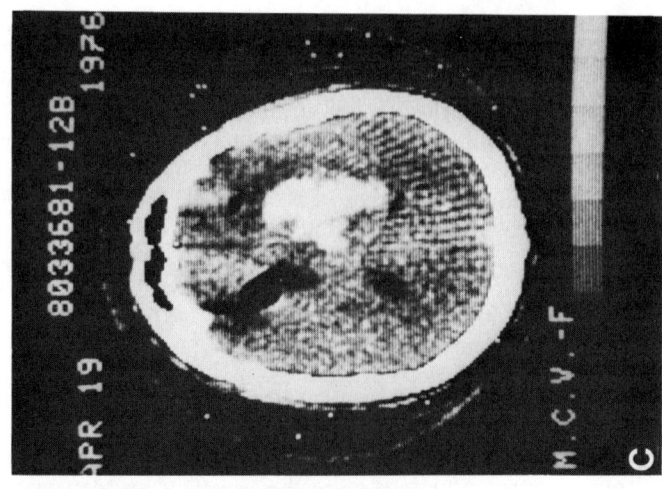
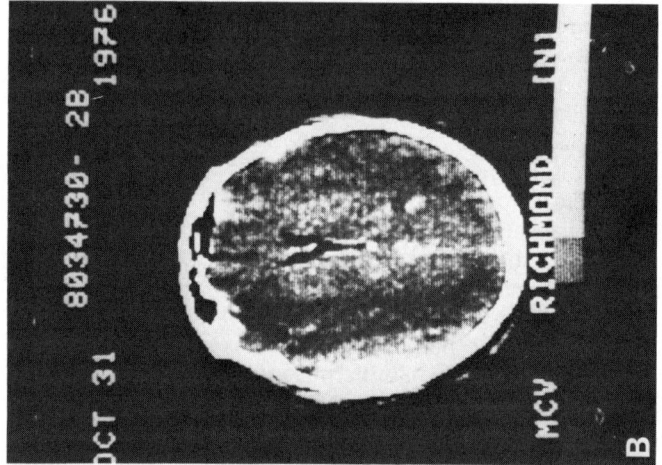
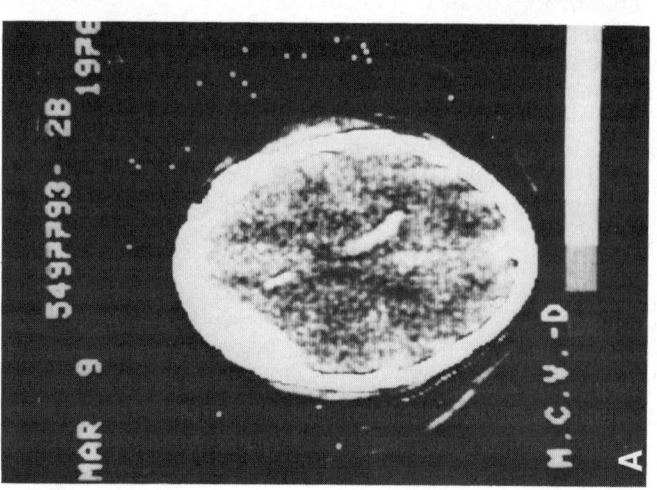

FIGURE 4-1. Computerized tomograms in three patients with severe head injury presenting in coma show (A) left frontal epidural hematoma; (B) left temporoparietal acute subdural hematoma; and (C) right intracerebral hematoma.

MANAGEMENT OF SEVERE HEAD INJURY

EARLY MEASURES AT THE SCENE OF THE ACCIDENT AND IN TRANSIT

Management of the patient with a severe head injury should ideally begin at the locus of injury and cover the transport of the patient to the hospital. All patients with head injury must be considered as having potential injuries to the cervical spine. Movement of the patient into the ambulance must be carried out with extreme care to avoid unrestrained movements of the head and neck. The most important single factor at this early stage is the establishment and maintenance of a clear airway. The mouth and throat must be cleared of blood, secretions, dentures, and foreign bodies. If circumstances dictate the patient should be transported lying flat on the back, then an adequate airway must be in position to prevent the tongue and lower jaw from falling back and occluding the airway. An oral or an esophageal occlusive airway is adequate for this purpose. If there is no airway present, the patient should be transported in the three-quarters prone position (patient is put on the side, then turned rather more prone, i.e., face down, with the uppermost leg drawn up so as to prevent the patient rolling onto the face, with head turned slightly to one side) so that the tongue and lower jaw tend naturally to fall forward and any vomitus or bleeding from the mouth drains away.

If oxygen is available, it should be administered during transport to the hospital in comatose patients because of the high incidence of hypoxemia (more than 30 percent) that has been recorded in such cases on arrival at the hospital. During transport, suction should be available to clear the oropharynx and nasopharynx of vomitus, blood, or secretions. Arterial blood pressure and the pulse rate should be checked. If arterial pressure is low, intravenous fluids should be given. Bleeding from the scalp can always be arrested by firm pressure. The consciousness level of the patient should be checked using the Glasgow Coma Scale. If it is possible to relay this information to the receiving hospital in advance of the arrival of the ambulance, then this should be done.

MANAGEMENT IN THE EMERGENCY ROOM

At this stage, the goals of management are normal levels of arterial oxygen tension and arterial blood pressure while assessment of neurologic status and extent of injuries is proceeding. In the comatose patient, an endotracheal tube should be inserted as soon as possible and the cuff inflated. This provides the best possible security to the airway. During insertion of the tube, it must be remembered that cervical spine injury is a possibility and excessive extension of the neck must be avoided. It may be necessary to perform nasotracheal intubation, and the task of inserting the tube should be handled by an expert. Intravenous lines must be established if not already in place.

The emergency room physician must then be in a position to declare whether the patient is safe for transfer for further diagnostic or therapeutic measures. The patient must not leave the emergency room until a secure respiratory and circulatory state has been attained.

Prophylactic treatment with anticonvulsants in comatose patients should be started early, while the patient is still in the emergency room, the aim being to achieve an anticonvulsant blood and tissue level as quickly as possible. If a decision has been made to treat this type of head-injured patient with steroids, these agents can also be begun as soon as the patient reaches the emergency room or even during transit to the hospital. There is currently no compelling evidence to support the use of steroids in either moderate or high dosages in the acutely head-injured patient, but it is a widespread practice. Mannitol solution should ideally not be given until the intracranial status of the patient is known. Intravenous mannitol will reduce ICP and may produce temporary improvement in the neurologic status of the patient. If it is given prior to full evaluation, the examining physician may be unable to determine the true urgency of the problem. If the CT shows an intracranial mass lesion that requires surgical decompression, mannitol is given at that point as a bolus of 1 g per kg body weight. This allows the beneficial effect of the mannitol to cover the patient through the relatively hazardous phase of transport from the radiology department to the operating room and induction of anesthesia. An exception to this policy is made in the case of patients who are admitted first to an outlying hospital and are thought to be developing signs of tentorial herniation such as deteriorating level of consciousness and unilateral pupillary dilatation. In such cases, it is recommended that the patient receive a bolus of mannitol (1 g per kg) to cover the period of transport to the next hospital.

OPERATIVE MANAGEMENT OF HEAD INJURY

There are two indications for surgical treatment of patients with head injury. The first is to provide relief from brain compression due to an intracranial hematoma or swollen hemorrhagic contusion. This is nearly always an emergency, and surgery must be carried out as soon as possible. This entails a full craniotomy with exposure of frontal, temporal, and part of the parietal lobes; evacuation of all hematoma; and, if necessary, resection of necrotic, swollen brain tissue. The use of mannitol solution is only a temporizing measure during the time taken to prepare for surgery. The second broad indication for surgery in patients with head injury is prevention of infection. This covers the debridement and toilet of compound wounds, repair of penetrating wounds to the scalp and dura, repair of persistent dural fistulas communicating with fractures at the base of the skull, and the surgical management of penetrating missile wounds of the head.

Although it is important that surgical measures for the prevention of infection from compound wounds be carried out relatively urgently, these need not be emergency procedures. In fact, it may be desirable to wait a few hours to permit the patient to be adequately ventilated and to take measures to reduce brain swelling and increased ICP prior to the surgical procedure. If operation is delayed for more than 24 hours, however, the risk of intracranial infection is increased.

There is no evidence that surgical treatment of depressed skull fractures or penetrating injuries of the brain affects the incidence of post-traumatic epilepsy at a later date. Prevention of post-traumatic epilepsy is, therefore, not an indication for surgery.

MANAGEMENT IN THE INTENSIVE-CARE UNIT

In the patient who is already comatose as a result of injury, the underlying principle of management is prevention of further deterioration. Since potential causes for such deterioration include hypoxemia, arterial hypotension, intracranial hypertension, fluid and electrolyte imbalance, infection, and elevations of body temperature, these factors must be monitored in the intensive-care unit and any adverse trends rapidly corrected.[12]

I have used artificial ventilation in all comatose head-injured patients via an endotracheal tube during the first week or two after injury. If artificial ventilation is required for a longer period, tracheotomy may be required. As a rule, however, it is safe to permit the patient to ventilate spontaneously after a week or so of artificial ventilation. In the critical 3 or 4 days after injury, we monitor arterial pressure continuously from an indwelling arterial catheter. This can also be used for the withdrawal of arterial blood for measurement of arterial Po_2, Pco_2, and pH.

A key factor in monitoring the patient with a severe head injury in the intensive-care unit is frequent assessment of clinical neurologic status. In patients who are less severely injured, this clinical assessment constitutes the only monitoring modality. The key factors recorded are the three elements of the Glasgow Coma Scale (eye opening, motor, and verbal

EARLY EVALUATION AND MANAGEMENT

response), pupillary reaction to light, eye movement reflexes (oculocephalic or oculovestibular), and comparison of limb power on the right and left sides recorded for both arms and legs (Table 4-2). All these items should be recorded hourly in comatose patients and at least once per shift for the alert patient. Results are noted on a neurologic watch sheet along with the blood pressure, heart rate, body temperature, and ICP, if this is recorded (Fig. 4-2). In this way, trends of improvement or deterioration in the head-injured patient can be clearly detected. When muscle relaxants or sedatives are used, neurologic evaluation becomes difficult or impossible, and considerable reliance must be placed on monitoring of ICP or brain electric activity (see Chapter 6).

Intracranial pressure can be monitored from a catheter in the lateral ventricle or from a screw in the skull inserted into the subarachnoid space. Another approach to measuring ICP is to insert a transducer directly into the epidural space. With all these methods, the ICP can be continuously recorded on a strip chart recorder or oscilloscope.

TREATMENT OF RAISED INTRACRANIAL PRESSURE

When ICP becomes elevated over 25 mm Hg mean or when any elevation of ICP appears to be accompanied by neurologic deterioration, measures should be taken to reduce the pressure. Hyperventilation is used first, bringing arterial Pco_2 down from 30 to 20 mm Hg. If this is unsuccessful in reducing ICP, CSF drainage is instituted, continuously venting the CSF line against a positive pressure of 25 cm H_2O. If CSF is aspirated or vented against atmospheric pressure, the ventricles will collapse, no further CSF will drain, and the ICP recording will be lost. If neither hyperventilation nor CSF drainage is successful, mannitol is given, using a starting dose of 1 g per kg body weight. If this produces a satisfactory reduction in ICP, the next dose of mannitol is half the initial dose. The effect of the mannitol solution is carefully monitored against the ICP record. The lowest effective dosage of mannitol is preferable. Prior to further administration of mannitol, serum osmolarity must be checked. If this is above 325 mOsm per liter, more mannitol is unlikely to be successful in reducing ICP and is likely to produce severe metabolic derangement.

There is much current interest in the role of barbiturate therapy in reducing raised ICP in head-injured patients. This is under study, and there is no present consensus as to the advisability of administering barbiturates to severely head-injured patients. The technique is not without its risks both because neurologic evaluation of the patient becomes impossible and because overly rapid administration of barbiturate may reduce the arterial blood pressure and cause cerebral ischemia in some patients.[24]

PROCESS OF RECOVERY FROM HEAD INJURY

In the comatose head-injured patient who is being managed in the intensive-care unit, orderly progress of the transition from dependence on life-support systems to independence is crucial if the best possible recovery is to be attained.

When ICP has been consistently below 20 mm Hg for 24 hours (including at least one overnight recording), the system can be discontinued. Artificial ventilation is continued until

TABLE 4-2. Neurologic Evaluation

Consciousness level	Glasgow Coma Scale
Other motor function	Best and worst response, comparison of limb power on right and left sides
Pupillary function	Response to light
Reflex eye movements	Oculocephalic and oculovestibular responses

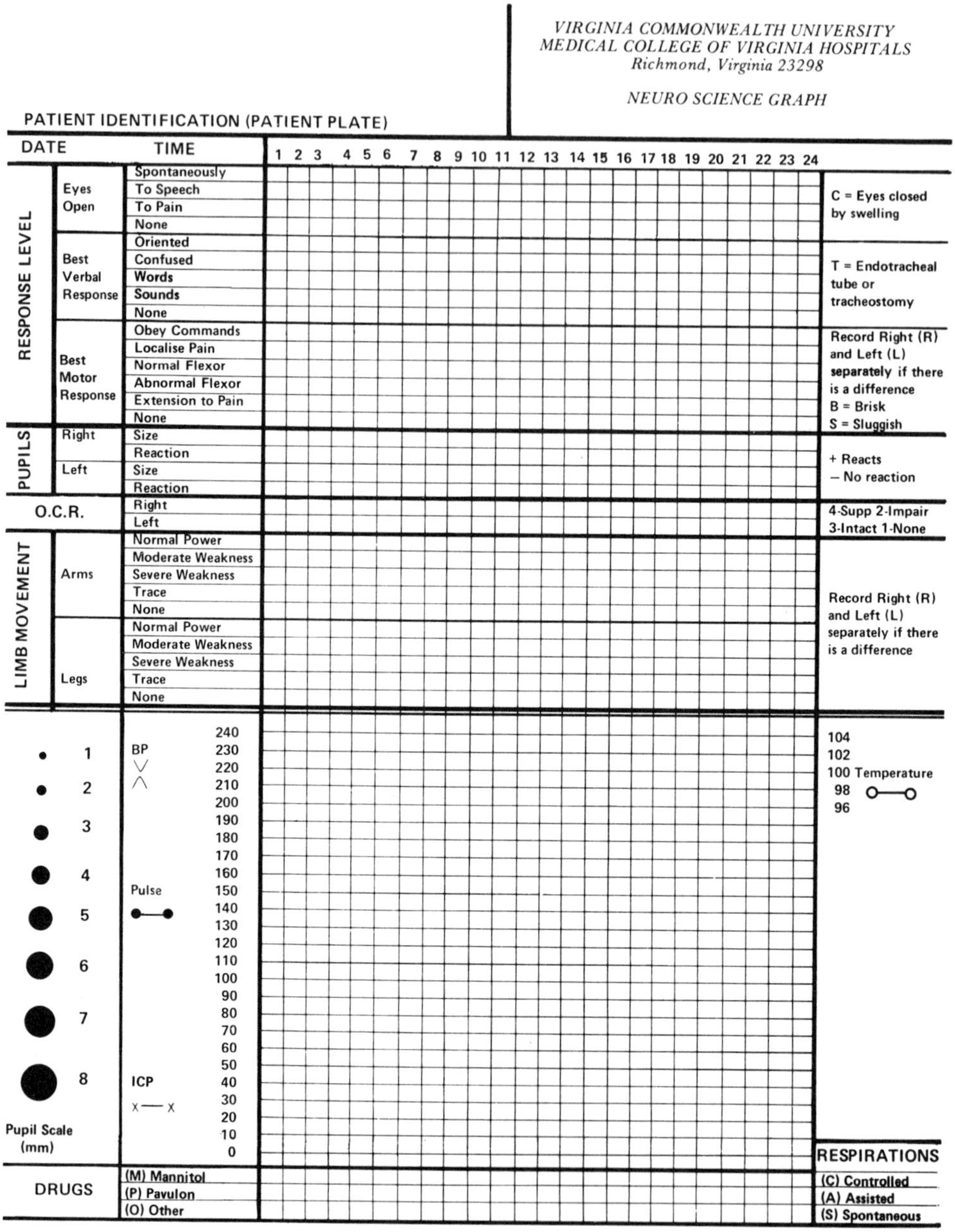
VIRGINIA COMMONWEALTH UNIVERSITY
MEDICAL COLLEGE OF VIRGINIA HOSPITALS
Richmond, Virginia 23298

NEURO SCIENCE GRAPH

PATIENT IDENTIFICATION (PATIENT PLATE)

DATE		TIME	1 2 3 4 5 6 7 8 9 10 11 12 13 14 15 16 17 18 19 20 21 22 23 24	
RESPONSE LEVEL	Eyes Open	Spontaneously		C = Eyes closed by swelling
		To Speech		
		To Pain		
		None		
	Best Verbal Response	Oriented		T = Endotracheal tube or tracheostomy
		Confused		
		Words		
		Sounds		
		None		
	Best Motor Response	Obey Commands		Record Right (R) and Left (L) **separately** if there is a difference B = Brisk S = Sluggish
		Localise Pain		
		Normal Flexor		
		Abnormal Flexor		
		Extension to Pain		
		None		
PUPILS	Right	Size		+ Reacts — No reaction
		Reaction		
	Left	Size		
		Reaction		
O.C.R.		Right		4-Supp 2-Impair 3-Intact 1-None
		Left		
LIMB MOVEMENT	Arms	Normal Power		Record Right (R) and Left (L) separately if there is a difference
		Moderate Weakness		
		Severe Weakness		
		Trace		
		None		
	Legs	Normal Power		
		Moderate Weakness		
		Severe Weakness		
		Trace		
		None		

Pupil Scale (mm): 1 2 3 4 5 6 7 8

BP ∨ ∧ ; Pulse ●—● ; ICP x—x

240 230 220 210 200 190 180 170 160 150 140 130 120 110 100 90 80 70 60 50 40 30 20 10 0

104 102 100 Temperature 98 o—o 96

RESPIRATIONS (C) Controlled (A) Assisted (S) Spontaneous

DRUGS (M) Mannitol (P) Pavulon (O) Other

FIGURE 4-2. Neurosurgical intensive-care watch sheet as used at the Medical College of Virginia.

normal blood gases can be maintained with spontaneous ventilation. The endotracheal tube is removed after adding dead space to increase depth of respiration. Feeding by nasogastric tube is increased until 3000 calories per day can be provided without aspiration.

Eye opening may recover through the stages of the Glasgow Coma Scale, but spontaneous eye opening usually begins, even in otherwise unresponsive patients, after about 2 weeks. Roving eye movements are common and may be wrongly interpreted as following movements. These usually appear within a few days in the recovering patient but not in the patient who remains in the vegetative state.

The best early indication of recovery is the motor response, which ascends through the stages listed in the Glasgow Coma Scale. In some patients who have had pronounced decorticate or decerebrate posturing, the early phase of recovery may be accompanied by the emergence of movement disorders consisting of dystonias or tremors. These subside spontaneously as a rule.[25]

Like the motor response, the verbal response usually returns through the stages noted on the Glasgow Coma Scale. The patient may go through a stage of shouting and uttering expletives, then through a stage of confusion and disorientation. At this stage, there may be florid delusions. Subsequent testing indicates that in this confusional state, which may last for several days, the patient is still within the period of PTA and will have no subsequent memory of conversation or events that occurred at this stage.

Emergence from coma is generally taken to be marked by obeying spoken commands and the return of speech or an equivalent signal from the patient. The end of PTA with return of continuous memory does not occur until later. Duration of PTA is commonly three or four times that of the period of unconsciousness. Until the patient has emerged from the period of PTA, the patient is not accessible for psychometric evaluation.[26] Other aspects of the rehabilitation process can, of course, begin at a much earlier stage.

FACTORS THAT HAVE A MAJOR INFLUENCE ON OUTCOME FROM SEVERE HEAD INJURY

As a result of several careful studies in which the clinical status of patients rendered comatose from head injury has been compared with outcome, there is a general measure of agreement concerning the major adverse significance of several clinical factors.[10,12,27-37]

One of the most important factors is the age of the patient. The younger the patient, the more likely he or she is to survive following head injury. The older the patient, the more likely he or she is to die. From my own studies, it appears that this increase of mortality with age is related mostly to the chances of dying from a medical complication of prolonged unconsciousness. The age of the patient does not seem to be a powerful predictor of severe disability or prolonged vegetative state after head injury. This is probably because older patients who might have suffered injuries severe enough to render them severely disabled or vegetative are more likely to die from pneumonia.

Another most important predictor of a poor outcome from injury is the presence of an intracranial, intradural hematoma requiring surgical decompression. The mortality and the rate of severe morbidity in head-injured patients are highest in those who have acute subdural or intracerebral hematomas, or both. These patients also tend to be older; they are more neurologically disabled to begin with and have the highest rate of postoperative intracranial hypertension.

The level of consciousness as determined on the Glasgow Coma Scale is also a powerful predictor of outcome. Of the three elements on the scale, the most powerful in predicting outcome is the motor response. There is a large increase in mortality and morbidity among patients who have abnormal (decorticate, decerebrate) or absent motor responses to painful stimulation as compared with those who are able to obey commands, localize, or even withdraw in a normal fashion. The presence of brain stem dysfunction as shown by bilateral pupillary abnormalities or abnormal eye movement reflexes is also associated with a much worse outcome from injury. The significance of these clinical factors, however, is that they predict an increase in mortality rather than any increase in the incidence of severe disability or vegetative state.

The CT scan not only is of value to indicate the presence of an intracranial hematoma requiring decompression but also has predictive value. Of most adverse significance is the presence on CT of lesions of increased density in the brain parenchyma, representing either hemorrhagic contusions or intracerebral hematoma.[22,38] Patients who have these lesions show an increased incidence of severe disability and intracranial hypertension, and high mortality. At a later stage, more than 2 weeks after injury, the presence of enlarged lateral ventricles on CT is associated with poor outcome. Most instances of ventricular enlargement represent compensatory ventricular dilatation consequent on loss of white matter related to extensive diffuse brain damage.[39] Focal lucent areas on CT may represent cerebral infarcts and correlate with focal neurologic abnormalities. Their appearance can indicate the need for early physical therapy. Sequential CT shows developing focal atrophy.

Intracranial hypertension is common after injury, particularly in those patients who have already required surgical decompression because of intracranial hematoma. In one-fourth of these patients and about 15 percent of all comatose head-injured patients, this intracranial hypertension cannot be controlled by conventional management measures and progresses until intracranial pressure is at the level of arterial pressure. Cerebral perfusion then ceases, and brain death occurs. Half of all head-injury deaths in the hospital are by this mechanism.[15]

Milder degrees of intracranial hypertension, 20 to 40 mm Hg, are also of adverse prognostic significance, even when the intracranial hypertension is controlled by treatment. Patients who suffer this type of treatable intracranial hypertension show a much higher proportion of severe disability than patients with normal ICP.

Based on the known outcome of many hundreds of patients with severe head injury, the combined influence of the abovementioned clinical variables can be assessed. In any individual patient in whom the various factors are known, it is now possible to predict with considerable accuracy the likelihood that the patient is going to survive or die as a result of head injury.[30,31,40] It remains to be seen whether adequate treatment of those factors that can be controlled or reversed will significantly improve the outcome. At present, it is unfortunately not possible to predict severe disability with the same degree of accuracy. Intracranial hypertension and the presence of dense intraparenchymal lesions on the CT scan are two factors that lessen the surviving patient's chances of good recovery from injury. Doubtless, more factors will be uncovered that have this predictive power. It may become possible within a day or two after injury to identify those patients who are likely to require prolonged and intensive rehabilitative measures and to start these measures as early as possible.

REFERENCES

1. Bricolo, A, Turazzi, S, and Feriotto, G: *Prolonged post-traumatic unconsciousness: Therapeutic assets and liabilities.* J Neurosurg 52:625, 1980.
2. Adams, JH: *The neuropathology of head injuries.* In Vinken, PJ and Bruyn, GW (eds): Handbook of Clinical Neurology, Vol 23, Injuries of the Brain and Skull, Part 1, Braakman, R (ed). Elsevier, Amsterdam, 1975.
3. Miller, JD and Jennett, WB: *Complications of depressed skull fracture.* Lancet 2:991, 1968.
4. Taylor, AR: *Post-concussional sequelae.* Br Med J 2:67, 1967.
5. Cartlidge, NEF: *Post-concussional syndrome.* Scott Med J 23:103, 1978.
6. Sullivan, HG, et al: *Fluid percussion model of mechanical brain injury in the cat.* J Neurosurg 45:520, 1976.
7. Povlishock, JT, et al: *The morphopathologic substrates of concussion.* Acta Neuropathol 47:1, 1979.
8. Russell, WR and Smith, A: *Post-traumatic amnesia in closed head injury.* Arch Neurol 5:4, 1961.
9. Miller, JD, et al: *Early insults to the injured brain.* JAMA 240:439, 1978.

10. MILLER, JD, ET AL: *Further experience in management of severe head injury.* J Neurosurg 54:289, 1981.
11. BUTTERWORTH, JF, ET AL: *Detection of occult abdominal trauma in patients with severe head injuries.* Lancet 2:759, 1980.
12. BECKER, DP, ET AL: *The outcome from severe head injury with early diagnosis and intensive management.* J Neurosurg 47:491, 1977.
13. GUDEMAN, SK, ET AL: *The genesis and significance of delayed traumatic intracerebral hematomas.* Neurosurgery 5:309, 1979.
14. ZIMMERMAN, RA, ET AL: *Computed tomography of pediatric head trauma: Acute general cerebral swelling.* Radiology 126:403, 1978.
15. MILLER, JD, ET AL: *Significance of intracranial hypertension in severe head injury.* J Neurosurg 47:503, 1977.
16. MILLER, JD: *Volume and pressure in the craniospinal axis.* Clin Neurosurg 22:76, 1975.
17. JENNETT, WB: *Epilepsy After Blunt Head Injuries,* ed 2. Heineman, London, 1975.
18. MILLER, D AND ADAMS, H: *Physiopathology and management of increased intracranial pressure.* In CRITCHLEY, M, O'LEARY, JL, AND JENNETT, B (EDS): *Scientific Foundations of Neurology.* Heineman, London, 1972.
19. GRAHAM, DI, ADAMS, JH, AND DOYLE, D: *Ischaemic brain damage in fatal non-missile head injuries.* J Neurol Sci 39:213, 1978.
20. ENEVOLDSEN, EM AND JENSEN, FT: *Autoregulation and CO_2 responses of cerebral blood flow in patients with acute severe head injury.* J Neurosurg 48:689, 1978.
21. GALBRAITH, S, ET AL: *The relationship between alcohol and head injury and its effect on the conscious level.* Br J Surg 63:128, 1976.
22. TEASDALE, G AND JENNETT, B: *Assessment of coma and impaired consciousness: A practical scale.* Lancet 2:81, 1974.
23. ROBERSON, FC, ET AL: *The value of serial computerized tomography in the management of severe head injury.* Surg Neurol 12:161, 1979.
24. MILLER, JD: *Barbiturates and raised intracranial pressure.* Ann Neurol 6:189, 1979.
25. GERSTENBRAND, F: *The course and restitution of brain injury in the early and late stages and rehabilitation measures.* Scand J Rehabil Med. 4:85, 1972.
26. MANDLEBERG, IA: *Cognitive recovery after severe head injury. 2. Wechsler Adult Intelligence Scale during post-traumatic amnesia.* J Neurol Neurosurg Psychiatry 38:1127, 1975.
27. BOWERS, SA AND MARSHALL, LF: *Outcome in 200 consecutive cases of severe head injury treated in San Diego County: A prospective analysis.* Neurosurgery 6:237, 1980.
28. BRUCE, DA, ET AL: *Outcome following severe head injuries in children.* J Neurosurg 48:679, 1978.
29. CARLSSEN, C-A, VON ESSEN, C, AND LÖFGREN, J: *Factors affecting the clinical course of patients with severe head trauma. Part 1: Influence of biological factors. Part 2: Significance of post-traumatic coma.* J Neurosurg 29:242, 1968.
30. CLIFTON, GL, ET AL: *Neurological course and correlated computerized tomography findings after severe closed head injury.* J Neurosurg 52:611, 1980.
31. JENNETT, B, ET AL: *Predicting outcome in individual patients after severe head injury.* Lancet 1:1031, 1976.
32. JENNETT, B, ET AL: *Prognosis of patients with severe head injury.* Neurosurgery 4:283, 1979.
33. MARSHALL, LF, SMITH, RW, AND SHAPIRO, HM: *The outcome with aggressive treatment in severe head injuries.* J Neurosurg 50:26, 1979.
34. OVERGAARD, J, ET AL: *Prognosis after head injury based on early clinical examination.* Lancet 2:631, 1973.
35. PAGNI, CA: *The prognosis of head injured patients in a state of coma with decerebrated posture.* J Neurosurg Sci 17:289, 1973.
36. PAZZAGLIA, P, ET AL: *Clinical course and prognosis of acute post-traumatic coma.* J Neurol Neurosurg Psychiatry 39:149, 1975.

37. VAPALAHTI, M AND TROUPP, H: *Prognosis for patients with severe brain injuries.* Br Med J 3:404, 1971.
38. SWEET, RC, ET AL: *The significance of bilateral abnormalities on the CT scan in patients with severe head injury.* Neurosurgery 3:16, 1978.
39. KISHORE, PRS, ET AL: *Delayed development of hydrocephalus in patients with severe head injury.* Neuroradiology 16:261, 1978.
40. STABLEIN, DM, ET AL: *Statistical methods for determining prognosis in severe head injury.* Neurosurgery 6:243, 1980.

BIBLIOGRAPHY

KALSBEEK, WD, ET AL: *The national head and spinal cord injury survey: Major findings.* J Neurosurg 53 (Suppl):S19, 1980.

KRAUS, JF: *A comparison of recent studies on the extent of the head and spinal cord injury problem in the United States.* J Neurosurg 53:(Suppl)S3, 1980.

Chapter 5

THE NEUROLOGIC EVALUATION

John J. Caronna, M.D.

The neurologic evaluation of the severely head-injured adult varies in detail and emphasis depending on how soon after the onset of illness or injury the patient is examined. The initial neurologic examination of the comatose patient in the emergency room or intensive-care unit aims to rapidly determine the cause of acute brain failure and its potential reversibility. The phase following the acute phase is characterized by the patient's neurologic condition stabilizing owing to prompt, appropriate medical or surgical treatment. In this postacute phase, the neurologic assessment seeks to define the extent of central nervous system (CNS) damage, and to identify prognostic indicants that predict eventual outcome.

Later during the recovery phase of illness, the clinical neurologic assessment aims to characterize the patient's rehabilitation potential and estimate the degree of eventual psychosocial adjustment.

In this chapter, the neurologic examination will be discussed in terms of these three phases of care for the head-injured patient: (1) an initial phase concerned with the differential diagnosis and acute treatment of coma; (2) postacute phase after stabilization in which prognostic indicants are sought; and (3) a later phase of rehabilitation in which the outcome achieved is assessed.

THE ACUTE PHASE

Diagnosis in the comatose patient represents a major challenge, even for the experienced clinician. Coma is not a disease in itself, but a product of a wide spectrum of life-threatening conditions that damage the CNS or depress its function. Even within the context of head trauma, coma may be due to neuronal or axonal injury, hypoxemia, or ischemia. Appropriate therapy, therefore, is dependent on accurate analysis of the underlying etiology and pathophysiology of the unconscious state. Often, the physician receives little information concerning the circumstances of coma or the patient's previous medical history. Nevertheless, the physical examination and the patient's response to simple diagnostic and therapeutic maneuvers will, in most cases, enable the physician to limit the differential diagnosis to one of several major categories and take appropriate measures to pursue the final diagnosis.

The management of coma depends on an accurate appreciation of clinical neurologic signs and an understanding of how coma and other disorders of consciousness occur. Familiarity with the neuroanatomic substrate of consciousness is a prerequisite of such an understanding.

REGULATION OF CONSCIOUSNESS

The human nervous system undergoes daily cycles of wakefulness and sleep characterized by striking changes in sensitivity to environmental stimuli and in motor activity. These changes in level of consciousness depend on a brain stem regulatory system called the reticular activating system (RAS).

Anatomically, the RAS consists of the paramedian regions of the tegmentum of the mesencephalon and the pons not associated with cranial nerves or specific ascending or descending pathways. Included in the RAS are the functionally related medial, intralaminar, and reticular nuclei of the thalamus.[1] By its location, the RAS has access to incoming sensory information and widespread connections to the cortical and subcortical motor systems.

Consciousness has two basic aspects: arousal and awareness.

Arousal is a crude function, which is simply wakefulness, and reflects activation of the RAS by somatosensory stimuli or innate motivational systems such as hunger. Natural sensory stimuli activate not only specific sensory relays to cortical sensory areas appropriate to the stimulus modality, but also the nonspecific projection system (RAS) that produces cortical arousal. Clinically, arousal is indicated by eye opening, either spontaneously or in response to stimuli. In some cases, arousal may occur in spite of complete destruction of the hemispheres.[2]

Awareness is manifested by cognition of self and environment and implies functioning cerebral hemispheres. The neocortex of the cerebral hemispheres is the site where intellectual processes are carried out and refinements in personality and behavior are developed. Clinically, awareness is marked by goal-directed or purposeful motor behavior, and the use of language.

Full consciousness implies that the patient is awake and normally aware of both internal and external stimuli. Mutually sustaining areas of both the RAS and the cerebral cortex are required to maintain full consciousness. Interaction between the cortex and RAS produces attention. Attention refers to the ability to concentrate or focus on a specific stimulus without being distracted by extraneous stimuli. Arousal is a more basic state in which the patient is awake and responsive to any environmental stimulus. Confusional states marked by alertness but inattentiveness can be produced by many pathologic conditions, of which metabolic and toxic encephalopathy, acute delirium, dementia, and diffuse cortical injury are but a few.

Coma results when a structural lesion or a toxic-metabolic process interrupts impulses from the reticular formation to the hemispheres, thereby preventing both arousal and awareness.

Clinically, the comatose patient maintains a sleeplike unresponsiveness from which the patient cannot be aroused. The definition of coma used in the International Data Bank Study of medical (nontraumatic)[3,4] and traumatic coma[5,6] is that "eye opening does not occur; no comprehensible speech is detected; and the extremities move neither to commands, nor appropriately to localize or ward off noxious stimuli." This definition corresponds closely to that proposed by the Head Injury Committee of the World Federation of Neurosurgical Societies: "an arousable, unresponsive state, regardless of duration, eyes continually closed."[7] This definition implies that there is no motor response to command and no speech. It is misleading, however, to define coma as an "unresponsive state" without qualification. A considerable range of reflex motor activity in the limbs can occur in response to noxious stimuli and is an indication of brain stem or spinal cord level responsiveness. Nonpurposive reflex movements such as flexor (decorticate) or extensor (decerebrate) posturing may be present. Stupor resembles coma except that the patient remains rousable if strong external stimulation is provided.

Coma induced by depressant drugs, anesthetics, or endogenous metabolic toxins may result from metabolic depression of the RAS or from acute damage to or depression of both

THE NEUROLOGIC EVALUATION

hemispheres. A unilateral lesion in a cerebral hemisphere does not cause coma until brain swelling impairs function, either of the opposite hemisphere (subfalcine or cingulate herniation) or, more frequently, of the rostral brain stem (central or uncal herniation)[8] (see below).

In some cases, particularly after severe head trauma or after anoxic-ischemic injury due to cardiac arrest, both hemispheres are severely damaged but the brain stem is preserved. After a period of coma, namely, eyes-closed unconsciousness lasting hours to days, wakefulness returns but without evidence of purposive behavior or cognition. This functionally decorticate state of eye-open unconsciousness is distinct from coma and has been termed the "vegetative state."[9]

PATHOPHYSIOLOGY OF COMA

All types of coma may be divided into three pathophysiologic categories: metabolic encephalopathy, supratentorial lesions, and infratentorial lesions. Each has a characteristic clinical evolution. The key to clinical diagnosis when the history is in doubt is to identify the initial anatomic distribution of the lesion and how it evolves.

Toxic-Metabolic Encephalopathy[10]

Noncerebral disease may affect consciousness by diffusely impairing metabolism of the cerebral cortex and brain stem. Brain metabolism may be depressed by exogenous toxins, as in the case of sedative drug poisoning, or by endogenous toxins, as occurs, for example, in uremia or hepatic failure. In hypoxia and hypoglycemia, the supply of extrinsic energy sources is insufficient for brain requirements, and coma occurs. Neuronal excitability also may be diminished by electrolyte and acid-base imbalances and by changes in serum osmolality.

Metabolic encephalopathy is the most commonly encountered cause of coma in a general hospital, and it frequently also exists as a complicating factor in patients with head injuries. For example, a comatose head-injured subject may have ingested toxic amounts of alcohol, sedatives, or anticonvulsants prior to having suffered cerebral trauma. The resultant comatose state may present with confusing neurologic signs and an unusual clinical evaluation because of the combined metabolic depression and structural damage to the CNS.

The typical clinical situation in primary metabolic encephalopathy is that the physician cannot localize the symmetric but patchy neurologic abnormalities to a regionally restricted lesion. Pupillary light reflexes are generally preserved (except in patients who have ingested glutethimide, atropine-like agents, or sedatives in high doses) even in the presence of signs of lower brain stem depression (e.g., apnea, absence of oculovestibular responses, and motor flaccidity with areflexia). In severe sedative drug poisoning, nearly all brain and spinal cord functions may be absent, including electrocerebral activity measured by a conventional electroencephalogram using scalp electrodes.

Supratentorial Lesions

Mass lesions of the cerebral hemispheres cause coma by herniating beyond the confines of the supratentional compartment and compressing the brain stem reticular formation. Clinically, two syndromes of herniation associated with supratentorial lesions are recognized.

Central Downward Transtentorial Herniation

Deep or midline masses, large-hemisphere infarcts, and subdural hematomas can compress and displace the supratentorial contents caudally through the tentorial opening in the subtentorial compartment. Unless herniation is checked by treatment, there will be a progressive failure of the rostral brain stem and then the pons and medulla.

Central herniation in its initial stages produces symmetric signs that may be mistaken for metabolic encephalopathy. Clinically, the first signs reflect failure of the diencephalon: reduced consciousness, 1 to 3 mm pupils with preserved reaction to light (bilateral central Horner syndrome), bilateral signs of corticospinal and extrapyramidal tract dysfunction, paratonic rigidity, grasp reflexes, decorticate posturing, and periodic Cheyne-Stokes respirations. At this state, rostral-caudal deterioration is potentially reversible by osmotic agents and surgery if a tumor or clot is present, but when signs of midbrain failure appear (fixed, dilated, or midposition pupils, or decerebrate rigidity), it is likely that distortion and compression have led to brain stem infarction.

Herniation of the Temporal Lobe Uncus

An expanding mass in the temporal lobe or lateral middle fossa may displace the uncus medially over the edge of the tentorial notch, and compress the third cranial nerve, the adjacent midbrain, and the posterior cerebral artery. The earliest sign of uncal herniation is unilateral pupillary dilation with a preserved or sluggish light reaction. As the uncus continues to compress the midbrain, the patient becomes deeply comatose and manifests an ipsilateral third-nerve palsy and contralateral decerebrate posturing. Bilateral decerebrate rigidity develops when the contralateral cerebral peduncle is compressed against the tentorial edge opposite the side of herniation. If treatment cannot halt brain displacement at this point, brain stem dysfunction will progress in a manner clinically indistinguishable from that caused by central herniation.

Subtentorial Lesions

Two types of posterior fossa lesions produce coma: lesions intrinsic to the brain stem that destroy the reticular formation, for example, pontine hemorrhage and paramedian infarction of the midbrain or pons; and lesions extrinsic to the brain stem that compress and distort it, for example, cerebellar tumor and hematoma.

Compressive lesions of the brain stem are often difficult to distinguish from intrinsic lesions, as cerebellar hematoma may mimic brain stem stroke clinically. In other cases, the caudal to rostral evolution of neurologic signs may resemble the patchy brain stem depression of sedative drug intoxication. Asymmetric motor signs and hypertension due to Cushing reflex[12] usually serve to identify brain stem compression.

Pathophysiology of Unconsciousness Due to Head Trauma

The traditional explanation for the brief or prolonged alterations of consciousness following blunt trauma has been primary brain stem concussion or damage, respectively.[13] An alternative explanation now in favor is that immediate coma that persists after head injury probably is due to widespread and severe damage to white matter, associated with disconnection of large areas of the cerebral cortex from subcortical structures including the RAS.[6,14] By contrast, delayed or deepening coma is associated with cerebral contusions, lacerations, and hematomas, which lead to increased intracranial pressure, brain shift, and herniation as described above.[15] In each case, the immediate or delayed coma after head injury results from disruption of the mechanisms that initiate and maintain cortical arousal.

IMMEDIATE MANAGEMENT OF THE COMATOSE PATIENT

MAINTENANCE OF RESPIRATION

The initial management of the comatose patient is directed toward stabilization. The steps taken in initial management will also be indispensable to eventual diagnosis of the underlying disorder.[16] The first step is to ensure an adequate airway, by intubation if necessary (Table 5-1). However, the rate and pattern of respiration should be noted before they are obscured by therapeutic measures such as intubation and mechanical ventilation, since disordered respiration is one of the best indicators of brain dysfunction. Depressed respirations usually accompany overdosage of opiates, sedative-hypnotics, and tranquilizers.

Severe hyperventilation ensues when acute brain damage, subarachnoid hemorrhage, or ingestion of acidic substances produces a lactic acidosis in the cerebrospinal fluid that in turn stimulates medullary receptors. Hyperventilation also can be of extracerebral origin, as is the case when neurogenic pulmonary edema complicates an intracranial catastrophe.

Periodic respiration implies bilateral hemisphere dysfunction, whereas ataxic breathing heralds impending medullary failure and apnea.

BLOOD CHEMISTRIES AND DEXTROSE ADMINISTRATION

Once adequate ventilation has been established, the following procedures are mandatory. Blood should be drawn for a determination of glucose concentration and routine chem-

TABLE 5-1. Management of the Comatose Patient

Immediate steps:
1. Ensure and protect airway patency.
2. In case of trauma, stabilize neck.
3. Institute resuscitative measures.
4. Draw blood for stat determinations of glucose, electrolytes, urea nitrogen, creatinine, complete blood count, prothrombin time, partial thromboplastin time, liver function tests, and osmolality; administer dextrose, 25 to 50 g, intravenously.
5. Monitor respiratory rate and pattern, blood pressure, pulse, rectal temperature, and cardiac function.
6. Obtain electrocardiogram and measure arterial blood gases.
7. Administer naloxone (Narcan) 0.4 to 0.8 mg intravenously, and thiamine 100 mg intravenously.
8. In case of recurrent seizures or status epilepticus, administer phenytoin in intravenous loading dose of 15 to 20 mg/kg (1000 to 1500 mg).
9. Briefly examine patient for signs of trauma and meningitis. Complete motor and neuro-ophthalmologic examinations; treat any metabolic derangements.
10. In suspected cases of bacterial meningitis, perform lumbar puncture.
11. If herniation present: hyperventilate; administer mannitol and corticosteroids; consult neurosurgeon.

Subsequent measures:
1. Insert nasogastric tube and Foley catheter.
2. Send blood and urine specimens for toxicologic screening.
3. If seizures continue, administer phenobarbital in intravenous loading dose of 10 to 15 mg/kg (750 to 1000 mg).
4. In case of toxic seizures or cardiac arrhythmia due to overdosage of anticholinergic or atropinic agents (e.g., tricyclic antidepressants, scopolamine, belladonna, antihistamines), consider physostigmine (Antilirium) 0.5 mg intravenously, every 30 to 60 min, to a maximum of 4 mg (adults) or 2 mg (children).
5. Obtain x-ray studies of chest, skull, cervical spine, abdomen, as indicated.
6. Perform computed axial tomography, angiography, to rule out space-occupying lesions, as indicated.
7. If no evidence of space-occupying lesions and diagnosis uncertain, perform lumbar puncture (cells, protein, glucose, glutamine, culture) to rule out subarachnoid hemorrhage, hepatic encephalopathy, herpes simplex encephalitis.
8. Obtain an electroencephalogram if metabolic encephalopathy or seizures are suspected.

istries, and for toxicologic analysis. Immediately afterward, 50 g of dextrose should be administered intravenously. Naloxone 0.4 to 1.2 mg and thiamine 100 mg should be administered intravenously to all patients regardless of whether opiate or alcohol abuse is suspected. At this point, arterial blood gases should be analyzed to confirm adequate oxygenation.

NASOGASTRIC INTUBATION

Placement of a nasogastric tube may be indicated to decompress the stomach and examine its contents. However, this procedure always places the patient at risk for aspiration, because the nasogastric tube dilates the gastroesophageal sphincter, permitting regurgitation of gastric contents around the tube. Therefore, in a patient who is comatose or has a depressed gag reflex, a cuffed endotracheal tube should be in place prior to passage of a nasogastric tube.

BLOOD PRESSURE

The blood pressure will often provide the first clue to the etiologic diagnosis of coma. Hypertension can be a reflex response to increased intracranial pressure (Cushing reflex) or brain stem ischemia. In rare instances, such as hypertensive encephalopathy, hypertension per se may be the cause of coma.[17] Hypotension may also indicate the presence of myocardial infarction, hemorrhagic shock, sepsis, or sedative-hypnotic drug overdosage.

PULSE

The pulse rate and rhythm may give additional clues to the cause of coma and should be recorded and monitored. Brachycardia associated with an elevated blood pressure is an ominous sign of brain stem compression. In such cases, reversible causes of transtentorial herniation such as subdural hematoma *immediately* should be considered and treated before cardiovascular collapse ensues.

TRAUMATIC INJURIES

During the initial stabilization and assessment of the vital signs, the patient should be checked quickly for signs of head trauma (scalp laceration, bleeding from the ears, cerebrospinal fluid rhinorrhea) and spontaneous movements (convulsions or posturing). When head trauma is a possible cause of coma, the presence of cervical spine injury should be assumed until the cervical spine can be examined radiologically. Therefore, the neck should not be flexed but should be stabilized immediately by sandbags or a headboard to prevent movement during physical and radiologic examinations.

HYPOTHERMIA

The patient's rectal temperature should not be neglected in the initial evaluation. Hypothermia[18] may be secondary to Wernicke syndrome, exposure, sedative overdosage, near-drowning, or hypothyroidism. This important sign often is not detected, either because the rectal temperature measurement is omitted or because an ordinary thermometer that cannot detect temperatures below 34°C is used. A body temperature below 26°C is enough in itself to produce coma; therefore, warming and resuscitative measures are indicated in all hypothermic patients, even when all vital signs are absent. Hypothermic patients have recovered even after prolonged cardiorespiratory arrests, presumably because of the protective effects of low body temperature and depressed cerebral metabolism.[19]

THE NEUROLOGIC EVALUATION

FEVER

The presence of fever in a comatose patient demands investigation for possible meningitis. If there is no history of trauma, the neck should be flexed to assess the presence of meningismus. Meningismus may indicate bacterial meningitis or subarachnoid hemorrhage, but in the latter case there is often a delay of up to 12 hours before blood in the subarachnoid cerebrospinal fluid pathways has produced enough chemical irritation of the meninges to be detected by neck flexion. In deep coma, meningismus may be absent despite the presence of bacterial or chemical meningitis. Other causes of fever include intracranial abscess and subdural empyema.

NEUROLOGIC EXAMINATION

Upon completion of the initial general assessment and treatment, the physician may be able to categorize the cause of coma as either metabolic CNS depression or structural cerebral damage. A systematic physical examination with attention to certain key neurologic signs should pinpoint the precise locus of CNS injury.[20]

The following neurologic examination has been derived from the practical scale developed for head injury by Teasdale and Jennett,[21] and the techniques for evaluating brain stem function described by Plum and Posner.[22] The examination consists of an assessment of the level of consciousness as determined by eye opening, verbal responses, and reflex or purposive movements in response to noxious stimulation of the face, arms, and legs; neuro-ophthalmologic function as indicated by pupillary size and response to light, spontaneous eye movements, oculocephalic (doll's eyes) and oculovestibular (ice-water caloric) responses; and vegetative function as reflected mainly by the respiratory pattern. This approach considers the brain in terms of its hierarchic, longitudinal organization into cortical and brain stem functions. Clinical neurologic signs can be correlated with specific anatomic sites to establish the severity and extent of CNS dysfunction (Table 5-2).

Level of Consciousness

Level of consciousness is best determined by the ease and degree, if any, of behavioral arousal. Attempts should be made to elicit a behavioral motor response by verbal stimulation alone. If no response follows even shouted commands, noxious stimulation can be applied to the face by digital supraorbital pressure, and individually to the arms and legs by compression of distal interphalangeal joints with a tongue blade or pen.

The significance of eye opening as an indication of activity of the RAS, and the correlation between verbal responses and hemisphere function have been mentioned above.

TABLE 5-2. Correlation Between Clinical Signs and Anatomic Substrate of Response

Neurologic Sign	Anatomic Region
Verbal responses, purposive behavior	Neocortex of cerebral hemispheres
Reflex limb movements; decorticate and decerebrate posturing	Brain stem
Eye opening spontaneously or to stimulation	Reticular activating system
Reactive pupils	Midbrain CN III
Corneal reflex	Pons CN V and VII
Doll's eyes and caloric responses	CN III, VI, VIII, and MLF
Breathing, blood pressure	Medulla
Deep tendon reflexes, triple flexion response, Babinski sign	Spinal cord

Motor Responses

The absence of motor response, especially if flaccidity and areflexia are also present, indicates severe brain stem depression and frequently is found in termination coma or in severe sedative intoxication.

Decerebrate or extensor responses correlate with destructive lesions of the midbrain and upper pons, but may also be present in reversible metabolic states such as hepatic coma[23] and anoxic-ischemic encephalopathy.[24] Decorticate or flexor responses occur following damage to the hemispheres, as well as in metabolic depression of brain function. Withdrawal and localizing responses imply purposive or voluntary behavior. Obeying commands is the most optimistic response and marks the return of consciousness.

Generalized or focal repetitive movements not affected by stimuli usually represent seizure activity. Focal seizures usually indicate a focal cortical lesion but may also occur in hypoglycemia, hyperosmolarity, and some drug intoxications (e.g., with aminophylline and tricyclic antidepressants).

Neuro-ophthalmologic Examination

The fundus of each eye should be examined for signs of increased intracranial pressure (papilledema and hemorrhage). Subhyaloid hemorrhage indicates the presence of subarachnoid or intracerebral hemorrhage, but may follow severe head trauma.[25]

PUPILLARY FINDINGS. The size, equality, and light reactivity of the pupils should be noted. In coma due to metabolic brain disease, the pupils generally are small but reactive to light. Similar pupillary response is noted in the initial phase of central herniation, and in the early phases of brain stem compression by a cerebellar mass. Small but reactive pupils are also a common finding in most elderly patients, and are present in normal persons during sleep. Very small, sluggishly reactive pupils that respond to naloxone administration are characteristic of an opiate overdose. Pinpoint pupils occur in pontine hemorrhage.

Bilateral dilated, fixed pupils indicate sympathetic nervous system overactivity, due to an endogenous sympathetic discharge (e.g., dopamine [Intropin]). Similar pupillary responses—dilation or mid-dilation—are seen in glutethimide-induced coma and overdosage of tricyclic antidepressants or other atropine-like agents. In coma secondary to amphetamine, cocaine, or LSD overdosage, the pupils are large but reactive. Midposition, fixed pupils indicate midbrain failure and loss of both sympathetic and parasympathetic pupillary tone, which can be caused by structural or metabolic disease. Such fixed and midposition—rather than dilated—pupils are seen in death.

A unilateral dilated, fixed pupil usually means damage to the parasympathetic fibers of the third cranial nerve as described under uncal herniation. If the patient has suffered head trauma, an ipsilateral epidural or subdural hematoma probably is present. If there is no evidence of trauma, an intrahemispheric mass lesion (hematoma, tumor, or abscess) is the probable cause of herniation.

EYE MOVEMENTS. Deeply comatose patients usually have no spontaneous eye movements. Spontaneous, roving, horizontal eye movements indicate only that the midbrain and pontine tegmentum are intact; they do not imply preservation of the frontal or occipital cerebral cortex. Conjugate lateral deviation of the eyes suggests the presence of either a massive hemispheric lesion (eyes look to the lesion) or a pontine lesion (eyes look away). Upward deviation may indicate seizure activity; downward deviation is characteristic of tectal compression by a thalamic hemorrhage or pineal tumor but also occurs in hepatic encephalopathy and other metabolic comas. Dysconjugate eyes are seen in all types of coma, both structural and metabolic.

DOLL'S EYES. Doll's eyes responses can be used to determine the integrity of the eighth, sixth, and third cranial nerves and their interconnecting brain stem pathways. The physiology of this reflex is presented in detail in standard texts.[26,27]

When the cortical influences are depressed but the brain stem mechanisms are intact (as in normal sleep and in coma), if the head is rotated horizontally to one side, the eyes will deviate conjugately to the opposite side. Brisk back-and-forth eye movements—like those of a doll in response to rocking the head to and fro—are characteristic of certain types of metabolic coma, especially hypoglycemia and hepatic encephalopathy. Doll's eyes indicate the integrity of proprioceptive fibers from the neck structures, the vestibular nuclei, and the nuclei of the third and sixth cranial nerves, as well as their interconnections via the medial longitudinal fasciculus. Unilateral lesions of the brain stem eliminate the oculocephalic response to the side of the lesion.

ICE-WATER CALORIC TEST. To determine the integrity of the eighth, sixth, and third cranial nerves when the doll's eyes are absent, it becomes necessary to perform the ice-water caloric test. In deep coma, the doll's eyes usually disappear before the ice-water caloric responses, because the latter are produced by a stronger stimulus. The caloric response is elicited in the comatose patient by irrigating the tympanum with 20 to 50 ml of ice water. When the patient is supine, with the head elevated 30 degrees, cold water produces convection currents in the lateral canals that inhibit the normal, spontaneous firing of the vestibular nerve. In the absence of cortical influences on the oculovestibular pathways (the same as those for doll's eyes), cold water produces tonic deviation of the eyes to the side of irrigation. Note that in a conscious patient, caloric stimulation produces imperceptible tonic deviation toward the ear irrigated (brain stem mechanisms) and marked nystagmus away from the side irrigated (cortical visual fixation mechanisms). Deep sedative-hypnotic drug coma, phenytoin overdosage,[28] and structural brain stem lesions (pontine hemorrhage, end-stage herniation syndromes, Wernicke syndrome)[29] eliminate the caloric response, as does end-organ (labyrinthine) disease.

Dysconjugate ocular deviation implies a unilateral lesion or metabolic depression of brain stem pathways. If one or both eyes fail to adduct, the lesion is in the medial longitudinal fasciculus or the third cranial nerve. The distinction between the two can be made by examination of the pupillary size and reaction to light, as previously discussed. Failure of abduction indicates a lesion of the sixth cranial nerve.

Further Diagnostic Assessment

Computed axial tomography (CT) or angiography should be performed before, or instead of, lumbar puncture whenever a cerebral mass lesion is suspected.

The information yielded by CT is particularly helpful in the head-injured patient. Swelling of the scalp and skull fractures can be identified; missiles and their tracks can be identified. Extracerebral mass lesions, such as epidural or subdural hematoma, are usually seen easily together with shift of the midline structures away from the offending mass. The midline is identified by the ventricular system and pineal gland, which is evident on CT even when not sufficiently calcified to be visible on plain x-ray films. More subtle indications of brain compression include effacement of the subarachnoid space and lateral ventricle on the affected side. Intraparenchymal lesions can be seen and the crucial differentiation made between hemorrhagic lesions (radiodense) and areas of infarct or edema (radiolucent). Finally, the volume of the ventricular system can be clearly seen. This may range from abnormally large in cases of hydrocephalus or post-traumatic brain atrophy, to completely absent on CT in cases of post-traumatic brain swelling.

Computed axial tomography is the procedure of choice whenever the physical examination is asymmetric or when there is a history of trauma, that is, whenever a space-occupying lesion is likely. The electroencephalogram usually is not part of the acute evaluation of the comatose patient but may be useful to assess the depth of metabolic encephalopathy and to rule out seizures.

If there is no evidence of a space-occupying lesion and the diagnosis is still uncertain, lumbar puncture should be performed to rule out subarachnoid hemorrhage, hepatic encephalopathy, and herpes simplex encephalitis.

Summary

Coma is a life-threatening complication of serious CNS injury, disease, or metabolic depression. Acutely, a careful neurologic examination is essential to the accurate etiologic and anatomic diagnosis of coma. The diagnosis of medical as opposed to traumatic coma depends heavily on clinical judgment, although laboratory tests may assist in the differential diagnosis of metabolic coma.

NEUROLOGIC ASSESSMENT IN THE RECOVERY STAGE

When the head-injured patient has recovered consciousness sufficiently to be able to speak and to obey complex commands, detailed neurologic assessment can begin and disability can be measured, but psychometric assessment must await the end of the period of post-traumatic amnesia.

Testing of cranial nerve function should include olfactory nerve testing. Anosmia is a common and underrated sequel of head injury. When present, it seldom recovers. Optic nerve testing should include a chart of the visual fields and accurate measurement of visual acuity. Eye movements must be fully tested—pupillary function and accommodation. Facial motor, auditory, and vestibular dysfunctions are not infrequently found in head-injured patients. Audiometry and electronystagmography are valuable in detecting minor degrees of auditory and vestibular dysfunction. Difficulties in swallowing are important to detect, as in the drowsy patient they are associated with aspiration of gastric contents and recurrent pneumonia.

Disorders of limb motor function are often quite subtle in head-injured patients, emerging with fatigue and requiring persistence and skill to elicit. Apraxia and incoordination are not uncommon but may emerge only when the patient returns home and attempts to resume normal activities.

PREDICTION OF OUTCOME IN COMA

Recent evidence indicates that extraordinary care of patients with severe brain damage adds substantially to medical costs but may do little to improve chances of functional recovery. This is particularly true for coma, for which studies indicate that despite the best treatment, about 40 percent of patients unconscious from head trauma[6] and only 15 percent of those unconscious from nontraumatic causes[4] made a satisfactory neurologic recovery.

Until recently, there were few attempts to determine in any exact way whether the presence or absence of particular neurologic abnormalities influenced the subject's prognosis. Several groups of neurologists and neurosurgeons have tried to identify and quantify early indicants that might correlate with prognosis. The results of parallel collaborative prospective studies of 1500 head-injured[5] and 500 medical-coma patients[4] indicate that within a few hours or days after the onset of coma, many patients show neurologic signs that differentiate, with a high degree of probability, the outcome extremes of death or vegetative state from good recovery.

HEAD INJURY

Head injury is frequent, predominantly affects young people, and produces huge financial, social, and emotional burdens. Thus, it is not surprising that great efforts have been directed at trying to predict outcome from head injury. The largest and most detailed studies of outcome after severe head injury are those of Jennett and collaborators in the United Kingdom, the Netherlands, and the United States.[5] They found that the age of patients and whether or not they had signs of brain stem dysfunction were the major factors at the outset that influenced prognosis. In general, younger patients can make a better recovery after deeper or more prolonged coma. Conversely, even when signs of brain stem dysfunction were absent, comatose patients in older age groups did badly.

Absence of pupillary responses, doll's eyes, or both at the time of first examination or at any point thereafter indicated a poor outcome in traumatic coma. In Jennett's series, 95 percent of patients died who, at 6 hours after onset of coma, had either nonreactive pupils or absent doll's eyes. If the pupils remained fixed at 24 hours after injury, 91 percent of 1000 patients died and only 4 percent made satisfactory recoveries.

Jennett and associates[5] found that by combining indicants such as motor signs and brain stem reflex responses, they could predict with an accuracy better than 95 percent between the extremes of death versus survival in many patients within the first 24 hours after injury. At 3 days, they could make 97 percent correct predictions of outcome in about half of the total patients still alive at that time.

MEDICAL COMA

The results of an international collaborative study of the correlation between clinical signs and outcome of medical coma have been published.[3,4] Five hundred patients in coma *not* caused by trauma or drugs were followed prospectively. The causes of coma were cardiac arrest or circulatory collapse (n = 50), stroke (n = 143), subarachnoid hemorrhage (n = 38), hepatic encephalopathy (n = 51), and miscellaneous, generally metabolic disturbances (n = 58). Overall prognosis was poor. Only 16 percent led an independent life at some point within the first year; the remainder either died without recovery from coma (61 percent), never improved beyond the vegetative state (12 percent), or regained consciousness but remained dependent on others for daily activities (11 percent).

Neurologic recovery did not depend on age. Prognosis related mainly to early clinical signs of neurologic damage and, to a lesser degree, to the cause of coma. Diseases causing structural brain injury produced the worst prognosis, and metabolic disorders carried the best prognosis.

Patients' levels of recovery at 1 year correlated strongly with the severity of clinical dysfunction observed during the first hours or days of coma. At admission to the study, absence of pupillary responses were each associated with less than 5 percent chance of achieving independent function. Only 1 of 120 patients lacking two of corneal, pupillary, and caloric responses ever regained independent function. By contrast, more than 25 percent of patients characterized by roving conjugate eye movements, withdrawal from pain, or eye opening to pain recovered independent function.

By the end of the first day, absence of any one of corneal reflexes, pupillary light reactions, caloric or doll's eyes responses, and motor responses was unfavorable and precluded a satisfactory recovery. Most patients recovered who spoke any words, who opened their eyes in response to noise, who had normal extraocular movement, who exhibited nystagmus on caloric testing, or who obeyed commands by 1 day after injury.

The studies referred to above have identified the clinical factors that are important in estimating prognosis in traumatic and nontraumatic coma. The next step is to assess the accuracy of these and other predictive schemes prospectively. Moreover, these investigations suggest a mechanism for identifying patients with relatively poor and relatively good prognoses. Therefore, future treatment trials might usefully stratify comatose patients in accordance with some of these findings.

The results of these collaborative data bank studies remove some of the uncertainty about what is accomplished by present applications of intensive care. A particular point of concern is that effort and costs often are greatest when chances of recovery are least, especially in delivering complex care to older persons with multisystem, chronic disease as well as profound CNS damage. Information provided by such studies of prognosis and outcome may enable physicians to direct maximal efforts to patients having the greatest potential for meaningful recovery.

ASSESSMENT OF OUTCOME

The outcome of patients who survive serious brain injury is a matter of concern for the patient, family, physicians, and society as a whole. Survival with brain damage is often prolonged and is usually associated with mental and physical deficits that have a marked effect on the quality of life.

A number of outcome scales have been devised to assess patients after cerebrovascular accident,[30] head injury,[31-33] and treatment for cancer.[34] Many are complex, involving either an analysis of various aspects of daily living or a score of muscle power limb by limb or joint by joint.

Others and I have used a scale based on the overall social integration—namely, independence—of the patient, which takes into account the combined effect of mental and neurologic deficits.[35,36] The scale has been used successfully in collaborative international studies of both head injury and nontraumatic coma. Five categories are recognized:

1. No recovery from coma until death.
2. Vegetative state, a state of functional decortication, namely wakefulness unassociated with evidence of cognition or psychologically meaningful activity, as judged behaviorally.
3. Severe disability. Patients in this category are conscious but dependent on others for some activities during every 24 hours.
4. Moderate disability. The patients are disabled but independent. The patients have been discharged from the hospital and are able to look after themselves, can travel by public transport, and some are capable of work.
5. Good recovery. Such patients can participate in normal social life and can return to work.

WHEN TO ASSESS OUTCOME

Most deaths occur in the first week after the onset of coma, but the process of recovery in survivors may continue for months. Division of patients into deaths and survivors can be made reasonably well at the time of discharge from intensive care, although there will be late deaths due to systemic complications among those who are vegetative or severely disabled.

On the collaborative international studies of nontraumatic[4] and head-injury coma,[5,6] outcome was assessed at 1, 3, 6, and 12 months after admission.

OUTCOME AFTER HEAD INJURY

In Jennett's study[5] of head injury, there were more than 500 survivors 3 months after injury, and their recovery was analyzed at 6 and 12 months. There were 376 survivors at 12 months, of whom 3 percent were moderately disabled and 50 percent had good recovery. Of those who made a good or moderate recovery by 12 months, two thirds had already reached this level within 3 months after injury and 90 percent had done so by 6 months. The implication of these results is that most recovery occurs within the first 6 months after head injury.

THE VEGETATIVE STATE AFTER HEAD INJURY

An important clinical question arises with reference to the vegetative state: Is recovery of consciousness or independence possible in patients diagnosed as vegetative? The answer to this question depends in part on the time of neurologic assessment.

In Jennett's study, 94 patients at 1 month after head injury were considered to indeed be vegetative (59 percent) or to be possibly vegetative or else very severely disabled. Of those confidently diagnosed as vegetative, 7 percent—as compared with 13 percent of those possibly vegetative—eventually achieved moderate disability. Such improvement was always apparent within 3 months after injury, and no patient diagnosed as vegetative 3 months after injury gained independence. Ten percent of patients diagnosed at 3 months as vegetative regained consciousness, but all of these remained severely disabled and totally dependent. These results indicate that in many cases the vegetative state can be recognized with confidence 1 month after injury, but that when there is doubt, the possibility of recovery to moderate disability may be entertained. In patients still vegetative at 3 months, the possibility of regaining an independent existence virtually can be excluded.

CONCLUSION

Thus, there remains the group of severely disabled head-injured patients about which there is most concern. Others who have made formal measurement of outcome after brain damage have stressed the need to take into account not only the degree of disability but also its duration. This is particularly true in the case of younger patients who have suffered head injury. Brain damage at age 25 is more devastating in its emotional impact on patient and family than is the same condition at age 65. Such patients face many years of continuing disability and reduced quality of life. There is no certain way to calculate the quality of life from the degree of disability since it depends largely on the personality and resources of the patient and family. In the end, the physician will best serve patients if he or she always tries to make a realistic yet sympathetic appraisal of the effect that the injury has had on the patient's quality of life in terms of present satisfaction and future prospects. It is in such cases that the neurologist and neurosurgeon must turn to others skilled in rehabilitation medicine to help. Continuity of care is important at this stage of rehabilitation, as is psychosocial counseling of the patient and family to help in their adjustment to the new realities of life.

REFERENCES

1. MORUZZI, G AND MAGOUN, HW: *Brainstem reticular formation and activation of the EEG.* Electroencephalogr Clin Neurophysiol 1:455, 1949.
2. BRIERLEY, JB, ET AL: *Neocortical death after cardiac arrest: A clinical, neurophysiological and neuropathological report of two cases.* Lancet 2:560, 1971.

3. BATES, D, ET AL: *A prospective study of nontraumatic coma: Methods and results in 310 patients.* Ann Neurol 2:211, 1977.
4. LEVY, DE, ET AL: *Prognosis in nontraumatic coma.* Ann Intern Med 94:293, 1981.
5. JENNETT, B, ET AL: *Severe head injuries in three countries.* J Neurol Neurosurg Psychiatry 40:291, 1977.
6. JENNETT, B AND TEASDALE, G: *Management of Head Injuries.* FA Davis, Philadelphia, 1981.
7. FROWEIN, RA: *Classification of Coma.* Acta Neuroklin 34:5, 1976.
8. JEFFERSON, G: *The tentorial pressure cone.* Archives of Neurolgy and Psychiatry 40:857, 1938.
9. JENNETT, WB AND PLUM, F: *The persistent vegetative state: A syndrome in search of a name.* Lancet 1:734, 1972.
10. CARONNA, JJ: *Encephalopathies.* In THOMPSON, RA AND GREEN, JR (EDS), *Critical Care of Neurologic and Neurosurgical Emergencies.* Raven Press, New York, 1980, p 101.
11. BIRD, TD AND PLUM F: *Recovery from barbiturate overdose coma with a prolonged isoelectric electroencephalogram.* Neurology (Minneap) 18:456, 1968.
12. CUSHING, H: *The blood pressure reaction of acute cerebral compression, illustrated by cases of intracranial hemorrhage.* Am J Med Sci 125:1017, 1903.
13. SYMONDS, CP: *Concussion and its sequelae.* Lancet 1:1, 1962.
14. STRICH, SJ: *The pathology of brain damage due to blunt head injuries.* In WALKER, AE, CAVENESS, WF, AND CRITCHLEY, M (EDS): *The Late Effects of Head Injury.* Charles C Thomas, Springfield, Ill, 1969.
15. PEVEHOUSE, BC, ET AL: *Ophthalmologic aspects of diagnosis and localization of subdural hematoma.* Neurology (Minneap) 10:1037, 1960.
16. CARONNA, JJ AND SIMON, RP: *The comatose patient: A diagnostic approach and treatment.* Int Anesthesiol Clin 17:3, 1979.
17. CUNEO, RA AND CARONNA, JJ: *The neurologic complications of hypertension.* Med Clin North Am 61:565, 1977.
18. REULER, JB: *Hypothermia: Pathophysiology, clinical settings, and management.* Ann Intern Med 89:519, 1978.
19. SIEBKE, H, ET AL: *Survival after 40 minutes submersion without cerebral sequelae.* Lancet 1:1275, 1975.
20. FISHER, CM: *The neurological examination of the comatose patient.* Acta Neurol Scand 45(Suppl 36):4, 1969.
21. TEASDALE, G AND JENNETT, B: *Assessment of coma and impaired consciousness: A practical scale.* Lancet 2:81, 1974.
22. PLUM, F AND POSNER, JB: *Diagnosis of Stupor and Coma,* ed 3. FA Davis, Philadelphia, 1980.
23. CONOMY, JP AND SWASH, M: *Reversible decerebrate decorticate postures in hepatic coma.* N Engl J Med 278:876, 1968.
24. CARONNA, JJ: *Diagnosis, prognosis and treatment of hypoxic coma.* Adv Neurol 26:1, 1979.
25. MULLER, PD AND DECK, JHN: *Intraocular and optic nerve sheath hemorrhage in cases of sudden intracranial hypertension.* J Neurosurg 41:160, 1974.
26. COGAN, DG: *Neurology of the Ocular Muscles,* ed 2. Charles C Thomas, Springfield, Ill, 1956.
27. BALOH, RW AND HONRUBIA, V: *Clinical Neurophysiology of the Vestibular System.* FA Davis, Philadelphia, 1979.
28. ORTH, DN, ET AL: *Ophthalmoplegia resulting from diphenylhydantoin and primidone intoxication.* JAMA 201:485, 1967.
29. GHEZ, C: *Vestibular paresis: A clinical feature of Wernicke's disease.* J Neurol Neurosurg Psychiatry 32:134, 1969.
30. RANKIN, J: *CVA in patients over the age of 60.* Scott Med J 2:200, 1957.
31. NAJENSON, T, ET AL: *Rehabilitation after severe head injury.* Scand J Rehabil Med 5:1, 1974.

32. ROBERTS, AH: *Long term prognosis of severe accidental head injury.* Proc R Soc Med 69:137, 1976.
33. STOVER, SL AND ZEIGER, HE: *Head injury in children and teenagers: Functional recovery correlated with the duration of coma.* Arch Phys Med Rehabil 57:201, 1976.
34. KARNOFSKY, DA, ET AL: *Triethylene melamine in the treatment of neoplastic disease.* Arch Intern Med 87:477, 1951.
35. JENNETT, B AND BOND, M: *Assessment of outcome after severe brain damage.* Lancet 1:480, 1975.
36. PLUM, F AND CARONNA, JJ: *Can One Predict Outcome of Medical Coma?* In *Outcome of Severe Damage to the Central Nervous System.* Ciba Symposium 34 (new series). Elsevier, Amsterdam, 1975, p 121.
37. LEVY, DE, KNILL-JONES, PP, AND PLUM, F: *The vegetative state and its prognosis following nontraumatic coma.* Ann NY Acad Sci 315:293, 1978.

Chapter 6

ASSESSMENT OF BRAIN FUNCTION WITH MULTIMODALITY EVOKED POTENTIALS

Pauline G. Newlon, M.S.
Richard P. Greenberg, M.D., Ph.D.

It is clinically important to assess the severity and extent of brain injury as quickly and accurately as possible after severe head trauma. However, this is a difficult task in comatose patients. Although advanced radiologic techniques such as computed tomography (CT) scan can disclose structural abnormalities that may require surgical intervention, they cannot provide information regarding the functional capability of the patient.

At present, the neurologic examination is the best tool available for evaluating neural function. But this technique does suffer limitations when the patient is unable to actively participate in the examination (see Chapter 5). In this instance, the clinician must depend largely on central nervous system (CNS) reflexive responses to assess brain function. Therapeutic barbiturate coma and muscle paralysis further compromise the value of the neurologic examination. Therefore, a need exists for complementary or alternative methods to assess the functional status of the CNS in comatose head-injured patients—ideally, methods that are immune to those variables that hinder the utility of the neurologic examination.

Sensory evoked potentials (SEPs) are another measure of brain function that can provide additional information about the neurologic status of comatose head-injured patients; SEPs are electrophysiologic recordings that represent discrete electric responses of the brain to specific sensory stimulation. These tests are noninvasive and, in most instances, do not require a conscious subject. Recent technical advances allow recordings of brain stem and spinal cord activity, as well as that of the cortex, to be made noninvasively. These factors enhance the applicability of the SEPs to evaluation of severely injured, comatose patients.

Sensory evoked potentials can be recorded from the scalp in response to stimulation of any sensory modality that can be peripherally activated, although the visual, auditory, and somatosensory systems are the most commonly employed in clinical settings. Figure 6-1 shows an exemplary schematic representation of a somatosensory evoked potential obtained from median nerve stimulation. Such an analog signal, obtained by computer averaging, shows characteristic voltage deflections occurring at particular time points after presentation of a stimulus (time zero). These waveforms are generally reproducible within a given subject and between different individuals, although some variability will be obtained. The peak deflections, or waves, are conventionally labeled according to their polarity (positive or negative) and the time after stimulation at which they occur (latency, usually expressed in milliseconds). Consideration of the normal appearance of any given SEP is usually based on a combination of four factors: (1) the presence or absence of particular peaks, (2) the latency of peaks, (3) the

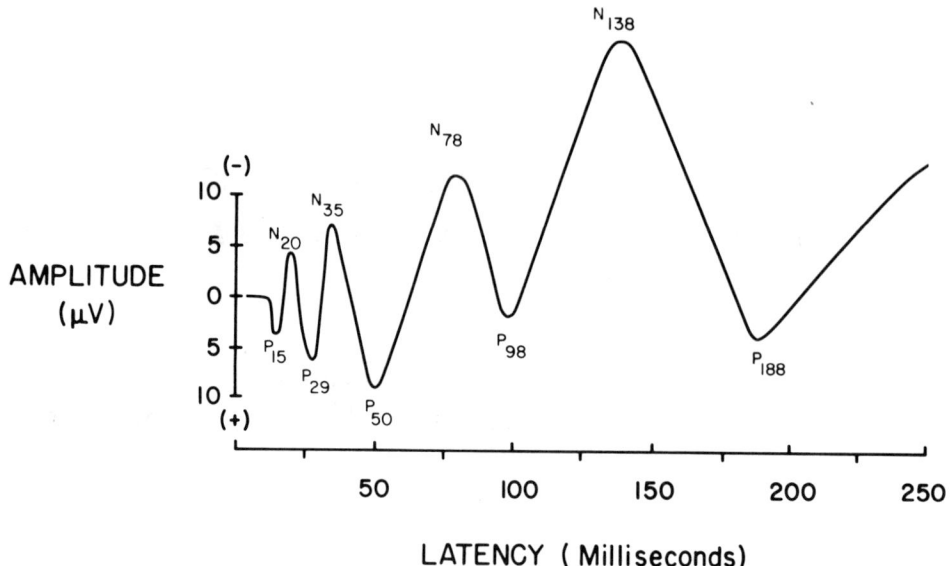

FIGURE 6-1. This schematic somatosensory evoked potential illustrates the characteristic waveform morphology. Similar waveforms can be obtained in many sensory modalities. The voltage deflections varying around 0 voltage are labeled according to their polarity (P or N) and the latency from time of stimulation at which the peaks occur. Positive waves are, by convention, presented downward.

peak-to-peak amplitude, and (4) the "duration" of a wave measured at its broadest point, parallel to the horizontal axis.

Since the normal elaboration of these potentials depends on the neural integrity of the pathway being stimulated, these tests can be used to assess disruption of specific sensory pathways or to generally evaluate the functional status of areas of brain tissue through which the pathway courses. For example, the somatosensory pathway runs a long course and allows one to examine neural activity through the limbs, spinal cord, medulla, pons, midbrain, and cortex. On the other hand, the visual system traverses a quite different extent of tissue, providing information about different substrates in the CNS (Fig. 6-2). Hence, abnormalities in SEPs may be indicators of functional compromise in various regions of the brain. The sensory modality most useful in a particular clinical situation will depend on the disease state and the brain region or function of primary interest.

Over the last decade, visual, somatosensory, and auditory evoked potentials have been reported to be clinically useful in a wide variety of neuropathologic states, including multiple sclerosis, cerebrovascular disease, brain death, supratentorial and infratentorial brain tumors, spinal cord disease or trauma, and others. In general, these studies have shown that particular clinical syndromes are often correlated with SEP abnormalities that reflect slowed central neural conduction, incomplete elaboration of sensory input, or, in some cases, total disruption of pathways at various levels of the CNS. The question of the potential value of SEPs in evaluating brain function in comatose head-injured patients arose concurrently with interest in the other clinical applications. In this chapter, we review our experience to date and that reported by others regarding the clinical value of SEPs in providing additional functional information concerning the severity and extent of brain injury, as well as in predicting potential for recovery. It is not within the intended scope of this chapter to provide details of the techniques used to perform these studies. The neurophysiologic mechanisms postulated for

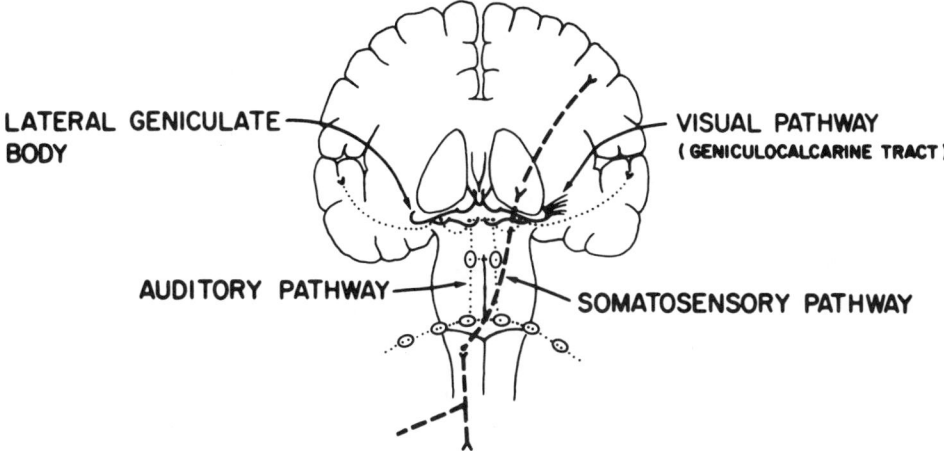

FIGURE 6-2. Schematic view of sensory pathways contributing to multimodality evoked potentials. The somatosensory system enters the brain stem at its most caudal portion. The auditory pathway enters at the pontomedullary junction, and the visual system traverses an area of brain more rostral than either of the latter two pathways.

the origins of particular waveforms are mentioned only where relevant. Readers desiring more information will find helpful references listed in the bibliography.

MULTIMODALITY EVOKED POTENTIALS

The particular sensory evoked potential chosen to test CNS function will ultimately depend on the goals of the study and the neuropathology under consideration. For example, auditory brain stem evoked potentials (EPs) can be used to assess subtle delays in central conduction in patients with multiple sclerosis because of the reliability of auditory brain stem response peak latencies in normal persons. Evaluation of spinal cord disease or injury requires the use of somatosensory EPs generated by stimulation of upper or lower limb peripheral nerves. Visual and auditory cortical potentials find particular relevance for assessment of higher-order cognitive function, as in processes involving attention, decision making, and so forth.

Since severe head injury often results in a diffuse insult to the brain, it would be ideal to evaluate all CNS tissue. This is not technically feasible. But the use of auditory, somatosensory, and visual evoked potentials together does enable a substantial proportion of the CNS to be tested, by virtue of the differences in location of the neuroanatomic pathways associated with these three sensory systems. The additional time involved in performing these studies is not overly burdensome. A majority of reports on SEPs in severe head injury use one or, at most, two modalities of stimulation. We have recorded multimodality evoked potentials (MEPs) in more than 300 comatose head-injured patients in the first few days after injury. This involves, in most cases, recording somatosensory cortical (SER) and brain stem responses (SBSR), auditory brain stem responses (ABSR), and visual cortical EPs (VER).

MULTIMODALITY EVOKED POTENTIALS IN COMATOSE PATIENTS

There are particular technical problems associated with recording MEPs in comatose patients in the intensive-care unit (ICU), but these have been discussed in detail elsewhere.[1]

It is important, in performing multimodal evoked potentials in comatose head-injured patients, to validate the integrity of peripheral receptors. For example, a falsely pessimistic judgment of brain function may be made if an absent SEP is recorded without verification of peripheral nerve depolarization. This can be determined with relative ease in most cases. With median nerve stimulation, a thumb twitch is produced. If this is absent, due to paralysis, the peripheral nerve action potential may be recorded over the arm or at Erb's point. Likewise, electroretinograms can be recorded from the eyelid, and eighth nerve potentials can often be checked at vertex leads or from wick electrodes placed near the tympanic membrane to verify visual and auditory receptor function, respectively.

It is doubtful that an evoked potential obtained from a comatose patient is comparable to that of an alert, awake, normal subject. The method of analysis used for responses of comatose patients when compared to SEPs from normal subjects must take this into consideration. Indeed, SEPs obtained in comatose patients often show an absence of activity occurring at long latencies (300 to 1000 msec) after the stimulus—activity that is generally associated with cognitive function or attentional factors. In the visual system, waves that can be seen in awake subjects after 250 msec often show changes in morphology during sleep. Although the neuroelectric correlates of the state of unconsciousness are certainly of interest in themselves, we have concentrated on evaluations of the CNS to detect areas of brain injury or dysfunction.

ANALYSIS OF DATA

We routinely record MEPs in head-injured patients in the first few days following injury and in serial studies up to 1 year later. When a study is performed, the results are recorded on magnetic tape and later analyzed off-line by computer that provides an analog printout and tables reporting latencies and amplitudes of appropriate peaks (Fig. 6-3). These data are then analyzed by the investigators, and a "grade" of abnormality is assigned to each SEP waveform. The grading system is composed of four categories of EP, based on commonly obtained abnormal responses recorded from these patients.[1] This system reflects waveform complexity primarily and ranges from grade I to grade IV for each SEP test. These grades denote waveforms of decreasing complexity such that a grade I response is nearly equivalent to that of normal subjects and grade IV is electric silence. Figure 6-4 depicts the characteristic waveform morphology associated with each grade for somatosensory, auditory, and visual cortical SEPs. Figure 6-5 provides the graded waveforms for somatosensory and auditory brain stem responses.

It is useful, for later reference, to discuss our interpretation of these waveforms from a neuroanatomic standpoint. A description of the brain areas that we believe to be compromised in the case of the different grades may be helpful in understanding the regional effects of head injury. The specific criteria for assigning these grades have been presented elsewhere.[1]

Somatosensory Cortical Response

The SER obtained from median nerve stimulation provides information about the brain stem, diencephalon, and cortex. We believe, as suggested by others, that the earliest components of SER (0 to 15 msec) arise from peripheral nerve, spinal cord, and brain stem, whereas the primary cortical response occurs at approximately 20 msec.[2-4] Potentials generated between 20 and 50 msec may be a result of information processing in the primary cortical areas of the precentral and postcentral gyrus.[2,3] The later potentials (50 msec and beyond) may be generated by areas of association cortex and indicative of higher-order integrative function.

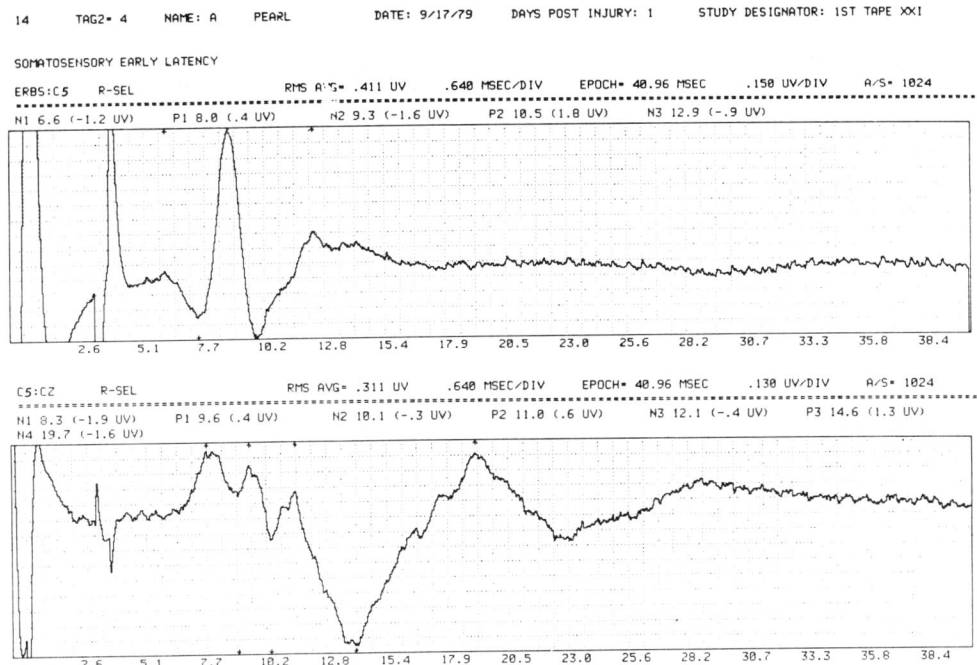

FIGURE 6-3. A typical computer printout of an SBSR obtained from right median nerve stimulation. The upper graph and table depict the Erb's point potential, and the lower tracing demonstrates the neck recorded brain stem response: positive is down. The small arrows designate peaks detected in the waveform by the computer: the latency and amplitude of each are provided in the tables above, in the order that they were detected. The horizontal axis equals 40 msec.

The graded potentials we assign for this modality show close correspondence with these neuroanatomic subdivisions. A grade I response consists of the presence of activity in all three latency periods, that is, brain stem, primary cortical, and secondary cortical components. This response, in comatose patients, would indicate "normal" integrative capability of cortical structures. A grade II response is made up of early and primary cortical components with a notable absence of potentials beyond 50 msec. This would suggest that information is reaching primary cortical areas but is not being processed further. Shifts in latency of the intermediate waves and decrements in amplitude are often seen when compared to waves in the grade I category. This grade is considered mildly abnormal. Grade III SER potentials are strikingly characterized by only two components: the first positive (P_{15}) and negative (N_{20}) waves. No later activity is discernible. This is interpreted as a severely abnormal response, indicative of failure in primary cortical function. A grade IV SER consists essentially of electric silence. However, we do record a P_{15} in the majority of these patients. This wave has been reported by others as well in patients who are considered brain dead by clinical and electroencephalographic criteria. This response is characteristic of significant diencephalic and/or brain stem dysfunction.

Somatosensory Brain Stem Responses

The early latency somatosensory response (SBSR) may be recorded from the skin overlying the seventh or second cervical vertebra, referenced to a frontal or vertex lead, or from parietal scalp referenced to the hand contralateral to the stimulated side. A period of

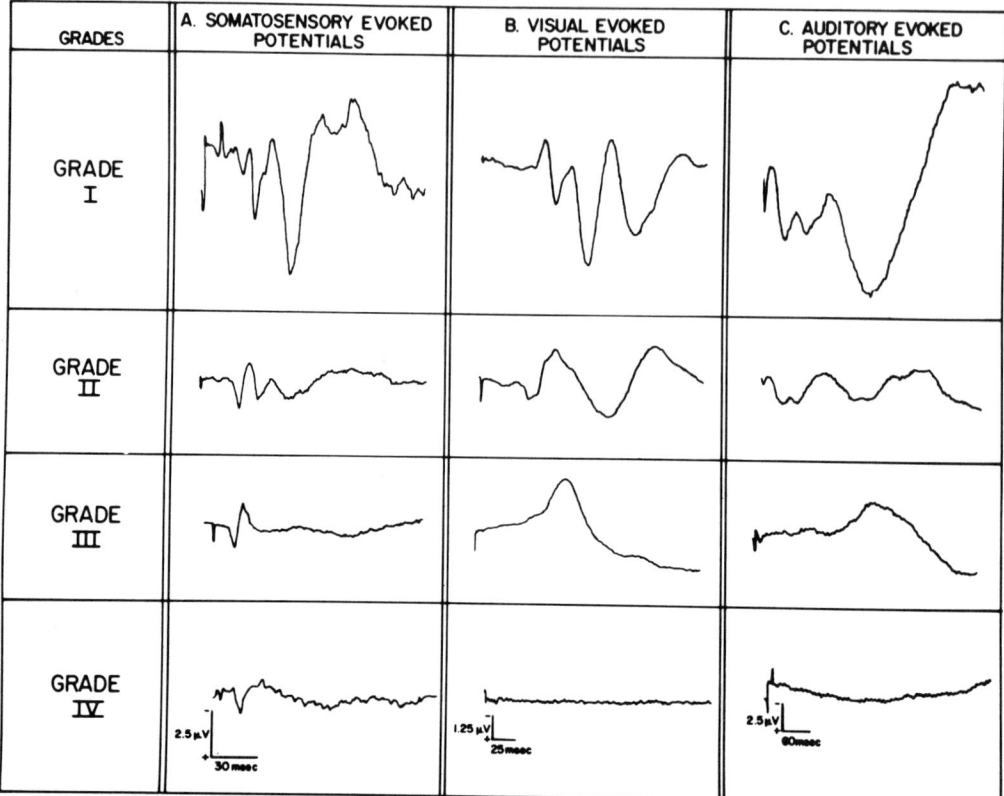

FIGURE 6-4. Graded cortical (long latency) evoked potentials. Four morphologically distinct responses can be identified for each modality in comatose head injury patients. These are arranged and labeled grades I through IV denoting decreasing complexity of waveform and increasing electrical abnormality.

only 30 to 40 msec is usually analyzed, allowing more refined resolution of the activity occurring very early after the stimulus. The neural generators of this response are the least understood of any of the SEPs discussed here, but there is some agreement as to the general origins of the four major peaks that are commonly recorded in normal persons. The apparent polarity of these peaks will differ depending on the chosen electrode configuration. In neck recordings (see Fig. 6-5), three of these peaks appear as negative and the fourth as positive. The first negative peak, which occurs at approximately 10 msec (N_1), is thought to arise from peripheral nerve. The generators of the second (N_2, 12 msec) and third (N_3, 14 msec) negative peaks and the positive peak (P_1, 18 to 20 msec) are more controversial, but the work of several investigators has suggested that these peaks arise from subcortical or cerebellar structures and that the positive peak may be the first arrival at cortex. In general, it is believed that activity between 10 and 20 msec probably represents activity in spinal cord, lemniscal tracts in the brain stem, thalamus, possibly cerebellum, and axons in the thalamocortical pathway. A grade I SBSR (see Fig. 6-5) indicates integrity of the entire brain stem. A grade II response is characterized by the presence of all waves, but with delays that are suggestive of conduction problems, which may be transient. A grade III SBSR shows a very definite N_3 but absence of the next positive deflection (P_1). This grade would indicate intact neural function in the caudal extent of the brain stem but irreversible damage to diencephalon or thalamocortical

ASSESSMENT OF BRAIN FUNCTION WITH MULTIMODALITY EVOKED POTENTIALS

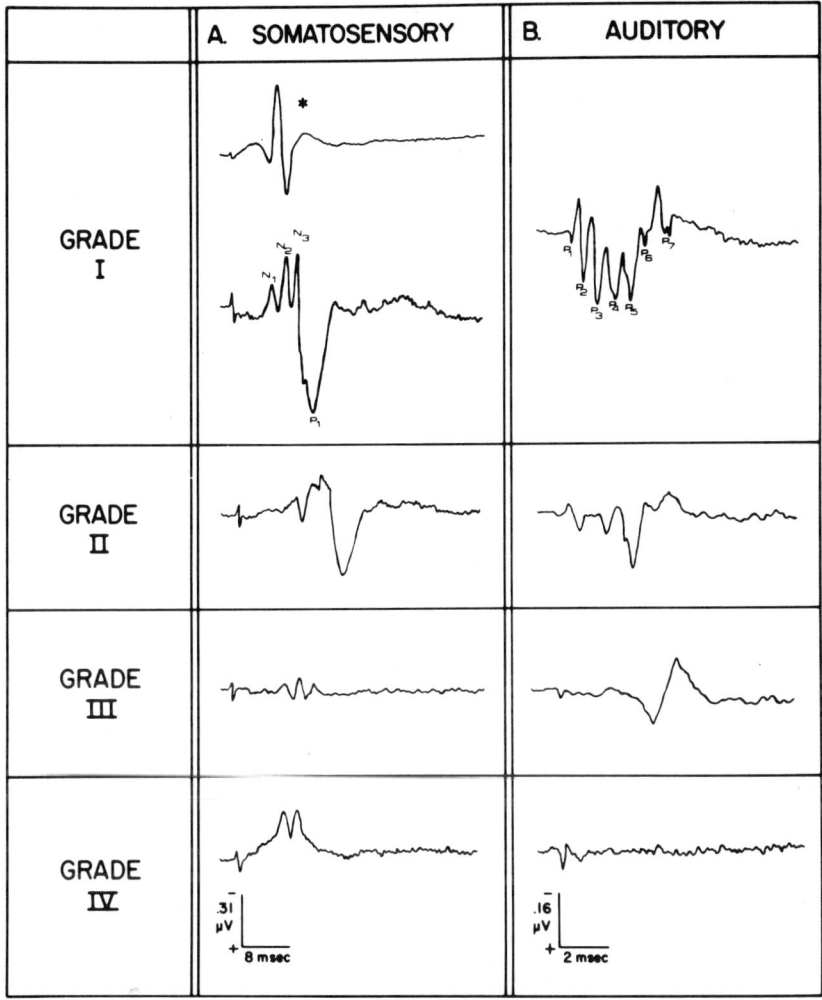

* ERB'S POINT TRIPHASIC ACTION POTENTIAL

FIGURE 6-5. Graded brain stem evoked potentials. Peaks that commonly appear in normal persons (grade I) are labeled by polarity and order of appearance rather than latency. As in cortical potentials, grades correspond to differences in waveform complexity representing dysfunction at various levels of the brain stem.

pathways. In a grade IV, the N_3 is absent as well, suggesting that even the lowest extent of the medulla has suffered injury.

Auditory Brain Stem Responses

The ABSR provides information primarily regarding subcortical function. Interest has been focused on the first 8 to 10 msec of activity following stimulation. In normal subjects, the first five or six waves of these potentials are quite consistent in latency regardless of state of consciousness. A grade I ABSR is indistinguishable from that seen in normal subjects with regard to morphology and latencies of waves. In grade II responses, only waves 1, 3, and 5 are clearly discernible, and delays in the latency of waves 1 to 5 may be seen, along with amplitude decrements. A severely abnormal waveform is seen in the grade III response. In this grade, only the eighth nerve potential (wave 1) has a normal latency and amplitude and is followed by a poorly defined positive wave occurring around 6 msec. This may be indicative of diffuse brain stem dysfunction at or above the level of the cochlear nucleus in the pontine brain stem. A grade IV response is one in which only wave 1 is present, and this wave is often itself abnormally prolonged.

Visual Cortical Evoked Responses

The majority of potentials recorded in response to light flash can be attributed to activity occurring in the hemispheres. Graded VERs are indicators of hemispheric function, mostly cortical, and can be normal even with brain stem dysfunction.[5] A grade I VER demonstrates integrity of the optic nerve, chiasm, and tract as well as primary and secondary cortical receiving areas. The grade II is a less complex response, presenting a pair of positive-negative deflections of longer duration than those seen in grade I, with electric silence beyond 200 msec. We interpret this to be evidence of intact function of primary areas with some compromise of secondary processing. The grade III VER consists of a single negative deflection occurring around 90 msec post-stimulus. This response suggests substantial compromise, even of the primary calcarine area and virtually nonexistent cellular function in surrounding tissue. Electric silence defines the grade IV response (assuming electroretinograms show retinal integrity).

DETECTING BRAIN DYSFUNCTION WITH SENSORY EVOKED POTENTIALS

Multimodality evoked potentials recorded early after injury in this sample of patients display a wide range of responses with respect to the severity and extent of neuroelectric abnormality. Hence, some patients show grade I SEPs in all modalities tested, whereas others may have some combination of abnormality, for example, mildly abnormal SERs and severely abnormal VERs. In the extreme case of brain death, no central activity is seen in any modality with the common exception of the P_{15} in the SER. Figure 6-6 shows an example of a 25-year-old patient who, on the first day after injury, demonstrated relative normality of MEPs while still comatose. This patient awoke within 14 days and went on to make an excellent recovery with no apparent residual sensory deficits.

Cortical Versus Brain Stem Dysfunction

Since MEPs assess pathways running through both brain stem and cortex, it is often possible to differentiate dysfunction which is primarily hemispheric from that which purely involves the brain stem. The great majority of patients we have studied demonstrate cortical or combined dysfunction, although pure brain stem injury has been indicated neuroelectrically and confirmed at autopsy in a few cases. Serious, diffuse cortical injury is manifest in MEPs by abnormality in SERs and VERs, while ABSRs and SBSRs remain normal. Figure 6-7 shows the MEPs recoded in such a case. This type of response is seen in patients with fairly substantial brain edema and greatly elevated intracranial pressure. In contrast, a focal right brain stem lesion is seen in Figure 6-8. Cortical SEPs show good elaboration of input in the SER obtained from stimulation of the left side of the brain stem and the VERs are intact bilaterally. However, the SBSR and SER for the right side of the brain stem are severely abnormal. Auditory brain stem responses for each ear are abnormal also, although the response that primarily involves the right brain stem (left ear stimulation) is more abnormal than that of the other side. Since

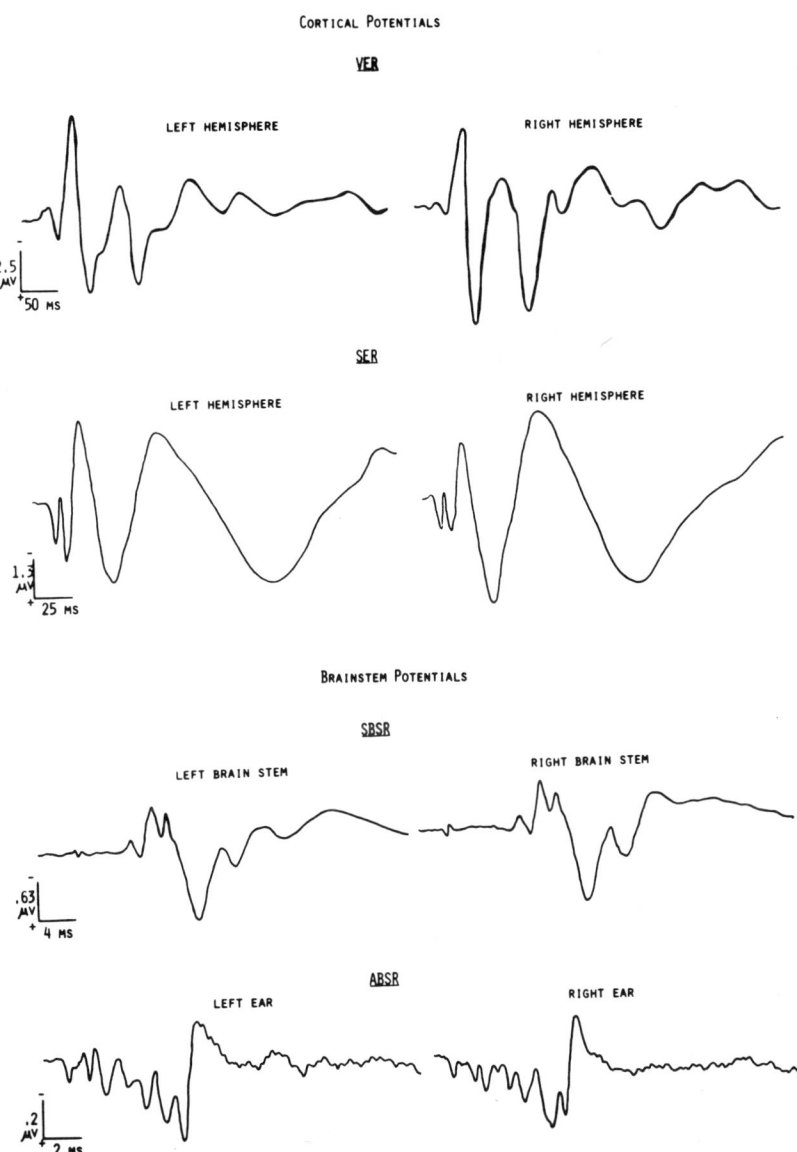

FIGURE 6-6. Multimodality evoked potentials obtained from a comatose 25-year-old man on the first day after injury. The neurologic examination could not be performed owing to neuromuscular paralysis (pancuronium) necessary to properly ventilate the patient. These potentials, obtained from unilateral median nerve stimulation, light flash, and monaural clicks, were all grade I. Based on these results, this patient was expected to make a good recovery and did so within 3 months.

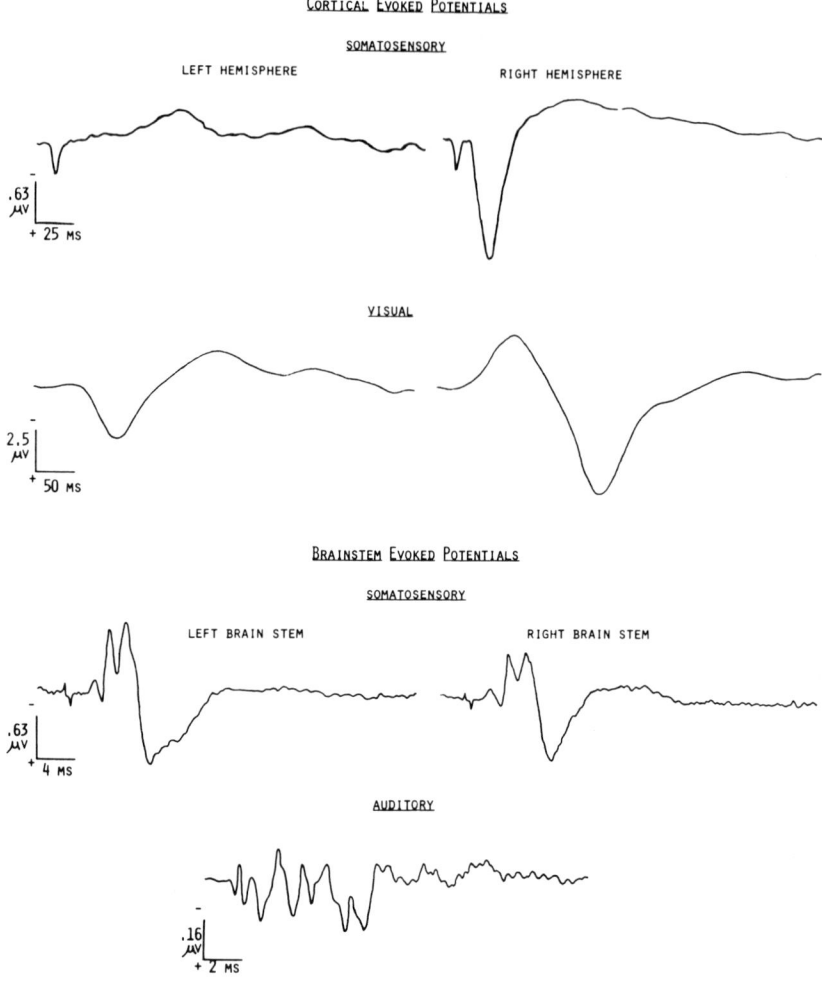

FIGURE 6-7. Multimodality evoked potentials obtained from a 3-year-old boy who was comatose following an auto accident. On day 1 postinjury, his cortical evoked potentials (SER and VER) indicated serious hemispheric dysfunction (more so on the left than the right), but the brain stem responses were normal bilaterally. Twelve months after injury he was severely disabled with a right hemiplegia, impaired motor strength in the lower limbs, and receptive aphasia.

the auditory pathway has substantial crossover and bilateral innervation of the brain stem, it is more difficult to localize discrete areas of dysfunction with this test. Abnormalities of the severity seen in these two examples, whether of cortical or brain stem etiology are usually associated with a poor outcome.

Focal Deficits

MEPs are useful in early detection of severe focal deficits in these three sensory systems.[5] Figure 6-9 provides an example of a patient who suffered cortical blindness as a result of

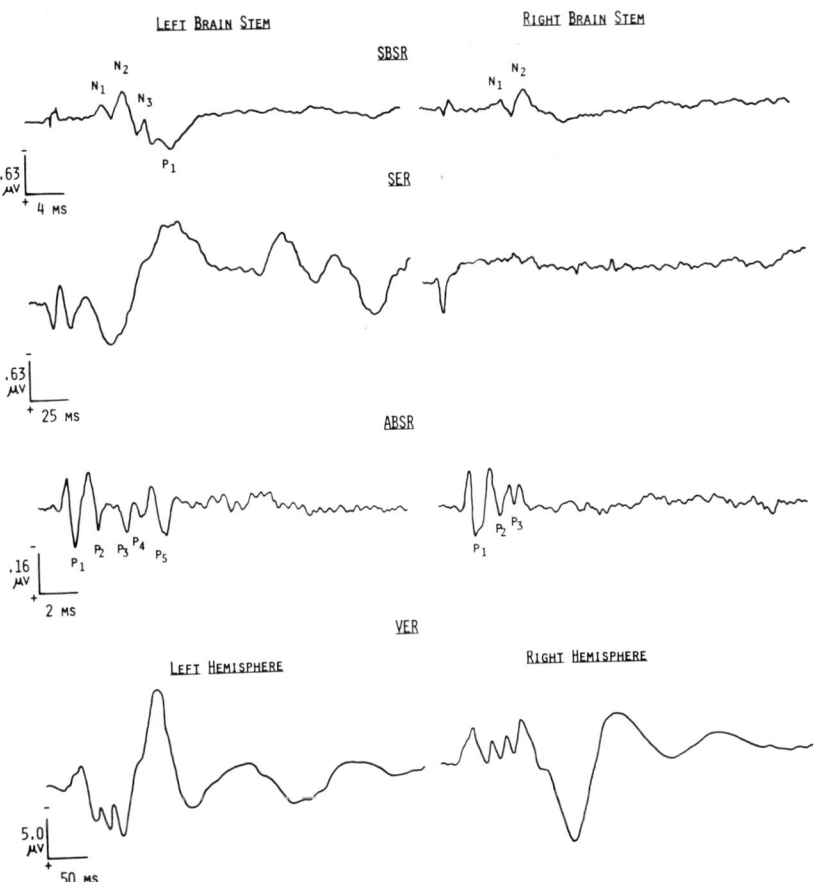

FIGURE 6-8. This 15-year-old patient who fell 70 ft from a tree demonstrated a fairly discrete lesion of the right brain stem. Note that with stimulation of the left brain stem via the right median nerve, three negative waves and one positive wave were obtained in the SBSR. However, when the other side was tested, only waves N_1 and N_2 were recorded. Similarly, the ABSR from left ear stimulation showed an absence of waves 4 to 6, whereas stimulation of the right ear produced a normal although somewhat delayed ABSR (grade II). Cortical SEPs from the visual pathway or from somatosensory stimulation of the intact side of the brain stem indicated hemispheric integrity. As late as 2 years after injury, this patient did not follow commands but did have spontaneous eye opening and spontaneous movement with spasticity.

injury. The auditory and somatosensory evoked potentials were intact, although no activity could be recorded in response to light flash except for the peripheral electroretinogram. Similarly, severe focal abnormalities in the somatosensory system have been associated with residual hemiparesis. However, by the same token, we have recorded relatively normal SERs from patients who demonstrate a hemiparesis early after injury, but in which case the clinically manifest weakness resolves, usually within a few months. Thus, it appears that when a particular functional sensory deficit presents early, MEPs can provide additional information regarding the transience or permanence of such a deficit.

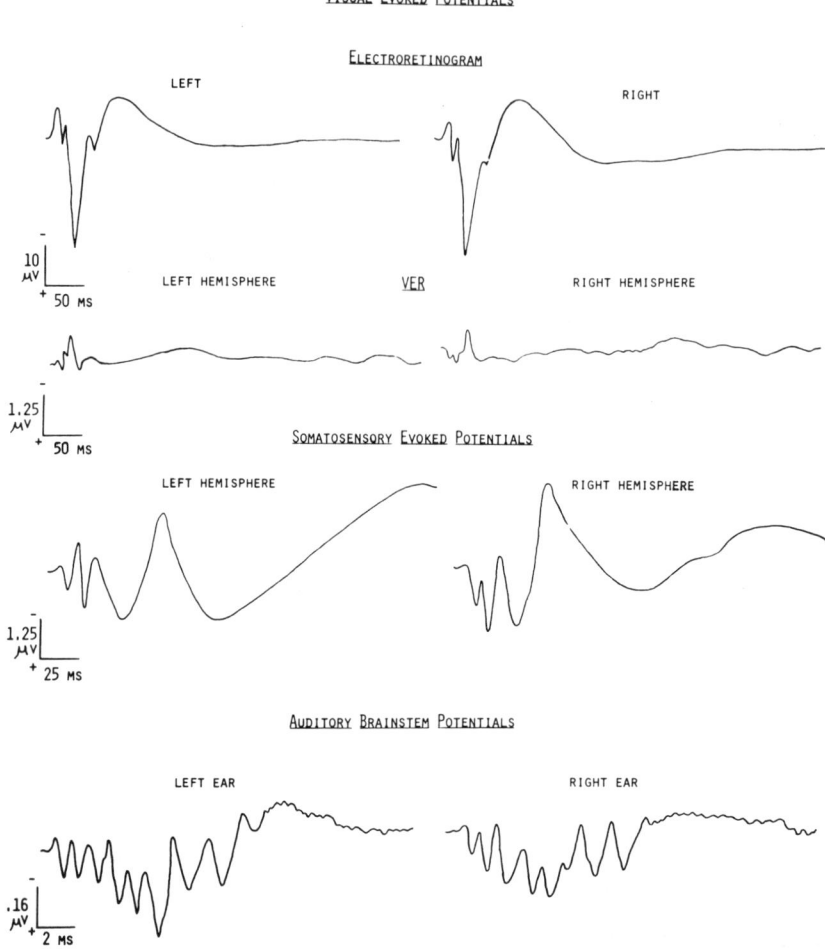

FIGURE 6-9. Neuroelectric evidence of cortical blindness in a 20-year-old man following an auto accident. Electroretinograms show peripheral activation of the visual system but no cortical activity could be recorded from occipital scalp. Somatosensory and auditory responses were within normal limits.

Correlation of Multimodality Evoked Potentials and Clinical Factors

The data obtained from MEP studies show an interesting relationship with some of the clinical signs that are considered to be key indicators of brain injury in comatose patients. Somatosensory and auditory EP abnormalities, particularly graded brain stem responses, correlate well with impaired oculocephalic responses and bilateral pupillary reactions.[5] On the other hand, VERs do not show this relationship. This difference in SEPs is consistent with the idea that impairment of these responses is due to dysfunction within the brain stem nuclei responsible for their control. Since the VER to light flash does not implicate this brain area, it is not surprising that no association is seen in this case. Uziel and Benezech[6] have reported a correlation between various levels of abnormality in ABSRs and "level of coma" in such patients, defined by oculocephalic reflexes and motor posturing. These authors reported that dysfunction determined to be at particular levels of the brain stem by these clinical signs was confirmed by a loss of waves in the ABSR that are generated above the level of presumed dysfunction.

Interestingly, we have found that presence or absence of motor posturing in this sample of patients shows a better correlation with the cortical or "nearfield" potentials than with brain stem SEPs. Our data suggest that this phenomenon is more closely associated with hemispheric dysfunction since it is often seen in patients who demonstrate normal brain stem function neuroelectrically and severe abnormalities in cortical SEPs.[5]

This also appears to be the case for duration of coma. Again, prolonged unconsciousness (more than 30 days) is generally associated with cortical rather than brain stem dysfunction. Patients with normal or mildly abnormal cortical responses are not unconscious as long as are those with severely abnormal cortical SEPs.[5] These findings may ultimately have implications for the heretofore postulated notion that prolonged coma and motor posturing are clinical reflections of brain stem injury. However, no one has yet been able to directly associate particular cortical SEP abnormalities with coma itself other than noting an absence of secondary cortical activity.

MULTIMODALITY EVOKED POTENTIAL AND PROGNOSIS

If a patient shows a particular level of evoked potential abnormality early after injury, what does this mean for recovery? That is, can we use the results of SEP studies to predict outcome? This issue has not been addressed adequately by many investigators in the literature, largely because of the small numbers of patients studied. Some authors have reported a few cases of patients whose post-traumatic SEPs were normal and who recovered or those with grossly distorted or absent SEPs who died. De La Torre and colleagues have reported, in a study of 17 comatose head-injured patients, to be able to discriminate "positive" versus "negative" recovery when SERs were analyzed according to the number of waves present in a particular period.[7] This analysis is quite similar to ours in that it reflects waveform complexity. Rappaport and coworkers[8] have shown that long latency auditory and visual SEPs were highly associated with functional disability determined by a 28-point rating scale. These authors studied surviving head-injured patients at fairly long post-traumatic intervals. They found that their tests correlated better with the upper ends of the disability range (excellent to moderately disabled) than with the lower ends (severe or vegetative), suggesting that long latency SEPs may be less able to discriminate more severe disability and probably indicate associative and integrating functions.

We have found MEPs to be quite valuable in predicting outcome. A recently concluded analysis of the prognostic accuracy of these tests in comparison with other clinical indices such as ICP, pupillary light response, motor posturing, extraocular motility, CT scan, and the Glasgow coma scale revealed that MEP data provided 91 percent accuracy of prediction—the highest obtained by any single indicant.[9] Furthermore, addition of MEP results to those of the other measures improved their accuracy of prediction and the confidence limits of prediction.[9] Hence, it appears that by themselves or in combination with other measurements, MEPs recorded early after injury are valuable tools with which to forecast patient outcome.

SEVERITY OF DYSFUNCTION

The primary variables of neuroelectric abnormality recorded early that play key roles in the ultimate recovery of the patient are the severity and extent of abnormality.[10] In general, patients with normal MEP studies (grade I) have a very good chance of making a good to moderate recovery (see Table 6-1, A). This is true for patients with, at worst, mild SEP abnormalities as well. However, the probability of good to moderate recovery drops impressively when severely abnormal or absent MEPs are obtained. If deaths that were judged to be due to nonbrain causes are eliminated from the analysis, as has been done in Table 6-1, B, a greater percentage of favorable outcomes in seen in grade groups I, II, and III, although no change is seen in the grade IV group. This implies that mild or, in some cases, even severe MEP abnormalities may represent neural substrates that are, for some reason, dysfunctional but do have potential to regain function. The absence of response (grade IV), however, seems to indicate cell death or irreversible damage. One point that emerges from these findings is that there are certainly measurable abnormalities seen early after injury in such patients which do not necessarily portend doom. Several authors have reported latency shifts or amplitude decrements in responses of comatose head-injured patients who ultimately do well and whose SEPs eventually return to normal. It appears that in the case of this traumatic condition waveform complexity may be more relevant for predicting recovery than are latency and amplitude criteria. In a study of central conduction time in 13 comatose head-injured patients by Hume and Cant[11] moderately abnormal somatosensory conduction times that returned to normal later were found in several cases. Likewise, Seales and colleagues[12] reported that in five head-injured patients who displayed "abnormal" ABSRs (defined by prolonged wave latencies) very early post-trauma, three of the five showed return to neuroelectric normality in follow-up studies and recovered clinically. The two patients who maintained abnormalities died. Even though these transient abnormalities may be associated with recovery of function, other factors must be considered as well when dealing with the individual case.

EXTENT OF DYSFUNCTION

For any given level of severity, abnormalities that are diffuse (appear in more than one modality) result in outcomes less favorable than those that are focal.[10] This can be seen in Table 6-2. A mild abnormality (grade II) in only one modality results in outcomes similar to those of patients with no deficit. However, a diffuse mild abnormality (grade II in two or more modalities) substantially reduces the probability of a good to moderate outcome. This is also the case for patients with grade III MEPs, although to a lesser extent. Hence, patients with focal deficits that are mild or, in some cases, severe may make a return to normal or near-normal existence. However, the presence of only one grade IV evoked response in a single modality indicates a poor prognosis. Four of the patients with focal absence of activity did survive (see Table 6-2). One patient with absent VERs suffered cortical blindness and bizarre mentation. Of the three who had absent SERs, two are severely handicapped in sensorimotor function and one is "locked in."

Diffuse abnormalities, particularly those in cortical SEPs, seem, anecdotally, to be associated with global events such as severe hypoxic insult, edema, or increased intracranial pressure; whereas focal deficits are often seen after a localized mass has been removed or with the presence of focal contusion. The interaction of severity and extent of dysfunction must be considered for each patient since both of these variables affect probability of recovery. Although patients with focal deficits tend to have better recoveries, intensive rehabilitative or occupational therapy is often a critical part of any success they obtain in returning to an independent life.

SECONDARY INSULTS

Mass Lesions

Approximately 50 percent of the patients admitted to our service present with a mass lesion. It is well known that the outcome of these patients is less favorable than that of patients

TABLE 6-1 Prognostic Value of Graded Evoked Potentials* in 100 Severely Head-Injured Patients

A. All Patients

	No of Patients	Good-Moderate		Severe-Vegetative		Dead	
		No	%	No	%	No	%
Grade I	31	27	87	1	3	3	10
Grade II	31	23	74	1	3	7	23
Grade III	17	9	53	1	6	7	41
Grade IV	21	—	—	5	24	16	76
TOTAL	100	59	59	8	8	33	33

B. Patients Who Died from Systemic Complications Excluded

	No of Patients	Good-Moderate		Severe-Vegetative		Dead	
		No	%	No	%	No	%
Grade I	28	27	96	1	4	—	—
Grade II	26	23	88	1	4	2	8
Grade III	14	9	64	1	7	4	29
Grade IV	17	—	—	5	29	12	71
TOTAL	85	59	69	8	9	18	21

*Outcome determined at one year; MEPs obtained on mean day 3.8

TABLE 6-2. Comparison of the Effect of Focal Versus Diffuse MEP Abnormalities on Patient Outcome

MEP Grade	No of Patients	Outcome					
		Good-Moderate		Severe-Vegetative		Dead	
		No	%	No	%	No	%
Grade I (No abnormality)	31	27	87	1	3	3	10
Grade II F	17	15	88	1	6	1	6
II D	14	8	57	—	—	6	43
Grade III F	10	6	60	1	10	3	30
III D	7	3	43	—	—	4	57
Grade IV F	14	—	—	4	29	10	71
IV D	7	—	—	1	14	6	86

F = focal dysfunction: abnormality in only 1 modality; D = diffuse dysfunction: abnormality in 1 modality.

without masses. We have found, however, that patients who demonstrate normal MEPs after having a mass evacuated do have a 70 percent chance of a good to moderate recovery—greater than the 35 to 40 percent probability that would be the case if this information were not available.[10] Hence, in this subset of patients, MEPs can provide supplementary data with which to make prognostic decisions.

Other Complications

The ability to forecast outcome with early MEP studies is compromised by the occurrence of secondary insult, whether it be neurologic or systemic.[10] Some complications have minimal effect on recovery, whereas others are disastrous. Pulmonary infection, meningitis, ventriculitis, and sepsis are quite serious in these patients. Patients with mildly or severely abnormal (grade II and III) MEPs may be particularly vulnerable to the effects of these complications, as seen in Table 6-3. The incidence of complication is not remarkably different across grade groups (total, percent). But the outcomes of those patients who develop these medical problems, particularly in groups II and III, are much less favorable than for those who do not. Hence, the effect of complication may well depend on the initial severity of brain dysfunction. Early detection and treatment of such insults would thus be critical in these patients. Also, this points out the importance in such circumstances of repeated MEP evaluation to assess any resultant changes in CNS function in the face of such factors. Sensory evoked potentials are sensitive to neurologic deterioration resulting from secondary insult and this sensitivity is seen in serial studies.

SERIAL EVALUATION: DYNAMICS OF RECOVERY

It is of value to know what happens to the MEPs of these patients over time in order to better understand recovery of function and to learn which of these abnormalities represent transient or reversible loss of function and which indicate irreversible damage to neurons. In Figure 6-10, the MEP grades for individual patients are plotted over the time intervals that serial studies are usually done. Grades I and IV MEPs do not change significantly up to 1 year after injury. But grade II and III SEPs do change considerably, for better and worse. Approximately 75 percent of those in grades II and III change. However, of those that change, 80 percent of grade IIs improve to grade I and 20 percent worsen to grades III and IV, whereas only 50 percent of grade IIIs improve, with the other 50 percent deteriorating to cell death. The deterioration seen in the grade II group is associated with the occurrence of secondary insult and, in some cases, is quite rapid. Also, the patients in the grade III group who show improvement are primarily those with focal deficits.[13]

EARLY MULTIMODALITY EVOKED POTENTIALS AND CLINICAL RECOVERY

The clinical manifestation of a prediction made from an early MEP study may not be realized until up to a year after injury.[10] It appears that a trend may exist between initial MEP abnormality and "clinical" recovery time defined by Jennett and Bond's outcome categories. In Table 6-4, initial MEP grade is compared with surviving patient outcome determined by follow-up neurologic examinations at 3, 6, and 12 months. There is a tendency for grade I patients to attain maximal recovery by 3 months. Grade II patients may take longer. For example, the four patients who were moderately disabled at 3 months reached "good" by 6 months. Also, three patients in the grade II group were clinically severely disabled at 3 months although MEP data from previous serial studies had actually shown improvement. They ultimately reached moderate disability, but not until 1 year, with intensive rehabilitation. Major problems in rehabilitation were restoration of controlled movement of limbs that had serious

TABLE 6-3. Prognostic Value of Early MEPs in Patients who Develop Secondary Insults*

	Good-Moderate		Severe-Vegetative		Dead		Total	
	No	%	No	%	No	%	No	%
Grade I								
Yes	11	73	1	7	3	20	15	48
No	16	100	—	—	—	—	16	52
Grade II								
Yes	11	58	1	5	7	37	19	61
No	12	100	—	—	—	—	12	39
Grade III								
Yes	1	13	1	13	6	75	8	47
No	8	89	—	—	1	11	9	53
Grade IV								
Yes	—	—	3	23	10	77	13	62
No	—	—	2	25	6	75	8	38

Yes = complication; No = no complication
*Complications include pulmonary infection/edema; meningitis, ventriculitis, GI bleed, inappropriate ADH, seizures, sepsis, and respiratory or cardiac arrest.

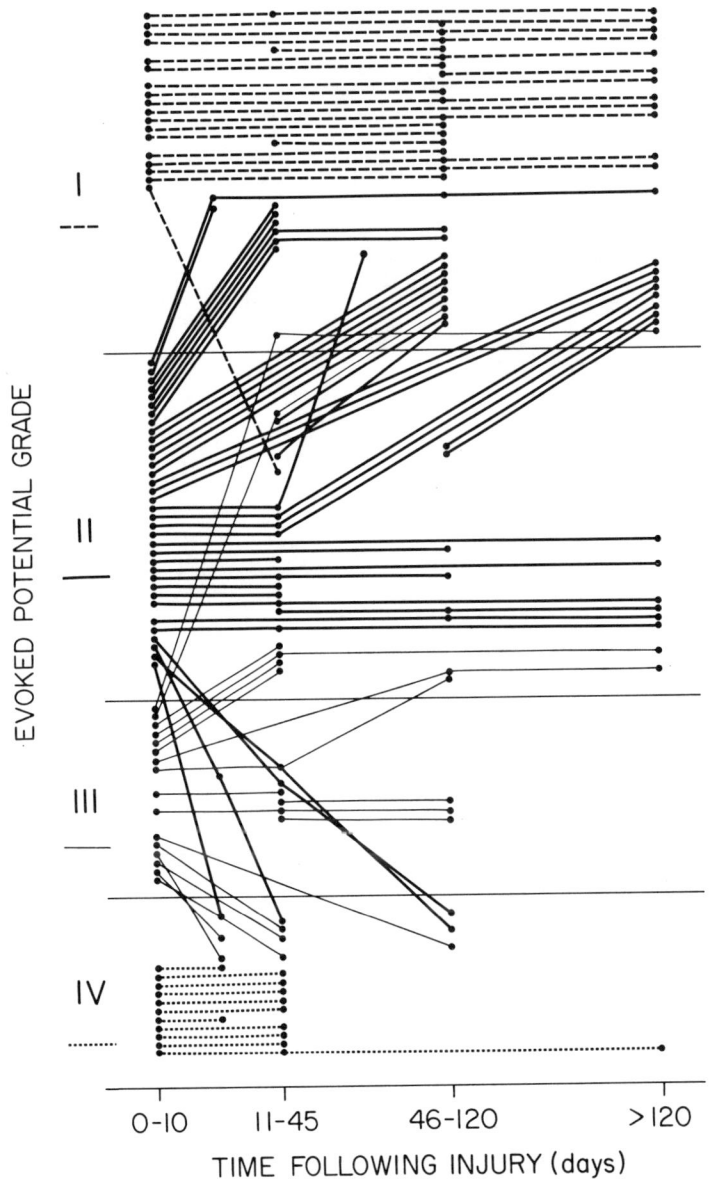

FIGURE 6-10. The recovery or deterioration of neuroelectric responses is seen when MEP results of 89 individual patients are plotted across the follow-up study time intervals. Patients were placed in grade groups based on the worst grade (most severe abnormality) obtained for any modality in the initial MEP evaluation.

contractures during coma. A similar result is seen in grade III patients although in a very small number of surviving patients. The fact that clinical recovery often lags behind that predicted by MEPs suggests that these tests may be able to pinpoint earlier than can be clinically determined patients with a potential for favorable recovery who may need rehabilitative programs to achieve that potential. This is particularly important for patients with mild dysfunction

TABLE 6-4. Clinical Recovery Time as a Function of Initial MEP Results in 42 Surviving Head-Injured Patients

	No of Patients	Good		Moderate		Severe		Vegetative	
		No	%	No	%	No	%	No	%
Grade I	17								
3 mo		13	76	3	18	1	6	—	—
6 mo		13	76	3	18	1	6	—	—
12 mo		13	76	3	18	1	6	—	—
Grade II	15								
3 mo		8	53	4	27	3	20	—	—
6 mo		12	80	—	—	3	20	—	—
12 mo		12	80	3	20	—	—	—	—
Grade III	6								
3 mo		3	50	2	33	—	—	1	17
6 mo		3	50	2	33	—	—	1	17
12 mo		4	67	1	17	—	—	1	17
Grade IV	4								
3 mo		—	—	—	—	1	25	3	75
6 mo		—	—	—	—	3	75	1	25
12 mo		—	—	—	—	2	50	2	50
Total group	42								
3 mo		24	57	9	21	5	12	4	10
6 mo		28	67	5	12	7	17	2	5
12 mo		29	69	7	17	3	7	3	7

and focal severe neuroelectric dysfunction since these are the most labile or "plastic" post-traumatic states.

SUMMARY

The post-traumatic clinical and rehabilitative management of severely head-injured patients can be facilitated by acquiring information about the functional severity and extent of injury and the reversibility of dysfunction. Evoked potential studies may provide such information, often earlier than clinical assessment can be made with confidence. The ability of these studies to identify neural pathways that are basically intact but transiently dysfunctional affords them a useful place among the other clinical indices of brain injury. The ultimate outcome of these patients certainly depends on a number of variables, some controllable and others not. But to the extent that the evoked potentials do reflect changes in the neurophysiologic status of the patient over time, the effects of these variables may be monitored.

The results of MEP studies are perhaps most useful in cases in which the clinical examination is unobtainable or shows inconsistencies leaving prognosis questionable. The patients who stand to gain from such information are particularly those who show dysfunction with potential to recover. The early identification of patients who will need and possibly be most responsive to rehabilitation programs can be quite important for efficient short- and long-term management.

The clinical use of SEPs in comatose head-injured patients is still in a fairly crude stage of development. Further study of the responses of these patients and careful analysis of the more subtle differences in waveforms may well enhance our understanding of the implications of particular abnormalities. We may find that these tests are restricted to discriminating viable from nonviable brain tissue in pathways of the brain subserving very basic sensory processes. But this ability in itself indicates substantial progress toward the knowledge of functional capability that is necessary to create an ideal clinical environment for recovery from severe head injury. Further research and development of the use of this technique in this context are certainly warranted.

REFERENCES

1. GREENBERG, RP, ET AL: *Evaluation of brain function in severe human head trauma with multimodality evoked potentials. Part 1: Evoked brain injury potentials, methods and analysis.* J Neurosurg 47:150, 1977.
2. ALLISON, T, ET AL: *On the neural origin of early components of the human somatosensory evoked potential.* In DESMEDT, JE (ED): *Progress in Clinical Neurophysiology, Vol. 7: Clinical Uses of Cerebral, Brain Stem and Spinal Somatosensory Evoked Potentials.* S Karger, Basel, 1980, p 51.
3. BROUGHTON, RJ: *The relationship of brain activity to scalp recordings of event related potentials.* In DONCHIN, E AND LINDSLEY, DB (EDS): *Average Evoked Potentials: Methods, Results and Evaluations.* NASA SP-191, US Government Printing Office, Washington, DC, 1969, p 79.
4. CRACCO, RQ AND CRACCO, JB: *Somatosensory evoked potentials in man: Farfield potentials.* Electroencephalogr Clin Neurophysiol 41:460, 1976.
5. GREENBERG, RP, ET AL: *Evaluation of brain function in severe human head trauma with multimodality evoked potentials. Part II: Localization of brain dysfunction and correlation with post-traumatic neurological conditions.* J Neurosurg 47:163, 1977.
6. UZIEL, A AND BENEZECH, J: *Auditory brain stem responses in comatose patients: Relationship with brain stem reflexes and levels of coma.* Electroencephalogr Clin Neurophysiol 45:515, 1978.

7. DE LA TORRE, JC, ET AL: *Somatosensory evoked potentials for the prognosis of coma in humans.* Exp Neurol 60:304, 1978.
8. RAPPAPORT, M, ET AL: *Evoked brain potentials and disability in brain damaged patients.* Arch Phys Med Rehabil 58:333, 1977.
9. NARAYAN, RK, ET AL: *Improved confidence of outcome predictions in severe head injury: A comparative analysis of the clinical examination, multimodality evoked potentials, CT and ICP.* J Neurosurg 54:751, 1981.
10. GREENBERG, RP, ET AL: *Prognostic implications of early multimodality evoked potentials in severe head injury patients: A prospective study.* J Neurosurg 55:227, 1981.
11. HUME, AL, CANT, MB, AND SHAW, NA: *Central somatosensory conduction time in comatose patients.* Ann Neurol 5:379, 1979.
12. SEALES, DM, ROSSITER, MA, AND WEINSTEIN, ME: *Brain stem auditory evoked responses in patients comatose as a result of blunt head trauma.* J Trauma 19:347, 1979.
13. NEWLON, PG, ET AL: *The dynamics of neuronal dysfunction and recovery following severe head injury assessed with serial multimodality evoked potentials.* J Neurosurg 57:168, 1982.

BIBLIOGRAPHY

CALLOWAY, E, TUETING, T, AND KASLO, SH (EDS): *Event Related Brain Potentials in Man.* Plenum Press, New York, 1978.

DESMEDT, JE (ED): *Clinical uses of cerebral brainstem and spinal somatosensory evoked potentials.* In *Progress in Clinical Neurophysiology,* Vol 7. S Karger, Basel, 1980.

Chapter 7

STANDARDIZED METHODS OF ASSESSING AND PREDICTING OUTCOME

Michael R. Bond, M.D., Ph.D., FRCS, MRC Psych., MRCP, DPM

WHY MEASURE OUTCOME?

Prior to 1965, very little was known about the complex physical, emotional, and social changes that contribute to the process of recovery from severe closed head injury. Nevertheless, there had been several approaches to devising methods of assessing the outcome of severe closed injuries, but they were based mainly on measures of physical handicaps and ability to return to work. In contrast, the problems posed by victims' mental difficulties for themselves and their families were neglected. Finally, assessments of outcome were often made only once, usually many months or even years after the injuries occurred. By this time, much of the recovery process had taken place and been missed, and the opportunity to develop indices of prognosis had been lost. Therefore, it is not surprising that there was uncertainty about the nature of recovery from injury in the minds of caring professionals and the families of the injured. For example, relatives were often told that they could expect the injured person to continue to recover for 2 years or more but were not given detailed information about the nature of the recovery they might expect. Vague statements of this kind, especially when made in the first few weeks after injury, are upsetting to relatives who later discover that many of the victim's deficits were established within a few months after injury and do not disappear later, as they had hoped.

The primary focus of head-injury research in the past 10 to 15 years has been to provide information for the prediction of the length and extent of the recovery process.

THE PROCESS OF MEASUREMENT

Because many persons are unclear about how to measure disability, it is worth considering the possibilities and the scientific restraints placed upon the one who measures. Measurements in head-injury research usually take one of two forms. Patients may be grouped in a general way according to a predetermined characteristic, for example, their level of "general dependency," a factor that forms the basis of the widely used Glasgow Outcome Scale[1] (Table 7-1). This is a global scale and as such has strength insofar as it gives a straightforward and readily understood picture of any group of patients studied; however, it reveals little about the subtle balance between physical incapacity and disturbances of behavior or of mental life.

TABLE 7-1. The Glasgow Outcome Scale in its Original Form and in Extended and Contracted Forms

Extended Scale		Original Scale	Contracted Scales		
Dead		Dead	Dead	Dead or vegetative	Dead
Vegetative		Vegetative			Survivors
Degree of disability:	5	Severely disabled	Dependent	Severely disabled	Conscious
	4				
	3	Moderately disabled	Independent	Independent	
	2				
	1	Good recovery			
	0				
Total categories	8	5	3		2

From Jennett, et al,[6] with permission.

The grades of the original scale are wide, and although not too precisely defined, the results gained are very useful for painting the broad canvas. An increase or decrease in sensitivity may be needed, and the means of achieving this are shown in Table 7-1. Detailed information is obtained differently by means of scales built on *carefully defined* items or questions that, for example, may assess individual components of behavior or attitudes and that, as a result, offer greater precision in rating deficits and the effects of treatments on them.[2] Further, psychologic tests used to assess these functions have items within their structure that may be identified according to their purpose as *instrumental* (i.e., measuring aspects of behavior), as *affective* (i.e., measuring emotional characteristics), or as *cognitive* (i.e., measuring aspects of intelligence).

When selecting tests, the experimenter must choose ones that will answer questions or hypotheses defined beforehand. Therefore, the tests selected must be *valid*. This means that they should measure what the experimenter wishes to measure or, in other words, actually predict the criterion of whatever is intended to be measured. Tests selected should also be *reliable*. This means that the observations made should be dependable, self-consistent, and stable. A test should yield results that are consistent, even when measured by more than one observer, and should be pertinent to the specific purpose the experimenter has in mind. As many of the physical and mental functions measured are part of a spectrum or range of functions, which in some cases are in continuity with normality, it is important to have information about the performance of normal individuals of comparable age, education, and perhaps sex. This enables the measurer to determine whether or not a group of head-injured individuals differs significantly from normal and, if so, to what extent. It is a general rule, therefore, that tests of this type must have been *standardized* in a normal population. Finally, each test should be within the capacity of the testee at the start of testing, thereafter increasing in difficulty to the point where limits of ability are reached. In the case of head-injured persons, tests should not be too lengthy because fatigue and impaired concentration interfere with performance and may invalidate results. It is commonly a fault among inexperienced researchers to design the "full and perfect" battery of tests, only to find that patients cannot

TABLE 7-2. Twenty-two Tests of Learning and Memory

Wechsler Memory Scale
Auditory-Verbal Learning Task (Rey)
Selective Reminding (Buschke)
Paired Associates Test (Inglis)
Babcock Story
Recurring Figures Test (Kimura)
Visual Retention Test (Benton)
Memory for Designs Test (Binet)
Memory for Designs Test (Graham-Kindall)
Rey-Osterrieth Complex Figure Test
Digit Symbol Test (WAIS)
Symbol Digit Modalities Test (Smith)
Facial Recognition Test (Milner)
Posner Task Test
Knox Cube Imitation Test
Block-Tapping Test (Corsi)
Recency-Primary Test (Corsi)
Boston Retrograde Amnesia Test
Tactile Performance Test
Tactile Nonsense Figure Test (Milner)
Memory Battery (Squires)
University of Wisconsin Memory Battery

and/or will not complete it. Selection of appropriate tests, especially of mental functions, may be very difficult simply because of the large number of tests available even for a single function, for example, memory (Table 7-2).

In general terms, the selection of tests depends on the kind of information required. Tests, or instruments (as they are often called), may be *structured, semistructured,* or *unstructured*. Structured instruments define exactly what is to be asked or read; semistructured instruments provide leading questions but rely on the interviewer to gain the needed information; and unstructured interviews may define only the area to be examined and allow complete personal judgment by the interviewer. The former are easy to score and provide standard, comparable information. The latter permit the interviewer to follow leads and explore a new area. They are also used to gain new ideas, whereas the structured instruments are used to test definitive theories. Finally, the instruments may be administered by a professional or trained interviewer, may be self-administered by the patient, or may be given to a close relative or friend, someone who knows the patient well and plays a significant part in the patient's life.

AIMS OF MEASUREMENT

The purpose of applying measurements to various aspects of the physical, emotional/behavioral, and social consequences of severe head injury are as follows:

1. Assessment of the severity of injury at the time of admission to hospital.
2. Assessment of the physical, mental, and social deficits during the process of recovery.
3. Assessment of global outcome and its relation to specific deficits mentioned in (2).
4. Assessment of the effects of the injury on family members.
5. All measures (1 through 4) may be incorporated into programs designed to evaluate rehabilitation techniques.

MEASURES OF OUTCOME

It is impossible to describe here all the instruments available for the assessment of head-injured patients; therefore, a small number have been selected because they are often used and fulfill most of the criteria of suitability described earlier, and because they illustrate recent discoveries about the process of recovery and means of predicting outcome. The measures have been selected from clinical neurologic, psychologic, and social assessment schedules in common use.

ASSESSMENT OF SEVERITY OF INJURY

Severity of injury is an important guide to short- and long-term outcome, although in the latter case it will be shown that so far our methods permit any given patient's prognosis to be drawn only in broad terms—especially with reference to the patient's ultimate possession and use of the higher social skills needed in everyday life, for example, to maintain a home, to maintain good relations with others, or to hold down a job.

ASSESSMENT OF POST-TRAUMATIC AMNESIA

In 1932, the late Professor Ritchie Russell[3] of the University of Oxford, England, proposed that the time taken to recover full consciousness is a measure of the quantity of brain tissue destroyed by a head injury. He based his observation on the fact that return of memory for day-to-day events on a *continuous* basis is the last stage in the restoration of full consciousness. *The time between injury and recovery of continuous memory is the period of post-traumatic amnesia (PTA).* Retrograde amnesia refers to the period of memory loss prior to injury and seems to be of less value as a measure of severity. When estimating PTA, which is a retrospective measure that can be used months or years after injury, it is important to establish when *full* memory for day-to-day events was restored; prior to this, patients may have isolated memories—for example, a visit from a relative or friend—but this is only an "island" in the midst of a "sea of forgetfulness." In many cases, the full return of memory is related to an important event in the patient's life, presumably reflecting a period of increased arousal—for example, movement from one ward or hospital to another, or to discharge home. In this context, it is interesting that full consciousness may be restored more quickly in children in whom it is prolonged by sending them home to a familiar environment. It has been suggested that in patients without dysphasia the duration of PTA is approximately four times the period taken to speak after injury. Relatives are able to date its end to the time the patient becomes lucid and clearly remembers recent conversations and events. The ability to recall recent events and the presence of correct orientation for time and place form the basis of tests recently designed to determine the end of PTA, in other words, tests that take us from retrospective to prospective assessment.[4,5]

In his original paper, Russell related the duration of PTA to the severity of injury in the following way:

PTA < 1 hr = mild injury
PTA 1–24 hr = moderate injury
PTA 1–7 days = severe injury
PTA > 7 days = very severe injury

In a recent study of 1000 severe head injuries in Glasgow, it was shown that all patients had a PTA greater than 2 days, 94 percent more than 1 week, 80 percent more than 2 weeks, and 60 percent more than 4 weeks.[6]

There is often concern about the accuracy of this method because it involves a retrospective assessment; however, all severe injuries have a PTA exceeding 1 day. The longer the period of amnesia, the less need there is for a precise estimation of its end—in fact, it is usually impossible to estimate PTA without accepting that the figure is within days or, in the case of the severest injuries, a week or two of its end. With regard to milder injuries, more precise estimations of PTA are possible, and Fortuny and others[4] have presented an expanded scale for minor injuries that may be used in association with their test for its duration. The gradings are as follows:

PTA < 10 min = very mild injury
PTA 10–60 min = mild injury
PTA 1–24 hr = moderate injury

Their study concerns patients who were admitted to an English hospital in a period of 6 months; the proportions in each of the three categories given were 46.7 percent, 17.3 percent, and 20.8 percent, respectively. Only 6.6 percent of patients had a PTA greater than 24 hours.

MEASUREMENT OF COMA DURATION

It should be remembered that an interest in measures of severity is related to a desire for one measurement that will predict immediate and late outcome with the highest possible accuracy from the time of injury onward, and that the use of coma duration has been perhaps the most popular universal measure of the severity of head injury. However, until recently, a satisfactory and universally acceptable means of defining coma was lacking, chiefly because agreement upon the hierarchy of physical signs indicating the depth of coma and reflecting the severity of brain injury had not been worked out. Unconsciousness and wakefulness are not two wholly different states. As the patient recovers, one state gradually shades into the other. Therefore, the process of return to awareness is continuous; during its course, a number of signs of specific neurologic dysfunctions may be detected, and each has significance in terms of the severity of brain damage.

Using the principle of the different significance for life or death of a number of the signs that may occur and for the degree of overall disability they predict later in recovery, Teasdale and Jennett[7] made the most significant contribution so far to our understanding of the assessment of disordered consciousness in the immediate postinjury period. They also developed, to a high level of accuracy, means of predicting the early outcome of injury, and both achievements were made through the construction of the Glasgow Coma Scale (Table 7-3). The attraction of the scale lies in the fact that those who use it—whether they be nurses, general surgeons, neurosurgeons, physicians, or junior or senior physicians—obtain consistent results. The instrument is relatively impervious to the effects of language and, therefore, has a high level of interrater and cross-cultural reliability. It enables us to define coma in descriptive terms without reference to supposed anatomic sites of dysfunctions or to levels that depend on the concurrence of certain degrees of responsiveness with other features such as pupil reactions or abnormalities of respiration. After considerable research involving all disorders of neurologic function that can be measured during unconsciousness and from which a hierarchy of responses can be obtained, three items proved to be the most sensitive measures of severity and predictors of outcome. They are *eye opening, motor response,* and *verbal performance;* each is graded independently. *Coma is defined as (1) not opening the eyes, (2) not obeying commands, and (3) not uttering understandable words.* The responses to testing are scored separately giving a total derived from $E+M+V$ with a range of 3 to 15 points. Conscious patients make the highest scores; 90 percent of those with scores of 8 or less are in coma,

TABLE 7-3. Glasgow Coma Scale

	Examiner's Test	Patient's Response	Assigned Score
Eye opening	Spontaneous	Opens eyes on own	E4
	Speech	Opens eyes when asked to in a loud voice	3
	Pain	Opens eyes when pinched	2
	Pain	Does not open eyes	1
Best motor response	Commands	Follows simple commands	M6
	Pain	Pulls examiner's hand away when pinched	5
	Pain	Pulls a part of body away when examiner pinches him	4
	Pain	Flexes body inappropriately to pain (decorticate posturing)	3
	Pain	Body becomes rigid in an extended position when examiner pinches victim (decerebrate posturing)	2
	Pain	Has no motor response to pinch.	1
Verbal response (talking)	Speech	Carries on a conversation correctly and tells examiner where he is, who he is, and the month and year	V5
	Speech	Seems confused or disoriented	4
	Speech	Talks so examiner can understand victim but makes no sense	3
	Speech	Makes sounds that examiner can't understand	2
	Speech	Makes no noise	1

Coma Score $(E + M + V) = 3$ to 15

TABLE 7-4. Outcomes Associated With Best Level of Responsiveness in First 24 Hours After Coma

Coma Response Sum	n	Dead or Vegetative (%)	Moderate Disability or Good Recovery (%)
11	57	12	87
8/9/10	190	27	68
5/6/7	525	53	34
3/4	176	87	7

From Jennett, Teasdale, and Braakman,[9] with permission.

while none of those with scores of 9 or more are in coma. This point in the scale is an important watershed because patients with scores of 8 or less are regarded as having had a *severe injury* given that the low score is maintained for a *minimum of 6 hours* from impact or the end of a period of postinjury lucidity during which the patient talked. Approximately 50 percent of these patients will die. Patients with scores more than 12 are regarded as having had minor injuries, although a significant number of them have residual deficits up to 3 months after injury (see Chapter 2). By exclusion, patients with scores from 9 to 11 have injuries of moderate severity. The critical reader will have realized that despite the effectiveness of the scale in giving a continuous measure of the features of coma, there is no *absolute* measure of what constitutes a severe injury. However, the definition given is widely accepted on the basis of the relationship between the score of 8 or less and the certainty of the presence of unconsciousness and the significance of scores below this level in terms of the chances of survival or death (Table 7-4).[9] The power of the coma scale is increased by use of scores of individual responses in the E, M, and V components. For further information, the reader should consult Jennett and Teasdale,[8] Chapter 14.

NEUROLOGIC ASSESSMENT OF OUTCOME

Until recent times, neurologic assessment was virtually the sole measure of the early and late outcome of brain injuries. As a result, there are many scales of widely varying complexity for the assessment of all aspects of neurologic functions encompassed by the broad areas of motor and sensory function, extrapyramidal activity, and higher-level mental activities, although in the last group interest has been confined chiefly to disorders of speech and consciousness. If the nature of the tests is examined in general terms, they appear to form three basic categories. First, there are tests based on a "points system" in which numerical values are assigned in a graded system to each physical parameter to be assessed. The total number of points gained either for an individual function—for example, the extent of motor dysfunction in a limb—or for all disabilities is used to represent the patient's neurologic status at any given time. Assessment of this type may be used to describe recovery, to predict the speed and eventual extent of recovery, or to evaluate the effects of treatment. A second approach was recently described by Roberts.[10] His large-scale retrospective survey of war veterans with head injuries depends upon very careful and detailed neurologic assessments. His analysis of the results gained leads to the formulation of patterns of disability, which in turn leads to the construction of central neural disability profiles. For example, Roberts identified the hemiparetic, brain stem cerebellar, and athetoid pseudobulbar patterns, and a fourth one that incorporates mental handicap—namely, decerebrate dementia. This is a familiar and traditional neurologic "grouping" process, but the validity of Roberts' "patterns of disability" awaits confirmation and acceptance by others. Finally, there are several methods of assessing neu-

TABLE 7-5. A Neurophysical Scale

Deficit		Score	
Motor Deficit			
Monoparesis		1	
Monoplegia		2	
Hemiparesis		3	
Hemiplegia		4	
Sensory Deficit			*Cranial Nerves*
One arm/leg, partial		1	Score 1 for each involved except:
One arm/leg, full		2	Vision. Score 2 for each eye.
One arm/leg and part trunk		3	Hearing. Score 2 for each ear.
Arm/leg and trunk		4	
Speech			*Physical Deficits*
Partial aphasia		2	Score 1 for mild/moderate.
Complete aphasia		4	Score 2 for severe.
Ataxia			
Each limb	Mild/moderate	1	
	Severe	2	
Dysarthria	Mild/moderate	1	
	Severe	2	
Dysphagia	Mild/moderate	1	
	Severe	2	

From Bond,[11] with permission.

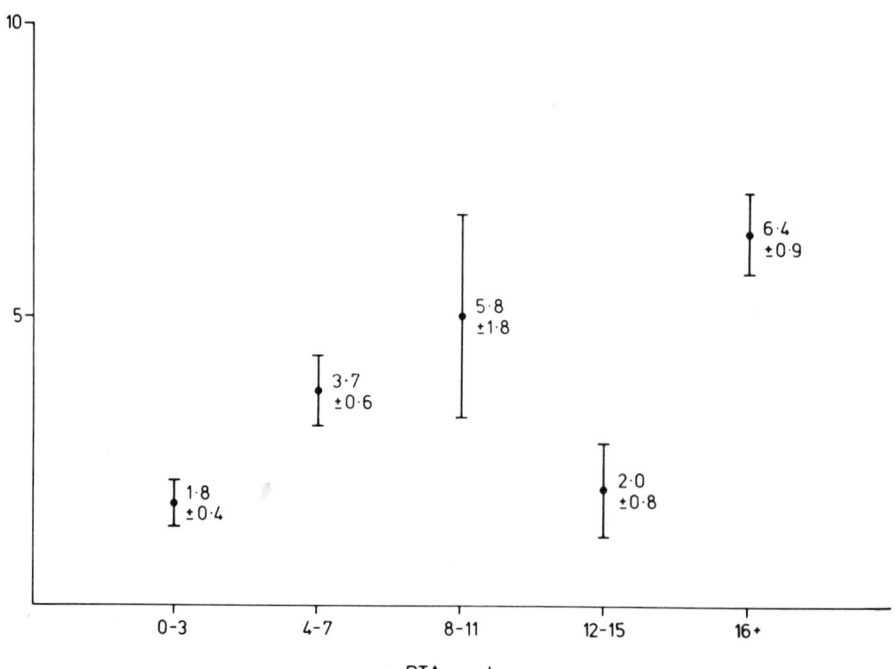

FIGURE 7-1. Changes in physical disability following severe head injury. (From Bond,[11] with permission.)

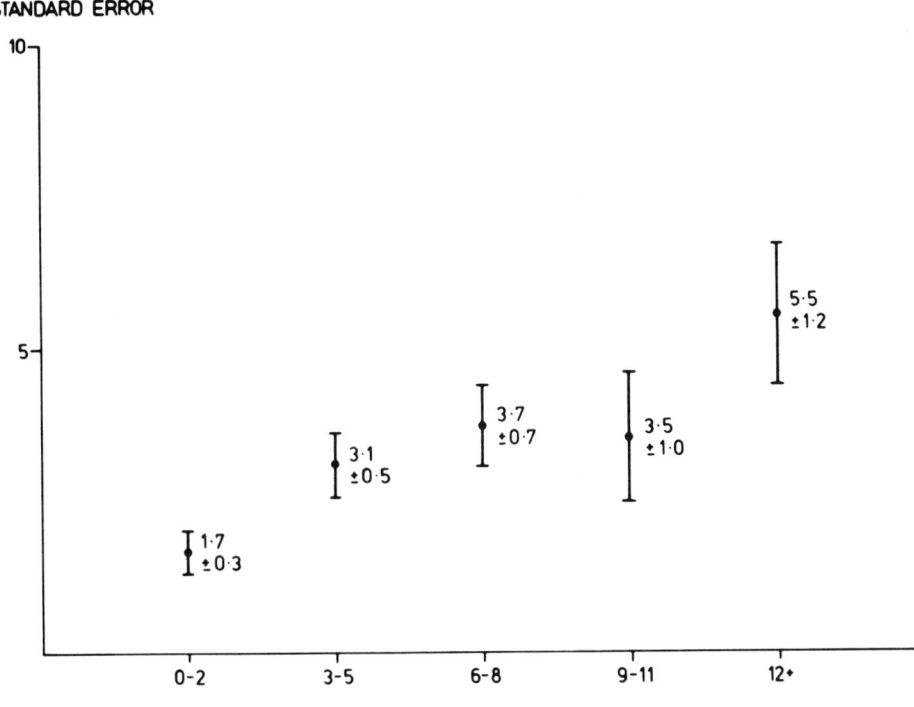

FIGURE 7-2. Relation between physical disability after severe head injury and social outcome. (From Bond,[11] with permission.)

rologic function by mechanical, electrical, or photographic techniques. For example, the first two of these are often used to assess muscle tone and power, and the latter—nowadays improved by the use of videotape equipment and computer analysis—to examine patterns of movements such as gait.

The question of which instrument to use depends on the objectives or aims of the assessor, but for everyday clinical use, relatively short scales that are reliable and easily performed by professionals with varying levels of experience are most acceptable. An example of a simple scale is given in Table 7-5[11] from which it will be noticeable that only the degree of deficit is rated and that there is no presumption about the central lesion responsible because "localization" is not of much value in studies of severe closed head injuries that cause widespread damage. However, the scale does make a number of judgments about the significance of each deficit for return to activities of daily life. The information gathered with this type of instrument has proven very useful in studies of the process of recovery from head injury. For example, scores of neurologic disability may be related to a measure of the severity of injury (PTA), as shown in Figure 7-1, and to overall levels of social disability (Fig. 7-2).[11]

ASSESSMENT OF MENTAL OUTCOME

COGNITIVE AND PERCEPTUAL FUNCTIONS

Psychologic measures of outcome are attractive because of the high degree of specificity, validity, and reliability. However, it is their very specificity that reduces their potency as predictors of the ways in which individuals will use their residual skills and adapt to changes in their personal lives. The best known of all instruments are those that measure cognitive functions. However, recent studies of tests of intelligence, perhaps the most widely used of all, reveal that residual intelligence levels relate only broadly to an individual's ultimate capacity to cope with work, except perhaps among those who earn their living chiefly by using their intellectual skills. It seems clear that memory and learning tasks are more sensitive measures of cognitive change, at least after closed head injuries, than conventional intelligence tests. In fact, performance on memory and learning tasks tends to correlate significantly with the severity of head injury. It is important to remember that measurements of intelligence are affected by the subject's educational level and age and that often tests must be completed within a given time. This means that patients may make lower scores than if given unlimited time to complete tests because mental slowness is one of the most common and persistent intellectual deficits of severe head injury. Other factors, including poor ability to sustain attention and the ease with which mental fatigue develops, influence performance on tests of all kinds; they also affect activities of daily living, perhaps accounting for the hesitancy and lack of confidence shown by many head-injured individuals. For this reason, increasing attention is being given to measuring these difficulties, and it has been found that levels of fatigue are often high in the early months of recovery but lessen with time.

Despite the problems mentioned and the discrepancies between performance in the laboratory and activities in everyday life, neuropsychologic tests of cognitive function have

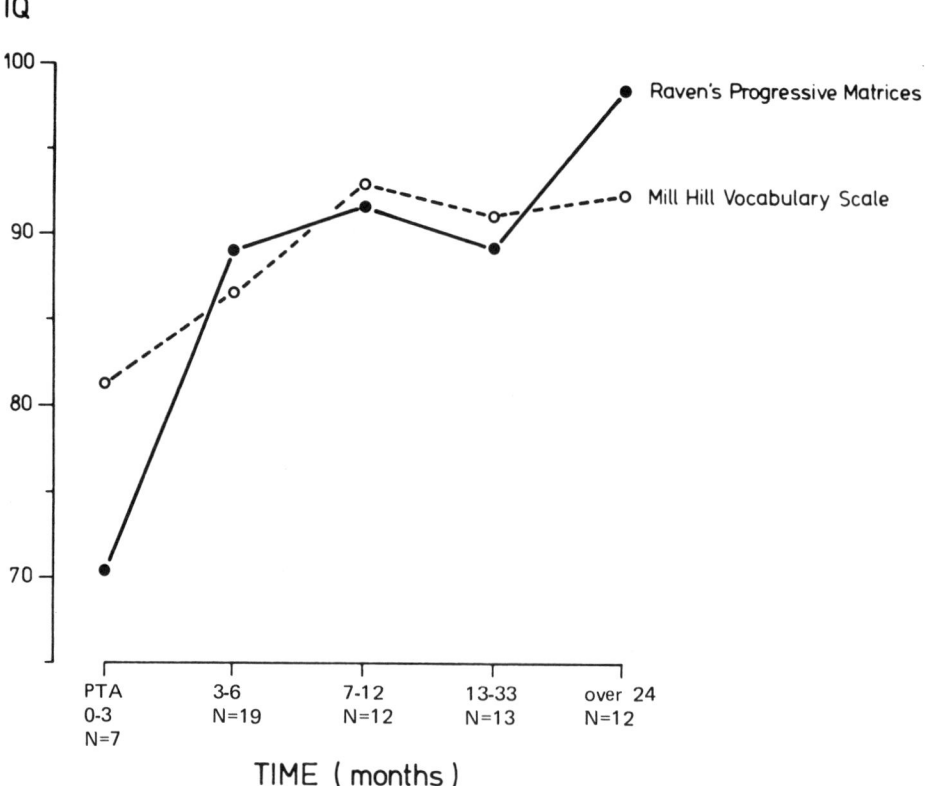

FIGURE 7-3. Recovery curves: changes in intellectual function after severe head injury. (From Bond and Brooks,[12] with permission.)

provided an immense amount of information about the way basic mental functions recover after injury. For example, they have been used to explore the concept of recovery curves, as shown in Figure 7-3.[12] These reveal the way in which verbal and nonverbal forms of intelligence measured by the Mill Hill Vocabulary Scale and Raven's Progressive Matrices tests, respectively, improve during the first year after injury. Although such measures are valuable in studying groups, it is clear that the results are applicable only in a general way and may not fit the progress of a given individual. This fact emphasizes the need for caution when attempting to extend general rules to individual cases and the desirability of constructing a recovery profile from the results of a carefully chosen battery of tests.

In addition to tests of cognitive function, assessments of perception are needed because it is known that perceptual deficits—for example, of visual-spatial orientation—often subtle in nature, may interfere quite substantially with practical activities of everyday life.[2] When severe, these deficits are very noticeable, leading to such difficulties as inability to dress or to locate one's body in space, thereby making even sitting or lying a task of great difficulty. However, they are almost certainly neglected in most "routine" follow-up examinations in surgical clinics. The full contribution of perceptual deficits to patient's difficulties has yet to be determined.

ASSESSMENT OF PERSONALITY AND BEHAVIOR

Of all the possible mental consequences of severe head injury, changes in personality and behavior are the most damaging of all in terms of their effects on family life and reintegration into society. The fact that changes in personality are a more serious barrier to effective rehabilitation and functional recovery than cognitive or intellectual changes was reported 40 years ago by Goldstein[13] and investigated again 20 years ago by Luria,[14] the famous Russian neuropsychologist. The latter described a lack of self-monitoring after frontal lobe damage, and clearly, changes of this type pose great challenges to rehabilitation. Therefore, means of accurately assessing alterations in personality and abnormal behavior are a central issue in rehabilitation research. So far, almost all published work on this subject has been based on a descriptive approach to the assessment of personality change; at this level, there is general agreement about the nature of the changes that may occur, and an account of them is given in Chapter 14. Apart from the use of the descriptive method, there are few scales for assessment of personality after head injury, although there are many for use among normal people and psychiatric patients. However, as these rely on an individual having insight into his or her own characteristics, they cannot be used where this facility is absent or distorted, as is often the case with head-injured patients. Moreover, the problem is compounded by the fact that there are many theories of personality but none that is universally accepted. Finally, several of the traits produced by brain injury are not constituents of normal personality, for example, the presence of apathy or persistent euphoria and loss of social restraint. Both characteristics do occur, however, in individuals with severe depression or hypomania, but instruments devised for assessing these clinical psychiatric problems contain many questions that are irrelevant when considering the syndromes produced by brain injuries.

In view of the difficulties described, it has become common practice to examine changes in personality by means of checklists devised with the possible complications of head injury in mind. These are completed by close relatives who provide information about the patient's current mental state and past character. Similar results may be achieved by means of analogue scales (Fig. 7-4), but these instruments may also be used to yield a measure of the extent to which a given characteristic is present, or by which it has changed as a direct result of injury.

Behavior rating scales are more practical instruments and are being developed in many rehabilitation centers. In brief, they are used to define broad areas of behavioral change and, within them, subbehavioral units which become the foci or targets for behavior modification

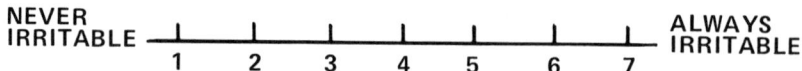

FIGURE 7-4. An analogue scale for assessment of personality characteristics.

therapies or shaping procedures. For example, one area might be "psychosocial behavior change"; within this, the identifiable subbehaviors include an individual's poor insight into one's own abilities, a poor reaction to criticism, inability to tolerate frustration, demands for excessive attention, feelings of persecution, self-abuse, and sudden changes of mood. Another area, "aggressive behavior," might be assessed in terms of violent or threatening behavior, offensive language, damage to property, impulsiveness, and premeditated attacks on others. By means of empirically defined grades of severity, usually involving a short numerical scale (for example, 0 to 4), behavioral profiles may be constructed and so form a basis for assessment of the effects of therapy, or an entirely different issue—namely, the natural history of any given behavior as part of a study to develop accurate means of providing a forecast of future events—in other words, a prognosis. The advantage of these techniques lies in their great flexibility of design and the fact that they can be assembled or packaged to suit individual patients in therapy and at the same time be made sufficiently reliable (eventually) to form the basis of a universally accepted range of instruments.

ASSESSMENT OF OVERALL OUTCOME

The final overall social outcome of severe head injuries has been defined in several ways. Terms such as good, fair, poor, acceptable, practical, worthwhile, and tolerable have been used by various writers. Others have taken a rather different view and expressed outcome in terms of ability to return to work—a matter that depends upon many factors other than the residual mental or physical deficits of the patient, availability of work and family attitudes to the injured person being only two that may have a marked effect. In order to overcome the uneven grading of many of the verbal scales used because most tended to emphasize the more severe effects of injuries (Table 7-6),[6] Jennett and Bond[1] removed value judgments as expressed in terms like "worthwhile" and "tolerable," and avoided the pitfalls of outcome based upon return to work, when they constructed the Glasgow Outcome Scale (see Table 7-1). In addition to avoiding the objections to earlier scales, this scale was also devised to facilitate multicenter studies on outcome and to predict outcome accurately. It is now widely used in Europe and North America. The scale is valid and has a high degree of interrater reliability; in a recent study, there was a 95 percent level of agreement between two observers rating 150 severely head-injured patients.[6] As Table 7-1 shows, the scale is flexible, which means that its three best categories may be expanded to six without loss of reliability if more closely defined groups are needed. It has proven to be valuable in studies of the natural history of recovery, and large-scale surveys have revealed that the greater part of recovery is achieved between 3 and 6 months from injury and that of those who by 12 months have made a good recovery, or who are moderately disabled, almost two thirds have already reached this level within 3 months after injury and 90 percent have done so by 6 months. Only 10 percent of patients who are severely or moderately disabled at 6 months will be in a better category 1 year after injury (Fig. 7-5).[12] These observations correspond with the pattern of recovery of many aspects of cognitive and physical function described earlier, thus adding to the accumulating evidence that the greater part of the recovery of those functions *directly attributable to activity of the brain* takes place within 6 months after injury. The overall picture of outcome after head injuries of all degrees of severity is shown in Table 7-7 from data obtained in Charlottesville, Virginia, 3 months from injury (see Chapter 2). Later im-

STANDARDIZED METHODS OF ASSESSING AND PREDICTING OUTCOME

TABLE 7-6. Classification of Disability Due to Brain Damage (Conscious Survivors)

Acute Brain Damage (Traumatic or Not)		Head Injury			Stroke	
Glasgow Scale Jennett and Bond		Najenson (1974)	Stover and Zeiger (1976)	Roberts (1979)	Rankin (1957)	Adams (1963)
(1975) 3 point	(1980) 6 point					
Severe disability						
	5		2	4		3
		2	3		4	
			4	3.5	3	2
	4		5	3		
Moderate disability						
3		3		2.5		
			6	2	2	1
2		4		1.5		
Good recovery						
1			7	1		
		5			1	
	0		8	0.5		

From Jennett et al,[6] with permission.

provements do occur, but to a lesser extent. On the other hand, considerable and increasing use of coping strategies of every kind, both mental and social, and the resultant interactions with others play an important role in late outcome. For this reason, measures of initial severity of injury, such as coma duration or the length of post-traumatic amnesia, weaken as predictors of psychosocial outcome if used later than 6 months after injury. However, this does not mean that PTA cannot be used to predict late outcome as measured by the Glasgow Outcome Scale. The relationship between these measures in patients, as reviewed by Jennett and Teasdale[8] at least 1 year after injury, is given in Table 7-8, from which it is clear that severe disability does not result unless PTA is greater than 14 days. Moreover, no more than 17 percent of patients with a PTA shorter than this will be moderately disabled; the remaining 83 percent will have made a good recovery despite the fact that they were all patients with severe injuries according to the criteria used at the time of admission. Thus it seems we have reached a position where measures of early severity primarily foretell the probability of life or death in the first days after injury (especially in the case of the Glasgow Coma Scale) or

TABLE 7-7. Outcome Among Survivors 3 Months After Head Injury

Outcome Grade GOS	% Total Population (n = 1248)
Vegetative	4
Severe disability	8
Moderate disability	22
Good recovery	66

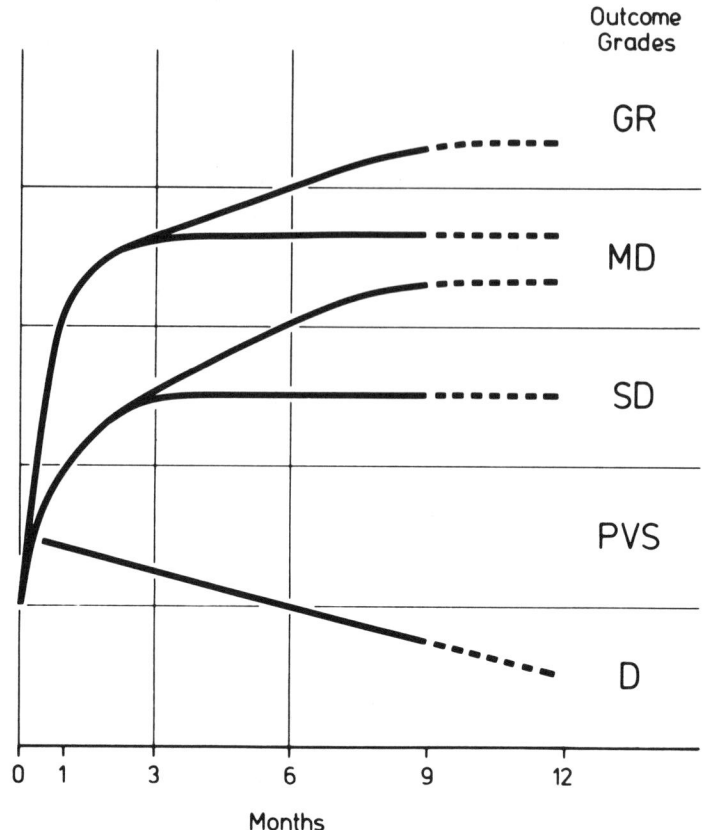

FIGURE 7-5. Outcome of severe head injury as measured by the Glasgow Outcome Scale. (From Bond and Brooks,[12] with permission.)

indicate the likelihood of damage to certain psychologic and neurologic functions that arise directly from activity in the brain. However, they do not forecast late outcome in other than broad terms.

A more detailed approach to assessment of the extent to which head-injured patients are able to cope with the basic functions necessary to everyday life, or what might be regarded as their quality of life, has several interpretations emphasizing that, as yet, the problem of the way in which this concept should be defined has not been solved. One approach that is commonly used centers on assessment of the efficiency with which an injured person can perform essential activities of daily life—in other words, cope with feeding, dressing, and

TABLE 7-8. PTA and Outcome at 6 Months

PTA	n	Severely Disabled (%)	Moderately Disabled (%)	Good Recovery (%)
<14 days	101	0	17	83
15–28 days	96	3	31	66
>28 days	289	30	43	27

From Jennett and Teasdale,[8] with permission.

toileting—using an activity of daily living (ADL) scale. As there are many instruments of this kind, the difficulty for the assessor lies in the selection of a valid and reliable scale.[15,16] This matter was recently reviewed by Sheikh and others[17] who produced an instrument with these qualities and one which gives scores in the hospital and at home that correlate significantly. As "life" is compounded of many elements, it might be argued quite reasonably that a single ADL scale does not give sufficient breadth because it gives only information about practical skills. In order to combat this objection, a different kind of battery may be used. It might include a psychiatric symptom checklist, an ADL assessment, an assessment of the patient's well-being by a close relative or friend, and a measure of social adjustment. The value and use of the last of these remain to be discussed.

ASSESSMENT OF SOCIAL ADJUSTMENT

In response to the therapeutic movements in the past two decades in psychiatry away from care in large institutions to an expanding concept of community care, a number of scales for the assessment of social adjustment have been developed. In the first instance, they were used with schizophrenic patients and their families, and for the evaluation of psychotherapy among outpatients. In 1973, a joint Food and Drug Administration–American College of Neuropsychopharmacology (FDA-ACNP) group was formed to develop guidelines for the evaluation of psychotropic drugs, which entailed examining social adjustment scales. The first review of the latter was produced by Weissman in 1975[18]; she described the reliability, validity, and use of 15 social adjustment scales. Since that time, many more have appeared, but only a small number might be of value in assessment of head-injured patients and their families.

Social adjustment has been defined by Weissman and Sholomskas[19] in broad terms as "the interplay between the individual and the social environment." These authors point out that an individual's major roles are the product of several interacting factors, including age, marital status, family constellation, and mental constitution. For example, a normal adult tends to fill an occupational, a marital, and a community role, at different times. In the case of those who are ill (mentally or physically) or disabled, symptoms often alter roles, but in some cases, the individual functions relatively normally despite their presence; this may happen in the case of those who make a good recovery where evidence of residual symptoms exists following a severe brain injury. On the other hand, as is well known, it is not uncommon for those who have had trivial injuries to function poorly. Thus, social adjustment is based on an individual's interactions with others and one's satisfaction and performance in roles that are molded by personality, family, and cultural expectations.

The instruments used to assess social adjustment may be of the self-report type. They depend on an interview or may be completed in the form of a postal or telephone assessment. A number of the tests are only for patients, but others may be completed by a relative or close friend. Although it is not the function of this chapter to review tests in detail, it is worth mentioning two in order to demonstrate the nature and purpose of instruments that may be of value in head-injury rehabilitation research and yet may be unfamiliar to readers.

The Katz Adjustment Scale—Relatives Form (KAS-R)[20] is a 205-item scale used to assess behavior and the life-situation adjustment of patients. Each item is rated on a 4-point scale. In more detail, there are five sections that cover (1) performance at socially expected tasks, (2) relatives' expectations for performance of the tasks, (3) free activities, (4) relatives' rating of performance, and (5) rating of symptoms and social behavior. The main weakness of the scale is its lack of coverage of marital, parental, and extended family relationships. Therefore, as a supplement, the Social Adjustment Scale—Self Report (SAS-SR) might be used. It measures instrumental and affective performance and the performance of various roles, which include social and leisure activities, relationships with the extended family, marital role, parental role, and family unit and economic independence. This is a stable, valid, and reliable test that has been used extensively in psychiatric and social research, where it has been shown that there is a significant correlation between self-reports and reports by others. This factor makes the test attractive for head-injury assessments.

CONCLUSION

In conclusion, it is clear that considerable progress has been made in recent years in defining ways of measuring the outcome of severe head injuries for the victims and their relatives. In the process, much has been learned about recovery from injury and the consequences for families of having an injured person among them. Although much has been achieved, there is a need for further research into the nuances of the emotional and social consequences of injury during the later stages of recovery, and the matter of designing and critically assessing methods of rehabilitation using valid and reliable tests has hardly begun.

REFERENCES

1. JENNETT, B AND BOND, MR: *Assessment of outcome after severe brain damage.* Lancet 1:480, 1975.
2. NEWCOMBE, F AND FORTUNY, LAI: *Problems and perspectives in the evaluation of psychological deficits after cerebral lesions.* International Journal of Rehabilitation Medicine 1:182, 1979.
3. RUSSELL, WR: *Cerebral involvement in head injury.* Brain 55:549, 1932.
4. FORTUNY, LAI, ET AL: *Measuring the duration of post-traumatic amnesia.* J Neurol Neurosurg Psychiatry 43:377, 1980.
5. LEVIN, HS, O'DONNELL, VM, AND GROSSMAN, RG: *The Galveston orientation and amnesia test: A practical scale to assess cognition after head injury.* J Nerv Ment Dis 167:675, 1979.
6. JENNETT, B, ET AL: *Disability after severe head injury: Observations on the use of the Glasgow Outcome Scale.* J Neurol Neurosurg Psychiatry 1981 (in press).
7. TEASDALE, G AND JENNETT, B: *Assessment of coma and impaired consciousness.* Lancet 2:81, 1974.
8. JENNETT, B AND TEASDALE, G: *Management of Head Injuries.* FA Davis, Philadelphia, 1981, p 317.
9. JENNETT, B, TEASDALE, G, AND BRAAKMAN, R: *Prognosis in a series of patients with severe head injury.* Neurosurgery 4:283, 1979.
10. ROBERTS, AH: *Severe Accidental Head Injury: An Assessment of Long-Term Prognosis.* Macmillan, New York, 1979.
11. BOND, MR: *Assessment of the psychosocial outcome after severe head injury.* In Outcome of Severe Damage to the Central Nervous System. Ciba Foundation Symposium 34 (New Series). Elsevier-Excerpta Medica-North Holland, Amsterdam, 1975.
12. BOND, MR AND BROOKS, DN: *Understanding the process of recovery as a basis for the investigation of rehabilitation for the brain-injured.* Scand J Rehabil Med 8:127, 1976.
13. GOLDSTEIN, K: *The two ways of adjustment of the organism to cerebral defects.* Journal of Mount Sinai Hospital 9:504, 1942.
14. LURIA, AR: *Restoration of Function after Brain Injury.* Pergamon Press, Oxford, 1963.
15. GARRAWAY, WM, ET AL: *Observer variation in the clinical assessment of stroke.* Age Ageing 5:233, 1976.
16. SMITH, ME, ET AL: *Measuring the outcome of stroke rehabilitation.* Occupational Therapy 46(3):51, 1977.

17. SHEIKH, K, ET AL: *Methods and problems of a stroke rehabilitation trial.* Br Med J 41:262, 1978.
18. WEISMANN, MM: *The assessment of social adjustment.* Arch Gen Psychiatry 32:357, 1975.
19. WEISMANN, MM AND SHOLOMSKAS, D: *The assessment of social adjustment by the clinician, the patient and the family.* In BURDOCK, EI, SUDILOVSKY, A, AND GERSHON, S: *The Behavior of Psychiatric Patients.* Marcel Dekker, New York, 1982, p 177.
20. KATZ, MM AND LYERLY, SB: *Methods of measuring adjustment and social behavior in the community: 1. Rationale, description, discriminative validity and scale development.* Psychol Rep 13:503, 1963.

CONCLUSION

J. Douglas Miller, M.D., Ph.D., FRCS Ed., FRCS Glas., FACS

Prompt clinical assessment and diagnostic studies are of the utmost importance in patients suffering from head injury. Urgent management measures must be undertaken as soon as possible after injury so as to provide the best possible milieu for neurologic recovery. As soon as the danger of imminent death recedes and survival seems likely, the attentive clinician should begin to think about rehabilitation, what the different disciplines can offer, what may be achieved, and the time when various rehabilitation measures should begin. This would be the ideal situation in the management of patients with head injury.

This section of the book has been devoted to descriptions of the means by which head-injured patients can be assessed and managed in the early stages and the ways by which an objective evaluation of outcome can be obtained. Through study of the relationship between clinical and laboratory findings and the final outcome, certain factors have been identified in the hours after injury as playing a major role in determining whether the individual patient is more likely to live or die after a head injury. It has proven much more difficult to predict survival with disability at an equally early stage. This is unfortunate because it is precisely the information needed for the early planning of rehabilitation. At the present time, two main factors point to an increase in the expected proportion of disabled survivors—moderate elevations of intracranial pressure (ICP) and the appearance of lesions of increased density on the CT scan lying within the brain parenchyma but insufficiently large to cause brain shift. It is unlikely that the moderately elevated ICP actually produces the disability. Rather, the raised ICP is an index of the widespread damage to the brain and resultant brain swelling. It is to be hoped that by further intensive study of clinical features and by the development of newer techniques based on CT and the measurement of evoked potentials, further and more specific early predictors of disability may be identified. In this way, it is to be hoped that head-injured patients may be directed early toward the most appropriate rehabilitative measures at a time when active postinjury changes are still occurring within the central nervous system at the cellular level. It is known, for example, that axonal sprouting is active in the injured brain in the first 7 days after injury.

It is extremely important to recognize the current problem of assessing outcome objectively and the related difficulty in making valid claims for the superiority of one management regimen over another in head-injured patients. Until this difficulty, which is discussed here, has been overcome, there will continue to be major problems in making comparisons of different modes or timings of rehabilitative measures. There is no reason for us to believe, however, that these difficulties cannot be overcome.

Finally, the management team must be realistic about the rate, extent, and final limits of neurologic recovery that will occur in a patient following head injury. When outcome measures that are acceptable in objective terms are used, most recovery takes place within the first 6 months after injury; after 12 months, little further improvement is likely. If finer outcome measures are used, it may be possible to record smaller improvements in outcome occurring at a later stage, but, of course, one can be much less certain that these are actually present. Knowledge of the presence of any pre-existing brain damage is crucial when counseling relatives of head-injured patients as to the expected outcome and fostering realistic expectations.

Clearly, after injury no person can be better than he or she was before and, to the relatives' knowing eyes, the patient's recovery often falls far short of people's hopes and expectations. Informed counseling is most likely to take place when the rehabilitation team members are involved in patient care and contact with the family occurs at an extremely early stage after injury, while the details of the accident and the pre-injury status of the patient are clear in everybody's mind. It is important for the members of the rehabilitation team to be familiar with the diagnostic measures and management methods that have been employed in their patient and to understand the underlying pathophysiology of head injury and the reasons various measures have to be instituted. The evolution of the patient's recovery must attain certain stages before various assessments and rehabilitative measures are appropriate or even possible. By involvement of the rehabilitation team from the outset, the appropriate measures may be applied at the soonest possible moment. This can only be to the patient's benefit. It is also to the benefit of the members of the acute-care and rehabilitation teams in appreciating, by practical example, the scope, limitations, and achievements that each other can provide.

Section 3

SPECIFIC PROBLEMS RELATED TO HEAD INJURY

Chapter 8

POST-TRAUMATIC EPILEPSY

Bryan Jennett, M.D.

Almost all the disabilities that follow head injury result from the incomplete resolution of deficits that are present soon after injury. Epilepsy is the only complication that can develop months or years after injury and that may lead to considerable handicap in a patient who has otherwise already made a good recovery. But it is much more common after more severe injuries, in patients who are already disabled to some extent in other ways. Only 5 percent of patients admitted to a hospital develop late traumatic epilepsy, but the incidence is more than three times as great in a series of severe injuries (more than 6 hours in coma); among these patients, epilepsy is twice as frequent in those who are severely disabled on the Glasgow Scale.[1]

Any brain will generate a seizure if it is sufficiently stimulated, as with suitable drugs or by an electric current (e.g., in electroconvulsive therapy). Whether or not epilepsy occurs with a lesser stimulus, such as injury, depends on the epileptogenic threshold of that particular individual and on the amount of brain damage. This epilepsy may occur during the first week after injury, in the phase of acutely changing pathophysiologic processes (early epilepsy). Or it may occur months or years after injury, when it is assumed that the scar of the injury is acting as a focus that triggers a seizure in certain circumstances. Some patients have seizures both in the first week and then later as well. In the context of rehabilitation, it is of course late epilepsy that matters; the significance of early epilepsy is that it indicates an increased likelihood that late epilepsy will occur, as will be explained later.

The significance of late epilepsy is that it is liable to persist, although the seizures may be infrequent if anticonvulsant medication is maintained. However, even after a remission of 2 years, it is quite common for seizures to return; this means that once a late seizure has occurred, the risk of recurrence remains. And it is this risk that constitutes the disability, quite apart from the actual embarrassment and, to a lesser extent, the hazard of the seizures themselves. In spite of the greatly lessened social stigma attaching to epilepsy nowadays, it still imposes considerable social restrictions. Many head-injured patients are young, and their career prospects are immediately restricted by epilepsy. The limitation that epilepsy imposes on driving affects the work and leisure activities of many people in westernized society, where mobility increasingly depends on private transport.

FEATURES OF EARLY (FIRST WEEK) EPILEPSY

Early epilepsy occurs most commonly in children under age 5, when it may follow mild injury. In adults, it seldom occurs except in association with depressed fracture, intracranial hematoma, or unconsciousness lasting several hours. In 60 percent of cases, the first (and often the only) seizure occurs within the first 24 hours; in half of these cases, it is within an hour of injury, occurring therefore in the ambulance or in the emergency room. Two thirds of patients have more than one seizure, and about 10 percent have status epilepticus (which is more common in younger children). About 40 percent have a generalized seizure, whereas another 40 percent have seizures that are confined to motor twitching in one area (commonly face or hand), a form of epilepsy rarely seen after the first week.

FEATURES OF LATE EPILEPSY

Epilepsy can take several forms, and many patients have more than one type of attack. There is some focal feature, at least at the onset of the attacks, in about half the sufferers from traumatic epilepsy; in most such cases, the seizures then spread and become generalized. But about half the patients have classic grand mal seizures, without a focal onset, and these are the most disabling of all. They cannot be concealed, nor can avoiding action be taken when they happen in potentially hazardous circumstances.

About one fifth of patients have only temporal lobe attacks; these take various forms, and some are frequently not immediately recognized as being epileptic in nature. The three main types are absences, psychic phenomena, and automatisms. In absences, the flow of speech is broken, the thread of conversation lost, and the patient is for a matter of seconds out of contact, yet only an observant onlooker might notice such an event. Psychic experiences by the patient may have no exterior component; there is a feeling of unexplained fear, of detachment from the surroundings, of deja vu, or of olfactory hallucination. Patients seldom volunteer information about such feelings, anticipating that they might be ridiculed or judged mentally ill; it is necessary, therefore, to ask them directly whether they have had any of these experiences. Automatisms are complex and often correctly executed motor activities, but of a stereotyped nature that makes them purposeless and inappropriate in the circumstances in which they are enacted. Moreover, patients are usually unaware of what they are doing, and are subsequently amnesic for the duration of the seizure. This period is normally only seconds or minutes—time to close a door, cross a room, clap the hands, or utter some stock phrase. Occasionally, it lasts hours, and then patients may carry out a whole series of complex activities that include responding apparently normally to social cues; they may, for example, travel across a city by public transport and then regain full consciousness in a place never visited before. Very occasionally, patients have a series of such episodes lasting several days, with some clear periods in between, and this may account for bizarre behavior that is interpreted as neurotic or even psychotic. There may be a clue to this in the form of epileptic activity in the temporal lobes on the electroencephalogram; but the best test is to give anticonvulsants, which in these circumstances often cause a dramatic improvement in behavior.

More than half the patients who develop late epilepsy have their first seizure within a year after injury, but the risk never quite disappears; more than one fourth begin their epilepsy more than 4 years later, and focal seizures related to depressed fracture have been recorded as starting 40 years after the injury.

PREDICTING LATE EPILEPSY

This potentially disabling complication affects only about 5 percent of all patients admitted to a hospital after head injury. This, and the frequent delay in its appearance, makes it very important to try to identify which patients are at risk, in order to offer advice about work and leisure activities in the future, and to take steps to minimize the risk of epilepsy by

TABLE 8-1. Risk of Late Epilepsy After Certain Injuries

	n	%
Acute intracranial hematoma*	128	35
No hematoma	854	3
After early epilepsy	238	25
No early epilepsy	868	3
Depressed fracture	447	17
No depressed fracture	832	4
In patients with neither hematoma nor depressed fracture:		
After early epilepsy	124	19
No early epilepsy	168	1

From Jennett,[2] with permission.
*Evacuated within 14 days of injury.

prescribing anticonvulsants. It used to be considered very difficult to anticipate which patients would develop epilepsy, but a large-scale study by Jennett[2] has indicated the few factors that do, in fact, influence the epilepsy rate. From a knowledge of these, it is now possible to calculate, soon after injury, the approximate level of risk in individual patients on the basis of various clinical features of the injury and its early course. There are three main factors that increase the likelihood that late epilepsy will develop: an acute intracranial hematoma, epilepsy in the first week after injury (early epilepsy), and a depressed fracture of the skull vault (Table 8-1).

In patients who have had an intracranial hematoma removed within 2 weeks of injury, the risk of epilepsy in the next 4 years is about 35 percent. Epilepsy more often occurs after intradural clots (45 percent) than after extradural hematoma (22 percent).

As for early epilepsy, it was once believed to be of little significance for the future. Actually, three fourths of such patients will not have another seizure, but the one fourth that do have further seizures in the future makes the overall risk of late epilepsy significantly greater than in patients who get through the first week after injury without a seizure. This increased risk applies even when there has been only a single early seizure whenever during the first week early epilepsy began, and whether the early seizures were focal or generalized.

Calculating the probability of late epilepsy after depressed fracture is more complicated. It depends on various combinations of other factors—whether the post-traumatic amnesia (PTA) exceeded 24 hours or not, whether the dura was penetrated, whether there were focal neurologic signs related to the fracture, and whether there was an early seizure. Except for early epilepsy, these are each indicators of the degree of brain damage suffered; it is to be expected that the more of them that occur, the greater the risk of late epilepsy. This risk ranges from less than 3 percent to more than 60 percent, according to various combinations of these factors (Fig. 8-1). Whereas it used to be considered that all depressed fractures were associated with an increased likelihood of epilepsy, it is now possible to reassure some 40 percent of patients that they have little chance of suffering from this delayed complication.

What are the chances that late epilepsy will develop in patients who have none of the predisposing factors? For those with neither a hematoma nor a depressed fracture, the risk is about 5 percent; if they also get through the first week without a seizure, then the risk falls to 1 percent; even if they have PTA of more than 24 hours, the risk is still less than 2 percent. On the other hand, if such patients do have an early seizure, then the risk of late epilepsy is almost 20 percent. It is therefore in this group of patients, in whom the risk of epilepsy is otherwise very low, that the occurrence of an early seizure is of the greatest significance for the future, because it greatly increases the likelihood that late seizures will develop.

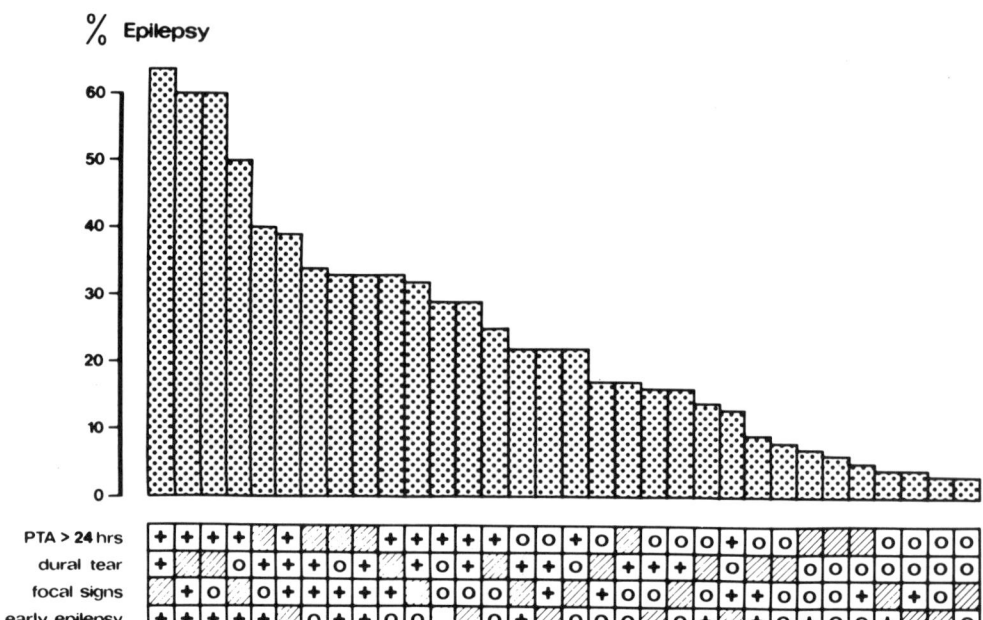

FIGURE 8-1. Late epilepsy after compound depressed fracture (three factors known).

The electroencephalogram (EEG) has proven to be disappointing in predicting the risk of epilepsy after head injury. Although patients with late epilepsy more often have an abnormal EEG than do patients without epilepsy, this abnormality largely reflects the degree of brain damage sustained at the time of injury; and this is already obvious from clinical features such as the occurrence of hematoma, different kinds of depressed fracture, and the duration of PTA. As a predictor, the EEG therefore adds little to what is evident from clinical features. Moreover, this difference is not evident until 2 years after injury, by which time most patients who will develop epilepsy have already had their first seizure (Table 8-2). As a *predictor*, therefore, the EEG adds little to what is evident from clinical features.

PREVENTION OF LATE EPILEPSY

There is no evidence that improved methods of treating head injuries in the acute stage have done anything to reduce the incidence of epilepsy. This is apparent from the incidence

TABLE 8-2. Frequency of Abnormal EEG Records at Varying Intervals After Injury

Time Since Injury	No Late Epilepsy	Late Epilepsy	p
4 mo	76%	83%	NS
4–12 mo	59%	67%	NS
1–2 yr	64%	71%	NS
2 yr	46%	73%	0.001

of epilepsy after head injuries sustained in combat in successive wars; with much more efficient medical care and dramatically reduced infection rates, there has been no difference in the epilepsy rate. Presumably, this is because epilepsy is related to amount of brain damage sustained at the time of impact, and this cannot be influenced by medical intervention.

Therefore, the only course open is the judicious use of prophylactic medication, and it might seem obvious that patients identified as having a high risk of epilepsy should have anticonvulsants. However, a survey of American neurosurgeons revealed that many of them did not attempt to protect their post-traumatic patients, giving as their reasons that they were uncertain which patients were at risk, or else that they believed that the overall risk was too low to justify medication.[3] Now that there are reliable statistics for calculating the risk in individual patients,[2] these excuses are no longer valid. It therefore becomes a matter of deciding what level of risk justifies the prescribing of drugs to a patient who has not yet had a late seizure (or perhaps has not had even an early seizure), and of agreeing what drugs should be used, when they should be started, and how long they should be continued.

Those involved with rehabilitation should help to see that patients on medication take their drugs regularly. Because of the mental changes after head injury, patients may be forgetful about their drugs, and they may also be untruthful when questioned about how carefully they have been maintaining their medication. The commonest reason that anticonvulsants fail to control epilepsy is that they are not being taken, or are not taken in sufficient dosage and regularly. This is why it is essential to measure blood levels at follow-up clinics before deciding that a change of drug is needed because of failure to control seizures. Sometimes the opposite problem arises, of patients (or their relatives) taking too much medication in an effort to control seizures; patients may then develop signs of toxicity that the rehabilitationist should be aware of. Ataxia and nystagmus are the side effects of phenytoin (Dilantin), the drug most commonly used; skin rashes may also occur.

As an early seizure is in any event an untoward complication, particularly in patients who are already suffering from significant brain damage, it is now often recommended that patients likely to have seizures should have anticonvulsants from the time they are first seen soon after injury. This would include all patients with depressed fractures, and those with intracranial hematomas; all those in coma should be treated initially, discontinuing the treatment once it became clear that no predisposing features had developed. This would also apply to many patients with depressed fractures who had been started on treatment before it was known whether there would be sufficient epileptogenic factors to justify continuing drug treatment.

It is certainly easier to insist on adequate treatment, with regular checks on the blood level of anticonvulsants, for 3 months than for a year or more. But in patients in the really high-risk groups (e.g., more than 30 percent), it would seem wise to maintain treatment for at least a year—until there is firmer evidence to support the contention that a briefer spell on drugs is effective.

EPILEPSY AND DRIVING

Most countries have clear regulations that specify the conditions under which patients at risk from epilepsy may or may not drive a car or fly an airplane. Such regulations are always more stringent for heavy goods vehicles and public service vehicles, and for commercial and military aircraft. Such regulations are based on a prescribed interval since the last recorded seizure, and this is commonly 2 years. However, some degree of discretion is allowed in some countries, and the extent and nature of this vary greatly. More controversial is what restrictions apply (or should apply) to patients who are in high-risk categories for developing epilepsy, but who have not so far had any seizures. In Britain, it is suggested that there should be a period of 6 to 12 months before such patients drive, but that still leaves open what level of risk is to be deemed high.[4]

It is clearly important that those responsible for the rehabilitation of patients with brain damage should be aware of the implications of epilepsy for the future, for both private and vocational driving and flying. There is no doubt that restrictions on driving are socially very frustrating in Western society, and that these can pose problems for rehabilitation. But the realities of the situation have to be faced, and it is essential not to set unrealistic goals that involve driving and that then have to be abandoned.

REFERENCES

1. JENNETT, B, ET AL: *Disability after severe head injury: Observations on the use of the Glasgow Outcome Scale.* J Neurol Neurosurg Psychiatry 44:285, 1981.
2. JENNETT, B: *Epilepsy after Non-Missile Head Injuries*, ed 2. Heinemann, London, 1975.
3. RAPPAPORT, RL AND PENRY, JK: *A survey of attitudes towards the pharmacologic prophylaxis of post-traumatic epilepsy.* J Neurosurg 38:159, 1973.
4. *Epilepsy after head trauma and fitness to drive.* Lancet 1:401, 1980.

Chapter 9

SPASTICITY

Ernest R. Griffith, M.D.

Although spasticity has been accorded much attention in scientific literature, there has been very little information specifically relating to spasticity associated with mechanical head trauma. Major differences in mechanisms and clinical manifestations between cerebral and spinal forms of spasticity have been recognized. However, the principal models for these two varieties of spasticity have been cerebrovascular accident and cerebral palsy versus spinal cord injury. It cannot be assumed that the mechanisms and clinical manifestations of spasticity are identical in cerebrovascular accident, cerebral palsy, and head trauma. I shall attempt, wherever possible, to point out the features of spasticity associated with head trauma that make its evaluation and management distinctive. At the same time, I will identify the similarities among these several types of spasticity related to brain or brain stem lesions, noting the implications of management techniques that have application regardless of the nature of the lesion.

The term spasticity has been variously defined. As a reference point for this chapter, the following definition and qualifying description are presented: Spasticity is a state of hypertonicity of striated muscle as manifested by increased resistance to passive stretch due to increased responses of static and often phasic stretch reflexes.[1] A principal characteristic of the reflex contraction is the so-called "clasp-knife" phenomenon, wherein the early and mid-period of stretch produces relatively greater contraction, whereas the later and terminal periods of stretch are associated with relaxation. Phasic stretch reflexes, as exemplified by increased deep tendon reflexes, are usually but not always increased in spasticity states. For example, hyperreflexia may be dampened by the coexisting presence of cerebellar lesions. When hyperreflexia is present, not only is there an increased response of the tendon reflex, but it appears at a lower stimulus threshold. Often, there is a radiating effect of reflex contraction of neighboring muscles. Clonus characteristically appears with spasticity but is not an invariable component. Spasticity should be distinguished from rigidity states of basal ganglion lesions and rigidity of abnormal posturings such as decerebrate or decorticate rigidity. Rigidity associated with basal ganglion disorders is exemplified by parkinsonian rigidity and dystonia. The hypertonicity of parkinsonian rigidity is characterized by increased resistance to passive stretch, which is either constant throughout the entire range of movement (so-called "lead-pipe" rigidity) or intermittent and rhythmic relaxation of the reflex contraction throughout the range of movement ("cogwheel" rigidity). Dystonia is a form of hypertonicity that occurs in association with sustained twisting movements or postures of the face, torso, and limbs. Decorticate and decerebrate rigidity are forms of hypertonicity in which characteristic postures accompanied by increased resistance to movement occur. In mechanical head-trauma lesions, these posturings may be mixed or may alternate from one form to the other in the same patient. Therefore, they might better be called abnormal posturings. Classic decorticate posturing is characterized by a flexion attitude of the upper limb with an extension attitude of the lower limb. Classic decerebrate rigidity is identified as an abnormal extensor tonus of the elbows and lower limbs. These rigidity states are not necessarily associated with hyperreflexia, and never produce clonus or the clasp-knife phenomenon unless spasticity is also present. Unlike spasticity, rigidity states do not produce increasing resistance that is directly related to the velocity of passive movement of the affected limb. It is critical that spasticity be differentiated from rigidity, states of failure of relaxation of voluntary contractions, and contractures since the management of each of these various disorders is quite distinctive.

ETIOLOGY AND PATHOPHYSIOLOGY OF SPASTICITY

Normal striated muscle "tonus" refers to the tension perceived as its resistance to passive stretch of the muscle-tendon complex. The basis for this tension is three sets of factors: the elastic properties of connective tissue within and surrounding the muscle as well as its tendon, the viscoelastic properties of the fibrillary proteins of each component muscle fiber with the muscles, and the active contraction force of the muscle secondary to either reflex or voluntary motor unit activity throughout the muscle.[2] The heightened tone of spastic muscle, then, is the result of an abnormal increase in reflex motor unit activity causing active contraction of the muscle. Any neurologic condition that alters the upper motor neuron pathways that directly or indirectly facilitate or inhibit alpha motor neuron activity may produce spasticity.

Multiple descending motor pathways project to the spinal cord so as to influence one or both motor neuron systems in the ventral horn (Fig. 9-1).[1] The major facilitatory pathways include direct tracts such as vestibulospinal and rubrospinal and indirect connections via the lateral reticulospinal tract. Inhibitory or suppressor pathways are indirectly projected to the cord via the medial reticular formations. Origins of these suppressor pathways include nuclei of the cerebellum basal ganglia and premotor cortex. Inhibition of alpha motor neurons may be direct or synaptic, presynaptic via stimulation of inhibiting internuncials or inhibition of stimulating internuncials, or postsynaptic by means of Renshaw cells that produce recurrent inhibition. Most corticospinal tract fibers project indirectly to the cord via either facilitatory or inhibitory interneurons. Less than 2 percent of corticospinal fibers directly terminate on alpha motor neurons as facilitatory pathways.[2] These independent parallel descending pathways

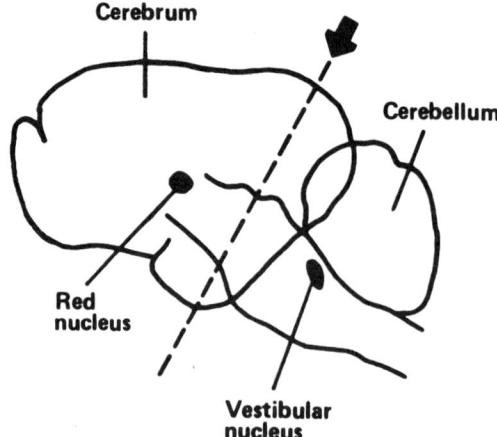

FIGURE 9-1. Facilitatory (+) and suppressor (−) areas of the brain. (From Bishop,[1] with permission.)

normally produce constantly varying activity in the alpha and gamma motor neurons in such a balance as to result in smooth, coordinated voluntary movement. Under these circumstances, gamma motor neuron activity produces varying degrees of contraction of intrafusal muscle fibers so as to render muscle spindle receptors more sensitive to stretch.

There are two types of gamma neurons: those mediating contraction of the nuclear bag fibers, which govern responsivity to the velocity of stretch; and those mediating contractions of nuclear chain fibers, which govern responsivity to the length of stretch (Fig 9-2).[3] The primary receptors emanate from both nuclear bag and chain fibers and thus respond to both velocity and length of stretch. The secondary receptors emanate mainly from nuclear chain fibers and are responsive only to length of stretch. The pathways of the primary afferents are monosynaptic to adjacent alpha motor neurons innervating the same muscle and its synergists. Long polysynaptic pathways synapse with motor neurons innervating antagonists of the primary muscle and with motor neurons of both synergists and antagonists on the opposite side with a reversal of the facilitation-inhibition relationship. The secondary axons are uniformly polysynaptic, connecting with motor neurons of synergists segmentally and intersegmentally,

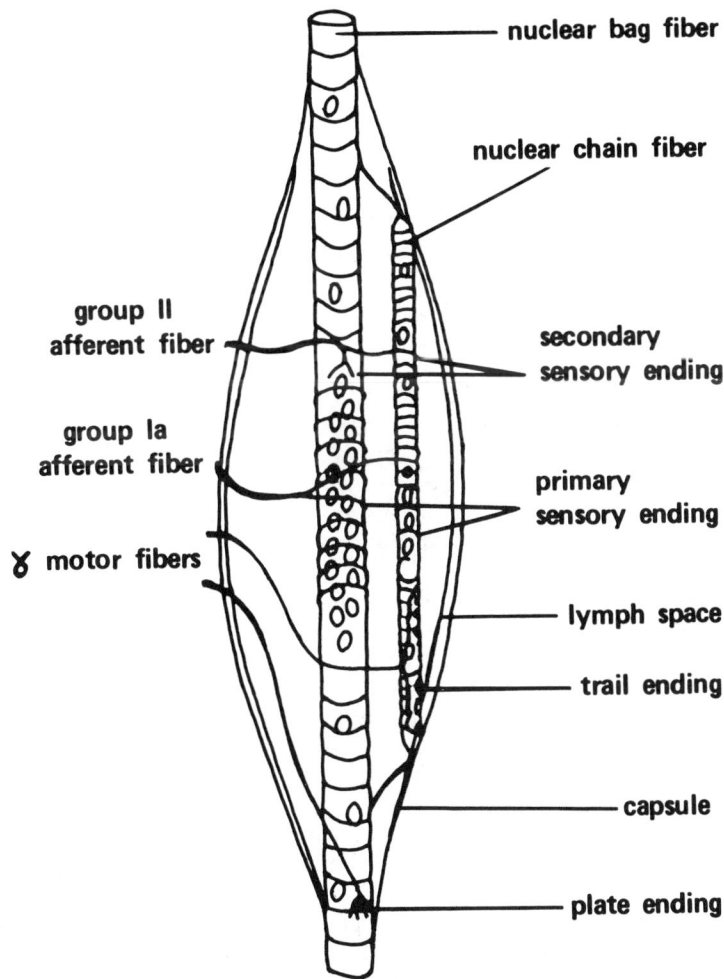

FIGURE 9-2. Diagram of muscle spindle (simplified). (From Bishop,[3] with permission.)

providing ascending axons to the reticular gray and thereby synapsing with gamma motor neurons. Thus the alpha motor neuron is influenced by two sensory systems emanating from the muscle spindle, one of which is sensitive to both velocity and length of stretch and the other which is sensitive strictly to length. The length-related component of the stretch is termed static or tonic, and the velocity-related component is termed dynamic or phasic. It is now seen that each of the two components of stretch is governed by two types of gamma motor neurons and two types of nuclear fibers. Three fourths of all gamma motor neurons are of the static type. It has become evident that different regions of the brain exert independent control over static and dynamic gamma motor neurons, hence controlling the stretch and velocity sensitivity of the spindle receptors.

In addition to this gamma feedback system to the alpha motor neuron, there are other major sensory influences at all levels of the central nervous system. Connections between sensory and motor cortex as well as afferent input to the lateral reticular formation involve most of the sensory systems. At the spinal cord level, the connections from exteroceptive and enteroceptive afferents to alpha motor neurons, usually by interneuronal connections, are well known. Cutaneous afferents that influence gamma motor neurons are the so-called gamma skin afferents. The receptors, apparently sensitive to pressure, appear to be especially populous near muscles and tendons. Their axons synapse with internuncial neurons that ascend to the reticular gray, thereby acting upon the gamma motor neurons.

Theoretically then, spasticity could be produced by any disorder that would result in an excessive stimulation of the alpha neurons. Disruption of the balancing influences of descending inhibitory and facilitatory tracts can be produced by either a destruction of inhibitory pathways or excessive irritation of facilitative pathways. These changes could occur in pathways that directly affect the alpha motor neurons, pathways that impinge on the gamma motor neurons, or a combination thereof. Other potential mechanisms of spasticity are conditions that have their direct effect on the internuncial systems that play upon alpha motor neurons or gamma motor neurons or both. Similarly, factors that cause direct stimulation of the motor neurons themselves could cause spasticity. Finally, an inappropriate and overwhelming overload of one or more of the sensory inputs might be a major determining factor if there were already some pre-existing lesion of the upper motor neuron systems.

Practically speaking, the commonest type of spasticity is that mediated by hyperactivity of the gamma motor neurons due to disinhibition, resulting from a destructive lesion or lesions involving one or more of the suppressive pathways.[1] Bishop[4] offers evidence to support the contention that dynamic gamma neurons are the more likely primary site of excitatory excesses. It has been postulated that the rigidity of parkinsonism is secondary to hyperexcitation of the static gamma motor neurons.[5]

Apparently, in widespread cerebral or brain stem lesions such as occur in mechanical head trauma, the lesions involve descending pathways that result in hyperactivity of both gamma and alpha motor neurons in a variable mix, depending on the segments of the cord under study.[6] Hence, a mixed type of spasticity results, with some muscles having characteristics of "gamma" spasticity and others the characteristics of "alpha" spasticity. Gamma spasticity has been defined as any spasticity decreased or stopped by interruption of the gamma spindle loop. Alpha spasticity has been defined as spasticity that is not decreased or stopped by interruption of the gamma spindle loop. These two types of spasticity are differentiated clinically by the application of cold to skin overlying affected muscles. In gamma spasticity, there is reduction of the degree of spasticity, whereas the alpha spasticity is either unaffected or enhanced by the application.

According to Wyke,[2] the only common type of spasticity due to primary hyperexcitability of alpha motor neurons is that produced by augmented nociceptive inputs, especially from painful muscles and joints or from viscera, resulting in enhanced spasticity in related (mainly flexor) musculature. Spastic states occurring in patients with tetanus infection and strychnine poisoning are due to alpha motor neuron hyperexcitability resulting from an antagonism of the inhibitory action of Renshaw cells that is normally exerted on these neurons. There appear to be examples of alpha spasticity associated with lesions selectively involving inhibitory descending pathways that predominantly synapse directly with alpha motor neurons.[3] We believe that pure alpha spasticity is a rare finding in mechanical head trauma. Our knowledge remains incomplete concerning these and other potential mechanisms of spasticity. Hence, the precision and efficacy of modern management leave much to be desired.

CLINICAL PICTURE

The salient signs of spasticity have been described in large part in the introductory remarks on definition and description of spasticity. The chief characteristic of the state is the clasp-knife response to passive stretch. Furthermore, the resistance to stretch is enhanced by increasing the velocity of stretch. Ordinarily, there is a threshold of velocity below which increased resistance is not apparent. In addition, tendon reflexes are usually enhanced and have lowered threshold. Often, muscles other than the one tapped respond. Clonus may be induced as part of the stretch reflex.

Some major points of differentiation may be made in contrasting cerebral and spinal cord forms of spasticity. Cerebral spasticity frequently is combined with other abnormal motor manifestations. In head trauma, rigidity states, ataxia, or both are often coexistent and may modify spasticity greatly. In the cerebrovascular accident hemiplegic, the usual distribution of spasticity adheres to the classic decorticate model of enhanced hypertonicity in antigravity muscles. Thus, the upper extremity musculature is positioned in a flexion attitude, accompanied by adduction and internal rotation at the shoulder and pronation of the forearm. The lower extremity is held in an extension pattern, accompanied by internal rotation and adduction of the hip, and equinovarus of the foot. Harris[7] has pointed out the interesting exception to the extension pattern of the lower extremity in the cerebral palsy patient. He notes a consistent attitude of knee flexion as contrasted to the knee extension of the stroke hemiplegic patient. My experience has been that the head-injured patient with this decorticate pattern adheres more closely to the stroke than the cerebral palsy model. Cerebral spasticity tends to be less violent than spinal cord spasticity, more regular, and more heavily influenced by such factors as postural changes, body positioning, and labyrinthine and tonic neck reflexes. Herman[8] has alluded to the spasticity of head trauma leading to contractures of antigravity muscles, which in turn decrease the manifestations of spasticity. The distribution of this type of spasticity is often more pronounced distally than proximally. Cerebral spasticity often partially or totally masks voluntary movement. When present, movements often occur as stereotyped, total or partial synergistic patterns associated with co-contractions of antagonist muscles. These patterns render the individual unable to produce selected isolated movements of limb or body segments. Spastic patterns may be related to primitive mass extension thrusts or flexion withdrawal reflexes. Association responses may be seen as a mirroring effect wherein voluntary contraction of the unaffected side is accompanied by similar movement of the spastic side. Where isolated movement is present, it is slow, stiff, and incoordinate. On maximal voluntary effort, the movement is often paradoxically opposite to that intended. Voluntary movement produces co-contraction due to stretch reflexes in antagonist muscles, then clasp-knife relaxation of antagonists and further exaggerated active motion in the same direction. Harris[7] has pointed to this common pattern of alternating extremes between flexion and extension synergies with poor voluntary control of movement between these extremes. Although his description was based on observations of individuals with spastic forms of cerebral palsy, the same phenomenon is observable in other forms of spasticity.

Spinal cord forms of spasticity are often more generalized patterns of either flexion or flexion-extension, with flexion often predominant in the latter pattern. Spinal forms of spasticity are frequently much more violent, associated with severe episodic muscle spasms, and often accompanied by crossed extensor and long spinal reflexes. Co-contraction does not occur with spinal level spasticity unless overwhelming sensory or suprasegmental inputs are present. Its course tends to be longer in duration, often intensified rather than improved by partial voluntary control, and as we shall see, it responds somewhat differently to antispasmodic drugs.

Wyke[2] has further differentiated several clinical types of spasticity. He describes an *immobility type* in which the affected muscles display the greatest evidence of spasticity in the absence of attempted movement. Examples of immobility spasticity include paraplegia associated with spinal cord lesions and hemiplegia due to cerebrovascular accidents. A *mobile type* of spasticity is enhanced on attempted movement of the affected part. Examples of this type include destructive lesions of the anterior cerebellum, cerebral palsy, and multiple sclerosis. A third form is characterized by *inability to relax* after performing a voluntary movement. This form may be seen in infantile cerebral palsy and various frontal lobe lesions including trauma. The spasticity of head trauma frequently combines the features of the immobile and mobile forms and may additionally demonstrate characteristics of the postmovement form.

Many influences affect spasticity of all types. Inciting factors include changes in external temperature, emotional stress, presence of infection, urinary calculi, heterotopic ossification, decubitus ulcers, fecal impactions, urinary tract obstruction, and trauma. Excessive sensory inputs of any or all modalities may enhance spasticity. Relaxation may result from muscle fatigue and drugs such as alcohol, sedatives, marijuana, and tranquilizers. Diurnal variations may cause wide fluctuations in the severity of spasticity.

Spasticity may be accompanied by disagreeable sensations of tightness, cramping, pain, sleeplessness, progressive contractures, subluxations and dislocations, postural deformities, trauma to self or others, damage to personal belongings and property, decubitus ulcers, triggering of fecal or urinary incontinence, and interference with postsurgical healing. The functional consequences of spasticity may include decrease or loss of balance, decreased mobility skills, interference with communications and vegetative functions, unacceptable cosmesis, decrease or loss of ADL skills, and interference with physical and occupational therapies. However, spasticity may have useful effects such as maintaining muscle bulk, decreasing the severity of osteoporosis, possible prevention of phlebothrombosis, decreasing stasis edema, and increasing the stability of standing, walking, and transfers.

EVALUATION OF SPASTICITY

The nature and the great degree of variability of the clinical manifestations of spasticity have made standardized measurements an elusive objective that has not fully been realized. The conventional neurologic examination provides a gross scoring system for deep tendon reflexes, differentiation between unsustained and sustained clonus, and a description of the degree of resistance to passive motion. A more detailed look at mobility functions entails an assessment of the effect of spasticity on posture, balance, transfer skills, ambulation, and other forms of movement. Goff[9] and Evans and colleagues[10] have described quantitative scoring systems of grading the effect of spasticity on patterns of movement. The grading system described by Goff relates spasticity to the degree of voluntary movement and degree of synergy of movement patterns in six categories, ranging from absence of voluntary movement to normal voluntary movement. Evans described a similar system of scoring of six categories, ranging from a total synergy pattern of either flexion or extension to normal voluntary movement. Movements of the four extremities are observed in the supine, prone, sitting, and standing positions. More indirect quantitative measures of the effect of spasticity on mobility may be obtained by the use of timed mobility tests, as described by Jebsen and colleagues,[11] or by other systems of scoring mobility in terms of degree of dependence.[12-14] Similarly, the quantitative scoring of ADL skills such as bathing, grooming, hygiene, and eating may be scored by any one of a number of systems that have been described and standardized.[12-15] Communication skills and swallowing function as well as positioning and seating capabilities must be included in these ADL evaluations when spasticity is under question. The problem with any of these functional measures is that they only indirectly measure the effect of spasticity, and many other variables may also be responsible for any of the specific dysfunctions. Nevertheless, they are essential for obtaining baselines and in following the efficacy of management of spasticity. The effect of local cold application on spasticity has already been mentioned as a method of determining alpha versus gamma type of spasticity. This is not an idle academic exercise, since gamma spasticity will more likely respond to systemic antispasmodic drugs as well as therapeutic application of local cold.[16] Careful clinical observation of the effect of various body and head positions and movements, such as elicitation of tonic and kinetic labyrinthine reflexes, symmetric and asymmetric tonic neck reflexes, and supporting reactions, has useful application in selecting specific management techniques. The modality of muscle vibration normally suppresses deep tendon and H reflexes.[4] In milder forms of spasticity, suppression may occur. However, in more severe forms, vibration has little or no effect upon these reflexes. The assessment of spasticity versus contracture is facilitated by use of either local or general anesthesia. Diagnostic peripheral nerve blocks using short- or long-acting local anesthetic agents will demonstrate the functional effect of ablation of focal spasticity. As indicated previously, spasticity may serve to maintain vital functional skills; therefore, the clinical assessment must include a determination of the contribution of spasticity to those skills. Transient ablation of the spasticity is an effective means of this determination. Some of the deleterious effects of spasticity are most readily identified by careful history taking. Discussions of mobility and self-care skills, sexual function, perineal hygiene, pain, and cosmetic effect are of critical importance. Finally, a musculoskeletal examination must be performed to determine the presence of contractures, dislocations, and progressive deformities.

A number of laboratory methods have been developed in an attempt to further evaluate spasticity.[4-6,17,18] Among these are simultaneous recordings of muscle contraction and the electromyographic response of a measured mechanical blow to the tendon or to the passive stretch of the muscle, controlled in speed, angle or extent of joint movement, and degree of force applied. The range of pendulousness associated with the deep tendon reflex response has been measured in terms of the degree and number of swings. Mechanical and electromyogram (EMG) responses of the muscle to electric stimulation of itself, its peripheral nerve, or skin afferents accompanying its peripheral nerve have been described. H reflexes and F responses[19] have been a source of considerable interest. Mechanical and EMG responses to mechanical nociceptive stimuli to skin are described. Micturition reflexes include electromyographic measurement of the external urethral sphincter or anal sphincter while detrusor contraction is simultaneously being recorded. Electromyographic responses of the muscle spindle afferent fibers in peripheral nerves are recorded during twitch concontractions stimulated electrically or mechanically. Most of these techniques have been used for research purposes; however, several have clinical application. Surface electromyography is readily performed as an adjunct in studying the effect of various factors on both spasticity and voluntary control. An example of its use is as a preliminary to electromyographic feedback. Micturition studies are of great value in patients with spinal cord injuries and deserve more extensive use in those head-injured patients who have clinical problems such as urgency, frequency, and incontinence.

MANAGEMENT

The presence of spasticity is not an indication for treatment per se. Certainly, many patients with mechanical head trauma who have spasticity do not require treatment. A thorough clinical evaluation should reveal whether sufficient indications exist for one or more methods of management. The major indicators are listed in Table 9-1. In considering indications for treatment, one must simultaneously regard what useful effects of spasticity will be interrupted by its treatment. These effects must not outweigh the primary beneficial effects of any procedure. Furthermore, the side effects of all forms of management must be carefully considered since they may, at times, negate the beneficial effects. The primary modalities of treatment are outlined in Table 9-2.

No matter what eventual combinations of therapy will be necessary to control spasticity, an educational program is a reasonable starting point. Early in the course of spasticity, the family rather than the patient may be the chief beneficiary of the educational program. Basic information as to the mechanism and expected course of spasticity, along with a review of factors that incite or alleviate spasticity, will allow the patient and family to fully participate in the regimen eventually selected, as well as to learn preventive techniques. Their appreciation of the role of anxiety, ability to assist in both physical and emotional relaxation, and reassurance based on adequate information are constructive elements of this program.

Not uncommonly as motor recovery proceeds, early rigidity and spasticity abate to the point where no further specific measures are required. Elimination or substitution of less noxious forms of inciting stimuli such as restraints, extraneous noise, tracheostomy tube, catheter, and nasogastric feeding tube abets this process. Ordinarily, several or more of the physical modalities should be assayed before consideration of antispasmodic drugs. A physical or occupational therapist is in a position to make critical observations as to the efficacy of a number of these techniques.

Routinely, spasticity that is resistant to therapeutic exercise should be tested as to its response to local cold. Ice massage, ice water immersion, or application of cold packs for 20 to 30 minutes directly overlying the affected musculature will provide information as to whether this modality will successfully relax muscle. Furthermore, spasticity that is reduced by cold will very likely respond better to both baclofen and diazepam than will cold-resistant spasticity. Relaxation of spastic musculature may persist for several hours, thus allowing other therapeutic activities to be facilitated. The relaxation is mediated via skin afferents before actual cooling of the muscle occurs.[20] Experimentally, cooling has the effect of decreasing or blocking nerve conduction, delaying transmission at the myoneural junction, increasing the duration of muscle contraction, and decreasing muscle spindle excitability. In cases of alpha spasticity, cooling may actually increase spasticity, a mixed effect of relaxation of some muscles, and either no relaxation or an enhancement of spasticity may occur in others.[19] Local heat may temporarily relax spastic muscle as a preliminary to other physical measures.

TABLE 9-1. Indications for Treatment of Spasticity

1. Improvement of voluntary motor control
2. Improvement of positioning and body stability
3. Improvement of balance and mobility spectrum of functions
4. Improvement of self-care spectrum of functions
5. Improvement of communication and swallowing functions
6. Prevention of contractures and deformities
7. Control of pain associated with spasticity
9. Facilitation of surgical procedures, particularly orthopedic procedures to correct contractures and deformities
10. Facilitation of nursing care such as perineal hygiene
11. Facilitation of therapeutic activities such as stretching, neuromuscular re-education, splinting, etc.
12. Improvement of cosmesis and body image

TABLE 9-2. Modalities of Management of Spasticity

A. Educational methods
  1. Avoidance of inciting factors
  2. General information about disorder
  3. Relaxation techniques
B. Physical modalities
  1. Cold
  2. Stretching techniques
     a. Manual
     b. Static
     c. Splints
     d. Casts
     e. Braces
  3. Positioning techniques
  4. Electrical stimulation
  5. Vibration
  6. Relaxation techniques
  7. Motor re-education techniques
C. Antispasticity drugs
  1. Diazepam
  2. Baclofen
  3. Dantrolene sodium
  4. Others
D. Chemical neurolysis
  1. Intramuscular
  2. Peripheral nerve
E. Surgical procedures
  1. Orthopedic
     a. Myotomy
     b. Myoplasty
     c. Tenotomy
     d. Tenoplasty
  2. Neurosurgical
     a. Peripheral neurotomies
     b. Implantation of peripheral nerve electric stimulators
     c. Dorsal cord electric stimulation
     d. Cerebellar electric stimulation
     e. Spinal cord procedures
        1. Posterior rhizotomy
        2. Anterior rhizotomy
        3. Radio-frequency anterior rhizotomy
        4. Cordotomy—Bischoff procedure and its modifications

Stretching techniques have been unnecessarily maligned as enhancing spasticity. Much of the basis for the avoidance of stretch procedures is their incorrect technique of application. Manual stretch may not produce increased spasticity if it is applied very gently and slowly so as not to exceed the threshold of velocity of movement that usually obtains. This type of stretch is not only necessary to maintain range of motion, but it often produces relaxation so as to facilitate therapeutic activities that immediately follow. Static stretching techniques using directly applied weights or force provided by pulley systems may be indicated for management of contractures as well as spasticity.[21] The effect of these methods must be individually evaluated to decide whether the post-stretch effect is one of relaxation or enhancement of tone.

Examples of lower extremity splints include spreader bars for the purpose of maintaining the thighs in abduction, posterior splints to maintain the ankle and foot in a neutral position with the most common positional abnormality being equinovarus, and knee-ankle-foot splints to maintain the knee in extension and the foot in neutral position for the occasional patient whose hamstring spasticity is predominant. Lower extremity splints may be made from plaster of Paris or molded plastic materials, or may be commercially available as air splints. In my experience, the more severely spastic limbs are not adequately held by such splints. In unresponsive or uncooperative patients, pressure areas rapidly develop and the devices are hard to maintain in proper position.

Snook[22] has described a spasticity reduction splint for the upper extremity, using the Bobath principle of maintaining a position that tends to reduce spasticity. This splint is applied dorsally in order to avoid palmar contact, which might elicit further spasticity. The usual position of the hand is in 30 degrees of wrist extension, with 45 degrees in metacarpal-phalangeal flexion, full interphalangeal extension, finger abduction, and thumb midway between abduction and extension. Based on very limited experience with this splint, I feel that it has merit in cases of mild to moderate spasticity of the upper limb, but in more severe cases of spasticity, the splint may provide more problems than benefits. Air splints may be useful in positioning the hand, wrist, or elbow with less severe degrees of spasticity.

The serial application of cylindric plaster-of-Paris casts for upper or lower extremities has been a source of recent interest at several centers treating head-injured patients. My own experience of lower extremity casting, primarily for control of equinovarus of the foot, is similar to that of Rancho Los Amigos Hospital. I believe that early short leg serial casting prevents severe ankle contractures and deformities. I change the cast every 7 to 10 days depending on the severity of the spasticity or rigidity and the improvement in range of motion. With contractures that have developed in the first 1 to 2 months after head injury, it is often possible to regain fully the lost range of motion. I see fewer skin problems with casting than I previously have with splinting procedures. A variation of the serial cast is the so-called dropout cast, which may be used to prevent movement in one direction while allowing it in the opposite direction.[23] This type of cast has been used in the management of knee and elbow contractures so as to allow passive or active movement of the limb, thereby decreasing the contracture. Unless the spasticity accompanying these contractures is concurrently managed, it may be enhanced, especially if there are skin complications.

Ankle-foot orthoses may be used for management of spasticity, particularly in an attempt to further control the foot position for weight bearing and ambulation. Severe spasticity may prove resistant to this form of management, causing breakdown of the sole of the shoe, escape of the heel from the shoe, curling of the toes in hyperflexion, exaggeration of ankle clonus, and so forth. Thus, these exaggerations of spasticity may require adjunctive treatment measures. However, at times, spasticity may be reduced by the proper positioning of the lower extremity in the brace. Less frequently, lower extremity bracing may be used to maintain knee flexion, hip extension, hip abduction, and hip external rotation. Long leg bracing has been rarely used for the control of spasticity alone in our experience. I have relegated its use primarily to postsurgical periods to maintain positioning after orthopedic procedures for corrections and contractures.

The effect of various positions on spasticity should be routinely assessed by therapists managing head-trauma patients. All assumptions about the effects of posture must be tested in each individual case. Steiskal,[24] in a study that included 20 subjects with cerebral type spasticity, demonstrated that the expected responses of the postural labyrinthine reflex did not usually occur. When prone, his subjects generally demonstrated increased activity of extensor limb muscles, whereas in the supine position, they displayed increased activity of flexors. These results, contrary to what would be expected in the case of tonic labyrinthine reflexes, were felt to be due to tonic stretch and exteroceptive reflexes. Steiskal's study included observations of the symmetric and asymmetric tonic neck reflex (TNR). The symmetric TNR usually demonstrated the expected response of increased upper limb extensor activity on neck extension, and increased upper limb flexor activity of neck flexion. The expected asymmetric TNR response appeared to be overcome by the effect of major deviation of the head and eyes in optic targeting. Most importantly, Steiskal applied these principles in subsequent motor re-education techniques and was strongly persuaded that facilitation or inhibition of flexors or extensors as well as inhibition of the asymmetric tonic neck reflex were of value in facilitating patients' voluntary motor control. Similarly, effects of various sitting, kneeling, and standing positions with head in midline and turned to each side may reveal valuable information with regard to control of spasticity and the unleashing of existing but masked voluntary movement. The principles of comfort, relaxation, adequate support, and proper alignment deserve equal attention. Close heed must be paid to the effect of the degree of the flexion and extension of each of the major limb segments in these various positions. A few further degrees of hip flexion may make the difference in comfortable sitting versus exaggerated back and hip extension that result in the patient sliding down and out of the chair. Adequate cervical support may require an orthosis. A forearm trough may provide added stabilization as an adaption to the arm rests of the chair. Other patients may benefit from upper limb slings as support and facilitators of voluntary control. A wedge cushion may provide the critical degree of hip flexion. Lower extremities may require stabilization with one or more types of strapping plus a thigh spreader bar. Methods of trunk support such as molded plastic vests incorporated to the chair might occasionally be called for. In ambulation, one should assess the effect of positioning the spastic upper extremity in extension and abduction at the shoulder plus extension of the elbow and wrist. This position may have a significant effect in decreasing flexor spasms during ambulation.[16]

Electric stimulation of spastic muscle may result in reduced spasticity that lasts for periods of up to several hours. Several possible mechanisms have been offered to explain this effect.[25] Stimulation might result in contraction of extrafusal fibers without contraction in the intrafusal fibers. Consequently, the spindles would be unloaded at the same time that the Golgi tendon organs were activated. Strong contractions of the muscle may produce a fatiguing effect which is similar to that occurring at the maximal voluntary contraction, thus producing relaxation of spasticity. If electric stimulation is found to be effective and of practical benefit, the patient may be equipped with a portable electric muscle stimulator to be used prior to therapeutic exercises.

Muscle vibration may occasionally have the effect of reducing mild to moderate degrees spasticity. More often, vibration is used as a method of neuromuscular facilitation but may be contraindicated if it enhances spasticity. At times, this or other methods of facilitation are used to stimulate contraction of antagonists of spastic muscles, thereby inducing reciprocal inhibition of spastic muscles.[26]

Relaxation techniques are frequently used concomitantly with motor re-education techniques. However, they may be effective alone or in conjunction with other modalities. Nonspecific relaxation methods not involving reflex inhibition principles may be taught the family as well as the patient by a clinical psychologist. The patients and their families may also learn local techniques such as "shaking-out" (i.e., passive shaking of affected limb so as to alternately stretch agonist and antagonist muscles) of the spastic extremity.

Motor re-education techniques are directed toward two major objectives: to enhance precise movement control and to improve coordination. When these objectives are attained, spasticity often abates. A number of systems of neuromuscular facilitation have been employed for these purposes.[27–30] Their efficacy remains controversial because of the lack of controlled studies as well as the doctrinaire attitudes held by some of their advocates. Several of these techniques, for example, the Bobath method, stress the use of postures that inhibit spasticity as starting points for attempting voluntary movements. The Kabat-Knott method of proprioceptive neuromuscular facilitation includes relaxation techniques. All these methods stress the assiduous control of various sensory inputs having the potential to modify internuncial activity, which plays upon either gamma or alpha neurons. Harris[31] has appropriated techniques from most of these systems in a unifying eclectic approach to neuromuscular education, as exemplified in the care of cerebral palsy patients. He describes a training program that is initiated by a period of gentle, slow, prolonged stretch in order to relax spasticity. He proceeds then to move the involved part to an active assisted movement, which is facilitated by a number of sensory inputs and verbal cues regarding the positioning so that the subject can feel movement. Then voluntary effort is attempted against resistance of a functional nature such as occurs when playing games or in performing activities of daily living. Activities proceed to independent exercises, standing, weight shifting, and progressive ambulation. Throughout this motor retraining, abrupt extremes of phasic movement are eliminated. Alternate desired motor behaviors are progressively shaped with gradual correction. This and other similar models have been the basis for management of motoric difficulties in head-injured patients with or without significant spasticity problems. We are impressed that as these motor skills return, the spasticity frequently abates. As mentioned previously, electric stimulation and vibration may be among the sensory inputs that are used as part of muscle re-education. Biofeedback in the form of electromyography[17] or joint position[32] have also shown promise in cerebral forms of spasticity. Topical electromyography has been used to both facilitate voluntary activity and relax spasticity.

The three systemic antispasticity agents now in greatest use are diazepam, baclofen, and dantrolene sodium. Diazepam (Valium) is believed to exert its action in three sites: It appears to inhibit the contraction mechanism of skeletal muscle in a manner similar to that of dantrolene sodium.[33] It enhances inhibitions mediated at the spinal cord and brain stem levels by enhancing gamma-aminobutyric acid (GABA) ergic presynaptic inhibition at the interneuron level.[34] In this respect, it acts very similarly to baclofen. At a third site of action, it depresses the reticular activation system.[26] The major side effects of the drug include drowsiness, dizziness, ataxia, muscle weakness, and habituation. The sedation effect may be accompanied by increased respiratory depression, hypotension, difficulties in handling secretions, and dysphagia. Abrupt withdrawal of the drug may severely intensify spasticity. Management of associated seizures may be complicated by the use of the drug. Diazepam, like baclofen, has proven to be more efficacious in spasticity due to brain stem or spinal cord injury.[35] However, it is occasionally quite beneficial, particularly where the sedating effect is desirable, as in some agitated patients. In adults, the usual starting dose, 2.5 mg once or twice a day, is cautiously advanced according to its primary and secondary effects.

Baclofen (Lioresal), a derivative of the neurotransmitter GABA, has as its primary site of action the same spinal cord and brain stem sites as does diazepam.[34] It often causes sedation, although generally less marked than that produced by diazepam. Other major side effects include anorexia, nausea and vomiting, constipation, dizziness, rebound intensification of spasticity, hallucinations on withdrawal, and dysphagia. Like diazepam, baclofen is predictably more effective in cold-responsive gamma type spasticity. The drug is particularly effective for flexor spasms seen with spinal cord types of spasticity.[5] The suppressant effect of baclofen on passive stretch reflex is largely extinguished by voluntary effort.[35] The drug proves more efficacious for spasms that impede voluntary effort. Despite the reluctance of its manufacturer to advertise its use for cerebral forms of spasticity, I have found it to be occasionally of benefit alone or in combination with dantrolene sodium. The usual starting dose for adults is 5 mg three times daily, with gradual increases in dosage every 3 to 4 days. Although the manufacturer's instructions indicate the upper level to be at 80 mg per day in four divided doses, there are reports of higher doses being used.[37]

Dantrolene sodium (Dantrium) has its main site of action in striated muscle, where it probably facilitates release of calcium from the sarcoplasmic reticulum, resulting in blocking of the excitation-contraction mechanism within the muscle fiber.[38] The most prominent side effects include drowsiness, general muscle weakness, liver toxicity, gastrointestinal complaints, and potentially, respiratory depression and dysphagia. Long-term use of the drug occasionally produces facial acne. Its propensity to photic sensitivity may enhance the effects of exposure to sunlight. Because of rare fatalities due to liver disease, routine hepatic function studies are necessary when using this drug. It is contraindicated in liver disease or dysfunction. Unlike the first two drugs, dantrolene sodium appears to be more effective in alpha types of spasticity.[6] I find it most useful in combination with one of the other two drugs in head-trauma patients so as to allow the lowest possible doses of each drug and the benefit of their additive (not synergistic) effects. The sedating effect of dantrolene sodium may become less striking with continued use. There is some indication that it is a more effective drug for spasticity associated with head trauma than for that produced by stroke syndromes.[38] The usual starting dose is 25 mg once or twice daily, with gradual increases up to 400 mg daily, if it can be tolerated.

Cohan and coworkers have described the use of chlorpromazine (Thorazine) and phenytoin (Dilantin) in 11 patients, three of whom had cerebral forms of spasticity.[39] These patients were initially given 200 to 300 mg of phenytoin daily. After 2 weeks, chlorpromazine was added, starting at 10 mg three times daily, and increasing up to the maximal tolerable dose of 65 mg three times daily. An additional 75 mg of chlorpromazine was given at night in sustained-release form. This preliminary report indicated that the combination worked better than either drug alone or a placebo. It was felt that several failures to improve were likely due to alpha spasticity.

Cendrowski and colleagues[35] reported on the comparative effects of clonazepam, baclofen, and placebo in the treatment of spastic patients, mostly with multiple sclerosis. Clonazepam was found to be relatively more effective in mild forms of spasticity due to cerebral lesions. A benzodiazepine derivative, clonazepam has many of the same side effects as its relative diazepam. The reports on these subsidiary drugs await confirmation by other studies.

I remain relatively unimpressed with the current usage of systemic antispasmodic agents in head-trauma patients. Although they often alleviate spasticity somewhat, they do so at the price of side effects that often create greater problems than the spasticity itself. Furthermore, the improvement may not be correlated by accompanying improved function in many cases.[40] Nevertheless, I believe that these drugs are worth a trial, usually in combinations of either baclofen–dantrolene sodium or diazepam–dantrolene sodium.

The value of diagnostic intramuscular or peripheral nerve anesthetic blocks has already been alluded to. A much longer period of observation of the effects of intramuscular or peripheral nerve neurolysis is afforded by the use of the neurolytic agents phenol and alcohol. Intramuscular neurolysis, as described by Halpern and Meelhuysen,[41] may be performed on a number of muscles at one sitting, using 5 percent aqueous phenol solution. The procedure provides varying degrees of muscle relaxation for periods averaging 4 to 6 months. Customarily, the spasticity returns, necessitating a repeat procedure or some other method of dealing with the recurrent spasticity. However, during that time, previously masked voluntary control can be enhanced, or bracing or surgery can be performed, as in the management of calf spasticity with attendant contractures. Neurolysis has had its greatest use for lower extremity muscles, although it is of occasional benefit for upper extremity muscles, as in the control of severe elbow flexion or finger flexion spasticity. Peripheral nerve neurolysis is most beneficial in predominantly motor nerves such as the obturator and musculocutaneous nerves. The procedure may be done transcutaneously[42] or by the open method.[43] Major side effects of the intramuscular procedure are transient muscle pain and formation of fibrotic nodules. Paresthesias and dysesthesias may result from the peripheral nerve procedure. There have been sporadic reports about the use of intramuscular alcohol, but there are no good studies in the literature concerning its use. The effects of intrathecal alcohol or phenol neurolysis are so unpredictable[44] and fraught with the hazards of altering neurologic function of the bladder and sexual reflexes that they should be abandoned for the management of this type of spasticity.

Orthopedic procedures involving muscle and tendon are usually directed toward the correction of contractures and attendant deformities, but may be combined with neurosurgical procedures such as peripheral neurotomies so as to deter spasticity and the recurrence of the deformities. Most often, these procedures involve the lower extremity, the commonest being some type of teno-Achilles lengthening with or without resection of one or more branches of the posterior tibial nerve. The tendon lengthening procedure may be combined with the transfer of a split anterior tibialis tendon laterally so as to provide an action of eversion of the foot.[45] Toe flexor and posterior tibialis releases may be performed in conjunction with Achilles tendon lengthening, or they may be performed as separate procedures. The Eggers procedure entails the reattachment of hamstrings (one or more) to the femur in order to reduce knee flexion and spasticity. Adductor tenotomies may be combined with obturator neurectomy.

Upper extremity procedures include releases of muscle or tendons to relieve contractures and spasticity at shoulder, elbow, wrist, and fingers. For the spastic flexed elbow, musculocutaneous neurectomy with or without soft tissue releases about the elbow followed by casting of residual contractures of greater than 30 degrees is a beneficial procedure.[23]

These and similar procedures have been well developed as a result of extensive experience with the management of spasticity and deformities in cerebral palsy. Ordinarily, one should wait 1½ to 2 years postinjury before considering this type of surgery. In the interim, intramuscular or peripheral nerve neurolysis may be done one or more times. Furthermore, chemical neurolysis at times produces sufficient relaxation to facilitate postoperative casting and bracing.

Neurosurgical procedures involving peripheral nerves include neurotomies, as already described, and implantation of electric stimulators. The primary use of such stimulators has been to induce dorsiflexion of the foot by means of stimulating the common peroneal nerve.[46]

Dorsal column electric stimulation has been described as being less effective for cerebral types of spasticity than for spinal cord–related spasticity.[47] Stimulators may be implanted at the cervical or upper thoracic levels endodurally after preliminary trial of stimulation epidurally. Limb paresthesias have been reported as a side effect. Judging from the literature, experience using this modality in head-trauma patients is extremely limited.

Several investigators have reported the use of cerebellar-implanted electric stimulators in head-trauma–induced spasticity.[48,49] Despite the optimism of these reports, experience with this method is still limited. Reports of complications such as mechanical failure, destructive changes of the cerebellum, infection, fluid leakage, and death are noteworthy. The basic mechanism of action and long-term effects of cerebellar stimulation are not yet fully appreciated.

The remaining neurosurgical procedures to be described are destructive in nature and therefore so drastic that they rarely merit consideration in head-trauma patients. These procedures should be considered as a last resort in extreme cases of spasticity where all other measures are unavailing. The most extensive experience with these procedures has been in spinal cord–injured patients who are nonambulatory. They include several techniques of anterior and posterior rhizotomy and several variations of myelotomy.

Percutaneous radio-frequency anterior rhizotomy is performed at the lower dorsal, lumbar, and sacral root level under fluoroscopy.[50] Unlike chemical rhizotomies, there is no compromise of pelvic visceral innervation, since control of the procedure is much greater.

Anterior rhizotomy may be performed as an open surgical procedure. As with radio-frequency rhizotomy, its chief indication is severe spasticity of the lower limbs where there is no significant residual voluntary motor function.[51]

Posterior rhizotomy is an open surgical procedure in which the entire root, or portion of the root, is severed. In an effort to selectively interrupt rootlets that are related to abnormal electric motor responses, a technique of functional rhizotomy has been developed, thereby sparing sufficient portions of the foot to minimize sensory losses.[52] This procedure has reportedly been used in cerebral palsy patients, but I am not aware of its use in spasticity associated with head trauma.

Myelotomy has also been employed as a last-ditch measure for control of severe spasticity of the lower extremities in nonambulatory patients, primarily those with spinal cord injury.[44,53] Essentially, the procedure is a transection of the gray matter between the ventral and dorsal horns, resulting in interruption of polysynaptic and monosynaptic reflex pathways. In addition to loss of motor function, there may be sensory deficits and changes in bladder function. With gradually increasing experience with electric stimulation methods, it appears that there is little, if any, indication for these drastic ablative procedures in head-trauma patients.

SUMMARY

Spasticity is a specific type of muscle hypertonus whose chief clinical manifestation is the clasp-knife phenomenon. In defining spasticity, careful distinction has been made from other states of hypertonia, as well as other causes of limitation of passive limb movement. A brief review of the neurophysiology of muscle tone and the mechanisms of spasticity has been presented. The distinction between alpha and gamma spasticity has been emphasized, noting that in many cases of head trauma, some muscle groups have characteristics of alpha and others those of gamma spasticity. The implications for management regarding response to cold and to the drugs baclofen and diazepam have been noted. The clinical characteristics of spasticity have been reviewed, pointing out some of the differentiating features of cerebral- and, specifically, head-trauma–induced spasticity. Clinical and laboratory methods of assessment were discussed, stressing the inherent difficulties of quantitative measurements of a disorder subject to many variations.

As the rehabilitationist considers the individual with spasticity due to head trauma, one must ask these fundamental questions: Does the spasticity compromise some specific function? Would its alleviation compromise some specific function, due to either reduction of the spasticity or a side effect of the treatment? Is there some inciting factor, the elimination or reduction of which would alleviate the spasticity? Primary indications for treatment were proposed, recognizing that spasticity in the head-trauma patient may require no specific therapy. A number of systems of management were outlined and described, ranging from educational strategies to radical ablative surgery. In more severe cases of spasticity, combinations of these systems may be necessary. It is felt that management techniques should be conservative in the first 1½ to 2 years, with the expectation that time and improving motor function will result in abating of the spasticity. Orthopedic procedures are directed primarily to the correction of contractures and deformities and, therefore, must be combined with other measures of spasticity control lest the musculoskeletal abnormalities recur. Of the neurosurgical procedures, the most promising appear to be the methods of electric stimulation. Physical modalities such as cold, therapeutic exercise, splints, casts, and braces combined with one or several systemic antispasmodic agents are usually sufficient to control more severe forms of spasticity in all but a small minority of cases.

REFERENCES

1. BISHOP, B: *Spasticity: Its physiology and management. Part I. Neurophysiology of spasticity: Classical concepts.* Journal of Physical Therapy 57:371, 1977.
2. WYKE, B: *Neurological mechanisms in spasticity: A brief review of some current concepts.* Physiotherapy 62:316, 1976.

3. BISHOP, B: *Spasticity: Its physiology and management. Part II. Neurophysiology of spasticity: Current concepts.* Journal of Physical Therapy 57:377, 1977.
4. BISHOP, B: *Spasticity: Its physiology and management. Part III. Identifying and assessing the mechanisms underlying spasticity.* Journal of Physical Therapy 57:385, 1977.
5. PEDERSON, E, ET AL: *Measurement of plastic and tonic stretch reflexes in antispastic and antiparkinsonian therapy.* Scand J Rehabil Med [Suppl] 3:51, 1974.
6. KNUTSSON, E AND MARTENSSEN, A: *Action of dantrolene sodium in spasticity with low dependence of fusimotor drive.* J Neurol Sci 29:195, 1976.
7. HARRIS, F: *Muscle stretch receptor hypersensitization in spasticity inapproprioception: Part III.* Am J Phys Med 57:16, 1978.
8. HERMAN, R: *The myotatic reflex: Clinicophysiological aspects of spasticity and contracture.* Brain 93:273, 1970.
9. GOFF, B: *Grading of spasticity and its effect on voluntary movement.* Physiotherapy 62:358, 1976.
10. EVANS, C, ET AL: *Rehabilitation of the brain damaged survivor.* Injury 8:80, 1976.
11. JEBSEN, R, ET AL: *Measurement of time in standardized test of patient mobility.* Arch Phys Med Rehabil 51:170, 1970.
12. MOSKOWITZ, E AND MCCANN, C: *Classification of disability in the chronically ill and aging.* J Chronic Dis 5:342, 1957.
13. SCHOENING, H AND IVERSON, I: *Kenny Self-care Evaluation.* Kenny Rehabilitation Institute, Minneapolis, Minn, 1965.
14. GRANGER, C, SHERWOOD, C, AND GREER, D: *Functional status measures in a comprehensive stroke care program.* Arch Phys Med Rehabil 58:555, 1977.
15. JEBSEN, R, ET AL: *An objective test of hand function.* Arch Phys Med Rehabil 50:311, 1969.
16. VARGHESE, G AND REDFORD, J: *Spasticity: Current concepts of management.* J Kans Med Soc 81:109, 1980.
17. BASMAJIAN, J: *Electromyographic investigation of spasticity and muscle spasm.* Physiotherapy 62:320, 1976.
18. SZUMSKI, A, ET AL: *Activity of muscle spindles during muscle twitch and clonus in normal and spastic human subjects.* Electroencephalogr Clin Neurophysiol 37:589, 1974.
19. FISHER, M: *Physiology and Clinical Use of the F Response.* Mimeograph No 13. American Association of Electromyography and Electrodiagnosis, Rochester, Minn, 1980.
20. MIGLIETTA, O: *Action of cold on spasticity.* Am J Phys Med 52:198, 1973.
21. KOTTKE, F: *Therapeutic exercise.* In KRUSEN, F, KOTTKE, F, AND ELWOOD, P (EDS): *Handbook of Physical Medicine and Rehabilitation,* ed 2. WB Saunders, Philadelphia, 1971, p 386.
22. SNOOK, J: *Spasticity Reduction Splint.* Am J Occup Ther. 33:648, 1971.
23. GARLAND, D, THOMPSON, R, AND WATERS, R: *Musculocutaneous neurectomy for spastic elbow flexion in non-functional upper extremities in adults.* J Bone Joint Surg [Am] 62:108, 1980.
24. STEISKAL, L: *Postural reflexes in man.* Am J Phys Med 58:1, 1979.
25. KNUTSON, E: *Physical therapy techniques in the control of spasticity.* Scand J Rehabil Med 5:167, 1973.
26. BISHOP, B: *Spasticity: Its physiology and management. Part IV. Current and projected treatment procedures for spasticity.* Journal of Physical Therapy 57:396, 1977.
27. BOBATH, K AND BOBATH, B: *The facilitation of normal reactions and movements in the treatment of cerebral palsy.* Physiotherapy 50:246, 1964.
28. ROOD, M: *Neurophysiological reaction as a basis for physical therapy.* Physical Therapy Review 34:444, 1954.
29. KABAT, H AND KNOTT, M: *Principles of neuromuscular re-education.* Physical Therapy Review 28:107, 1948.
30. BRUNNSTROM, S: *Methods used to Elicit, Reinforce, and Coordinate Muscular Response—Upper Motor Neuron Lesions.* APTA-OVR Institute Papers. American Physical Therapy Association, New York, 1956.

31. HARRIS, F: *Correction of muscle imbalance in spasticity: Inapproprioception, Part IV.* Am J Phys Med 57:123, 1978.
32. BROWN, D, DEBACHER, G, AND BASMAJIAN, J: *Feedback goniometers for hand rehabilitation.* Am J Occup Ther 33:458, 1979.
33. LUDEN, H AND ROBERT, F: *The action of diazepam on human skeletal muscle.* Eur Neurol 11:345, 1974.
34. DAVIDOFF, R: *Pharmacology of spasticity.* Neurology 28:46, September 1978.
35. CENDROWSKI, W AND SOBCZYK, W: *Clonazepam, baclofen, and placebo in the treatment of spasticity.* Eur Neurol 16:257, 1977.
36. MCLELLAN, D: *Co-contraction and stretch reflexes in spasticity during treatment with baclofen.* J Neurol Neurosurg Psychiatry 40:30, 1977.
37. DELANEY, J: *Medical treatment of spasticity.* Curr Probl Surg 17:245, 1980.
38. PINDER, R, ET AL: *Dantrolene sodium: A review of its pharmacological properties and therapeutic efficacy in spasticity.* Drugs 13:3, 1977.
39. COHAN, S, ET AL: *Phenytoin and chlorpromazine in the treatment of spasticity.* Arch Neurol 37:360, 1980.
40. JONSON, B, ET AL: *The effects on spasticity in hemiplegic patients.* Acta Neurol Scand 51:385, 1975.
41. HALPERN, D AND MEELHUYSEN, F: *Phenol motor point block in the management of muscular hypertonia.* Arch Phys Med Rehabil 47:659, 1966.
42. KHALILI, A AND BETTS, H: *Management of Spasticity with Phenol Nerve Blocks.* Final Report RD-2529-M. Department of Health, Education and Welfare, Social and Rehabilitation Service, Washington, DC, 1970.
43. MOONEY, V, FRYKMAN, G, AND MCLAMB, J: *Current status of intraneural phenol injections.* Clin Orthop 63:122, 1969.
44. LAHA, R, DUJOVNY, M, AND OSGOOD, C: *Dorsal longitudinal myelotomy.* Paraplegia 14:189, 1976.
45. ROPER, B, WILLIAMS, A, AND KING, J: *The surgical treatment of equinovarus deformity in adults with spasticity.* J Bone Joint Surg [Br] 60-B:533, 1978.
46. DAVIS, R AND GESINK, J: *Evaluation of electrical stimulation as a treatment for the reduction of spasticity.* Bull Prosthet Res: 302, 1974.
47. SIEGFRIED, J, ET AL: *Electrical spinal cord stimulation for spastic movement disorders.* Applied Neurophysiology 41:134, 1978.
48. MCLELLAN, D, SELWYN, M, AND COOPER, I: *Time course of clinical and physiological effects of stimulation of the cerebellar surface in patients with spasticity.* J Neurol Neurosurg Psychiatry 41:150, 1978.
49. DAVIS, R, ET AL: *Control of spasticity and involuntary movements: Cerebellar stimulation.* Applied Neurophysiology 40:135, 1977–1978.
50. DUJOVNY, M, LAHA, R, AND YONAS, H: *Surgical management of spasticity.* Curr Probl Surg 17:249, 1980.
51. CUSICK, J, LARSON, S, AND SANCES, A: *The effect of T-myelotomy on spasticity.* Surg Neurol 6:289, 1976.
52. FASANO, V, ET AL: *Surgical treatment of spasticity in cerebral palsy.* Childs Brain 4:289, 1978.
53. IVAN, L AND WILEY, J: *Myelotomy in the management of spasticity.* Clin Orthop 108:52, 1975.

Chapter 10

DEFICITS IN ACTIVITIES OF DAILY LIVING

Robin McNeny, O.T.R.

Any activity necessary to an individual's function can be categorized as an activity of daily living, whether it be dressing oneself in the morning, managing basic financial matters, or reading a bus schedule. An individual's time is consumed with the pursuit of activities of daily living that satisfy needs and maintain the effectiveness and quality of life.

Traumatic brain injury, however, has a devastating effect on an individual's ability to perform activities of daily living. The prolonged periods of acute care and rehabilitation, as well as the often severe residua of the head injury, limit and may even preclude many activities of daily life. This involves more than just self-care skills. Advanced living skills vital to an individual's independence—such as meal planning, social and leisure interests, and communication skills—may also be affected.

In addressing these special deficit areas, the rehabilitation professional must be cognizant of the individual's premorbid life tasks, interests, and social roles. There should be an understanding of which skills contributed to a pleasurable and productive existence in order that they be incorporated directly and indirectly into the treatment program.

Activities of daily living may be divided into basic skills and advanced skills. The basic skills include the areas of self-care, such as feeding, dressing, and hygiene; whereas advanced skills involve higher-level tasks, such as financial management, social skills, and driving. Though certain therapeutic activities mentioned below will be described as being performed by certain members of the rehabilitation team, it should be recognized that many procedures can be performed by a variety of rehabilitation professionals.

BASIC ACTIVITIES OF DAILY LIVING

FEEDING

Intake of a properly balanced, nutritious diet is vital to recovery from any serious illness or injury. However, traumatic head injury frequently causes problems that interfere with dietary intake. The problems include oral dysfunction, specific physical limitations, and behavioral changes.

Oral Dysfunction

Dysphagia, drooling, aspiration, and general weakness of oral structures are common sequelae of many conditions, including head injury. Thorough evaluation by the physician, occupational therapist, speech pathologist, and nurse yields information regarding the extent and severity of the oral deficits. Once the deficits are defined, the goals of a remediation program should be to (1) inhibit primitive reflexes while facilitating weak reflexes, (2) improve swallowing patterns, (3) increase strength and coordination of oral structures, and (4) encourage adequate dietary intake.

Griffin[1,2] has outlined a program she has found successful in treating the problem of dysphagia in the head-injured population. This approach can be incorporated into any standard oral facilitation program, as needed.

In assessing oral dysfunction, several key areas need to be considered:

1. The peripheral speech mechanisms.
2. The quality of the swallow: whether it is present or absent and whether it is reflexive or volitional.
3. The quality of the patient's taste receptors.
4. The ability of the patient to manage foods of varying textures.
5. The presence or absence of necessary reflexes.

Recommendations for inclusion in a dysphagia training program are made on the basis of this evaluation. The training proceeds from the achievement of a saliva swallow to introduction of semisolid and solid foods. The initial training phases should be performed in occupational and speech therapy. Collaboration between the two professionals should be directed toward facilitating the best swallowing pattern possible.

As swallowing improves, drooling usually lessens. Drooling is further reduced as the patient becomes involved in an oral strengthening program. This program should include the following:

1. Imitation of facial expression: smiles, puckers, and frowns to strengthen oral muscles.
2. Straw-sucking activities.
3. Lip-strengthening activities, such as holding a piece of paper between the lips tightly.
4. Blowing activities.
5. Repetitive sounds, such as pa, pa, pa or la, la, la.

The speech pathologist, occupational therapist, and registered nurse collaborate to treat any oral dysfunction present in a head-injured patient. The role of the nursing staff is vital, since they are with the patient at mealtime and can reinforce a program designed in speech therapy and occupational therapy. The observations made at mealtime regarding carry-over of instruction, success with various food substances, and family participation in the program are of particular value and are best made by the unit nurse. Changes in the program are then based on the success achieved by the patient on the unit.

Physical Limitations

Traumatic head injury can create certain physical problems that make self-feeding difficult or impossible. Visual problems, poor head control, upper extremity injuries or dysfunction, jaw fractures, dental problems, and decreased balance all complicate feeding.

The rehabilitation team works on different aspects of the patient's physical problems simultaneously. In physical therapy, the patient with severe physical deficits should be involved in a comprehensive exercise program. This program may include passive range of motion exercises to stretch contractures, strengthening exercises to improve available musculature, and balance training.

The occupational therapist will consider the need for splinting to improve positioning or functional use of the hands. Adaptive feeding devices such as extended or weighted utensils, suction plates, or cup holders may be suggested to minimize physical deficits. In addition, the physical and occupational therapists may need to work with the physician and rehabilitation engineer, if available, to devise special seating apparatus or head control devices. At times, upper extremity orthoses are necessary. Once the best combination of devices and aids is determined, the head-injured patient is trained to use adaptive equipment and works to increase tolerance to feeding.

These feeding skills developed in therapy are carried over onto a ward feeding program involving the patient, family, and nursing staff as well as the occupational therapist. With supervision, patients feed themselves, using whatever adaptive devices they need, and the nursing staff and the family are given suggestions they may use to improve patients' success at subsequent sessions. Because endurance is likely to pose a problem initially, the family and nurses should be given guidelines as to when to offer assistance.

Behavioral and Cognitive Problems

Though oral dysfunction and physical limitations are largely responsible for difficulties in feeding in the head-injured population, behavioral and cognitive disturbances may affect the success of the feeding process. Lethargy, poor attention span, distractability, disorientation, and agitation, as well as poor body scheme, diminished visuo-spatial skills, and right/left confusion, can all be limiting factors when feeding is impaired. When these are coupled with the problems already discussed in oral dysfunction and physical impairment, it is easy to understand that the success of training programs initiated is much more doubtful when cognition is impaired.

The severity of such a problem is best illustrated by this case example:

Case Example: R.W.

R.W., a 30-year-old married woman, was admitted to the neurosurgical ICU following an automobile accident during which she suffered a severe head injury. After a period of several weeks, R.W. was admitted to the rehabilitation unit. She was highly agitated, severely disoriented, and continually in motion, unable to remain still for more than seconds. Her balance was severely impaired. These behaviors created problems at mealtimes, as R.W. could not be coaxed to sit and feed herself. She refused food and sought ways to avoid eating such as hiding her tray under linen on the linen cart. Because of her extended period of coma, nutrition was a particular problem for R.W.; she had lost 30 lb during her stay in the ICU. Therefore, the nurses, her family, and the dietitian concentrated on improving R.W.'s feeding patterns and nutritional status using several techniques.

1. A family member, usually her husband, was always present at mealtime to provide encouragement to the patient and stress the importance of good nutrition in her recovery.
2. A plate, silverware, and table linens from home were brought to the hospital to make R.W.'s surroundings more familiar.
3. The nurse and dietitian assessed R.W.'s premorbid eating patterns, discovering that she was a perpetual dieter and had always been interested in her appearance. Therefore, they selected a diet low in calories but high in nutrition to increase the appeal of food to R.W. Her family assisted by bringing favorite foods from home.

4. Distractions were minimized; R.W. ate in her room away from other patients, the television, and staff. She was to concentrate on the meal before her. Limits were set at first, such as a requirement that she complete the entire tray before she leave the room.

These strategies were successful. After approximately 3 weeks on the rehabilitation unit, R.W. was completing full meals with a minimum of supervision. As her orientation improved, she was able to verbalize the rationale for her current diet and its contribution to her recovery.

Techniques such as those used with R.W. have been successful with other head-injured patients. Consistency of approach is a key element; hence, family and new staff need to fully understand the program before it is begun.

DRESSING

The newly admitted head-injured patient on the rehabilitation unit may experience problems in dressing. The patient may still be wearing pajamas or may appear disheveled, with clothes on backward, fastenings undone, or colors mismatched. This most likely results from a lack of interest in appearance, a decreased attention span, perceptual problems, impulsivity, or lethargy. The head-injured patient is often oblivious to dressing concerns in the early stages of rehabilitation.

Of early concern to the staff is the effect physical residua of the head trauma have on the ability to manage clothes. Of all the areas of deficit, the physical limitations are probably the most quickly overcome through modified techniques, practice sessions, and adaptive aids. Techniques used are familiar to most rehabilitation professionals, especially occupational therapists and nurses, and are those used with individuals with other types of physical disability.

The patient who has problems with perception following head injury may find dressing more difficult and progress slower than will the patient whose limitations are chiefly physical. Good visual-spatial skills are needed to distinguish parts of clothing, to line up buttons, and to get socks on straight. Intact body scheme is needed to understand the relationship between clothes and one's body parts. Sequencing skills are necessary so that clothes are applied in a logical order, as well as for the successful completion of higher-level tasks, such as shoe-tying.

Several steps may be taken to facilitate dressing independence with the perceptually disabled patient:

1. Recommend that the patient wear simple, solid-colored clothing with a minimum of fastenings to reduce visual stimuli. Just locating the sleeve is hard enough, without having to deal with a multicolored, geometrically designed fabric.
2. If the patient cannot learn to discriminate between front and back, or left and right, use visual cues, such as the neckline label, to aid in locating clothing parts. Also, marking a part of clothing with a safety pin or inconspicuous thread can serve the same function.
3. To alleviate sequencing problems, place a chart by the patient's bed to instruct in the correct sequence for dressing. This also helps staff keep their instructions to the patient consistent.
4. Everyone working with the patient should be aware of the perceptual deficits and the techniques employed to remedy them.

During the dressing training program, the head-injured patient will need to learn to refocus attention on appearance. Staff and family need to make the patient gently aware of disheveled or dirty clothes. It will require patience, a consistent approach by the team, and an increased self-awareness by the patient. This increased awareness will often coincide with improved orientation and an enhanced insight into the patient's current condition.

DEFICITS IN ACTIVITIES OF DAILY LIVING

A few suggestions are given to aid staff and family in dealing with this problem:

1. Monitor the patient's daily dressing routine. Call attention to buttons the patient failed to fasten or mismatched socks.
2. Place a mirror in the room if one is not already available, and encourage the patient to check carefully appearance after dressing to detect errors.
3. If the patient's interest during dressing wanders, redirect attention and help the patient continue to work.
4. Family and staff should provide positive reinforcement for a neat appearance.

HYGIENE SKILLS

Today's society places great value on the well-groomed, freshly washed, and pleasingly perfumed body. Dirty hair, body odor, and sour breath are labeled undesirable and unacceptable. However, after traumatic head injury, many patients will present with an inferior level of hygiene. During the recovery process, this unkempt appearance is excused, as are the patient's failures to perform other functional skills. During the rehabilitation process, the focus changes, with reintegration into the community a goal; inadequate personal hygiene can be a barrier to such reintegration.

If the patient physically cannot perform some hygiene skills, adaptive equipment may improve the level of function. Extended toothbrushes, combs, and hairbrushes help the patient with limited range of motion and/or strength. Suction scrub brushes and suction nail clippers that adhere to firm surfaces facilitate dental and nail care for the one-handed patient. In many cases, the patient is well motivated to upgrade hygiene skills but has such severe physical limitations that independence seems unlikely. The case of P.B. demonstrates that intensive therapy can help a patient surmount tremendous problems.

Case Example: P.B.

P.B. was a 43-year-old woman who suffered a severe head injury in an automobile accident. Because of the nature of her injury, P.B. experienced a severe loss of visual acuity in both eyes. Hygiene skills were particularly difficult for her, but she desired treatment to assist her in performing hygiene tasks as independently as possible. The areas of most importance to her were:

1. Developing a mechanism to help her accurately part her hair and assure herself it was neatly combed.
2. Overcoming safety problems inherent in her practice of using a safety razor on her legs and underarms.
3. Practicing shampooing her hair.

In occupational therapy, P.B. practiced shaving her legs with a safety razor. She concentrated on using light, uniform pressure. She was encouraged to develop greater tactile sensibility in her fingers so that she could determine whether her hair was parted correctly or if she had unshaven areas on her legs. Though at the time of discharge P.B. still required close supervision for these tasks, she had a greater sense of self-satisfaction and eventual independence seemed likely.

Just as with dressing, the staff and family need to encourage the poorly groomed patient to take more interest in appearance. Frequently, the problem is that the patient lacks sufficient initiative to schedule hygiene tasks into the day, and they are left undone. This problem can be addressed in several ways. First, inclusion of the patient in a regular hygiene session with other patients where skills such as nail care, shaving, and make-up application are reviewed can be useful. Families should be encouraged to bring in the patient's own hygiene aids. In addition, if the family is willing, they should be encouraged to devote a portion of their visiting time to special hygiene tasks such as polishing nails. As the patient begins to show more initiative, increased safety awareness, and less need for supervision, a hygiene schedule can be hung in the room outlining the specific tasks the patient needs to perform and when they must be done. The chart provides structure the patient still needs while allowing greater opportunities for independence.

The amount of time required for the reacquisition of these basic daily living skills differs from patient to patient and is dependent on many variables. Nevertheless, these are important areas that need early attention by the professional rehabilitation staff. Recovery of these skills should not be left to nature, time, or chance.

ADVANCED LIVING SKILLS

Advanced living skills include a wide range of activities that require high-level skills and are considered vital to the individual's independent living. Traumatic head injury interrupts the performance of these skills, frequently for a considerable time. As a result, life roles are changed, dependence on others is increased, and self-esteem may be lessened. A thorough understanding of the patient's limitations by the entire rehabilitation staff is necessary to help the patient, family, and friends cope with the alterations inherent in the patient's life style. While realistically outlining areas where the patient cannot function alone, the team should be available for emotional support and assistance.

As a patient on the rehabilitation unit, the head-injured adult undergoes evaluation in many areas to determine the severity of deficits resulting from the head injury. Particular emphasis should be placed on skills the patient performed routinely as part of the life role. For the high school student, these skills might include the ability to speak and write intelligibly; while for the homemaker, an important skill might be the ability to safely supervise the children and meet their needs. During evaluation, each member of the team should assess all areas of competency and, in conjunction with the patient, set goals and design treatment.

COMMUNICATION SKILLS

Traumatic head injury may cause speech and language deficits such as aphasia or dysarthria. Vocal cord paralysis or scarring is often encountered, resulting in diminished voice volume. Comprehension of written and spoken material may be impaired. The patient may provide too little information during conversation, omitting words and sentences vital to one's understanding of the remark, or the patient might talk excessively, perseverating on a thought, unable to divert oneself.

Speech pathologists address the speech and language dysfunction, often offering alternate forms of communication to those patients for whom vocalization is not possible. Many head-injured patients also have difficulty with writing skills resulting from a specific physical limitation, cognitive impairment, or perceptual problems. In speech and occupational therapy, the deficits are identified and intervention provided. Dominance retraining may be necessary if writing with the dominant hand is no longer feasible. To overcome incoordination, special writing aids or weights might be used to improve legibility. Perceptual training may help the patient develop better use of space for writing, as the perceptually disabled patient may tend to overshoot the edge of the paper when writing or may fail to start writing at the left-hand margin. In addition, difficulty with letter formation may be the result of visual-spatial deficits.

The patient should be encouraged to participate in conversation with other patients and with staff. Informal conversation is beneficial in improving speech and language skills as well as orientation, and it encourages appropriate social interchange. (See Chapter 11 for further discussion of communication deficits.)

HOME LIVING SKILLS

In our modern age, men as well as women are assuming the homemaker role. These responsibilities include meal planning and preparation, cleaning, and laundry. The head-injured adult often lacks the ability to physically perform these jobs; however, physical ability is usually less of an issue than is the patient's ability to perform them safely and judiciously on an independent level. Unfortunately, independent performance is frequently not possible.

Actual observation of the patient performing these tasks in a simulated situation should be arranged in occupational therapy as soon as it is feasible. Principal goals of the evaluation and training process should include (1) improving safety awareness, (2) determining judgment skills, (3) increasing competency in skill areas, and (4) delineating areas where supervision is required. All information gathered during training sessions as well as specific recommendations for supervision should be shared with the family to ensure follow-through after discharge.

It cannot be stressed enough that thorough evaluation of homemaking abilities is necessary with head-injured adults. The behaviors displayed by this population of individuals are unique to them, and observation of them engaged in activities is the best method of evaluation. A head-injured client often "looks better than he or she actually is," and this is often borne out in performance. Consider the case of N.H.

Case Example: N.H.

N.H. is the 15-year-old son of working parents. Admitted to the rehabilitation unit after a severe head injury, N.H. experienced physical impairment, including right-sided weakness and diminished coordination. He demonstrated moderate to severe visual spatial deficits but was independent in his self-care skills.

Because N.H.'s parents worked, he had been at home alone for extended periods of time before and after school prior to his accident. He occasionally prepared light meals. Therefore, as part of his occupational therapy program, N.H. was asked to engage in kitchen activities, including the preparation of a frozen pizza. Significant deficits were uncovered during the evaluation. N.H. had difficulty opening the box as a result of his right-sided weakness. He was unable to locate the temperature setting for the oven in the written box instructions. He failed to note the baking time and neglected to check the pizza's progress at an appropriate interval. He did remember to turn the oven off after use and safely removed the hot pizza pan from the oven.

As a result of his poor performance, it was determined that N.H. lacked sufficient safety awareness to be trusted at home alone.

FAMILY RELATIONSHIPS

Related to home-living skills are the care of children by a head-injured parent and the husband-wife relationship. The relationship between family members is special and needs particular attention from the professional staff.

Physical, perceptual, cognitive, and behavioral changes all lead to alterations in the patient's role as parent and spouse. All too frequently, the patient is regarded as a child. Authority as a parent is undermined; the patient is seen as unable to carry out parenting responsibilities.

The individual's physical capabilities must be addressed early in the rehabilitation process. We should consider whether the patient can manage the role of spouse and parent, given the physical disability. If not, can modifications be made or adaptive skills be taught to facilitate greater independence?

If there are perceptual or cognitive problems, we should determine in which areas these deficits lie and how they affect safety awareness, judgment, and competency. Evaluations in neuropsychology and occupational therapy are essential in this determination.

Healthy family relationships are encouraged during the rehabilitation process. The family is made as integral a part of the team as possible; it is believed that their support and participation demonstrate their continued interest in and love for the patient. Children are encouraged to visit, and care is taken to help them with anxieties that naturally arise during recovery.

Home passes allow a break from the hospital routine and setting and are valuable in promoting family relationships. The pass allows the patient to interact with the children on familiar ground. There is time for the patient to test the skills the patient feels are important in maintaining an effective relationship with the offspring. Problems that arise should be discussed with staff members, and some resolution of the problem is sought.

Family nights sponsored by the nursing staff provide an evening of socialization that involves patients and families. The evening can include a shared supper for the entire family and then a planned activity in which everyone may participate. The staff is able to observe the interaction of family members and note signs of stress, uncertainty, rejection, or anxiety. These problems are then addressed with the patient, family, and appropriate staff.

Family days are structured to maximize the family's involvement in all aspects of the treatment program. The family is asked to accompany the patient through an entire day in the hospital and to ascertain what the therapies are concentrating on during their daily sessions. Methods for enhancing the in-clinic programs during visits in the evenings and on weekends are given by each therapist. The family gets a clearer picture of the patient's abilities and disabilities.

TIME MANAGEMENT

There is the need in every individual's life for components of work, play, and rest. To maintain this balance, an adult has to budget time, set priorities, and work efficiently. The disorientation and cognitive deficits that frequently result from brain injury hamper one's ability to manage time.

Structuring the environment will help the head-injured patient's orientation and time-management skills. A daily schedule that includes meals, hygiene tasks, and family visits will aid the patient in establishing a daily routine. The entire staff should reinforce adherence to the schedule and help the patient deal with schedule changes.

Participation in a 24-hour reality orientation program is beneficial for the disoriented patient. Good orientation is crucial for effective time management. Clocks, calendars, and a large schedule board available on the unit aid in increasing the patient's awareness of time. Reminders from staff as to the patient's individual schedule are also helpful. (See Chapter 24 for further discussion of reality orientation.)

As the patient improves, involving the patient in the scheduling process creates a greater sense of autonomy and control. With the patient's input, breaks for rest or to watch a favorite television show can be worked around therapy.

Initially, free time, such as evening and weekend hours, may require strict structuring by the staff to prevent aimless wandering or excessive sleeping. Physical, occupational, and speech therapy can send evening and weekend work assignments to the unit for the patient to complete. Recreational programs should be available, and the patient may be involved in a ward task designed to let the patient assist a staff member with a routine job, such as clearing the table in the dining room of trays after meals.

The head-injured adult may still have problems with time management after discharge. It is therefore important to equip the family with mechanisms to help them deal with the problem. Most of the techniques used in the hospital are easily adapted to home; instruction from the staff will aid the family in their use.

FINANCIAL MANAGEMENT

Most adults are capable, to a reasonable degree, of managing their income, budgeting expenses, and disbursing cash as needed. However, the imposition of a head injury alters one's ability to judiciously manage financial affairs. This may be a result of difficulty with mathematical and monetary skills, or behavioral changes, such as poor quality control, impulsivity, or a lack of sound judgment. As a result, a family member will frequently need to assume control of the patient's finances. The magnitude of this problem may be compounded by a loss of income and large hospital bills.

The occupational therapist should work with the head-injured adult in increasing the level of competency in money management. Certain critical areas should be addressed: (1) the ability to complete simple computation; (2) the ability to recognize coinage and bills and to compute the value of money; (3) the ability to use money correctly to purchase needs, incorporating skills in making change; (4) the ability to budget, including an understanding of the difference between needs and wants, principles of saving money regularly, and the ability to control impulse buying; and (5) the ability to manage banking skills, including writing checks, maintaining balances and checking registers, and managing a savings account.

Specific problem areas receive concentrated treatment. Deficits that persist are discussed with the team and the family. The goal is to create as little dependency as possible while still protecting the patient's financial security.

SOCIAL ROLES

Needless to say, one's roles in the family and society undergo significant stress and change after head injury. Within the family, the head injury produces stresses that affect all intrafamilial relationships. The friends and acquaintances of the head-injured adult are even less well equipped than the family to cope with the changes they perceive in the individual. The physical changes alone may cause discomfort for them. When the aberrant behavior associated with head trauma is added to this, they feel even more uncomfortable.

In recent years, rehabilitation personnel have been developing a greater sensitivity for this problem. There needs to be a greater integration of interested friends who will become participants in the program; their participation can ease their anxieties. A greater emphasis needs to be made on the patient's postdischarge status. Outpatient treatment programs, day-care programs for head-injured adults, residential facilities, and patient-centered and family groups are all viable alternatives for the head-injured adult. However, they are only sporadically available.

During the hospitalization, the groundwork for the resumption of social roles needs to be laid. Interaction between patients is vital; appropriate behavior needs to be developed, and inappropriate behavior needs to be controlled. Success in social situations needs to be achieved by every patient, whether it is in a structured patient milieu or during a group therapy session. Recreational activities provide the ideal setting for head-injured patients to test their social skills.

DRIVING

A traumatic head injury renders most of its victims incapable of operating a motor vehicle. This limitation may last only a year or two or may be permanent. Certain factors determine the restrictions placed on driving: (1) medical problems, such as paralysis, ataxia, and seizures; (2) medications that slow responses or impair consciousness; (3) poor judgment and altered mental status; (4) perceptual problems; and (5) visual disturbances.

Driving skills should be addressed as early as the patient's medical condition and mental status will allow. This frequently occurs months after discharge from the inpatient program. Despite this factor, referral to a driving evaluation program, often available in occupational or physical therapy, should be made by the physician.

A thorough driver evaluation program for the head-injured adult should encompass several skill areas:[3]

1. *Physical skills.* Can the patient physically handle the mechanics of driving? Does the patient require special adaptions to promote ease of handling or safety?
2. *Visual skills.* Is peripheral vision within the normal range? Does the patient scan the roadway well for hazards? Does the patient require corrective lenses?
3. *Perceptual skills.* Does the patient judge depth and distance well? Does the patient use space on the roadway adequately? Can the patient recognize colors and shapes of traffic signs with relative ease? Is there evidence of right/left confusion? Can the patient follow verbal directions to get to a destination?
4. *Speed of motor responses.* How quickly does the patient respond when the patient needs to brake quickly, or change lanes or travel directions?
5. *Judgment.* Is there any evidence in the patient's driving to indicate impulsivity or lack of quality control? In an emergency situation, how well does the patient exercise decision-making skills?

Based on a comprehensive evaluation that may include the use of a driving simulator, the physician and evaluator can make a decision regarding the patient's suitability for driving. It is a decision that should be made after careful consideration and a complete analysis of the driving evaluation.

OTHER ISSUES

Many deficits in activities of daily living are addressed while the head-injured adult is still on an inpatient service. Still other areas cannot be addressed until much later because of the patient's lack of readiness for training prior to discharge. For these individuals, the training program should be available on an outpatient basis, and the physician should be sensitive to changes in the patient that indicate a need for additional treatment.

Follow-up therapy is traditionally given on an individual basis. The therapist spends a brief, concentrated session several times weekly with the patient. However, individual treatment is not always ideal.

An alternative to one-to-one treatment is the group treatment session. It usually involves four to six head-injured adults at similar functional levels who engage in therapeutic activity simultaneously. There are distinct advantages inherent in this treatment approach. First, it provides an opportunity for socialization with others that many head-injured adults lack. Second, the group offers support to one another when problems or frustrations surface. In addition, the group members' feelings that they alone are different and isolated from society are challenged when they begin to meet one another and discuss their concerns. For these reasons, the group treatment approach may be preferred by many professionals for this population.

The head-injured adult's altered life roles and personality, functional limitations and new dependencies, and own frustrations with self tax the family's coping mechanisms. These problems certainly affect the individuals involved as well as the family structure as a whole and must be considered during the period of outpatient follow-up. They may affect the patient's level of performance of activities of daily living. Consider the case of R.D.

Case Example: R.D.

R.D. sustained a head injury at age 17 and spent several months in a rehabilitation program. He left the service with significant physical and mental residua, including a left hemiparesis, left homonymous hemianopsia, inappropriate affect, and dysarthric speech.

At the time of hospital discharge, R.D. returned home with his parents, both of whom are employed outside the home. R.D. has, since discharge, had several unsuccessful placements in sheltered workshops and vocational programs, all designed either for the physically or mentally impaired. His failures in these programs were chiefly due to his inaccurate perception of his abilities and liabilities, his poor memory, and his inadequate social skills. He was able to care for his personal needs well but lacked skill in advanced areas. He refused outpatient treatment to improve deficits in social skills. Unfortunately, there was no other option for R.D. within his locale.

CONCLUSION

Head injury presents a complex challenge for rehabilitation professionals. If head-injured adults experienced severe though predictable physical deficits—as do patients with cerebral palsy—or only significant mental impairment—similar to that found in mental retardation—then there would be little difficulty encountered working through these problems in a traditional manner. However, head injury yields an unpredictably mixed array of deficits, and there is no way to predict the types of functional limitations that might result from a given injury. The rehabilitation team then must face the problem of exactly how to cope with these individuals and reintegrate them into a satisfying life style.

REFERENCES

1. GRIFFIN, K, STUBBERT, J, AND BRECKENRIDGE, K: *Teaching the dysphagic patient to swallow.* RN Sept 1974:60.
2. GRIFFIN, K: *Swallowing training for dysphagic patients.* Arch Phys Med Rehabil 55:465, 1974
3. HOFKOSH, J, SIPAJLO, J, AND BRODY, L: *Driver education for the physically disabled.* Med Clin North Am 53:685, 1969

Chapter 11

COMMUNICATION DISORDERS

Michael Groher, Ph.D.

Loss of the ability to communicate effectively can be a frequent finding secondary to severe head trauma. Only in the past decade has the importance of speech and language come to the fore as a crucial determinant of the patient's acute and future health status. As Najenson and colleagues[1] have pointed out, communication may play the pivotal role in determining the quality of survival.

Most of the literature has dealt only with the medical management of the patient, treating communication and its role in total rehabilitation in an accessory manner. The importance of speech and language deficits after head trauma has been minimized, partly from failure to agree on an accepted set of terminology that accurately describes the deficits, partly from the lack of empirical data relative to the treatment of communication disorders, and partly from the failure to believe that communication deficits secondary to head trauma deserve special attention because they represent a unique speech and language symptomatology.

The difficulty in describing the exact nature of the speech and language deficits is in part due to the variability in the acute communication symptomatology and in the eventual course and outcome of recovery. Patients who are rendered unconscious or who are semi-comatose rarely are able to communicate. Less severe injuries may produce clinically normal speech and language skills, but the patient may not be aware of events that transpired immediately before or after the accident. Between these two extremes, there may be any manner of deficit in the patient's communication skills, or in the patient's awareness of or responsiveness to the environment, which provides the basis for communication. Therefore, the exact nature of the patient's communication status may depend on when the examiner completes the assessment. Failure to delineate when communication measures are made during the course of recovery is part of the reason much of the earlier literature[2-5] relative to communication deficits after trauma lacked agreement as to the exact nature of the pathology and its progression over time. Patients clearly manifest a different set of communication deficits at different stages in their recovery. The problem of accurate description is compounded by the failure of many investigators to use either a repeatable or a standardized testing procedure, creating gaps and irregularities in the interpretation of the accumulated data. To report that a patient evidenced a naming deficit or a problem with auditory comprehension, without knowing the level of severity or complexity, opened the door for different interpretations of the patient's communicative abilities and led to subsequent confusion over the nature of the deficit.

Further difficulty in understanding the nature of the communication deficits after head trauma arises from the inconsistencies in the terminology used to describe the disorder. Early reports[2,3] focused on the issue of post-traumatic amnesia and the accompanying loss of memory as the primary mechanism to explain poor communication skills. Russell and Espir[6] stated that these severe losses of memory that may be part of post-traumatic amnesia often amount to a mild form of aphasia. London[7] described communication losses as changes in intellectual functioning due to forgetfulness, poor concentration, and slow wits. Luria[8] felt that those communication deficits after head trauma definitely were consistent with aphasic language symptomatology. Halpern, Darley, and Brown[9] concluded that language disturbance secondary to trauma was most consistent with a pattern of confused language which was clearly different from that of patients who had aphasia secondary to etiologies other than trauma. After investigating a sample of 14 patients with closed head trauma, Groher[10] concluded that the patients evidenced both elements of aphasic and confused language disturbance in the acute stages of recovery, but that the specific aphasic component quickly resolved, leaving the patient with what Halpern, Darley, and Brown[9] termed "the language of confusion." More recently, Hagen, Malkmus, and Burditt[11] have taken the stance that language impairments after head trauma should be diagnosed and treated as part of an underlying cognitive disorganization.

These seemingly apparent differences in the use of descriptive terminology lead one to question whether or not investigators are describing truly identical groups of patients, using recognized repeated measures over time.

Descriptions of communication disorders after trauma may be at odds due to a number of often-ignored methodologic considerations. Answers to some of the following questions may help to clear some of these discrepancies. First, one must consider the nature of the traumatizing act. Did it produce an open or closed head injury? Missile wounds, for instance, are more likely to produce open head injuries, whereas automobile accidents typically produce closed head injuries. If there is a communication deficit secondary to the traumatizing act, is there a difference between these two groups? Secondly, are age and a previously positive neurologic history important in determining the effects of trauma on communication? Thirdly, has the investigator selected patients who were comatose or not comatose following trauma? Does this affect recovery? What radiographic and/or neurologic evidence is presented? That is, are we dealing with patients who have diffuse or focal lesions, and are the lesions localizable? And finally, are patients who present with communication disorders secondary to trauma appropriately grouped and studied with those patients who suffer communication impairment secondary to vascular disease?

OPEN VERSUS CLOSED HEAD TRAUMA

Much of the early literature that discussed communication disorders and head trauma dealt with patients who had suffered open head injuries, usually from fragment penetration during war.[8,12,13] These descriptions usually sought to connect a particular speech or language disorder to a specific lesion site in the central nervous system. Invariably, postmortem analysis revealed that these penetrating lesions producing speech and language disorders were generally confined to the frontal, temporal, and parietal lobes of the left cerebral hemisphere. Patients were then divided into groups using typologic systems for classifying aphasia. Dresser and associates[14] concluded that in left hemisphere lesions, the deeper the penetration, the poorer the eventual outcome of communication skills. The prevalence of communication disorders in large groups of patients with open head trauma ranges from 14 to 23 percent, with a median of 20 percent.[15,16,17]

Hagen, Malkmus, and Burditt[11] have suggested there may be clinical differences in communication symptomatology between open and closed lesions because of the varying nature of the pathology. They chose to divide trauma patients into four categories: closed head trauma, depressed skull fracture, penetrating wounds, and brain stem/cerebellar pathology, all of which have the potential of creating different and varying effects on communication. In some cases, the resultant deficits may overlap among groups.

Luria's work[8] remains as the only investigation that sought to compare the speech and language deficits of open- and closed-head-trauma patients. After reviewing 800 cases, Luria concluded that there did not appear to be any significant differences in the language capabilities of both groups immediately after trauma; however, the two groups did differ in the residual period (1 to 3 months). Incidence of aphasic disturbances following trauma to the left cerebral hemisphere decreased from 75 to 38 percent in closed head injuries, while they went from 88 to 68 percent in open head injuries. Open-head-injury patients also displayed aphasic symptomatology longer than did closed-head-trauma patients. In addition, closed-head-injury patients in the initial period suffered fewer communication deficits as a group than did the penetrating-wound patients. The implication from Luria's work is that patients with closed head injuries and communication deficits not only improve more following trauma than patients with open head injuries, but also at a faster rate.

Currently, no published statistics document the percentage of communication disorders in consecutive cases of closed head trauma, although my experience suggests that, like open head injuries, the prevalence of communication disorders following closed head injuries ranges from 15 to 25 percent.

DURATION OF UNCONSCIOUSNESS

It is generally accepted that the medical prognosis for recovery from head trauma becomes poorer as the duration of unconsciousness increases. By implication, if the patient is to survive, the prognosis becomes poorer for successful communication. After following 15 open- and closed-head-trauma patients for 1 year, Najenson and others[1] concluded that even after prolonged coma communication recovery was possible. Groher[10] measured the relationship between language and memory test scores and the number of days unconscious in 14 patients who had suffered closed head trauma. He concluded that a positive relationship did exist for those patients who were unconscious for 6 or fewer days, and for 32 or more days. That is, patients who were unconscious for fewer than 6 days had better initial language and memory skills than other patients, and patients who were unconscious for more than 32 days had the poorest communication. These relationships remained the same for 6 months after regaining consciousness. Owing to the small number of patients in these studies and the lack of other empirical evidence relative to communication deficits and the length of unconsciousness, it is difficult to be sure that the duration of unconsciousness plays a direct role in either the initial communication deficits or their eventual outcome.

EFFECTS OF FOCAL AND DIFFUSE DAMAGE ON COMMUNICATION

Trauma to the skull is capable of producing focal, multifocal, and diffuse effects in any part of the central nervous system at any particular level with varying degrees of decompensation of communication. Usually, the location and extent of the lesion, together with the patient's age and premorbid medical history, will dictate the accompanying speech and language deficits. However, because head trauma can produce lesions at the trauma site, opposite it, and anywhere in between, it may be difficult initially, as Wertz[18] pointed out, to classify the resultant symptoms. Luria[8] suggested that it was too difficult to localize the pathology immediately after the trauma (both open and closed) but that localizable signs could be forthcoming after a 1-month period when brain edema had subsided.

It is generally accepted that closed head injuries tend to produce more diffuse pathology,[18,19] whereas open head injuries produce more focal pathology.[11,14]

Luria[8] found that actual localization of pathology—whether it was focal or diffuse—was easier in closed head injuries because the dura remained intact. Understanding the implications for diagnosis and treatment of whether or not a patient has a communication disorder secondary to a closed (diffuse) or open (focal) head injury is well known. Focal left cortical pathology usually results in aphasia, whereas diffuse pathology results in disturbances of awareness, attentiveness, memory, perception, and orientation, of which aphasia is a part.

APHASIA SECONDARY TO TRAUMATIC AND VASCULAR ORIGINS

Many investigations of aphasia in the past 30 years have selected their subjects without regard to whether the etiologic factor producing the aphasia was vascular or traumatic. In those patients who had suffered from closed head trauma, there usually is no neurologic evidence to support a unilateral focal lesion. In light of the present knowledge about the effects of trauma on communication, the wisdom of grouping trauma and vascular patients with communication disorders into one empirical investigation is highly suspect.

Alajouanine[20] argued that traumatic language problems did not differ from those of vascular etiology because both had localizable damage; however, their prognoses may be different because trauma patients tended to be younger. It was not clear in this study whether or not Alajouanine meant closed or open head trauma. In their discussion of recovery, Kertesz and McCabe[21] acknowledged the uniqueness of trauma patients by providing a separate analysis of their recovery, noting that their recovery was better and faster than that of patients with vascular disease and communication disorders. They also alluded to the young age of the trauma patients as a variable that may play an important role in recovery.

One of the first studies to separate patients with aphasia secondary to vascular insults and trauma was completed by Heilman, Safron, and Geschwind[22] in 1971. It is one of the first efforts to systematically study a group of patients, all of whom evidenced speech and language pathology secondary to closed head trauma. Although their evaluation of the patients selected focused on types of aphasia, these authors did note that the most common form of aphasia in this group (anomia) was often associated with other higher cortical functions.

The differences between the types of speech and language performance of trauma patients and patients with vascular disease were also a part of the investigation by Halpern, Darley, and Brown.[9] They tested a group of 40 patients with neurologic involvement, using 10 parameters of speech and language performance. The pattern of performance in the trauma group was clearly different from that in patients who suffered impairment from vascular etiologies. As summarized earlier, Halpern, Darley, and Brown[9] felt that the pattern of performance by the trauma patients was most consistent with confused language, wherein patients evidenced specific language impairment (not as severe as those with vascular insults) and a generalized disorientation that affects the structure and relevancy of language.

The literature of the past 5 years has begun to suggest that patients who suffer head trauma—in particular, closed head trauma—may have aphasia but that they also may have additional cognitive deficits, including memory and perceptual disorders, disorientation, difficulty relating to the environment, faulty judgment and reasoning, difficulty in open-ended language situations that produces irrelevant responses and confabulation, and problems with so-called higher-level and more abstract uses of language.[10,11,18,23] Such behaviors are usually not found in patients with aphasia secondary to cerebrovascular disease.

The fact that it is difficult to account for the poor communication skills of trauma patients based upon only a description of aphasia has been most recently explored by Hagen, Malkmus, and Burditt,[11] who argue that the language impairments seen in trauma patients are part of an underlying cognitive disorganization and are, therefore, apart and separate from other language disturbances that are neurologically based. Moss[24] has summarized the cognitive approach to diagnosis and treatment by noting that what have been damaged are the supportive processes for communication, of which speech and language are just one part. The theoretical underpinnings of the cognitive approach in understanding the communication deficits of trauma patients are most useful because they allow one not only to explain specific speech and language deficits, but to link these deficits to the oft-observed disorders of memory, orientation, perception, and abnormal behaviors, which have received special attention in other sections of this book.

SPECIFIC SPEECH AND LANGUAGE DEFICITS

Luria[8] divided the aphasic symptomatology of both open- and closed-trauma left hemispheric lesions into three major categories: (1) total aphasia, which was a severe loss in the powers of expression and reception of language and was accompanied by loss of ability to attend—this form usually lasted for the first 2 to 3 weeks; (2) typical aphasic symptomatology, including disorders of auditory comprehension, naming, word-finding, and reading and writing disturbances, not accompanied by other disorders of cognitive function such as attention, perception, or memory; and (3) subtle and slight loss of language in which expressive output was less smooth, articulation impairment on difficult or more unusual words, and poor comprehension of more difficult grammatical constructions, all of which were not equally apparent at all times, especially when fatigued.

Leischner,[5] in a group of 55 patients with open head trauma, found that the majority evidenced deficits in both the expression and reception of language secondary to lesions in the left parietal and temporoparietal lobes. The second most common finding was an expressive aphasia, followed by sensory aphasia and anomias. In addition, most patients evidenced agraphias, alexias, finger agnosia, constructive disorders, and apraxias.

Heilman, Safron, and Geschwind[22] studied 13 patients with closed head trauma and aphasia. Using the Boston Test for Aphasia, they divided their subjects into two major groupings based on expressive and receptive language scores. Nine of the 13 patients demonstrated anomic dysphasia that was characterized by mostly fluent speech with verbal paraphasias and circumlocutions. Their comprehension and repetition abilities were good, but they evidenced abnormal naming skills, especially to confrontation. Six of these nine had additional defects not unlike those found by Leischner, including right-left confusion, finger agnosia, dyscalculia, and dyslexia. The remaining four patients demonstrated Wernicke aphasia.

Five of the 10 patients studied by Halpern, Darley, and Brown[9] who evidenced confused language skills were patients suffering from trauma of less than 3 months' duration. These patients were measured in 10 categories of intellectual and language functioning. Confused patients evidenced deficits in all 10 categories. The highest percent of impairment for this group was arithmetic, followed by reading comprehension, writing to dictation, and relevance. The least affected areas were fluency, auditory retention, naming, and syntax. The category of language relevance separated this group from those with aphasia, general intellectual impairment, and apraxia. The authors also commented on the fact that these patients gave bizarre responses to the testing stimuli, leading them to conclude that clarity in thought process and accuracy of memory were impaired. Such irrelevance in their responses was not evident to the patients, and they made no attempts to correct them. Lack of relevance in language output has been frequently mentioned by other investigators as one of the hallmarks of patients suffering from head trauma.[10,11,23]

Groher,[10] using the Porch Index of Communicative Ability (PICA), measured the speech and language characteristics of 14 closed-head-trauma patients immediately after regaining consciousness and at monthly intervals up to 6 months. Patients initially showed a marked reduction in all language modalities when compared with other aphasics. Verbal skills were the strongest (33rd percentile), while graphic (12th percentile) and gestural (6th percentile) skills lagged behind. Most difficulty on the PICA was noted on subtests 2 and 3, which require the patient to show the examiner what to do with common environmental objects. In addition, comprehension of reading material was poor, a finding both Heilman, Safron, and Geschwind[22] and Halpern, Darley, and Brown[9] reported. All subjects initially had a marked anomia, with both literal and nominal paraphasic errors during production. Patients were unable to write the names of objects and could not write to dictation. By the end of the fifth month, all language skills were at the 70th percentile level. Patients were able to make their needs known verbally and could sustain an informal conversation. In fact, most observers felt that their communication skills were normal. However, standardized testing revealed that patients continued to show delays in simple and complex auditory processing tasks, irrelevance in language output, and difficulty in spelling and sentence construction.

Kaplan, Phillip, and Halper[25] followed six patients with closed head trauma for a period of 2 to 6 months, rating their cognitive function upon admission and discharge. Part of this evaluation included general communication status, oral expression, reading, writing, and dysarthria. Other aspects of cognitive functioning included memory and visual perception. All patients had impairments on all language tasks ranging from moderate to severe. After discharge, most patients had mild reading and moderate writing disturbance. Four of the patients' overall communication dysfunctions were judged as moderate impairment, while the remaining three patients evidenced mild impairment. None of the seven reached the communication level of minimal impairment.

Kriendler, Michailescu, and Fradis[26] studied verbal fluency in 8 closed-trauma and 12 open-trauma patients immediately after suffering the insult and 1 to 3 months later. Their speaking rate compared with that of normal persons was low in 10 cases and normal in nine, while one had complete loss of speech. Re-evaluation of speaking rate showed the rate had increased in 18 patients. The speaking time and the number of utterances had also risen significantly by 3 months postinjury.

Hagen, Malkmus, and Burditt[11] list some of the more typical language problems that usually all occur at some time during the patient's recovery. These include word retrieval problems, decreased auditory comprehension, poor visual and reading comprehension, expressive language that may be characterized as jargon, linguistically intact statements that lack relevancy, confabulation, circumlocution, tangential expressions, failure to inhibit the flow of language, and problems with verbal and graphic syntax.

THE PROBLEM OF DYSARTHRIA

The prevalence and type of dysarthria following head trauma are not well known. In general, the type and its effect on speech intelligibility will be reflected by the locus of damage in the central nervous system. Diffuse upper motor involvement produces pseudobulbar effects, whereas brain stem contusions produce flaccid effects. During the acute stages of recovery, both systems may be involved.

Rusk, Block, and Lowman[4] reported that in a group of 93 trauma patients, approximately one third (30) evidenced dysarthria in their acute illness. In follow-up studies between 5 and 15 years, 15 patients were unchanged, while 14 patients had significantly improved. Specific measures of improvement were not discussed. Dresser and associates[14] reported that 8 percent of 864 Korean veterans who had suffered head trauma (closed and open) continued to show signs of dysarthria after 15 years. Hagen, Malkmus, and Burditt[11] acknowledge the presence of dysarthria in trauma patients secondary to both neurologic systems damage and cognitive (failure to monitor articulation) deficits. They reported such symptomatology as articulatory imprecision, reduced or accelerated rates, reduced audibility, and monopitch and monoloudness, which they feel is part of the voice of confusion. Najenson and coworkers[1] also have noted the prevalence of the harsh and monotonous voice quality with reduced breath support. They found that the dysarthric symptomatology continued to be present after language skills had approached normal levels. Malkmus[23] has estimated that 20 percent of her patients with language deficits also evidenced either mixed, flaccid, or spastic forms of dysarthria, which initially produce severe intelligibility scores. However, her experience suggests that good intelligibility returns after 12 months. All 14 of the closed-head-trauma patients studied by Groher[10] evidenced dysarthria after regaining consciousness. Nine of the 14 had spastic (pseudobulbar-type) dysarthria, and five had spastic-ataxic involvement. Six of the nine patients with spastic dysarthria completely resolved within 6 months, while the remaining eight continued to evidence only minimal intelligibility problems, none of which significantly interfered with communication. Kaplan, Phillip, and Halper[25] reported similar improvement in their patients, noting that all seven patients initially had dysarthria ranging from severe to moderate, while the majority had only mild effects at discharge 2 to 6 months later.

RECOVERY OF COMMUNICATION

In the acute stages of recovery from head trauma, maintenance of vital life functions is the primary concern of the medical staff. As the patient achieves medical stability, attention is focused on the evaluation of motor and sensory systems and failure to communicate with the environment. Establishing a viable communication system between patient and staff greatly enhances the ease with which medical care can be provided. Communication can become an important barometer for assessing change in the patient's acute medical status. Therefore, it can help provide a valuable dimension in the physician's prognostic statements to the family. As the patient improves, documentation of positive changes in communication may be most important in determining the quality of survival, many times dictating future social and vocational goals.

Many acutely ill trauma patients are able to function only at vegetative levels. Early communication assessment is not possible using traditional standardized testing measures that require patient responsiveness and a sufficient attention span. The use of the communication evaluation in the acute patient as a tool for prognostication has received little attention. Teasdale and Jennett[27] felt that an evaluation of verbal functioning is an important variable in the early phrases of medical management. Miller[28] listed lack of verbal responsiveness in the acute stages as the least important prognosticator out of 12 factors in determining eventual outcome.

Recognizing the need to describe acute communication recovery accurately, Hagen, Malkmus, and Durham[29] developed eight descriptive categories that aid in describing communicative recovery. This categorization is important because it is able to link communication recovery with cognitive recovery. Therefore, it relies not only on charting the patient's communication skills but on observation of behaviors other than communication that are important prerequisites for meaningful communication. The scale ranges from level 1 (no response), in which the patient is unaware of any external input; to level 4, (confused-agitated) where the patient responds primarily to one's own internal confusion with inappropriate verbalizations and confabulation; to level 8 (purposeful and appropriate), where the patient is now able to communicate effectively by integrating recent and past events although social, emotional, and intellectual capacities may still be reduced in situations involving the use of more complex and abstract language strategies.

Ideally, information on the recovery of communicative function in trauma patients should include not only the amount and kinds of functions recovered, but also data on how fast the recovery occurred. In general, investigators have found that patients with communication disorders secondary to head trauma recover more communicative skills at a faster rate than patients with vascular etiologies. Verbal and comprehension skills tend to parallel each other in their recovery and begin to peak at 6 months, although recovery past this period has been documented.

Residual language deficits past 6 months are usually found on more abstract aspects of communication, especially reading and writing.

Najenson and associates[30] studied a group of 40 closed- and open-trauma patients who had been rendered unconscious, all regaining consciousness within 3 months. The age range was 19 to 45. Using the Functional Communication Profile (FCP), they found that after the initial evaluation, 20 of the 40 showed signs of aphasia. After 6 months, six patients were not aphasic. During the 6-month period, they observed a great deal of variability in recovery of functions, although patterns of recovery did exist. All subjects showed progressive improvement, more in listening and reading skills than in oral expression and writing. After 6 months, most language difficulty was on higher-level reading tasks and narrative writing. No patient after 6 months remained in the severe category of impairment on the FCP.

Najenson and associates[1] studied the recovery pattern of another group of 15 patients, mostly with closed head injuries. The mean age was 33, and nine of the 15 underwent craniectomy. Nine of the 15 functionally recovered, while six remained vegetative. Recovery of this group was similar to that of the first group. Visual and auditory comprehension returned first, followed by oral expression. However, this group showed later recovery of reading and writing skills. The first signs of recovery after regaining consciousness ranged from 3 weeks to 5 months, with complete recovery ranging from 4 to 9 months. The authors noted that communication recovery paralleled locomotor recovery.

Using the PICA, Groher[10] measured the speech and language characteristics of patients with closed head trauma immediately after regaining consciousness (mean time 9 days) and each month for a period of 5 months. All subjects were male veterans, and the mean age was 31. Unlike the recovery patterns reported by Najenson and associates,[1,30] Groher found that verbal skills were the first to return and were superior to comprehension capabilities up to the first month. Significant improvement in comprehension, verbal, and graphic skills was noted at 2 months after onset. Verbal skills improved significantly up to the fourth month. After 4 months, comprehension abilities were as good as verbal skills. Writing performance was just becoming functional after 4 months. As language improved, so did negative behavior patterns such as striking out during nursing care and uncooperative behavior during therapeutic rehabilitation sessions. All patients were capable of making their needs known verbally after 5 months but still evidenced signs of aphasia characterized by processing delays and word-finding difficulty. After 6 months, patients scored well on most standardized measurements for aphasia but still evidenced problems of relevancy, inhibition of verbal output, and sequential organization of ideas into logical outcomes. After 6 months, six of the 14 patients returned to work. All six had difficulty with job assignments, primarily related to continued ineffective problem-solving using communication, poor memory, and poor judgment.

Reporting on their experience with 2000 head-trauma patients over a 17-year period, Hagen, Malkmus, and Burditt[11] found that recovery of communication skills was closely allied to, and even dependent upon, the patient's cognitive recovery. Levels of cognitive function during recovery serve as important determinants of communication recovery. It is these authors' contention that cognitive (and therefore communicative) recovery is hierarchical, beginning with the recovery of attention mechanisms (both internal and external), discrimination, seriation, recovery of memory, categorization, association, and finally skills involving analysis and synthesis of input and output.

Six of the seven trauma patients presented by Kertesz and McCabe[21] had achieved Aphasia Quotient scores of 90 and above on the Western Aphasia Battery after a period of three months. Initial Aphasia Quotient scores ranged from below 30 to 88. One patient continued to show improvement after 2 years. Porch[31] also has presented data suggesting that the recovery of trauma patients can continue past 2 years. He found that their recovery pattern was characterized by a series of recovery spurts followed by plateaus. Gradual improvement was seen up to 32 months after onset.

There are little specific data on the speech and language characteristics of trauma patients beyond the sixth month of recovery. Groher[10] reported that although patients were not typically aphasic, they continued to be unable to use their language to solve problems at home and at work.

Malkmus[23] confirms this impression, commenting that most patients at 6 months have intact language skills as tested by standardized aphasia test batteries; however, their language capabilities are only sufficient for more concrete and simple tasks. For instance, auditory and graphic retention of material beyond one sentence may be difficult, especially if the requirement is to focus on one specific bit of information. In general, the retention and integration of auditory and graphic information become poorer as the amount and complexity increases. Malkmus[23] found that expressive language skills after 6 months are intact for most daily conversational needs but, when patients are asked to formulate specific responses, began to deteriorate. Patients often continue to evidence ideational perseveration, with difficulty shifting from topic to topic, continued word-retrieval problems, disorganization of thought content with incompleteness of expression, and reduced abstract verbal reasoning capacity. Groher[32] has found that this type of language performance interferes with patients' psychosocial recovery because their language is often interpreted not as organically impaired, but as part of a personality disorder.

Difficulty with higher-level language skills past 6 months was also noted by Thomsen.[33] In a follow-up study of 12 patients with aphasia secondary to closed head trauma, Thomsen found that four had no characteristics of aphasia but had aphasic traits like poor verbal learning. Patients also showed continued difficulty on language problems involving analysis of synonyms, antonyms, metaphors, and picture description.

Groswasser and colleagues[34] studied a group of 20 patients with closed and open head traumas with aphasia at admission, at 6 months, and at 30 months after onset. After 6 months, 14 of the 20 remained aphasic; at 30 months, nine remained aphasic, with the majority of scores on the Functional Communication Profile ranging between 51 and 74.

In a 15-year follow-up of 864 open- and closed-trauma patients, Dresser and associates[14] found that 53 of the 88 who were aphasic were now employed. This implies that their communication deficits did not significantly interfere with their employment. In comparison with the group without aphasia, these authors felt that the presence of aphasia was a significant predictor of unemployment.

SUMMARY

The study of communication disorders secondary to head trauma is only in its initial stages. The importance of the communicative act in the rehabilitative process cannot be underestimated, as the constructs of language are closely tied with other cognitive dimensions such as perception, memory, orientation, attention, and psychosocial behavior, all of which are frequently impaired. Because of the frequent involvement of more than one cognitive system, the treatment of specific language, perceptual, or memory deficits should be interdependent, and, as such, places demands on all professionals of the rehabilitation team to coordinate their efforts. Prerequisite behaviors for successful communication—including environmental awareness, selective attention, and auditory and visual discrimination—are often impaired acutely and need to receive the special attention of the speech/language pathologist.

Patients must be directed through these early stages of recovery if they are to receive the maximum benefits from communicative remediation efforts.

The evidence presented suggests that communication disorders that result from head trauma are different from those whose etiology may be vascular, neoplastic, or metabolic. Trauma patients with communication disorders tend to be younger, display multiple cognitive system involvement, recover more language at a faster rate, improve for a longer period of time, and have the opportunity to return to some type of work setting more often than patients with vascular disease and aphasia. These differences suggest that the approach to treatment of trauma patients may be different from that used with other aphasic patients. While more traditional aphasia rehabilitative techniques may be used at some point in the patient's recovery, other types of treatment strategies must also be initiated. These include structuring the patient's environment to aid in orientation and communication; providing constant, organized language inputs at appropriate levels of complexity; providing tasks that develop selective attention and discrimination of incoming stimuli; developing environments that allow the patient to respond in his or her strongest expressive modality; and eventually providing treatment to assist the patient in solving life's everyday problems that are dependent on language.

Even though most patients recover basic language skills by 6 months, they continue to show deficits in the analysis and synthesis of receptive and expressive language skills. These skills are necessary for any successful communication beyond more automatic and social conversation levels, in the performance of job assignments, and in the learning of new information. Patients need continued speech and language rehabilitation even though their performance may appear normal to most observers. Remediation should be directed toward assisting the patient in retaining specific bits of critical information gathered from larger pieces (auditorily and graphically), analysis and/or summarization and categorization of language inputs, organization of expressive outputs into logical sequences, and concentration on shifting topics without significant delay. All tasks should be oriented toward focusing the patient to perform in a way that is relevant to the stimulus input, be it self- or environment-stimulated. Success in job performance and in psychosocial adjustment will depend on how well the patient is able to perform on these more abstract tasks of language use.

REFERENCES

1. NAJENSON, T, ET AL: *Recovery of communicative functions after prolonged traumatic coma.* Scand J Rehabil Med 10:15, 1978.
2. RUSSELL, WR: *Cerebral involvement in head injury: A study based on the examination of 200 cases.* Brain 55:549, 1932.
3. GLASER, MA AND SHAFER, FP: *Skull and brain trauma: Their sequelae: Clinical review of 255 cases.* JAMA 98:271, 1932.
4. RUSK, HA, BLOCK, JM, AND LOWMAN, EW: *Rehabilitation of the brain-injured patient: A report of 157 cases with long term follow-up of 118.* In WALKER, E, CAVENESS, W, AND CRITCHLEY, M (EDS): *The Late Effects of Head Injury.* Charles C Thomas, Springfield, Ill, 1969.
5. LEISCHNER, A: *The pathological brain syndrome in the brain injured.* In WALKER, E, CAVENESS, W, AND CRITCHLEY, M (EDS): *The Late Effects of Head Injury.* Charles C Thomas, Springfield, Ill, 1969.
6. RUSSELL, WR AND ESPIR, MLE: *Traumatic Aphasia: A Study in War Wounds of the Brain.* Oxford University Press, London, 1961.
7. LONDON, PS: *Some observations on the course of events after severe injury of the head.* Ann R Coll Surg Engl 41:460, 1967.
8. LURIA, AR: *Traumatic Aphasia: Its Syndromes, Psychology and Treatment.* Mouton, The Hague, 1970.

9. HALPERN, H, DARLEY, FL, AND BROWN, JR: *Differential language and neurologic characteristics in cerebral involvement.* J Speech Hear Disord 38:162, 1973.
10. GROHER, M: *Language and memory disorders following closed head trauma.* J Speech Hear Res 20:212, 1977.
11. HAGEN, C, MALKMUS, D, AND BURDITT, G: *Intervention Strategies for Language Disorders Secondary to Head Trauma: Short Course.* American Speech-Language and Hearing Association, Atlanta, 1979.
12. GOLDSTEIN, K: *After-Effects of Brain Injuries in War: Their Evaluation and Treatment.* Grune & Stratton, New York, 1942.
13. HOOK, O: *Comments on rehabilitation of the brain-injured.* In WALKER, E, CAVENESS, W, AND CRITCHLEY, M (EDS): *The Late Effects of Head Injury.* Charles C Thomas, Springfield, Ill, 1969.
14. DRESSER, AC, ET AL: *Gainful employment following head injury: Prognostic factors.* Arch Neurol 73:111, 1973.
15. PENSE, F: *Diagnosis and therapie der neurosen bei hir neurletzten.* In REHWALDIED, E (ED): *Das Hirntrauma.* G Thieme Verlag, Stuttgart, 1956.
16. HILLBOM, E: *Delayed effects of traumatic brain injuries, neurological remarks.* Acta Psychiatr Scand 137:7, 1959.
17. TEUBER, HL: *Recovery of function after brain injury in man.* In *Outcome of Severe Damage of the Central Nervous System.* Ciba Foundation Symposium. Elsevier-North Holland, New York, 1975.
18. WERTA, R: *Neuropathologies of speech and language: An introduction to patient management.* In JOHNS, DF (ED): *Clinical Management of Neurogenic Communicative Disorders.* Little, Brown & Co, Boston, 1978.
19. BROOKSHIRE, R: *An Introduction to Aphasia.* BRK Publishers, Minneapolis, 1973.
20. ALAJOUANINE, T, ET AL: *Etude de 43 cas d'aphasie post-traumatique.* Encephale 46:1, 1957.
21. KERTESZ, A AND MCCABE, P: *Recovery patterns and prognosis in aphasia.* Brain 100:1, 1977.
22. HEILMAN, K, SAFRON, A, AND GESCHWIND, N: *Closed head trauma and aphasia.* J Neurol Neurosurg Psychiatry 34:265, 1971.
23. MALKMUS, D: Personal communication, 1980.
24. MOSS, C: Unpublished material, 1980.
25. KAPLAN, P, PHILLIP, P, AND HALPER, A: *Recovery of self-care activities in patients with traumatic brain damage.* Presented at the 3rd Annual Post-Graduate Course on the Rehabilitation of the Traumatic Brain-Injured Adult, Williamsburg, Va, 1979.
26. KRIENDLER, A, MICHAILESCU, L, AND FRADIS, A: *Speech fluency in aphasics.* Brain Lang 9:199, 1980.
27. TEASDALE, G AND JENNETT, B: *Assessment of coma and impaired consciousness.* Lancet 2:81, 1974.
28. MILLER, JD: *Early diagnosis and management of severe head trauma: Implications for rehabilitation.* Presented at the 3rd Annual Post-Graduate Course on the Rehabilitation of the Traumatic Brain-Injured Adult, Williamsburg, Va, 1979.
29. HAGEN, C, MALKMUS, D, AND DURHAM, P: *Levels of cognitive functioning.* In *Rehabilitation of the Head Injured Adult.* Professional Staff Association, Downey, Calif, 1979.
30. NAJENSON, T, ET AL: *Prognostic factors in rehabilitation after severe head injury: Assessment six months after trauma.* Scand J Rehabil Med 7:101, 1975.
31. PORCH, B: *Recovery from Aphasia.* PICA Workshop, Albuquerque, NM, 1976.
32. GROHER, M: Unpublished material, 1979.
33. THOMSEN, IV: *Evaluation and outcome of aphasia in patients with severe closed head trauma.* J Neurol Neurosurg Psychiatry 38:713, 1975.
34. GROSWASSER, Z, ET AL: *Re-evaluation of prognostic factors in rehabilitation after severe head injury: Assessment thirty months after trauma.* Scand J Rehabil Med 9:147, 1977.

Chapter 12

COGNITIVE DEFICITS

Yehuda Ben-Yishay, Ph.D.
Leonard Diller, Ph.D.

The assessment of cognitive disturbances after traumatic brain injuries is a critical feature in the understanding of the nature of the underlying processes, the planning of remedial interventions, prognostication about the future potential for recovery of functions, and the postrehabilitation management of the patient. The assessment is guided and limited by (1) the definition of the problems encountered by the patient, (2) the level of analysis of the behavioral disturbances, (3) the methods of measurement employed, and (4) the specific objectives of the inquiry.

The overall orientation of this chapter is a remedial-interventional (i.e., rehabilitation-relevant) one. Viewed from this perspective, it is futile and simplistic to reduce the problem of cognitive deficits in the head-trauma patient to the level of routine psychologic testing. The understanding of cognitive disturbances in head-trauma patients in a remedial-rehabilitation setting is focused by two major questions: What does a clinician diagnose and what does a clinician treat? It takes place in a context of a consideration of questions such as, What is the nature of the complaint? What is the specific purpose of the examination? At what particular stage of the patient's recovery following the trauma is the examination undertaken? What is the overall context of the examination (i.e., is the patient an inpatient, undergoing multiple treatments, or an outpatient)? What type of brain injuries did the patient sustain; what are the patient's history, present personal status, and the network of "significant others?" In short, the assessment of a head-trauma patient is a dynamic, multidimensional, clinical process that is buffeted by many considerations external to the narrow act of testing.

Before articulating our rehabilitation-focused approach to the definition and the assessment of cognitive deficits in head-trauma patients, we shall briefly (1) review some of the influences and considerations that helped formulate the current trends in clinical neuropsychologic practices; (2) point out some of the main points of convergence and divergence between ours and the more traditional neuropsychologic approaches; and (3) indicate the existing gaps in knowledge as well as methodology that necessitated the development of our (the Institute of Rehabilitation Medicine [IRM], New York University) particular approach.

DIFFERENT APPROACHES TO DEFINING COGNITIVE DEFICITS

Cognitive disturbances are difficulties in information processing due to brain damage, which alter the ways in which the person experiences and responds to stimuli and interface with everyday living. While it is readily apparent even to the naive observer that changes in mental life can occur after brain damage, students of the problem have generally interpreted these changes in terms of the dominating analogies or metaphors of a given time. Contemporary students of cognition view mental life as a system of information flow. Problems in information processing account for why people fail to respond adequately to the demands of their environment and why they are unable to use or organize their environment in the most effective way.

Approaches to the definition and the assessment of cognitive disturbances come from several traditions. It is useful to briefly point out the underlying thoughts that guided these traditions, because psychologic terms and their referents, which are used in assessment, may appear to be esoteric and somewhat removed from the realities of the patient's day-to-day problems and the management of these problems. We note four traditions.

PSYCHOMETRIC TRADITION

Assessment of cognitive deficits is viewed as an extension of clinical psychometric testing to a population of head-injured people. The psychometric approach has its origins in early 20th-century psychology when it was discovered that children's responses to standard types of questions and problems could be scored and the results compared with those of other children. These comparisons were used to identify differences in academic proficiency among individuals. The psychometric tradition has thus produced the well-known standard intelligence tests, which have been applied in a wide variety of settings outside the school system. Less well known, but equally important to our field, are two additional contributions of the psychometric tradition—one methodologic, and the other clinical.

Methodologically, it was discovered that the various tests yielded different scores that could be intercorrelated with each other. The result of such analyses that led to the further discovery of various clusters of correlations, which were called "factors." The statistical factors, in turn, then provided a way of looking at the organization of the various skills that constitute mental life. The factorial analytic approach led the way to envisioning mental life as being organized by a structure of factors, or clusters of skills and subskills. Indeed, a leading current psychometric theorist, Guilford,[1] postulates the presence of 128 basic abilities in humans, of which 88 are already known, while the others remain as yet to be identified.

The psychometrists' search for hypothesized abilities, or the attempts at detecting cognitive deficits after head injury on the basis of deviations from the presumed normal patterns of skill structure, is similar in spirit and style of approach to the attempt of 19th-century chemists who sought to understand the nature of matter by postulating a table of elements of a finite number and then proceeded to identify these elements empirically.

The factorial approach to the study of the organization of mental life has been used among others to examine the decline of mental life with aging or as a basis for the development of educational programs.

On a clinical level, it was pointed out that profiles of psychometric test results could be compared. It was reasonable to expect that profiles derived from brain-damaged people would differ from those obtained from normal people. Over the past 50 years, a voluminous body of literature has been developed in support of this tradition.[2] Although there is some dispute as to whether standard psychometric tests are in themselves sufficient, the logic of profile analysis remains. In brief, the expectation that test profiles of brain-damaged people would resemble each other in ways in which they did not resemble those of normal people is based on the idea of a structural like-mindedness appearing in patterns of test scores.[3]

CLINICAL NEUROLOGIC APPROACH

In a clinical neurologic examination, the examiner is looking for behavioral expressions of central nervous system damage. An attempt is made to describe specific deficits as well as overall patterns of deficits to arrive at a syndromal account of the problem. As part of this account, the neurologist tries to rule out competing explanations for failure on a given task. For example, before concluding that a task was failed because of a visual perceptual problem, one would first have to rule out the presence of other problems, such as poor visual acuity or inability to execute required movements, which might be the primary cause for the failure of the specific performance; and, second, one would also have to demonstrate that a failure in performance would occur as well in other tasks that have visual perception but no other abilities in common. The examination is a means of hypothesis testing to establish, more precisely, the nature of the deficit. In this method of reasoning where facts are tested by double disassociation,[4] a syndrome is not viewed as a statistical aggregate of deficits but as a precise description of a pattern of deviations.

The clinical neurologist capitalizes on some of the tools and the ways of reasoning of the experimental psychologist. Behavioral neurology, for example, received a great impetus from the work of Geschwind,[5] who showed how studies of the behavior of brain-damaged animals and people under different kinds of experimental conditions could be used to identify behavioral deficits in highly precise terms and thereby deduce the localization of brain damage in syndromes of aphasia and other disorders involving higher-level mental functions.

The clinical neurologic method provides a useful conceptual and methodologic tool for clinical investigation. It too is rooted in an approach based on 19th-century science. The model is basically that of the biologist who is trying to account for the purposeful nature of behavior, its development with age, and its breakdown in functions in various pathologic states. The relevance of normative considerations to neurologic assessment of cognitive deficits is a hotly debated issue. Some authors[5,6] have criticized the use of norms in neurologic diagnosis, arguing that neurologic diagnosis is not really based on statistical considerations, since a syndrome is a pattern that is determined by the inner organizations of symptoms. The syndrome constellation is a unique expression of a disturbance and not a statistical composite. Accurate prediction from one element in the syndrome to the next via a prediction that certain findings will covary and others will not confirms a neurologic diagnosis.

LEARNING THEORY APPROACH

A third approach to the understanding of cognitive deficits after head injury is via the examination of a head-injured person's ability to learn and to assimilate new information. This includes the examination of the patient's ability to respond to various types of modifications of the stimulus or response properties of the task, various types of cueing designed to elicit optimal behaviors, and different types of reinforcements. The use of various techniques for assessing the learning potential of the individual—that is, the study of the individual's capacity to modify behavior in response to systematically altered and controlled environmental contingencies—can be used as a clinical tool for the detection of the presence of brain injury as well as for insights into the kinds of strategies that might be useful for improving behavior. It has been advocated by a number of investigators,[7-10] studying a wide variety of patient populations. But the most systematic development in this area is the series of recent studies[11-14] showing that (1) there is a lawfulness in the stimulus condition, which can be quantified and scaled in a manner which makes some tasks easier and some harder to perform; (2) head-injured people can be trained and profit from progressive cueing, based on such ordering of tasks according to level of difficulty; (3) individuals with different levels of competence require different amounts of cueing, where a more capable person requires fewer cues than a less capable one to pass a task that is outside their respective "zones" of competence; (4) a number of hitherto described "qualitative" differences in style of performance between head-injured and non-head-injured people can be quantified and predicted; and (5) systematic remedial training can improve one's overall competence in the given task, but not necessarily alter the difference in style of approach to the task.

REHABILITATION APPROACH

Because of the basic concern in rehabilitation is with the disabled person's behaviors in daily life, the tendency is to focus on functional behaviors. Hence the expressions of the disability in the patient's naturalistic world—self-care, competence in daily life activities, work—become the ultimate data base for rehabilitation. For this reason, measures of impairment yielded by the three previous approaches are used in rehabilitation only insofar as they serve to elucidate the underpinnings of deficits in functional terms.[15] The functional orientation in rehabilitation has therefore molded the ways in which a patient's competence, or the lack of it, is being assessed. Thus, for instance, whether a person can grasp and release is measured in terms of whether or not the person could grasp and release a cup or other utensils rather than a contrived object. The concept of motoric competence in executing a series of self-care activities in daily life is measured in terms of how much assistance the person would require to perform that task. In regard to employment, the emphasis has not been on standard tests of generic skills or of overall aptitude but on "job samples," or on-the-job trials.

Thus, cognitive disturbances may be assessed from four different standpoints: (1) psychometrically, in terms of deviations from expected single test scores or from expected (theoretically assumed) patterns of underlying skill structures; (2) neurologically, as syndromal formulations that trace and relate the behavioral deficits to the underlying disturbances in the mechanisms of behavior, which short-circuit the orderly flow of information processing; (3) remedially, in terms of sampling the individual's ability to acquire, retain, and assimilate new information, that is, to learn and to modify one's behavior; and (4) functionally, in terms of sampling basic or compound daily life functional competencies. Each of the above approaches to the assessment of cognitive deficits following a brain injury starts off from a different basis and, therefore, asks a different set of questions; each may have developed different methods of assessment, which in many instances may address the same or different contents. Our approach to assessment of cognitive deficits, which will be outlined further below, draws on all four of these standpoints, for each has something valuable to contribute, not only from a methodologic point of view, but also in terms of content.

Two important aspects of the assessment of cognitive deficits after head injuries require further comment in this context: the issue of the use of norms for comparisons and the problems of assessing functional limitations. Each of these will be briefly examined.

USE OF NORMS

Three types of normative comparisons are pertinent—comparisons of the brain-damaged person's performance with that of normal persons, with the performance of other brain-damaged people, and with the level of functioning of the person prior to the brain injury. All three are pertinent for different kinds of questions, but they may be differentially salient. For example, with regard to diagnosis all are pertinent. With regard to employment, data on normal persons are most relevant. With regard to prognosis, data on other traumatically brain-damaged populations are most pertinent. With regard to questions relating to the individual patient's own future goals, data on premorbid functioning may be most pertinent. Most tests that are standardized on normal persons may be insensitive to differences at the lower ends of the normal range on a given task, so that important distinctions between different individuals or changes within the same individual may be lost. On the other hand, tests standardized on brain-damaged populations might have ceilings that are too low for normal persons. Also, with regard to norms for the head-injured populations, there are as yet no bodies of norms that might serve the multiple purposes of assessment, such as serving as markers for training by gauging the extent of recovery in given functions or as guidelines in the management of patients. The establishment of such norms is limited by the fact that basic demographic factors such as age, sex, education, ethnic background, type of injury, and duration since injury are known to influence the patterns of psychometric tests. Hence, one would require vast bodies of such data to be available for the proper comparisons.

PROBLEMS IN ESTABLISHING THE LONG-TERM MENTAL SEQUELAE OF TRAUMATIC HEAD INJURY

By now it has been established with virtual certainty[16] that the long-term mental sequelae outstrip the physical as a cause of difficulties with the vocational and personal rehabilitation of the patient and with the problems encountered in the areas of living arrangements, social readaptation, and strains on family life. Similarly, as empirical evidence is accumulating, there is a growing realization that many of the mental sequelae of severe traumatic head injury resemble those encountered in varying degrees in patients with diffuse structural brain disorders of nontraumatic origin, such as aging or arteriosclerosis,[17] or patients with brain damage resulting from cerebrovascular accident, postinfectious diseases, or postsurgical sequelae.[18,19]

There is, however, still no agreement among students on which of the person's behaviors should be considered under the rubric of "physical," when assessing the sequelae of brain injury, and which should be assessed as part of the "mental" sequelae. It may be said, in general, that those who concentrate the study on the effects of head injury on the functional behaviors of the total person (which unfold within "naturalistic" settings and are the expressions of the person's "coping"—adaptive solutions to the particular demands of particular situations) tend to view the study of single isolated symptoms, or of one-to-one relationships between focal areas of cerebral impairment and specific, circumscribed behavioral deficits, as being not particularly relevant to the concerns of the clinician, whose major interest lies in assessing the functional aftermath of the brain injury and the possibilities of restoration of functions.[16,17,20]

Moreover, as has been recently pointed out,[21] the assessment of functional disorders in the head-injured patient must be comprehensive in nature and should encompass in its scope a wide spectrum of measurements that do not belong in the current repertoire of any single clinical discipline (e.g., neuropsychiatry, neurology, traditional clinical neuropsychology, and clinical psychology). A convenient scheme is to divide the behaviors that are to be singled out for careful scrutiny into three broad categories.

The first category is what was traditionally termed the "content" areas. Under this rubric belong (1) measures of the ability to imitate and to execute, with one hand alone or with both hands in synchrony, simple motor actions, including acts involving simple coordination, strength, and steadiness of hand control; (2) measures of integrative functions, involving the varieties of perceptual, perceptual-motor, and sensory-motor interactions; (3) assessment of the various (acquired) skills possessed by the individual; and (4) a wide spectrum of measures of acquired intelligence.

The second category includes the various "process" areas. The term refers to areas of functioning such as (1) attention, concentration, and psychomotor persistence; (2) memory functions; (3) problem-solving abilities, including the ability to learn, retain, and assimilate new information; and (4) judgment.

The third category includes aspects of performance which, in a strict sense, do not qualify as either content or process parameters, but which contribute or modify, to a significant degree, the overall functions that are subsumed under the former two categories. This category includes basic psychophysical underpinnings of more complex functional behaviors, such as (1) the capacity to voluntarily assume the mental and physical set described as "initiative," "spontaneity,"[20] or "dynamia"[22]; (2) physical and mental stamina and endurance[21]; and (3) the basic, physiologic-vegetative components of emotions, which, along with the expressive (i.e., body manifestations) and the associated imagery components, form the basis for the normal emotional reactions in a person.[20]

In the more classic tradition of neuropsychology, the basic concern was more with establishing specific brain-behavior relationships, or the elucidation of theoretical notions, than with the comprehensive "mapping" of the many blatant and more subtle forms in which mental sequelae of head injury impinge on and manifest themselves in the various functional life domains of the patient. But even the more recent, clinically oriented studies tend to be delimited to certain aspects of behavior only, such as memory and orientation problems,[23] cognitive disorganization or deficits in acquired and process intelligence,[24–27] subtle impairments of language,[28] problems in auditory attention,[29] memory deficits,[30] perplexity, fatigue, distractability,[31] and disturbances in emotional responses.[32]

Thus, as we have pointed out earlier, a rehabilitation-oriented approach to the study of mental sequelae of head injury requires the careful "mapping" of the individual patient's deficit areas, along the entire continuum of behaviors that are comprised of the three categories of measurement mentioned above, for the understanding of cognitive defects in head injury is incomplete when it is confined to the higher-level intellectual and symbolic functions alone. And from the standpoint of a total organism approach, it is "not at all appropriate to omit the symptoms belonging to defects in the lower level functions, the so-called motor and sensory instrumentalities, which are necessary for realization of the symbolic functions"[17] of the patient.

In assessing the head-injured individual, it would therefore be very useful for the clinician to have a comprehensive listing of the critical—that is, representative—areas of deficits. Such a listing, which should be cast in a descriptive language, could then serve as a checklist of functional "descriptors" against which, as a first step only, the patient's various mental and cognitive sequelae could be "mapped." Then, a more precise, in-depth, dynamic assessment would follow, culminating in a differential diagnosis with specific, operationalized recommendations for remedial intervention.

PROBLEMS IN THE ASSESSMENT OF FUNCTIONAL LIMITATIONS DUE TO MENTAL SEQUELAE OF HEAD INJURY

During the past 10 years, the field of rehabilitation has begun to address issues such as progress in rehabilitation, outcomes, the relationships between these and severity of the disability, and questions relating to goal setting in individuals who have chronic disabling conditions. Such issues are dictated by pragmatic considerations, and to deal with them in an adequate fashion requires the methodical and systematic gathering of much information that relates to the individual's day-to-day functioning in naturalistic settings. The traditional way of assessing cognitive deficits in terms of psychometric tests or circumscribed clinical observations will simply not suffice. Hence, rehabilitation workers, as indicated above, felt impelled to develop the tools and to broaden the scope of their investigation, to include among their diagnostic tools measures of functional competence in a wide variety of naturalistic settings.

The recent advances in the assessment of functional limitations have not as yet been applied to the situation of the person with cognitive deficits due to brain damage. When one approaches the question of the effects of cognitive defects on the person's functional life domain, many important generic questions begin to surface: How does memory loss that is identified by a psychologic test manifest itself in everyday life? How do cognitive deficits impact on interpersonal relations? How do cognitive deficits affect the person's communication skills in everyday life? What is the specific impact of various deficits on the person's work abilities? The patient who performs well on a battery of memory tests but cannot remember being tested on repeated occasions is a good example. In short, the interface between cognitive deficits, as measured by specific psychometric tests, and the quality-of-life issues has not been well explored.

To adequately transpose cognitive deficits, as measured by specific behavioral and psychometric tests and observations, into functional and quality-of-life units of observation requires yet another step. Three concepts are implicit in this process and bear a brief discussion in this context. These concepts are capacity levels, statuses, and roles. Of the three, the concept of capacity levels needs little further explanation since it actually refers to the data base that is obtained from the various tests and behavioral assessment procedures discussed above. But the place of status and role evaluation in a rehabilitation context is removed from traditional thinking in clinical neuropsychology, and these concepts therefore need some clarification.

The following example will illustrate the use of status evaluation as part of the assessment of functioning in the head-injured patient. Take, for example, two status items from the current intake evaluation report of a 42-year-old head-injured, married man, the father of two teen-aged sons, whose injury occurred 3 years prior to this assessment. The intake report stated that (as of 1 month before this evaluation was undertaken) "the patient has been living with his parents" (no longer with his wife and children) and that his "current legal status was 'separated.'" Careful evaluation revealed that the two statuses, cited above, were causally related and could be traced to a multidimensional spectrum of causes, wherein, due to a "spillover" effect, the total level of pre-existing pathology (e.g., due to recent increases in either the quality, or intensity, or frequency of occurrence of such varied symptoms and behavioral deficits as distractibility, confusion, added need for supervision in daily life activities, irritability, outbursts, inappropriate personal and interpersonal behaviors, exacerbated "deviations" from pre-injury family roles, and so on), the above drastic changes in the patient's status have occurred. Statuses, in short, are "Polaroid" pictures of momentary constellations of a multitude of deficits that interact with one another and with the particular circumstances of the patient's family and social milieu. They are not immutable entities. Under some circumstances, a worsening situation could be reversed through therapeutic interventions to a more desirable state. Under a different set of circumstances, statuses can become drastically altered for the worse.

Clinical neuropsychology has used neurologic syndromes as its reference points. These reference points may be necessary for the understanding of the underlying deficit, but they are not sufficient for the rehabilitation of the individual. Another concept is the concept of role. Role generally refers to those learned "scripts," or "algorithms," for different functional and interpersonal situations. Roles account for a great deal of the variance in behavior, but they also possess, especially in the more instrumental and "universalistic" realms of behavior (such as "worker-boss" transactions), a degree of lawfulness and predictability of the pattern of responses, some explicit and implicit "rules of the game," and expectations and assumptions. Thus, role refers to the person's ability to actually respond adequately and reliably in a variety of multiply determined and context-bound situations, and that involves more than the intactness of a set of skills. The three major roles that are pertinent to rehabilitation are (1) family roles (i.e., to be a "spouse," "sibling," "child," "relative"); (2) vocational/educational roles (including the possession of required skill-bands, persistence, efficiency, and work-relations); and (3) "fitting in" in one's intimate and the larger, universalistic, social contexts. Hence, roles have a bearing on the question of whether an individual will be capable of readjusting to family life and living at home, whether or not one will prove employable again (and with what degree of competitiveness), and whether or not one will become again an autonomous social being.

With the foregoing in mind, we now present a tentative outline (Table 12-1) of major areas of deficit that can be observed in severely head-injured people, in various degrees and permutations, and which ought to be sampled, as was mentioned in an earlier section.

TABLE 12-1. A Tentative Outline of Areas of Deficit That May Affect the Cognitive Functions of Severe Head-Trauma Patients

Area of Functioning	Specific Subclasses of Dysfunctions, Presumed to Be Caused by Interactions Among Generic Underlying Deficits in This Area
Initiative; activity level; emotional "tone"	Inability to self-initiate or self-induct into even simple, familiar acts/routines/communications/"thoughts," without the help of an "other"; plus the inability to independently sustain (any of the above) without constant re-induction by an "other." Inability to self-initiate (as above), but once inducted by an "other," a demonstrated ability to independently sustain/persist in such activities. Various manifestations of behavioral "lag" or delay of responses, abnormally slowed down "rhythm" of response . . . Various manifestations of abnormal reduction in the rate of activities (or "passivity"); manifestations of "lack of stamina" . . . Various manifestations of inability to become emotionally "involved" in/with (e.g., "flatness" of affect, or "remoteness") . . .
Basic motor and sensory functions	Various problems in the imitation/execution of simple motor sets on command (one-handed; with two hands in synchrony, and with two hands in competition) . . . . Various specific deficits in the sensory, auditory, visual, and tactile modalities Various problems in the integration of sensory-motor, or tactile-kinesthetic, or perceptual-motor skills involved in the execution of basic (e.g., daily self-care) activities; or difficulties in the more complex forms of integration (e.g., driving, athletic activities)
Attention and concentration	Problems in maintaining attention and concentration (or freedom from distractions) during the performance of even the simplest psychomotor tasks (e.g., sort a pile of objects into large and small categories, press elevator button at the right time) Problems in maintaining attention and concentration during the performance of (higher-level) integrative functions (e.g., organizing, assembling, sequencing routines) Problems in maintaining attention and concentration during the performance of various structured, higher-level reasoning and/or learning activities Problems in maintaining attention and concentration in the course of (circumscribed and structured) interpersonal communications or interactions Problems in maintaining attention and concentration in "open-ended," unstructured situations (e.g., a noisy "cocktail" party) Various problems associated with abnormal "stimulus boundedness" (distractability); disinhibition (impulse control problems); hyperresponsiveness (problems in the modulation of responses).
Memory	Time span: Problems with recall/retention/recognition of events that occurred in the immediate past (0 to 60 sec, processed through either the auditory, visual, or tactile modalities) Problems with recall/retention/recognition of events that occurred in the short-term past (1 min to 1 hr): as above

COGNITIVE DEFICITS

longer than recent days/weeks). . . .
Problems with recall/retention/recognition of events that occurred in the remote past. . . .

Content:
Problems in the retention of even short and simple instructions/assertions. . . .
Problems in the retention of basic routines of daily life. . . .
Problems in the retention of simple assignments/"chores" (e.g., to be done that day, or a day later). . . .
Problems in the retention of significant, personally relevant and meaningful, material (e.g., the "gist" of an important resolution, or commitment made by the patient, in the presence of/with a "significant other". . . .

Learning and assimilation of new information:
Problems in retaining/recalling material which was learned in various systematic practice sessions; and which, at the time, was mastered to criterion levels. . . .

Language, thinking, communications

Problems in speech involving defects in the instrumentalities of language (e.g., dysarthria; word substitution or word finding difficulties; anomia; verbal apraxia; certain types of grammatical errors)
Problems in thinking; ranging from deficits in the simple exposition (articulation) of thoughts, variants of higher-level abstraction disorders, such as inability to comprehend the main idea; to weigh alternatives; to formulate a logical course of action; to arrive at conclusions; to draw inferences; to think in symbolic terms; etc.
Problems in the oral and/or written processing and communication of (a) written material, (b) audiovisual materials, and (c) interpersonal discursive material.

Problem solving

Problems in carrying out routine self-care and household chores. . . .
Problems in carrying out basic adaptive behaviors/routines (e.g., making a phone call; asking for directions; routine shopping; using public transportation). . . .
Problems with higher-level, moderately complex problem-solving situations:
  involving convergent reasoning; i.e., the ability to clearly formulate a problem, the objective sought, the relevant factors to be considered. . . .
  involving divergent reasoning; i.e., systematically considering the alternatives, choosing a strategy of approach to the solution. . . .
  involving "executive" abilities; i.e., formulating an operational plan of action, orchestrating and prioritizing details, executing the plan, monitoring the performance, and verifying the solution obtained against the original problem
Note: A head-trauma patient may be impaired in all aspects of the problem-solving cycle, as shown above, or in certain aspects of the problem-solving cycle only.

Judgment

Problems involving the inability to exercise good judgment concerning what is appropriate in the manner of dressing, the use of verbal and nonverbal expressions or gestures, and in general a loss of awareness of what "fits" various occasions. . . .
Problems involving the loss of propriety concerning matters of one's own "privacy," "invasion" of other people's privacy, and inability to maintain "friendliness" or "chumminess" within proper bounds. . . .

Roles

Problems with inadequacy or loss of basic family "role"-playing ability. . . .
Problems with inadequacy or loss of "universalistic," work-related role-playing ability. . . .
Problems with inadequacy or loss of "universalistic," social role-playing ability (e.g., "traveler" on crowded train, bus; "customer" in a store; "theater-goer" in the lobby; "patient," or "pupil").

IRM APPROACH TO ASSESSMENT OF COGNITIVE DEFICITS IN HEAD TRAUMA

The IRM approach to the assessment of cognitive deficits in head-trauma patients is a rehabilitation-relevant approach. It recognizes the need for enlarging the overall scope of inquiry beyond the boundaries of the traditional psychometric approach and the need for (1) developing an overall conceptual framework capable of defining the full scope of the inquiry as well as the specific dimensions of behavior to be singled out for measurement; (2) developing specific tools, that is, the various measures capable of differentially assessing deficits in skills and in abilities to learn and to integrate; and (3) pinpointing the common barriers that prevent persons with head injury from functioning normally, as a step toward defining the treatment objectives and the tools required to activate those objectives. In this section, we will outline in brief the salient aspects of our approach.

BARRIERS TO FUNCTIONAL NORMALCY

Figure 12-1 illustrates what appear to be the three principal barriers that must be overcome in the rehabilitation of the head-injured patient. These barriers are problems in attention,

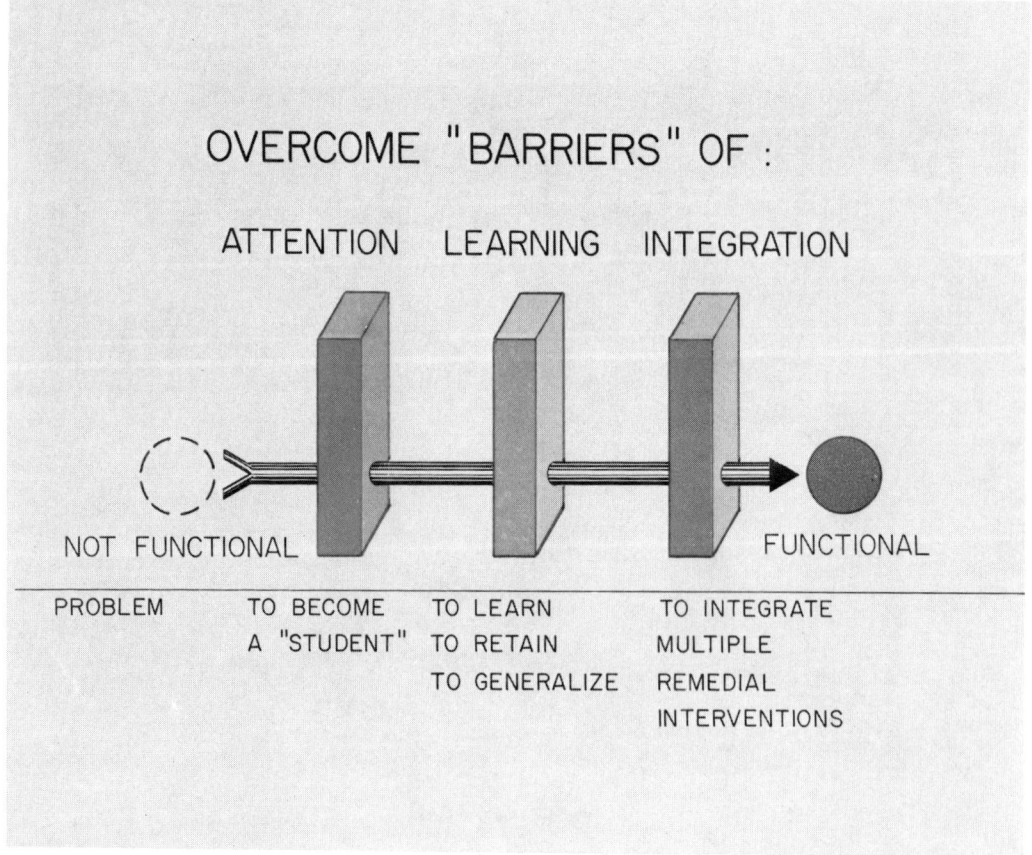

FIGURE 12-1. Defining the cognitive-remedial tasks in the rehabilitation of severely head-injured persons.

problems in learning, and problems in the integration of what has been learned. With regard to the attentional "barrier," our early experience in working with head-injured people suggested that it was difficult to obtain a valid assessment of deficient as well as intact skills on standard psychologic tests because the patient often did not adequately pay attention or follow instructions. If one wishes, therefore, to reliably assess the patient's deficits and assets, or to engage the patient in any type of instructive remedial activity, the first barrier must be effectively overcome.

A second set of problems evolves around the learning barrier. The issue here pertains to questions such as (in view of the combined effects and the interactions of the patient's attentional, memory, and thought-processing deficits) what is the patient's potential for absorbing new information? What is the relationship between current degree of dysfunction and the capacity to benefit from various teaching interventions? What is the relationship between the foregoing and the ability to retain newly learned material?

The third barrier pertains to the question of assimilation and integration of what is learned and the ability to apply what is learned effectively and appropriately in different situations. Integrating what is taught in order to solve problems in practical situations is a long-term concern in education. If a student has two deficits and is provided training to compensate for both areas of deficit, how are the effects of the separate training combined? Many issues concerning the acquisition, transformation, and application of knowledge in the service of the person's functional life have been ignored by all the different approaches to the assessment of cognitive deficits in head-injured persons, which have been cited above.

The state of the art of cognitive assessment of head-injured patients does not permit a response to the challenges posed by these barriers in a simple or easy way. Our approach, which is presently in its empirical validation stage, is evolving gradually. In the following, we summarize the salient features of this system.

A Working Hypothesis Concerning the Core Deficits in Severe Head Trauma

On the basis of our cumulative experiences over the past few years with many head-injured patients undergoing active rehabilitation, we have arrived at a tentative formulation of a parsimonious hypothesis. The hypothesis is illustrated in Figure 12-2. Accordingly, we hypothesize that in the severely head-injured patient, the post-traumatic problems can be traced to essentially five basic (generic, core) underlying deficit areas; that these deficit areas, while overlapping and influencing one another to some extent, can and do occur relatively independently from one another as well; and that they appear in various permutations and in a differential manner from individual to individual. The five areas of basic deficit are (1) problems in basic arousal and attention; (2) impairments in the underlying skill structures; (3) memory disturbances; (4) language and/or thought disturbances; and, as is clearly evident in certain patients with a bifrontal syndrome, (5) inadequate feeling tone (or, a defect in the basic neuropsychologic underpinnings of the emotive processes).

Our hypothesis, as the figure indicates, implies further that the patient's dysfunctions in both the rational, problem-solving domain and the emotive, imaginative, and empathic domain are affected by these core deficits differentially; but whether or not—and the degree to which a single behavior, which is embedded in a particular situational context, will be normal or pathologic—will depend on the interactions between the two domains, as well as on the specific content of the behavior.

Hence, it should be quite obvious that a system for the assessment of cognitive deficits in head-injured patients, if it is to be relevant for rehabilitation, must be a comprehensive one. It should encompass the entire range of the patient's behaviors, which have a direct bearing on the assessment of the patient's initial competencies, on capacities for benefiting from various systematic remedial interventions, and on predicting final outcomes.[33,34]

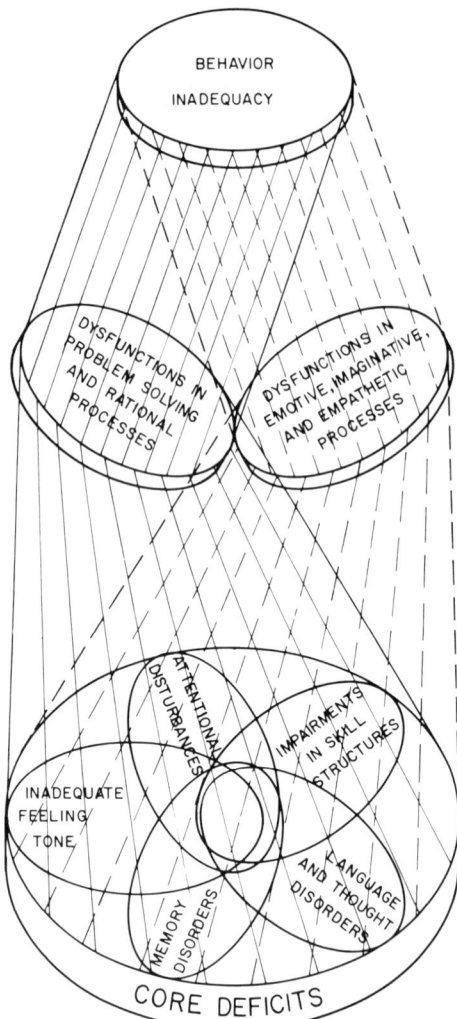

FIGURE 12-2. A schematic presentation of a hypothesis concerning the cause-effect relationship between generic deficits and behavior dysfunctions in severe head injuries.

Comprehensive System of Assessment of Cognitive Deficits in Head-Injured Patients

Figure 12-3 is a schematic outline of the IRM system of assessment. It consists of (1) a range of measures of baseline competence, along a multidimensional functional continuum, (2) a structure, including uniform procedures and programmatic elements which permit the systematic derivation of several process measures (i.e., measures of ability to respond to various remedial interventions), and (3) measures of outcome. We will consider each one in turn.

BASELINE MEASURES

The baseline measures are tentatively divided into five areas. These include the (1) psychomotor, (2) integrative, (3) verbal ideations, (4) personal, and (5) interpersonal areas.

COGNITIVE DEFICITS

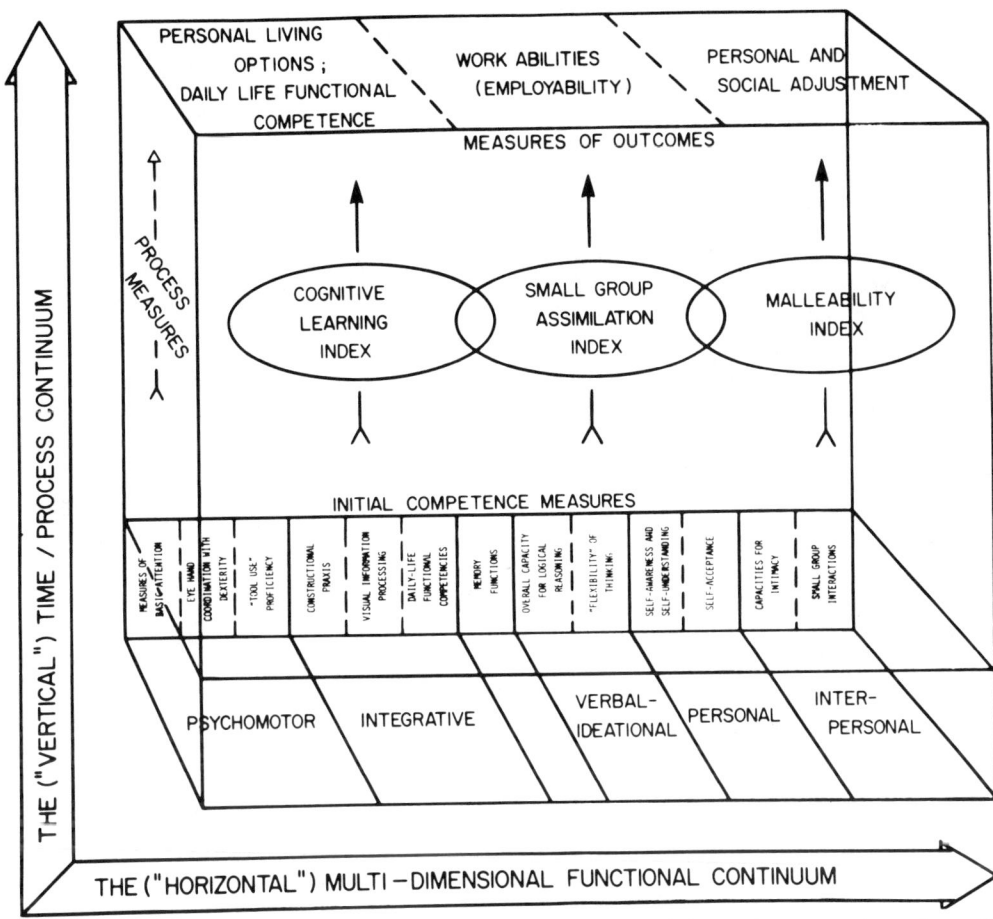

FIGURE 12-3. A schematic presentation of the IRM system for defining the parameters of cognitive deficit in severe head injuries.

We regard the present division as tentative and perhaps somewhat arbitrary—tentative in the sense that it awaits empirical confirmation, and arbitrary in the sense that it implies relatively clear-cut distinctions between abilities and functions, which may not indeed turn out to be the case. For each of these areas, a family of measures (to be described below) was used. These measures combine some standard testing procedures commonly used in neuropsychologic assessment, and some special tests that we devised to meet our special concerns. In addition, we developed measures of behavior in interpersonal situations and measures of functional adaptive behaviors pertinent to head injury. Since the latter two are not part of the traditional assessment strategies, we will comment on them briefly. Traditional testing in both the psychometric and the clinical neurologic approach has assayed competence in terms of ability to respond to words, to solve verbal problems, to deal with numbers and letters, and to manipulate objects. The traditional methods have not ventured into the area of interpersonal skills or competence in handling interpersonal situations. While there are no suitable tests for head-injured people with norms in this area, we felt it necessary to develop such tasks, which could be quantified in terms of their stimulus and response parameters, in order to provide us with a basis for assessing competence in an area of vital interest.

The formal IRM assessment battery, which is administered both at baseline (i.e., before the commencement of remedial interventions) and after the cessation of the remedial interventions phase, has been described in detail in a series of monographs.[35] In the present context, we merely wish to identify these measures and to briefly describe their underlying logic.

The psychomotor area contains three families of tests. The first group of tests consists of different (operationalized, developed, electronically monitored) measures of basic alertness, attention, concentration, psychomotor persistence, and speed of reaction with modulated responses. Included among these are measures of reaction time, visual-motor anticipation, ability to perceive auditory and visual rhythms and to synchronize motor responses accordingly, time estimates, and the like.

The second group of psychomotor tests consists of three standard measures of eye-hand integration with finger dexterity, the Purdue Peg Board test series. And the third group of psychomotor tests consists of a number of calibrated "tool use samples" that were developed in our setting. The purpose of these tool use measures is to gauge the patient's functional proficiency in the use of simple tools.

The second area of testing involves a series of tests in the integrative perceptual-cognitive domain. These include various (standard and/or specially developed) measures of constructional praxis and perceptual motor processing; measures of visual discrimination and visual information processing, including sequentially presented and simultaneously presented visual-spatial materials; a variety of perceptual cognitive tasks involving various degrees of stimulus processing difficulty; special measures of navigation and orientation in space; and a specially developed procedure for assessing the patient's behavior in a series of 19 parameters of daily life functions.

The Behavioral Competence Index (BCI) consists of 19 ratings of behaviors, which are based on the report of a significant other or a staff observation. In most instances, the rater is asked to assess behavior(s) in terms of a premorbid standard, the degree of supervision required to complete the behavior, and the frequency of occurrence of pathologic responses. Unlike traditional measures of activities of daily living, which are expressed in terms of whether the individual can perform the act, the BCI is concerned with what the person actually does in one's naturalistic milieu. Traditional measures assess skill; BCI assesses activities and role adequacy. Among the behaviors sampled are (1) performing daily tasks in and outside the house; (2) interpersonal activities; (3) personal activities reflecting autonomous appropriate behavior, for example, orientation, self-regulation of affect, and planning a day; and (4) appreciation of the consequences of the disability.

We also included in our battery five standard, well-known neuropsychologic measures of immediate and short-term recall (WAIS, Digits forward and backward tests, NCCEA, sentence repetition, and Benton Visual Retention Test). These standard measures were included in order to enable the determination of the relationships of each of these separately and a number of—as yet to be finalized—measures of memory deficit expressed in various daily-life, "naturalistic" situations.

The third area, the verbal ideational domain, is assessed by a series of standard and specially developed tests. The first group consists of a series of standard measures of academic skills (verbal comprehension, numerical reasoning, reading mechanics, spelling, and spatial reasoning skills). The second group consists of the standard WAIS intelligence scales, which measures general intellectual aptitude. And the third group in this category consists of a series of tests of higher-level abstract reasoning that were developed in our setting, specifically for head-injured patients. These include special measures of the ability to generate precise categoric formulations by using either verbal concepts or by sorting objects; measures of the ability to flexibly shift one's categoric "set," while engaging in either verbal or object categorization tasks; measures of the ability to abstract the central focal point or idea, in special context-bound situations and to articulate these ideas in a concise and precise manner, as exemplified by the capacity to self-generate "telegram" messages, to fit specific sets of circumstances, or to identify the relevant "messages" when they are presented embedded in irrelevant materials.

The fourth area of assessment includes two special, operationalized indexes of "personality": self-esteem and self-appraisal. Responding to precisely and uniformly administered instructions, the patient is called to demonstrate, in front of a small group of staff and peers, ability and willingness to (1) make a statement concerning which of two personal qualities the patient esteems the most and why; and to (2) provide a well-articulated statement of self-appraisal that starts with the words, "I am a person who . . ." The patient's performances, which are recorded verbatim, are then scored according to an explicit weighting system by a term of "judges."

The fifth area includes three specific measures of various aspects of interpersonal skills. These were also devised in our setting. The measures are administered in a small group setting, according to precise and uniform testing procedures. The first of these is a measure of the person's empathic abilities, specifically, the ability to (1) role play according to a precise "scenario" an interaction with two "friends," in which the patient's assignment is to ascertain the facts and the reasons for a mild dispute between friends; and, following that, to (2) analyze and articulate his or her understanding of the nature of the dispute and the relationship between the two "friends." The second is a measure of the patient's personal repertoire and style of interaction with a small group. The measure, which is a cumulative index, is derived by rating the content of assertions, the style of communication, and the physical gestures and mannerisms displayed by the patient during the unfolding of a uniform "scenario" for introducing oneself to the group (according to specific stimuli provided by a designated leader). And the third and last measure, which consists also of cumulative ratings, is an index of the patient's "social cooperation" during an (uniformly administered) assignment to jointly plan a party.

PROCESS AND OUTCOME MEASURES

As indicated in Figure 12-3, the IRM system includes three different indices which reflect the ability to profit from the remedial intervention program. These measures include (1) the Cognitive Learning Index, a measure of the patient's ability to profit from remedial cueing; (2) the Small Group Assimilation Index, a measure of the patient's capacity to assimilate personally relevant and meaningful information, during the small-group exercises, designed to improve interpersonal skills; and (3) the Malleability Index, a measure of the patient's "tractability," or openness, willingness, and ability to significantly modify, or eliminate from the repertoire, certain pathologic behaviors that were specifically targeted by the staff for vigorous, explicit, and directive intervention at the beginning of the treatments. Similarly, the IRM system of measurements also includes a number of outcome criterion measures, which are the functional targets of the program of intervention. These measures, while properly belonging in a system of assessment of the cognitive and functional sequelae of severe brain injury, are outside the scope of the present chapter and will therefore not be elaborated on.

SUMMARY

This chapter outlines the principal concerns of a rehabilitation-relevant approach to defining the mental and cognitive sequelae of severe brain injury; briefly summarizes the main contributions of various traditional systems of assessment and points out the still existing gaps in knowledge; calls to attention the problems in establishing the long-term mental and cognitive sequelae of severe head injury and points out the need for a comprehensive approach to the task; suggests a tentative outline of the principal areas of deficit that ought to be sampled in head-injured patients within the context of a rehabilitation focused inquiry; and briefly outlines the IRM system of assessment, remediation, and prognosis of functional recovery following severe head injuries.

REFERENCES

1. GUILFORD, JP: *The Nature of Human Intelligence.* McGraw-Hill, New York, 1967.
2. KLOVE, II: *Validation studies in adult clinical neuropsychology.* In REITAN, RM AND DAVIDSON, LA (EDS): *Clinical Neuropsychology: Current Status and Applications.* John Wiley & Sons, New York, 1974.
3. REITAN, RM: *A research program on the psychological effects of brain lesion in human beings.* In ELLIS, NR (ED): *International Review of Research in Mental Retardation.* Academic Press, New York, 1966.
4. TEUBER, HL: *Perception.* In FIELD, J, MAGOUN, HW, AND HALL, VE (EDS): *Handbook of Physiology: Section 1, Neurophysiology III.* American Physiological Society, Washington, DC, 1965, p 1595.
5. GESCHWIND, N: *Disconnection syndromes in animals and man.* Brain 88:237, 1965.
6. GESCHWIND, N AND KAPLAN, E: *A human cerebral disconnection syndrome: A preliminary report.* Neurology 12:675, 1962.
7. SIDMAN, M, ET AL: *Behavioral studies of aphasia: Methods of investigation and analysis.* Neuropsychology 9:119, 1971.
8. WILLIAMS, M: *The effects of past experience on the elderly.* Journal of Mental Science 104:783, 1960.
9. ZARIT, JH, COLE, KD, AND GUIDER, J: *Memory training strategies and subjective complaints of memory in the aged.* Gerontologist 21:158, 1981.
10. MILLER, M AND ROHR, ME: *Verbal mediation for perceptual deficits in learning disabilities: A review and suggestions.* Journal of Learning Disabilities 13:319, 1980.
11. BEN-YISHAY, Y, ET AL: *Relationships between initial competence and ability to profit from cues in brain damaged individuals.* J Abnorm Psychol 75:248, 1970.
12. BEN-YISHAY, Y, DILLER, L, AND MANDLEBERG, I: *The ability to profit from cues as a function of initial competence in normal and brain injured adults: A replication of previous findings.* J Abnorm Psychol 76:378, 1970.
13. BEN-YISHAY, Y, ET AL: *Similarities and difference in block design performance between older normal and brain-injured persons: A task analysis.* J Abnorm Psychol 78:17, 1971.
14. BEN-YISHAY, Y, ET AL: *Differences in matching persistence behavior during block design performance between older normal and brain-damaged persons: A process analysis.* Cortex 10:121, 1974.
15. BOLTON, B AND COOK, DW (EDS): *Rehabilitation Client Assessment.* University Park Press, Baltimore, 1980.
16. LISHMAN, WA: *Organic Psychiatry.* Blackwell Scientific, Oxford, 1978, chapter 5.
17. JENNETT, B AND TEASDALE, G: *Management of Head Injuries.* FA Davis, Philadelphia, 1981, chapter 12.
18. REITAN, RM: *Psychological testing after craniocerebral injury.* In WALKER, AE, CAVENESS, WF, AND CRITCHLEY, M (EDS): *The Late Effects of Head Injury.* Charles C Thomas, Springfield, Ill, 1969, p 84.
19. FAHY, TJ, IRVING, NH, AND MILLAC, P: *Severe head injuries: A six year follow up.* Lancet 2:475, 1967.
20. GOLDSTEIN, K: *Functional disturbances in brain damage.* In ARIETI, S (ED): *American Handbook of Psychiatry,* Vol. 1. Basic Books, New York, 1959, p 770.
21. BOLL, TJ, O'LEARY, DS, AND BARTH, JT: *A quantitative and qualitative approach to neuropsychological evaluation.* In PROKOP, CK AND BRADLEY, LA (EDS): *Medical Psychology.* Academic Press, New York, 1981.

22. LURIA, AR: *Restoration of Function after Brain Injury.* Macmillan, New York, 1963, chapter 7.
23. LEVIN, HS, O'DONNELL, VM, AND GROSSMAN, RG: *The galveston orientation and amnesia test: A practical scale to assess cognition after head injury.* J Nerv Ment Dis 167(11):675, 1979.
24. LEVIN, HS AND GROSSMAN, RG: *Behavioral sequelae of closed head injury.* Arch Neurol 35:720, 1978.
25. MANDLEBERG, I: *Cognitive recovery after severe head injury.* J Neurol Neurosurg Psychiatry 38:1127, 1975.
26. MANDLEBERG, I AND BROOKS, DN: *Cognitive recovery after severe head injury: 1. Serial testing on the Wechsler Adult Intelligence Scale.* J Neurol Neurosurg Psychiatry 38:1121, 1975.
27. BOND, MR AND BROOKS, DN: *Understanding the process of recovery as a basis for the investigation of rehabilitation for the brain injured.* Scand J Rehabil Med 8:127, 1976.
28. LEVIN, HS, ET AL: *Linguistic recovery after closed head injury.* Brain Lang 12:360, 1981.
29. GRONWALL, DMA: *Paced auditory serial addition task: A measure of recovery from concussion.* Percept Mot Skills 44:367, 1977.
30. LEVIN, HS, GROSSMAN, RG, AND KELLY, PJ: *Short-term recognition memory in relation to severity of head injury.* Cortex 12:175, 1976.
31. LEZAK, MD: *Subtle sequelae of brain damage: Perplexity, distractibility, and fatigue.* Am J Phys Med 57(1):9, 1978.
32. PRIGATANO, G: *Dealing with the emotional-motivational disturbances of the traumatically head injury patient.* Invited symposium, Rehabilitation of Post-Traumatic Brain Damaged Patients. APA Convention, Los Angeles, Calif, 1981.
33. DILLER, L, ET AL: *Studies in cognition and rehabilitation in hemiplegia.* NYU Medical Center, Rehabilitation Monograph #50. NYU Medical Center, New York, 1974.
34. BEN-YISHAY, Y, ET AL: *Prediction of rehabilitation outcomes from psychometric parameters in left hemiplegics.* J Consult Clin Psychol 34:436, 1970.
35. BEN-YISHAY, Y, ET AL: *Working approaches to remediation of cognitive deficits in brain damaged.* NYU Medical Center, Rehabilitation Monographs #59, 1978; #60, 1979; #61, 1980; #62, 1981. NYU Medical Center, New York, 1978–1981.

Chapter 13

DISORDERS OF MEMORY

Neil Brooks, Ph.D.

After severe head injury, patients commonly complain of disturbance of memory. Indeed, nearly 40 years ago, Tooth[1] reported 61 percent of his 100 "postconcussional" patients complaining of difficulties in memory and "absentmindedness," and in a recent study of 55 severe head injuries in Glasgow, 69 percent of relatives felt that memory disturbance was still a problem in the injured patient 12 months after injury.[2]

In view of this, it is not surprising that the literature contains an increasing number of studies of memory disturbance after head injury, including a recent excellent review by Schacter and Crovitz.[3] Following that review, it is clear that a number of major questions remain about the nature of the memory disorder. These are shown below and will be used to structure the content of the chapter.

The main questions about memory disturbance are:

1. What kinds of memory deficit will a patient suffer?
2. What is the reason underlying deficits in memory?
3. Can the deficits be predicted at an early stage knowing the severity of injury?
4. How rapidly, and to what level does memory performance recover?
5. Does memory test performance relate in a clear way to everyday life memory performance?
6. How may memory functions be improved?

WHAT KINDS OF MEMORY DEFICIT WILL A PATIENT SUFFER?

DEFICITS FOUND EARLY AFTER INJURY

Immediately after injury and for some time thereafter, patients may be unable to retain information from one day to the next. The characteristics of this early amnesia—post-traumatic amnesia (PTA)—have been well described by Russell,[4] and reviewed by Schacter and Crovitz,[3] but it is still unclear whether patients are storing any new information during PTA. Studies of memory during PTA are rare, and the two known to me[5,6] contain flaws that make interpretation difficult. Fodor's paper[5] contains inadequate information about the precise procedures that were used to measure memory, but she concluded that head-injured patients in PTA had "a disturbance in the retrieval of related stimulus material relative to a control group." They could retain *some* material immediately after presentation but were unable to organize it sufficiently coherently to retrieve it later. My pilot study[6] also investigated memory organization during PTA, but using only small numbers (five head-injured patients and five controls). The patients were presented with 3 lists of 12 words organized acoustically, semantically, or randomly, and were tested on free and cued recall, being asked in cued recall, for example, "what words sounded alike?". Head-injured patients could use this structure, as evidenced by better performance on clustered than on random lists; and a comparison of free and cued recall differences suggested that head-injured patients may have difficulty in *retrieving* semantically stored information.

The patchy evidence reviewed here suggests that patients may store some information during PTA, but this will be limited in quantity and of doubtful accessibility for retrieval.

MORE DELAYED DEFICITS

After PTA, the patient may recover cognitive functions completely, although even after a short PTA, some patients still complain of persisting memory difficulties. After a longer PTA (anything over a week), memory disorders may be more severe and persistent; this has been documented in a large number of studies.[7-14] Conkey[7] studied mildly injured patients early after injury and noted severe difficulties in new learning. The early study by Tooth[1] concerned more severely injured patients than those seen by Conkey. Twenty-nine percent of Tooth's patients had a PTA of more than 1 day (classified as "severe" by Russell[3]), and 60 percent had a PTA longer than 1 hour. Tooth's "postconcussional syndrome" patients were seen at different times after injury (many longer than a year); of the 100 patients, 61 complained of some subjective disturbance of memory. Many patients (the exact number was not specified) reported relying on a notebook to record essential information. Few of Tooth's cognitive tests involved memory directly: one simple test, Digit Span (the recall of a series of digits), did show rather poorer performance in head-injured patients than in uninjured controls, but the differences were not large. Furthermore, Tooth found no significant differences in digit recall between patients who did and those who did *not* spontaneously complain of memory disturbance.

Following Tooth's account, there is a gap in the literature[11,12] until the early 1970s, when interest rekindled in this area. More recent studies[9,13] support the early conclusions of Conkey and others, showing marked difficulties in new learning often persisting long after the injury.

Brooks[14] used the Wechsler Memory Scale[15] to investigate memory within 2 years after severe injury and found that head-injured persons had particular difficulty in new learning. The recall of premorbidly acquired information was much less impaired. Other workers have also used the Wechsler Memory Scale.[16,17] However, Black[16] gives no details of exact scores or patient severity, so his results are difficult to interpret, as they are in the methodologically flawed study of 70 patients reported by Kear, Colwell, and Heller.[17] In this study, the only information given about the severity of injury is that "the injuries varied from the mild to the very severe"—a less than helpful description.

Further recent evidence of severe learning and memory deficit has been provided by Brooks and Aughton,[9] who tested 89 severely injured patients within 2 years of injury, using a simple measure involving learning three unrelated word pairs. Inglis[18] reported that head-injured patients were found to be highly significantly worse than non-head-injured orthopedic controls on this test, both on initial testing and when retest was carried out without warning after 1 hour.

WHAT IS THE REASON UNDERLYING DEFICITS IN MEMORY?

That head injury may cause severe learning and memory difficulties persisting long after the end of PTA cannot be doubted. However, the reasons underlying these impairments are not easy to ascertain. Many writers have commented on slowness and attention deficits following head injury,[8,19,20] and it is possible that an attentional disturbance underlies a poor performance on other cognitive tasks, including learning and memory.

Other writers have assumed that the learning and memory deficit is primary, and then have tried to identify precisely which measures of learning and memory show impairment and why. A number of different processes have been examined, as follows.

LONG- AND SHORT-TERM MEMORY

Brooks[21] found that on a test of short-term memory (Digit Span), severely injured patients were relatively unimpaired, but this was not the case with a measure of long-term memory. This study also used a test involving free recall of 20 lists, each comprising 10 unrelated words. On immediate recall, no difference was found between head-injured and control patients on recall of words at the end of the list (words thought still to be in short-term memory), but head-injured patients had a slight deficit in recall of words at the beginning of the list (words thought to have been transferred into long-term memory). On delayed recall (representing retrieval from long-term memory), and on other measures,[22] head-injured patients were significantly worse than controls.

STORAGE OR RETRIEVAL?

A further approach to understanding the deficit is to attempt to distinguish between new learning (storage) and retrieval of stored information. This question was reviewed succinctly by Schacter and Crovitz[3] and was considered briefly in the previously cited study by Brooks.[21] In addition, Levin and Peters[23] reported a single head-injured patient who was tested on recognition of nouns both immediately after presentation and after a 30-minute delay. Immediate performance was normal, but the patient showed a larger memory loss than controls after the delay, as was found in an earlier study by Brooks.[24]

The Brooks[21] study also examined intrusion errors (an error where a word from a *previous* list is incorrectly recalled). Although an error, this gives evidence that information has been stored but retrieved incorrectly. Head-injured patients made significantly fewer intrusion errors than controls, and this was interpreted by Brooks as faulty storage, on the assumption that the information had never been stored adequately in the first place. However, this finding must be interpreted with caution, as Schacter and Crovitz[3] point out, for only after all other means of demonstrating retrieval have been exhausted—for example, cued recall, recognition, and so forth—could this be unequivocally interpreted as evidence for defective storage alone.

MEMORY SENSITIVITY

A quite different approach to understanding the learning and memory deficit was attempted by Brooks,[25,26] although it was later criticized by Richardson.[27] Brooks used signal detection theory (SDT) to analyze errors made by head-injured patients on a continuous recognition learning task. The SDT enables the separation of memory sensitivity (how good the memory system is) from decision criteria (how certain the subject will be before identifying a memory item). In this study, head-injured patients made fewer correct recognitions and also more false-negative errors (failing to recognize a recurring item) than non-head-injured controls, whereas they did not differ on false-positive errors (falsely recognizing a nonrecurring item). Head-injured patients appeared, therefore, to have a twofold memory problem, showing both a reduced memory efficiency and an increased caution.

CAN THE DEFICITS BE PREDICTED?

Attempts to predict the severity of the subsequent deficit in head-injured patients have been a constant feature of the neurosurgical head injury literature. An ability to make accurate predictions has important implications for the management of individual patients and for the allocation of scarce rehabilitation resources. As a rough general rule, the simpler the criterion behavior that one is attempting to predict, the easier the prediction. Therefore, predicting the likelihood of physical recovery by 3 or by 6 months after injury is relatively easy,[28] but prediction of psychologic recovery is not so easy unless very crude predictions of the "deteriorated/not deteriorated" type are attempted. The problem in predicting psychologic recovery is that patients vary widely in cognitive capacity before injury, and a given memory performance after injury may represent either no memory deterioration, or a mild, moderate, or severe deterioration depending on the patient's level before injury.

Notwithstanding these difficulties, attempts have been made at psychologic prediction using early indices of severity of brain damage. In addition, later prediction has been attempted by comparing psychologic performance of persons with and without varying indices of severity of damage. A range of different indices has been proposed, reflecting broadly either duration of impaired consciousness level or measures of focal damage. The measures of duration of impaired consciousness level have comprised either coma or duration of PTA, and measures of focal damage have involved the presence of focal neurologic signs, the presence of an early operated intracranial hematoma, or a skull fracture.

DISTURBANCE OF CONSCIOUSNESS LEVEL

Russell[4] first used PTA duration (rather than coma) to assess severity of diffuse damage. He found a relationship between PTA duration and the subsequent severity and duration of disability (in a very broad sense). Russell used clinical analysis rather than psychologic tests but found a strikingly increasing incidence of complaints of memory deficit with increasing PTA duration.

Many workers have reported the effects of PTA or some similar index on subsequent cognitive performance. Tooth[1] found that the longer the PTA, the poorer the patient's digit span performance when tested many months after the end of PTA. Patients with PTA longer than 24 hours were particularly poor when compared with those with shorter PTA.

Studies in Glasgow have frequently found an association between PTA and cognitive performance, in patients tested within 2 years of severe injury.[9,10,13,14,24,25] On the Wechsler Memory Scale, Brooks[14] found a strong association between increasing PTA and decreasing learning and memory scores, and this was also the case with other learning and memory measures.[9,10,13] An interesting feature was observed on a simple measure of word learning[18] that involved learning three unrelated pairs of words.[9,10,13] This test was given twice, the second test given without warning 1 hour after the first. The scores for the immediate test showed the expected gradation from short to long PTA, but the effect just failed to reach significance. However, on the delayed testing, the effect was large and highly significant. These results, therefore, suggest an interaction between delay and severity, with the effects of severity becoming more marked as the length of time over which memory is tested increases. In retrospect, however, a much better statistical test of this would have been a repeated measures analysis of variance.

Coma rather than PTA has also been frequently reported.[8,13,29] The early study by Ruesch[8] incorporated a measure of coma, but as is often the case in this area, no simple, clear definition of coma criteria was given. Ruesch felt that coma significantly predicted cognitive outcome at 3 months after injury in a group of patients with mild injuries. Klove and Cleeland's study[29] examined duration of coma (defined as length of time to become responsive to verbal commands) as a predictor of performance on a large number of cognitive tests within 2 years of injury. The results are difficult to interpret due to the small number of cases seen and to the contradictory results of different methods of statistical analysis used. However, when the effects of other potentially important variables such as skull fracture, electroencephalographic abnormality, or presence of neurologic signs were factored out, the relationship between coma and memory dysfunction dropped to a insignificant level.

The Glasgow group[13] examined the influence of coma in their 1980 study in 62 patients who had been monitored on the Glasgow Coma Scale[30] during the first days after injury. Memory performance was compared across three coma subgroups using analysis of variance; on a variety of learning and memory measures, there was no significant or discernible relationship between increasing coma duration and decreasing memory performance.

SIGNS OF FOCAL BRAIN DAMAGE

The relationship between the presence of focal neurologic signs and cognitive performance has often been assessed, either by examining the significance of early neurologic dysfunction as a predictor of subsequent cognitive performance or by comparing the cognitive performance of patients with and without neurologic signs at the time of psychologic testing. Tooth[1] showed that the performance on digit span of patients still showing signs was slightly poorer than that of patients who were sign-free, but as he pointed out, there was a direct association between length of PTA and presence of abnormal signs. Furthermore, the patients with a longer PTA were more likely to have skull fracture, and it is known that patients with a fracture are more likely to have an intracranial hematoma. Separating out any single cause or clinical factor is, therefore, not easy, although it has been attempted.[29,31] Klove and Cleeland[29] found only a weak relationship between the presence of neurologic signs and general cognitive performance within 2 years after injury, although in their large battery of tests, the strongest influence was on measures of memory. This relationship was not, however, found by Brooks on tests of short- or long-term memory[21] or recognition memory.[25] However, Levin and coworkers[31] felt that early neurologic signs could be a significant predictor of later memory deficit, with one sign in particular—the presence of oculovestibular deficit—being very significantly associated with poorer memory performance. Oculovestibular deficit probably reflects the general level of diffuse damage to the brain as a whole rather than a specific brain stem dysfunction, as usually only a very severe injury will cause damage to structures as far down the neuraxis as the upper brain stem.[32]

As with neurologic signs, the possible significance of a fracture or a hematoma as a predictor of memory disturbance is difficult to interpret, as it is not an independent index.[13,33] Ruesch and More[33] examined their patients within 24 hours of injury, and found that patients untestable during that period were more likely to have intracranial hematoma and (to a rather lesser extent) skull fracture. Tooth[1] also assessed the possible significance of skull fracture for memory performance. On his simple memory test, the fracture patients were slightly (but not significantly) worse that nonfracture patients, but it is always possible that any difference represents diffuse rather than focal damage, as 62 percent of his 39 fracture patients had a PTA of more than 24 hours.

Klove and Cleeland[29] compared 20 fracture patients with 20 nonfracture patients and found absolutely no difference on memory performance between the two groups. Brooks and coworkers[13] also examined the significance of fracture and of hematoma: the 65 fracture patients (bilateral in nine patients) were compared with 24 patients in whom no fracture had been diagnosed. With the exception of one rarely administered memory test, there were no significant memory differences between the two groups. The analysis was then carried further to investigate reports[34,35] that the site of impact (usually measured by site of fracture) would predict cognitive performance many years later. Smith[34] and Roberts[35] found that patients with a right-sided impact (hypothesized to cause left-sided brain damage via contre coup) performed significantly worse on verbal than nonverbal learning and memory tests, whereas left-sided impact and right parietal impact cases performed worse on visual-spatial learning. These deficits were thought to be independent of PTA. In view of this finding, Brooks and colleagues compared the memory performance of 32 left-sided fracture patients with that of the 23 right-sided patients and found no differences between these groups on learning and memory performance; nor were there any differences between patients with a linear and those with a depressed fracture. A further analysis examined the possible significance of hematoma. The 52 patients who had been operated on for an intracranial hematoma were compared with patients in whom no operation had been carried out, and it was found that the operated patients performed significantly better on at least one measure of learning (the recall of stories). This was felt to be due to the less severe diffuse damage in the hematoma patients (PTA = 16.2 days) than in the remaining cases (PTA = 21 days); $t = 1.98$, $p < 0.05$.

Although the analysis by Brooks and coworkers failed to replicate the Smith and Roberts hypothesis[34,35] that contre coup mechanisms give purely focal cognitive deficits, other workers have reported specific memory disturbance related to localized and lateralized damage, evidenced by neurologic or radiologic findings.[36-38]

Despite these reports, it is preferable to view severely head-injured patients as suffering diffuse rather than focal damage. This would accord with the neuropathologic evidence and with the experimental work of Ommaya and Generelli.[32]

HOW RAPIDLY DOES MEMORY RECOVER, AND TO WHAT LEVEL?

Memory outcome after severe injury is variable, with some patients showing a rapid return to full functioning, others a slower progression toward the same result, and some patients never reaching their premorbid level. Not only do patients differ in the final level reached, but they also differ in the rate at which they reach that level. An understanding of recovery rate is important clinically and theoretically, although an adequate analysis of memory recovery raises many formidable methodologic and practical problems.[39]

The first large-scale attempt at assessing psychologic recovery was reported in 1938 by Conkey.[7] She used mildly injured patients examined during the first 12 months after injury, and a large battery of tests, including measures both of new learning and of recall of premorbid information. Her patients were seen five times if possible, but patient attrition was a major problem, and Conkey was able to examine on all occasions only four patients, despite beginning her first assessment on 25 cases. In summarizing her results, Conkey noted that whereas performance on recall of premorbidly acquired information was relatively unaffected even early after injury, this was not the case with measures of new learning, on which performance consistently lagged behind that of all other functions. By the end of the first year, the performance of the four patients seen on all occasions was just reaching a normal level, when the mean scores for all four patients were compared with the mean scores of uninjured control groups. However, Conkey described the individual recovery patterns in her four patients, showing how remarkably variable these were and showing implicitly how much information mean scores on groups of patients will conceal about the performance of individuals.

Within the last 10 years, a series of recovery studies have been reported, but many of them, including my own, have added relatively little to Conkey's early report.[10,37,39-41] The common strategy has been to use a large battery of cognitive tests, and in order to try to control for practice, a retested control group has been used if at all possible. However, other approaches are being tried.[19,43]

Parker and Serrats[40] examined recovery in 118 patients tested frequently during the period 1 to 24 months after injury on the free recall of lists of 12 words. Different lists were used at each session, thereby reducing practice effect, the authors hoped. The duration of coma was stated to show little relationship with time taken for memory recovery, although the duration of "post-traumatic disorientation (PTD)" was felt to be important in terms of predicting the rate and extent of recovery. In the shortest PTD cases (1 day or less), 32 percent had recovered to a normal level by 12 months; whereas in the longest PTD cases (over 1 month), only 50 percent had reached normal by 2 years. In the shortest PTD group, 50 percent were normal by 1 month.

Groher[41] tested patients serially, using the Wechsler Memory Scale, and found Conkey's pattern of recovery,[7] with the ability to perform tasks resting on the use of "old" information recovering long before that on tasks requiring new learning. However, although the general trend in memory functioning was toward continuing improvement, it seemed that if memory skills *were* going to recover fully, they would do so by 2 months after injury. Furthermore, despite finding insignificant correlations between memory performance and duration of unconsciousness, Groher did point out that the two patients with the longest coma did have by far the worst initial and final memory performance, and he went on to suggest that the relationship between severity and subsequent memory performance may be nonuniform, being stronger at the extremes of severity and weaker in the middle of the severity range.

Lezak[37] addressed much the same issues as those raised by Groher and found that fewer than half of her 24 severely injured patients showed a memory performance within normal limits by the third year after injury, with a consistent recovery effect found on only the two simplest measures. This pattern was found in virtually all her patients, with site of injury having very little influence. On all measures, the more severely injured patients (those with more than 2 weeks of coma) performed worse than other patients at each occasion. Lezak also described individual differences in recovery, and found on some measures a deterioration of memory performance between 2 and 3 years after injury.

The study by Brooks and Aughton[10] assessed memory recovery over the first year after injury. Twenty-four severely injured patients were tested at 3, 6, and 12 months on a large battery of tests, which included measures of memory. The latter measures were found to show more prolonged and slower recovery than did measures of perception, intelligence, or language—so much so that by the third assessment, the only measures on which head-injured patients were still significantly worse than non-head-injured controls were those of memory. A replication of this study involved a cooperative effort among psychologists in Glasgow, Rotterdam, and Groningen, and the results were substantially the same.[39] An analysis of recovery in terms of severity (PTA) showed that the patients with the longest PTA performed worse at first and final test, but there were no signs of differentially slower rates of recovery in the most severely injured patient.

Gronwall and Wrightson[44] assessed head-injured patients weekly on a paced serial addition task until performance was normal. The number of days to reach normal was found to be related to PTA and also to the presence of a previous concussion. In patients with a PTA less than an hour, it took an average 27 days to reach normal; whereas patients with PTAs of 1 to 24 hours took 41 days to reach this level. Within these two PTA groups, the presence of a previous concussion was a significant factor: previously concussed patients with a PTA less than 1 hour took 31 days, compared with the other similar PTA cases taking 23 days. In the longer PTA cases, the times to reach normal were 47 and 35 days, respectively.

To summarize the work on memory recovery, it is evident that the recovery of psychologic functions involving memory lags behind that of other functions. The recovery rate of learning and memory is slower than on other measures, and the final level reached is likely to be much lower. The severity of injury appears to affect mainly the level of recovery rather than its rate, although unfortunately many of the studies reported have used rather small numbers of patients, which does make it difficult to draw firm conclusions.

DOES MEMORY TEST PERFORMANCE RELATE TO "EVERYDAY" MEMORY?

To a large degree, the clinical significance of memory deficits identified by means of memory tests has been taken for granted, despite the fact that every clinical neuropsychologist must have seen patients with complaints of severe memory deficit who show adequate memory test performance, or those who show few complaints concerning memory yet obtain very poor scores on memory tests. Some of these patients may be identified as "functional" or as lacking in insight, but there still remain patients for whom the relationship between everyday memory performance and memory test performance is not strong.

Few investigations of this relationship have been reported, and those that have appeared tend to concern normal volunteer subjects. One reason for the dearth of studies is probably the limited understanding we have of the requirements of day-to-day memory as was shown in the symposium on Practical Aspects of Memory.[45] A number of contributors to that symposium addressed themselves to this problem.[46-48]

Wilkins and Baddeley[46] used normal volunteer subjects and found, if anything, a negative relationship between free recall of word lists and a measure of "absentmindedness." In addition, 30 percent of subjects who had failed to carry out a task were quite unaware of their omission. This important finding led Wilkins and Baddeley to comment that not only do laboratory tests generalize rather poorly to the real world, but also studies relying on subjects' reporting of failure to recall may miss a substantial proportion of failures.

In Glasgow, an attempt was made at a simple analysis of the relationship between day-to-day memory and memory task performance in head-injured patients.[48] A close relative of the patient filled in a simple questionnaire about the patient's memory. The questionnaire dealt with items such as forgetting to do things at specified times, forgetting where things had been left, forgetting peoples' names, and so forth, and the four memory tests were conventional clinical ones involving associate learning, story recall, and design reproduction. The questionnaire had been devised by Sunderland, now of the Applied Psychology Unit at Cambridge. In addition to filling in the individual items of the questionnaire, the relative was encouraged to summarize on a 5-point scale the overall severity of the patient's deficit. At 3 months, this rating bore a significant relationship only to delayed performance on the recall of stories, but not to immediate performance or to performance on the recall of a complex design. At 6 months, the relationship between the overall rating and all four clinical memory tests was highly significant at less than 0.001, but at 12 months the correlation had reduced, being significant (at $p < 0.003$) only for the delayed performance on the design. Caution should be used in interpreting these results, as different forms of the psychologic test were used at each time of assessment.

HOW MAY MEMORY FUNCTIONS BE IMPROVED?

The management or treatment of memory disorders is now under active study, with reports of therapeutic programs beginning to appear. The reports mainly involve training patients to use simple mnemonics or organizational strategies, for example, bizarre interactive visual imagery or forming words into meaningful sentences; and often assume that a memory skill taught in one situation or to solve one problem will necessarily generalize to other situations or problems.

In 1972, Patten[49] reported briefly on the use of a memory system that involved teaching the patient to form visual images and connect these with the items to be remembered. The patient is taught a specific list—for example, 1 = bun; 2 = shoe; 3 = tree, and so forth—and any list of items to be remembered in the future is paired in order with the visual images in this list by using as striking and bizarre an interactive image as possible. Patten describes seven patients whom he tried to help using this system, of whom four (all with left-sided temporal lesions) improved in terms of reported memory performance and general everyday morale. The three patients who did not benefit had either a presenile dementia or, in two cases, severe memory defects probably amounting to an amnesic syndrome. These patients had no awareness of the defect, and their deficit is known to be very resistant to treatment.[50,51]

Other reports of the use of imagery and similar methods have appeared.[52,53] Glasgow and associates[52] described a single head-injured patient who benefited from instructions in the use of imagery, and subsequently Lewinson and coworkers[53] examined 19 patients suffering vascular brain damage who were taught the use of visual imagery in the recall of word lists. These patients were compared with those not taught the method and were found to have superior performance at 30 minutes' recall but not at 1 week after initial learning. Lewinson comments that "the particular utility of imagery mnemonics remained to be validated."

Attempts at a more detailed validation were reported recently.[54] The Gianutsos study[54] involved a classic individual case-study methodology of four head-injured patients using multiple baseline assessments. The training sessions comprised instruction in semantic processing involving forming stories to link words, and the results over prolonged training demonstrated some improvement in aspects of memory task performance in all four patients. However, only one patient achieved striking gains, and she also showed a spontaneous remission of motor deficits before beginning the study. One patient showed an initial gain followed by a relapse; in another patient, improvement was slow and slight.

An alternative approach was reported by Fowler, Hart, and Scheehan[55] in a single head-injured patient with severe memory disturbance. These workers used behavior modification in which an operational definition of memory was made in terms of day-to-day behavioral goals, for example, reaching target activity by specified times. The patient was given a detailed daily schedule in which all activities were listed, together with a timer, and was rewarded for achieving a given goal within a specified time. Failure to achieve this goal resulted in social disapproval. The patient showed enormous improvement. During baseline testing, he missed all daily appointments unless specifically directed by a staff member, whereas at the end of his first week of the study he missed three out of a possible 24, and during the second week he missed only two appointments. Finally, the timer was removed, and using the schedule alone, the patient missed only two out of a possible 42 appointments over a 2-week period, and subsequently he went on to obtain for himself a diary that he used spontaneously.

Undoubtedly, many clinicians with widely differing backgrounds are using memory retraining techniques with brain-damaged patients. Little is known about the range of such techniques, as many clinicians may be reluctant to publish on often small numbers and using techniques that involve many components which may be difficult to specify or control. An attempt has been made to find out what is being done in Britain at the present time. Psychologists working at the Medical Research Council's Applied Psychology Unit at Cambridge (Harris, Sunderland, and Baddeley) have sent out a questionnaire to 49 rehabilitation units thought to be likely to be dealing with brain-damaged patients who were suffering cognitive difficulties. The questionnaire was fairly open-ended, aimed at finding out who was attempting to retrain memory, what was being done, and whether the treatment was aimed at a specified memory problem or a generalized memory performance. Twenty-two questionnaires were completed by 10 psychologists, 6 medical doctors, 5 occupational therapists, and 1 speech therapist.

Analysis of the results showed that the patients being treated by these workers included those with head-injuries, stroke, "senility," multiple sclerosis, tumor, and Korsakoff/amnesic syndrome. Many respondents commented spontaneously on the lack of effective techniques, although many different techniques and materials were being used. However, some material being used by respondents as a test (e.g., the Wechsler Memory Scale) was used for training by others. No respondents felt that they were "very effective," although seven felt themselves to be moderately, nine marginally, and one not at all effective. Nine respondents reported that they were attempting to treat a particular memory disturbance, and five were attempting to improve memory generally.

SUMMARY AND CONCLUSIONS

That head injury causes memory impairment is well known. The impairment on memory is more severe than on other cognitive functions and is certainly longer lasting. Furthermore, the more severe the diffuse injury, the more severe the memory impairment, although the relationship between purely focal damage and memory impairment is much less strong. In cases where focal or lateralized damage has been related to increasingly severe memory impairment, it is always difficult to know whether the focal sign merely gives a further indication of the severity of the diffuse damage; and as far as psychologists are concerned, blunt head injury should be considered to be a diffuse lesion.

Memory recovers slowly compared with other cognitive functions, and even at the end of a 2-year period, many patients are still complaining of memory difficulties and have poor memory test performance. However, the precise impact of such deficits on the performance of "everyday memory" tasks is often not known. Finally, it is important to note that treatment of memory disturbances is still at an early stage, although more papers are now appearing in this area. The techniques currently used largely involve visual imagery or other elaborative forms of semantic coding. Further work in this area is needed.

REFERENCES

1. TOOTH, G: *On the use of mental tests for the measurement of disability after head injury.* J Neurol Neurosurg Psychiatry 10:1, 1947.
2. MCKINLAY, WW, ET AL: *The short term outcome of severe blunt head injury as reported by relatives of the injured persons.* J Neurol Neurosurg Psychiatry 44:527, 1981.
3. SCHACTER, DL AND CROVITZ, HF: *Memory function after closed head injury: A review of the quantitative research.* Cortex 13:150, 1977.
4. RUSSELL, WR: *The Traumatic Amnesias.* Oxford University Press, London, 1971.
5. FODOR, IE: *Impairment of memory function after acute head injury.* J Neurol Neurosurg Psychiatry 35:818, 1972.
6. DUNN, J AND BROOKS, DN: *Memory and post traumatic amnesia.* Journal of International Research Communications 2:1497, 1974.
7. CONKEY, RC: *Psychological changes associated with head injuries.* Arch Psychol (Frankf) 33(232), 1938.
8. RUESCH, J: *Intellectual impairment in head injury.* Am J Psychiatry 100:480, 1944.
9. BROOKS, DN AND AUGHTON, ME: *Psychological consequences of blunt head injury.* Int Rehabil Med 1:160, 1979.
10. BROOKS, DN AND AUGHTON, ME: *Cognitive recovery during the first year after severe blunt head injury.* Int Rehabil Med 1:166, 1979.
11. CRONHOLM, B AND JONSSON, I: *Memory functions after cerebral concussion.* Acta Chir Scand 113:263, 1957.
12. DENCKER, SJ: *Closed head injury in twins.* Arch Gen Psychiatry 2:569, 1960.
13. BROOKS, DN, ET AL: *Cognitive sequelae in relationship to early indices of severity of brain damage after severe blunt head injury.* J Neurol Neurosurg Psychiatry 43:529, 1980.

14. BROOKS, DN: *Wechsler Memory Scale performance and its relationship to brain damage after severe closed head injury.* J Neurol Neurosurg Psychiatry 39:593, 1976.
15. WECHSLER, D: *A standardized memory scale for clinical use.* J Psychol 19:87, 1954.
16. BLACK, FW: *Cognitive and memory performance in subjects with brain damage secondary to penetrating missile wounds and closed head injury.* J Clin Psychol 31:441, 1973.
17. KEAR-COLWELL, JJ AND HELLER, M: *The Wechsler Memory Scale and closed head injury.* J Clin Psychol 36:782, 1980.
18. INGLIS, J: *A paired associate learning test for use with elderly psychiatric patients.* Journal of Mental Science 105:440, 1959.
19. GRONWALL, D AND SAMPSON, H: *The Psychological Effects of Concussion.* Auckland University Press, Auckland, NZ, 1974.
20. VAN ZOMEREN, AH AND DEELMAN, BG: *Long-term recovery of visual reaction time after closed head injury.* J Neurol Neurosurg Psychiatry 41:452, 1978.
21. BROOKS, DN: *Long and short term memory in head injured patients.* Cortex 11:329, 1975.
22. TULVING, E AND COLOTLA, VA: *Free recall of trilingual lists.* Cognitive Psychology 1:86, 1970.
23. LEVIN, HS AND PETERS, BH: *Neuropsychological testing following head injuries: Prosopagnosia without visual field defect.* Dis Nerv Syst 68:21, 1976.
24. BROOKS, DN: *Memory and head injury.* J Nerv Ment Dis 155:350, 1972.
25. BROOKS, DN: *Recognition memory, and head injury.* J Neurol Neurosurg Psychiatry 7:794, 1974.
26. BROOKS, DN: *Recognition memory after head injury: A signal detection analysis.* Cortex 10:224, 1974.
27. RICHARDSON, JTE: *Signal detection theory and the effects of severe head injury upon recognition memory.* Cortex 15:145, 1979.
28. JENNETT, B, ET AL: *Disability after severe head injury: Observations on the use of a practical scale.* J Neurol Neurosurg Psychiatry 44:285, 1981.
29. KLOVE, H AND CLEELAND, CS: *The relationships of neuropsychological impairment to other indices of severity of head injury.* Scand J Rehabil Med 4:55, 1972.
30. TEASDALE, G AND JENNETT, B: *Assessment of coma and impaired consciousness: A practical scale.* Lancet 2:81, 1974.
31. LEVIN, HS, ET AL: *Long term neuropsychological outcome of closed head injury.* J Neurosurg 50:412, 1979.
32. OMMAYA, AK AND GENNARELLI, TA: *Cerebral concussion and traumatic unconsciousness.* Brain 97:633, 1974.
33. RUESCH, J AND MOORE, B: *Impairment of intellectual functions in the acute stage of head injury.* Archives of Neurology and Psychiatry 50:165, 1943.
34. SMITH, E: *Influence of site of impact upon cognitive performance persisting long after severe closed head injury.* J Neurol Neurosurg Psychiatry 37:719, 1974.
35. ROBERTS, AH: *Severe Accidental Head Injury.* Macmillan, London, 1979.
36. THOMSEN, IV: *Verbal learning in aphasic and non aphasic patients with severe head injury.* Scand J Rehabil Med 9:73, 1977.
37. LEZAK, MD: *Recovery of memory and learning functions following traumatic brain damage.* Cortex 15:63, 1979.
38. UZZELL, BP, ET AL: *Lateralised psychological impairment associated with CT lesions in head injured patients.* Cortex 15:391, 1979.
39. BROOKS, DN, ET AL: *Problems in measuring the process of psychosocial recovery after head injury* (submitted for publication).
40. PARKER, SA AND SERRATS, AF: *Memory recovery after traumatic coma.* Acta Neurochir (Wien) 34:71, 1976.
41. GROHER, M: *Language and memory disorder following closed head trauma.* J Speech Hear Res 20:212, 1977.

42. KLONOFF, H, LOW, MD, AND CLARK, C: *Head injuries in children: A prospective five year follow up.* J Neurol Neurosurg Psychiatry 40:1211, 1977.
43. ESON, ME, YEN, JK, AND BOURKE, RS: *Assessment of recovery from serious head injury.* J Neurol Neurosurg Psychiatry 41:1036, 1978.
44. GRONWALL, O AND WRIGHTSON, P: *Cumulative effect of concussion.* Lancet 2:995, 1975.
45. GRUNEBERG, MM, MORRIS, PE, AND SYKES, RN: *Practical aspects of memory.* Academic Press, London, 1978.
46. WILKINS, AJ AND BADDELEY, AD: *Remembering to recall in everyday life: An approach to absent-mindedness.* In GRUNEBERG, MM, MORRIS, PE, AND SYKES, RN: *Practical Aspects of Memory.* Academic Press, London, 1978, p 27.
47. HERRMAN, DJ AND NEISSER, U: *An inventory of everyday memory experiences.* In GRUNEBERG, MM, MORRIS, PE, AND SYKES, RN: *Practical Aspects of Memory.* Academic Press, London, 1978, p 35.
48. BROOKS, DN: *Psychological deficits after severe blunt head injury: Their significance and rehabilitation.* In OSBORNE, DJ, GRUNEBERG, MM, AND EISER, JR: *Research in Psychology and Medicine,* Vol II. Academic Press, London, 1979, p 470.
49. PATTEN, BM: *The ancient art of memory: Usefulness in treatment.* Arch Neurol 26:25, 1972.
50. CERMAK, LS: *The encoding capacity of a patient with amnesia due to encephalitis.* Neuropsychologia 14:311, 1976.
51. JONES, MK: *Imagery as a mnemonic aid after left temporal lobectomy: Contrast between material-specific and generalized memory disorders.* Neuropsychologia 12:21, 1974.
52. GLASGOW, RE, ET AL: *Case studies on remediating memory deficits in brain damaged individuals.* J Clin Psychol 33:1049, 1977.
53. LEWINSOHN, PM, DANAHER, BG, AND KIKEL, S: *Visual imagery as a mnemonic aid for brain injured persons.* J Consult Clin Psychol 45:717, 1977.
54. GIANUTSOS, R AND GIANUTSOS, J: *Rehabilitating the verbal recall of brain injured patients by mnemonic training: An experimental demonstration using single case methodology.* J Clin Neuropsychol 1:117, 1979.
55. FOWLER, RS, HART, J, AND SHEEHAN, M: *A prosthetic memory: An application of the prosthetic environment concept.* Rehabilitation Counselling Bulletin December:80, 1972.

Chapter 14

BEHAVIORAL SEQUELAE

Mitchell Rosenthal, Ph.D.

The behavioral manifestations of head injury are perhaps the most difficult to understand, measure, predict, and treat of all of the disorders that accompany traumatic brain injury. Therefore, it is not surprising that this category of residual dysfunction is considered by rehabilitation staff, as well as the relatives of head-injured patients, to be the greatest obstacle to the successful restoration of the patient to a productive status within the family and community.[1,2] The identification and management of behavioral problems within the acute, subacute, and extended phases of rehabilitation have begun to receive greater attention within comprehensive prospective research protocols.

To understand the nature of behavioral dysfunction, it is first necessary to state an operational definition. For the purposes of the present discussion, behavioral dysfunction will be defined as "those overt actions that result in socially maladaptive interactions between the patient and environment." To provide further clarification, the range of behavioral problems that will be discussed is often referred to as the emotional or personality changes that result from head injury. This definition is restrictive in the sense that it would not include the majority of cognitive disorders, which include defects in thinking, information processing, learning ability, memory, visual perception, and so forth. It should be stated, however, that so-called cognitive deficits often accompany behavioral problems and can create socially maladaptive behaviors. (For further information about the nature of cognitive dysfunction, the reader is referred to Chapters 12 and 13.)

FACTORS THAT CONTRIBUTE TO BEHAVIORAL DYSFUNCTION

Kretschmer[3] was among the first researchers to discuss the behavioral effects of head injury. He described three factors that need to be examined to understand behavioral changes: (1) characteristics of each patient prior to the head injury; (2) changes in psychic traits that may be attributable to the brain damage itself; and (3) psychologic difficulties in life. The latter category would likely refer to the problems confronting the head-injured person when the person returns to the home environment and must live with the altered state imposed by the injury. Goldstein[4] termed this the "catastrophic reaction," which was characterized by anxiety, restlessness, and overorderliness, and represented the injured person's attempt to adjust to the environment.

PREMORBID FACTORS

In discussing the significance of premorbid personality, Symonds[5] noted, "It is not only the kind of injury that matters, but the kind of head." One can infer from this statement that the sum total of characteristic ways of behaving, level of cognitive functioning, and methods of coping with stress would be an important determinant of the ultimate behavioral changes resulting from head injury. Tobis[6] and Field[7] noted the high frequency of premorbid maladaptive behavior patterns that characterize the head-injured patients in their study populations. Lishman[8] extended this concept by including the pre-existing family history in this regard, by noting that a history of familial psychiatric instability tended to increase the probability of behavioral disturbance. Cronholm[9] also recognized that the pretraumatic coping strategies of the patient will be an important determinant of the manner in which the patient deals with the effects of brain injury. He proceeded to describe a formula for conceptualizing the post-traumatic behavior of the head-injured patient as follows:

$$\text{Coping strategy} = f(\text{Cerebral injury, mental trauma, environmental factors, social structure, premorbid personality, etc.})$$

It should be noted that the factors noted above must be considered as interacting with each other. Moreover, in any individual case, the relative significance (or weighting) of any single factor may be disproportionate to the others. For example, the patient who sustains massive bifrontal injury and subsequent behavioral changes will be greatly limited in social interaction by the injury itself, independent of any other factors. In another case, a victim of closed head injury with a history of asocial behavior, impulsivity, impaired interpersonal relationships, and a chaotic family life may be likely to exhibit marked behavioral maladjustment, irrespective of the severity of the lesion and other factors.

SITE OF LESION

In recent years, there has been much speculation as to the correlation between site of injury and subsequent behavioral manifestations. The greatest consensus regarding the correlation of locus of injury and observed behavioral consequences is found in the literature describing the "frontal lobe syndrome." In general, this category of behavioral dysfunction usually refers to a constellation of symptoms including decreased drive, lack of goal-directed behavior, apathy, lethargy, social disinhibition, childish behavior, poor judgment, inappropriate sexual and aggressive behavior, and dull or flat affect. A classic example of such behavior abnormalities is well illustrated by the celebrated case of Phineas Gage,[11] who sustained a penetrating head injury as a result of an explosion that catapulted a crowbar through the frontal lobe. Though he was premorbidly considered to be a well-balanced, socially appropriate individual, the effects of the penetrating injury left him with intact formal intellect but great changes in his personality:

> He is fitful, irreverent, indulging at times in the grossest profanity, manifesting but little deference for his fellows, impatient of restraints or advice. . . . a child in his intellectual capacity and manifestations, he has the animal passions of a strong man. . . .

After the injury, he survived for 12 years but never returned to his premorbid personality and life style, and tended to wander aimlessly without direction or goal until his death.

In the case of traumatic brain injury, damage to the frontal lobes is of particular significance due to the high frequency of cases in which the frontal lobes are affected. This is perhaps related to the primary etiology of closed head injury, that is, automobile accident, in which the front of the head is so often injured. The most severe manifestations of frontal lobe behavior are usually seen in cases of bifrontal injury to the orbital surface. In these cases, the entire range of symptoms previously described is observed, especially antisocial conduct and behavior.

It has also been observed that the frontal lobes appear to fulfill an "executive" function; that is, the role of the frontal lobes would appear to be one of regulation and integration of behavior. Perhaps that is why patients with frontal lobe injuries tend to behave without rhyme or reason. The ability to attend, persist, and engage in purposeful, goal-directed behavior is impaired. Their sense of identity and self-esteem often appears to be nonexistent. These patients often behave "for the moment only," failing to acknowledge the relationship of their action to its consequence. The following case illustrates the unusual world of the frontal lobe patient:

> W.B. was a 48-year-old, black, married man with four children employed as an assembly worker in an automobile plant. He sustained a bifrontal injury in an automobile accident. His physical recovery proceeded quite rapidly, with little apparent overt physical residua at 4 weeks postinjury. Yet his behavior was greatly changed from his premorbid status. Upon discharge to his home, his wife reported that he exhibited a complete lack of drive, interest, and motivation. His daily routine consisted of sitting alone in a room, staring at the TV, not attending to his children or wife. He would not speak unless spoken to. When asked to perform a household chore, he would begin to wipe the dishes and, within 5 minutes, cease the activity, sit down, and stare into space. At times, he would wander outside the house and be found walking in the road. If asked where he was going, he was unable to provide an answer.

Blumer and Benson[10] described this behavioral pattern as "pseudodepressed," attributing its origin to destructive lesions of the prefrontal convexity, basal ganglia, and thalamus, and their connections. The antisocial, childish, euphoric behavioral patterns are said to constitute a "pseudopsychopathic" personality. The case of Phineas Gage, described above, would be more likely to be in this category, which is attributable to injuries to the orbital surface of the frontal lobe.

As may be obvious, the prognosis for social and vocational recovery of patients with frontal lobe injury is quite poor. In his extensive studies of head-injured veterans of World War II, Luria[12] noted that of all the types of head injury, those with frontal lobe involvement are least likely to return to work and experience a successful readjustment to the family environment. Perhaps the biggest obstacle to rehabilitating these patients is their profound lack of insight into the origin of the maladaptive nature of their behavior. Indeed, a neurologic concomitant of the injury has been described as "lack of foresight and judgment." In addition, these behavioral abnormalities have proven to be largely insensitive to psychopharmacologic intervention. Stern[13] has reported the successful use of dextroamphetamines in 11 frontal lobe patients in decreasing fatigability, improving the ability to attend and concentrate, and promoting a greater awareness of themselves and their immediate environment. However, to date, there have been no long-term studies that have attested to the success of environmental manipulations, psychotherapeutic intervention, or pharmacologic management in altering the unusual constellation of behaviors that comprise the frontal lobe syndrome.

Other structures within the brain have been implicated in the manifestation of behavioral change after head injury. Lishman[14] noted an observed relationship between focal electroencephalographic abnormalities in the temporal lobe and disinhibition of aggression. This phenomenon of disinhibition is seen in violent outbursts in response to minor stresses experienced by the head-injured victim. It may take the form of verbal outbursts or actual physical violence. Sweet and colleagues[15] have associated the presence of such behavior with damage to medial temporal lobe structures. The aggressive behavior seen in traumatic head injury bears some similarity to the behavioral abnormalities associated with temporal lobe seizures. However, it should be noted while post-traumatic epilepsy does occur in cases of head injury, the relative occurrence is statistically quite minimal (5 percent) and may or may not take the form of temporal lobe seizures in their classic form. Further research is needed to clarify the relationship of temporal lobe damage and behavioral abnormalities.

Hypothalamic and basilar branch injuries have been noted to create a variety of behavioral problems, including sluggishness, mood fluctuations, marked irritability, sleep disturbances, and appetite irregularities.[16]

Sleep-wakefulness alterations and excessive cravings for nourishment often present themselves in the early stages of recovery from head injury. In my clinical experience, these behavioral problems tend to be relatively short-lived but can be especially troublesome for staff and family members to comprehend and manage. The following illustrates this problem:

> John was a 15-year-old boy who was struck by an automobile while walking in the street and suffered a closed head injury. Computerized tomography (CT) failed to reveal any hematoma or localized cortical damage. He was unconscious for 4 days and remained in the neurosurgical unit for 2 weeks, when he was transferred to the rehabilitation unit. Shortly after arrival, John, who had achieved the ability to ambulate without assistance, made hourly visits to the kitchen, begging for food. In addition, he called his parents and told them to bring in food, as he was not getting enough to eat. This insatiable appetite persisted day and night and was unfortunately reinforced by his family. Finally, amphetamine therapy was started, and the family was instructed to ignore all requests for food. His intense craving for food rapidly diminished.

It was difficult to determine whether the cessation of the behavior was caused by the institution of the amphetamines or the tighter environmental controls. In other cases, however, despite all modes of intervention, this insatiable drive for nourishment has been known to persist for months and even years after the injury.

In many instances, the presence of behavioral dysfunction cannot be correlated with evidence of focal neurologic evidence of destructive lesions. As Jennett[17] and others have noted, most head injuries result in diffuse brain damage, which may be seen in normal CT scan and only microscopic widespread white matter damage upon autopsy. Problems such as fluctuating depression, irritability, poor frustration tolerance, inability to deal with stress, and sexual dysfunction are often seen in head-injured persons, irrespective of the neuropathology of their injury. These behavioral changes may be attributable to the diffuse and widespread organic damage, the presence of pre-existing emotional and behavioral problems, or perhaps the response of the "environment to the newly head-injured" person.

ENVIRONMENTAL FACTORS

Upon discharge from the rehabilitation center, the head-injured patients often return to an environment—consisting of relatives, friends, and colleagues at school or at work—that may facilitate or inhibit recovery. The presence of some of the aforementioned behavioral deficits is often a tremendous burden on the family,[18] which should not be underestimated. The manner in which the family members (often spouse or parents) respond to the observed changes in their loved one can create conditions that maintain dysfunctional behavior or create additional emotional distress. It often takes months or years for the family to recognize and accept the permanence of the personality changes that are so frequently in evidence.

It is not surprising that Lezak and coworkers[19] in a study of the long-term psychologic consequences of head injury in 39 patients (up to 5 years postinjury) found that the most persistent psychologic consequences of the injury were in the areas of social contact, work/school, and leisure, as measured by the Portland Adaptability Inventory. The experience of most clinicians working with head-injured persons is that although some behavioral symptoms improve over time (e.g., poor impulse control, hostility, impaired judgment), the inability of the patient to recover to the premorbid level of activity because of mental sequelae often creates additional emotional/behavioral problems, such as anxiety, depression, irritability, social isolation, decreased self-esteem, and impaired social relationships. It is paradoxic and ironic that as the head-injured patient becomes more able to function (from a cognitive and behavioral standpoint), the increased perception of behavioral alterations imposed by the injury itself impairs the patient's ability to make a satisfactory return to social, economic, and vocational productivity.

To summarize the foregoing discussion on the various factors that contribute to behavioral dysfunction following head injury, it would seem that three factors have primary significance in determining behavioral outcome from head injury: (1) the nature of the premorbid behavior of both patient and family; (2) the location of the lesion and its corresponding effect on behavior, and whether the damage appears to be focal or diffuse; (3) and the environment the patient returns to—in effect, the consequences of living with a severe head injury. In the case of the latter, investigators have only recently begun to recognize its significance and attempt to study the manner in which it may affect outcome.

COURSE OF RECOVERY

Certain behavioral sequelae of head injury appear in a fairly predictable, but not invariant, sequence after the injury. During the initial phase of emergence from unconsciousness, the head-injured victim is likely to be disoriented (to time and place more often than to person), quite agitated, potentially violent, and totally unaware of the nature of the injury and the need for hospitalization. At times, episodes of delirium and hallucinations may occur.[13] It is as if the patient moves back and forth between a dream-like state of unreality and a fearful, anxious, disjointed state of experience. These feelings are complicated by the presence of post-traumatic amnesia (PTA), which is an absence of day-to-day memory of events or people. During this period, the patient's behavior is likely to be unpredictable, bizarre, and impulsive, often necessitating chemical or physical restraints. Intensive monitoring and supervision of behavior by nursing and therapy staff are required.

As the patient moves out of PTA, the patient displays better orientation to the environment and a limited recognition of the state of physical and/or mental disability. This period of recovery, which may be termed "subacute," is usually in evidence when the patient is transferred from the neurosurgical unit to the rehabilitation center. At this point, the bizarre, psychiatric-like behaviors typically subside. The patient is likely to remain impulsive and display poor judgment. The patient is easily frustrated and may show episodic outbursts in response to minor frustrations. Since the patient does not yet fully comprehend the nature of the injury and cannot recall how it occurred, the patient is likely to perceive the world as threatening. Perseverative responses, either verbal or motor, are present. The patient appears stimulus-bound, unable or unwilling to adapt to minor changes in the daily schedule or environment. Family members are often surprised to observe the childlike dependence that begins to be prominent. The head-injured patient may show an extraordinary attachment to relatives and friends and become extremely upset when they leave. Another manifestation of this dependency may be seen in the number of telephone calls made by the patient on a daily basis to home, much to the consternation of staff members and friends. The following brief case example illustrates a common reaction of the family to this behavior:

> Paula H. was a 17-year-old girl who suffered a closed head injury in an automobile accident on Christmas Eve, 1976. After 2 weeks on the neurosurgery unit, she was transferred to the rehabilitation unit. When her parents would visit her, she was unusually affectionate, continually kissing and hugging her parents. When they started to leave the hospital, she would walk with them,

begging them not to leave her alone in the hospital. Prior to the injury, Paula was quite independent of family rule and tended to argue frequently with her mother. She was described as a typical, rebellious teenage girl. In discussing her postinjury behavior, Mr. and Mrs. H. expressed ambivalence about the behavior—concern that she was acting like a young child, but pleased about the affection and intimacy in their new relationship.

It is my experience that this state of childlike dependence may continue for an extended period, though it is rarely the case that the intensity of the dependency will persist, unless it is reinforced by the family.

During the third phase of recovery, the patient may yet be hospitalized in the rehabilitation center, transferred to a long-term rehabilitation program, or at home with the family. This phase (often starting 3 to 6 months postinjury and continuing beyond) is usually marked by a considerable improvement in both cognitive and language functions. The patient can recall day-to-day events, reliably recognize people, and show more appropriate interpersonal relationships. Often, patients have a greater awareness of their physical limitations, and a growing awareness of some of their mental deficits. Impulsive behavior is less frequent; thus, less intense supervision of daily activities is required. Irritability, impatience, and poor frustration tolerance are still common. The denial of disability is manifested in statements by patients such as, "I'm as good as I was before; why won't you let me go home, or return to school?" This feeling of return to normality is often reinforced by the frequent appearance of physical integrity, ability to ambulate independently, and capacity to perform most daily activities. During this period, which may continue indefinitely, head-injured patients must come to terms with their new identity, which is invariably less desirable than their previous identity. They are often confused and upset by the restrictions placed on their behavior. When fuller acceptance of disability occurs, the result is often anxiety, depression, and anger. Fears about the permanence of brain damage and its implications are expressed. Rejection by peers or family members is often perceived. The unfortunate consequence of adapting to head injury is the disquieting realization that the remainder of one's life will be a difficult struggle.

OUTCOME STUDIES

Since the measurement of long-term outcome from head injury was reviewed earlier in this book (see Chapter 7), this section will briefly highlight only a few reports that have systematically studied the behavioral sequelae resulting from trauma.

The work of Levin and colleagues at the University of Texas at Galveston is certainly a good model for the examination of behavioral residuals of brain injury. Levin and colleagues[20] followed 27 patients with closed head injury for approximately 1 year postinjury. These patients were all considered to be severely injured, as indicated by a score of 8 or less on the Glasgow Coma Scale. Behavioral outcome was assessed by the completion of the Glasgow Outcome Scale and Brief Psychiatric Rating Scale (BPRS). The BPRS consists of 18 scales of emotional/behavioral function, which are rated on the basis of a semistructured interview by a trained examiner. A major finding of the study was the presence of marked behavioral dysfunction of those patients classified as severely disabled. In these cases, behavioral deficits were characterized by two general factors identified as Thinking Disturbance and Withdrawal/Retardation. These patients had very little comprehension of their cognitive deficits and would tend to deny any appreciable deficits attributable to the injury. Motor slowing and aspontaneity in behavior were also observed. Four of the subjects had severe psychiatric disturbance, with two being diagnosed as psychotic. There was a generally shorter duration of coma for those patients who made a good recovery, though considerable variability was observed among the various groups classified by outcome.

Roberts and colleagues[20] in England reported the results of a long-term follow-up of 291 patients admitted to the Accident and Neurosurgical Services of the Radcliffe Infirmary between 1948 and 1961. These patients and their families were interviewed between 10 and 24 years post-trauma. Assessment of personality dysfunction was made on the basis of observations and interviews with the patient and family members (usually spouse) and clinical assessments made during the interview. Severity of dysfunction was measured on an eight-category scale, which ranged from no disability to inaccessibly psychotic. The authors found that the most frequently occurring pattern of behavioral problems (50 cases) was that of euphoria and disinhibition combined with irritability and defective memory—termed *fronto-limbic dementia*. On the basis of this personality disorder, these patients were considered to be severely disabled. Their behavioral problems greatly limited their ability to perform normally in household, social, vocational, or family activities. In the 26- to 34-year-old age group, another complex of symptoms was identified as *frontal dysmnesia* (34 cases), which consisted of childish behavior, loss of initiative, euphoria, disinhibition, and slight memory defect. Irritability was noticeably absent in this group.

Ota[21] studied 1168 adults with closed head injury between 1952 and 1961 in both the early and chronic stages of recovery from injury (1 day to 21 years postaccident). The author performed psychiatric examinations on each patient and classified patients according to traditional psychiatric nosologic categories. In his investigation, 22 percent of the patients were identified as having neurotic complaints—which were attributed primarily to the organic brain damage itself. He identified 52 cases of psychoses, with approximately one third of this group having psychogenic origin. In examining the incidence of organic psychoses, he noted the difficulty in showing a causal relationship between the structural damage imposed by the injury and the manifestation of a persistent psychotic state. He identified 80 cases of character changes related to brain damage resulting in a complex of behaviors including aspontaneity, apathy, euphoria, irritability, emotional callousness, and increased spontaneity. In this group, the vast majority of patients primarily displayed aspontaneity and apathy. Though most patients studied had little insight into their physical and mental disturbances, gradual improvement in function appeared to be correlated with a greater understanding of deficits and was accompanied by irritability, anxiety, and depression.

SECONDARY BEHAVIORAL DISTURBANCES

Thus far, the discussion has focused primarily on the emotional and behavioral changes that would appear to have their origin in the structural damage accompanying severe closed head injury. In addition to these problems, there would appear to be several behavioral disturbances that are more a result of the stress of adapting to the trauma and its devastating effects upon the patient's life style and daily existence. In this section, brief descriptions and clinical examples will be presented to illustrate the nature and impact of these so-called secondary behavioral disturbances.

DENIAL

The inability to acknowledge the effects of head injury is often observed in the treatment of these patients. As in the case of other catastrophic disabilities (such as spinal cord injury), denial seems to be most pronounced in the early stages of the recovery period (first few months postinjury). Though it often poses major problems for rehabilitation staff, denial may, in fact, be an adaptive mechanism initially if the patient is avoiding a major emotional disorder through the selective use of denial. In the case of head injury, it is rarely the case that the patient denies the injury itself or even the physical sequelae. Most often, the mental sequelae (which are less observable and apparent to the patient) tend to be minimized or dismissed as nonexistent or transient. In most cases, the patient will cooperate with the treatment team in submitting to examination and therapy designed to remediate the mental deficits, despite the fact that the patient overtly denies their existence and significance.

The maladaptive effects of denial are often experienced after the patient returns to the community. In some cases, living with the disability in the home environment makes the patient more aware of the mental deficits and facilitates a more realistic adaptation to the disability. Yet, in others, the tendency to block out the reality of the situation is reinforced by well-intentioned family and friends who are struggling to display an optimistic, hopeful outlook that life will eventually become as normal as it was prior to the injury. The adverse consequences of this strategy can be demonstrated in the following case illustration:

> Peter sustained a severe closed head injury in an automobile accident at age 21. At the time, he was a senior in college, achieving high grades, and planned to attend law school after graduation. After 3 months of hospitalization, he returned to college and managed to complete his BA degree in Economics. Physically, he was left with mild left-sided weakness but could ambulate independently without assistive devices and was totally independent in activities of daily living. Neuropsychologic examination revealed that his IQ returned to the bright-normal range, somewhat below his estimated premorbid level of function. Memory assessment resulted in the finding of mild short-term memory defects. Reading skills were good, though slower than normal, and comprehension was at a 10th grade level. Despite advice to the contrary, he persisted in pursuing law school entrance immediately. His performance on the Law School Admission Test was marginal. Nevertheless, he did not acknowledge the possible persistence of mental deficits and proceeded to enter a law school program. Within four weeks after entry, he dropped out, claiming that his professors were unfairly grading him. He searched for another law school which would accept him but failed in this effort and became quite despondent.

Though Peter's mental sequelae were milder than those of many head-injured patients, his refusal to accept their presence led to severe discouragement and emotional distress. This pattern of ill-advised resumption of premorbid educational and vocational activities is frequently seen in head-injured patients, despite the fact that only about 50 percent of severely injured patients are capable of returning to their previous vocation.[20]

DEPRESSION

As stated previously, head injuries most frequently affect the young (aged 15 to 30) and result in major changes in their daily lives for many years. Head-injured persons usually experience a feeling of loss due to the changes necessitated by the injury. They are less able to perform physically, more dependent socially, and often feel a sense of impotence in trying to reconstruct their lives. Social relationships are less rewarding and often diminish, vocational prospects are dim, and life becomes less interesting. On account of diminished mental abilities, they may be more dependent on spouse or parents and feel less of a person. This form of reactive depression should be contrasted with depressive illness, which is quite rare after closed head injury.[20]

During the subacute (rehabilitative) phase of recovery, depression may be viewed as a positive event, in that it signals the lessening of denial and usually reflects the patient's growing understanding and insight into the realization of the extent of the disability. Often, this insight will be more related to the acknowledgment of the physical impairments caused by the injury, rather than the mental sequelae. Because physical recovery usually proceeds quite rapidly during the first 6 months of the recovery period, the depressed mood does not necessarily inhibit the patient's performance in the rehabilitation program. As with other behavioral sequelae, this problem of depression becomes more troublesome when the patient is returned to the community. At this point (usually 3 to 6 months post-trauma), physical recovery starts to plateau, and a recognition of mental deficits is forthcoming. Inability to resume premorbid educational or vocational activities, dependence on family, loss of friends, and a limited schedule of daily activity cause a heightened amount of anxiety, frustration, sadness, and anger, which results in a chronic state of depression. Suicidal ideation may appear. Occasionally, the depressed state will be masked by a tendency to overreact to minor frustration and exhibit restlessness and agitation.

DEPENDENCE UPON OTHERS

In the young head-injured adult, the net effect of the mental and physical sequelae is to cause the patient to become more emotionally dependent on others. This pattern of behavior is characterized in remarks by family members who note the emotionally regressed and childish nature of their relative's behavior. The patient tends to be more physically affectionate, demanding, egocentric, in need of constant attention, and lacking in the ability to delay immediate gratification. This set of behaviors is especially difficult for the spouse of the head-injured patient, who may unwittingly reinforce the behavior for fear of aggravating the loved one or exacerbating the emotional distress. On account of the patient's childish dependency, the spouse feels as if he or she is caring for a young child, as opposed to interacting with a grown-up partner. Problems are also created when head-injured persons return to their parents and siblings. Conflicts arise in parent-child and sibling relationships. Since the behavior is assumed to be related to the brain damage, family members are often reluctant to place limits on behavior or reprimand the patient, since the patient is not considered to be truly responsible for and aware of the behavior. Two brief case examples are presented below to illustrate this problem:

> Richie B. was a 19-year-old victim of head trauma with bilateral frontal lobe injury. Severely defective memory, disinhibition, apathy, and childishness were primary sequelae of the injury. After approximately 1 year of hospitalization, he returned home to live with his brother, mother, and stepfather. He was unable to engage in any meaningful vocational pursuit. Therefore, he spent most of his time at home with his family. He became excessively demanding of his mother's attention, displaying anger, irritation, and jealousy whenever the mother would spend time with his younger brother. On occasions when the mother would leave the home to visit her friends, he would telephone her every 10 minutes to ask when she would be returning home and why he couldn't be with her. The problem eventually extended to the relationship between his parents—he was unable to tolerate his mother's attention toward his stepfather and demanded attention and physical displays of affection from his mother almost constantly.

> John R. had a closed head injury in 1972 resulting in left temporal lobe damage. Despite memory deficits, he made an excellent recovery and was able to return to his job as a foreman in an automobile assembly plant within 2 years after injury. Prior to the injury, Mrs. R. reported that their marriage was quite satisfactory and home life with their two young children was ideal. Since the injury, John has become extremely "clingy," continually asking for verbal and physical reassurance of her love. He refused to go out in the evening because he didn't want to "share her with anyone." He seemed suspicious of her activities during the day while he was working and asked her for a complete report of how she spent her day. He accused her of having relationships with other men while he was at work. In addition, he tended to withdraw from the children and resented any attention his wife gave to the children.

MINOR HEAD INJURY

Although the primary focus of this chapter is the behavioral sequelae of severe head injury, a few words should be mentioned about so-called minor head injury. In these cases, there is either transient or no loss of consciousness, and rarely is there a need for extensive neurosurgical or rehabilitative interventions. This is usually known as a concussion and rarely results in any apparent physical impairment. Symptomatology is usually based on subjective report and may not present until days or weeks after the injury. The most frequent complaints are headaches, dizziness and vertigo, irritability, seizures, memory deficits, impaired concentration, easy fatigability, oversensitivity to auditory and visual stimuli, and depression. This constellation of problems is referred to as the postconcussion syndrome (PCS). Often, these symptoms subside within a few weeks or months; in other cases, they may persist up to several years after injury and create vocational disability and family stress.

Several investigators have noted the presence of neurophysiologic data which is correlated with PCS. Taylor and Bell[23] examined patients with PCS within 2 months postinjury and compared mean cerebral circulation time with that of control subjects. Their findings indicated a 20 percent longer mean cerebral circulation time for the PCS group. Other evidence of neurophysiologic dysfunction is found in the work of Harrison,[24] who has documented the presence of benign positional nystagmus in patients who complain of vertigo. Electronystagmography has been found to be a useful diagnostic tool in demonstrating vestibular dysfunction in head-injured persons. Problems related to impaired concentration, memory defect, irritability, depression, and chronic headaches have not been shown to directly correspond to any specific neurologic dysfunction.

Much has been written about the psychogenic aspect of the postconcussion syndrome, especially in regard to what has been termed "accident neurosis."[25] Miller noted that 50 percent of all patients admitted to a British hospital because of head injury have pending claims for financial compensation. This is perhaps due to a high proportion of cases that are related to industrial accidents or pending liability litigation (in the case of automobile accidents). Miller also reports that there is an exaggeration of postconcussional symptoms for a prolonged period (up to 2 years postinjury) and a rapid resolution of symptoms once a financial settlement is reached. It is of interest that most of these cases are settled out of court.

As time proceeds from injury, the severity of PCS symptoms usually diminishes. The longer symptoms remain, the stronger the possibility that psychogenic factors play a role in their persistence and that compensation is a motivating factor. As Alexander[26] points out, one must be aware that two types of PCS exist: one that is time-limited and primarily related to the neurophysiologic effects of trauma, and another type (accident neurosis) that may be more related to psychogenic causation.

CONCLUSION

In this chapter, a review of the major emotional and behavioral sequelae of traumatic brain injury has been presented. A variety of factors contribute to the presence and persistence of these problems, including extent of brain damage, site of brain damage, premorbid personality function, response of the environment, and financial compensation. Of these factors, the relationships between the site of lesion and the observed behavioral changes have received the greatest amount of investigation in past research. Injury to the frontal lobes results in an identifiable complex of deficits, including decreased drive and initiative, dull or flat affect, disinhibition, disregard for social mores, exacerbation of appetite drives, apathy, lethargy, lack of goal-directed behavior, inability to regulate behavior, and an impaired sense of self-identity. Other investigations have found a relationship between lesions to the temporal lobe and episodic violent behavior, which may accompany the presence of a seizure disorder. Hypothalamic insults may create disturbances in sleep-wakefulness, appetite irregularities, and alterations in mood.

The presence of a premorbid history of behavioral abnormalities, not uncommon in head-injured persons, often predisposes the victim to an exacerbation of these traits. For example, the person who has a history of antisocial conduct and poor impulse control may show an even stronger tendency to exhibit such behavior after a head injury. The individual who exhibited a passive-dependent personality may become yet more withdrawn and introverted after the injury. In recent years, the response of the environment to newly head-injured persons has been receiving greater attention by clinicians and researchers alike. Despite recent advances in the long-term rehabilitation of head-injured persons, few programs provide adequate services that effectively resocialize, re-educate, and retrain the patient to assume a satisfying role within the family, work, and community environments. In the absence of such programs, behavioral sequelae are likely reinforced and maintained for an indefinite duration. Thus, the family bears the burden of coping with their relative whose behavior and personality function contribute to high levels of family stress and emotional distress.

At present, our ability to identify and describe the likely behavioral residua of head injury is reasonably good. Some progress has been achieved in correlating neurologic focus of trauma with observed behavioral alteration. To date, however, adequate instruments that objectively measure deficits and predict severity and duration have not been developed. It is incumbent upon members of the neurologic and rehabilitation professions to address behavioral dysfunction from the early stages of recovery to the later phase of reintegration into the community. Priority should be placed upon early intervention with patient and family to modify the expression of primary behavioral dysfunction (resulting from the neurologic insults) and minimize the possibility for secondary disturbances that are created, in part, by our inability to successfully reintegrate the patient into society.

REFERENCES

1. Jennett, B and Teasdale, G: *Management of Head Injuries.* FA Davis, Philadelphia, 1981.
2. Bond, MD: *Assessment of the psychosocial outcome after severe head injury.* CIBA Foundation Symposium 34:141, 1975.
3. Kretschmer, E: *Uher psychogene Wahnbildung bei traumatischer Hirnschwache.* Z Ges Neurol Psychiat 45:272, 1919.
4. Goldstein, K: *Aftereffects of Brain Injuries in War.* Grune & Stratton, New York, 1948.
5. Symonds, CP: *Mental disorders following head injury.* Proc R Soc Med 30:1081, 1937.
6. Tobis, J, Pure, K, and Sheridan, J: *Rehabilitation of severely brain injured patients.* Presented at the American Congress of Rehabilitation Medicine, San Diego, Calif, November 1976.
7. Field, JH: *Epidemiology of head injuries in England and Wales: Report from Research Division.* Department of Health and Social Security, London, 1978.
8. Lishman, WA: *The psychiatric sequelae of head injury: A review.* Psychol Med 3:304, 1973.
9. Cronholm, B: *Evaluation of mental disturbance after head injury.* Scand J Rehabil Med 4:35, 1972.
10. Harlow, JM: *Recovery from the passage of an iron bar through the head.* Publications of the Massachusetts Medical Society 2:329, 1868.
11. Blumer, D and Benson, DF: *Personality changes with frontal and temporal lobe lesions.* In *Psychiatric Aspects of Neurologic Disease.* Grune & Stratton, New York, 1975, p 151.
12. Luria, A: *Higher Cortical Functions in Man.* Basic Books, New York, 1966.
13. Stern, JM: *Cranio-cerebral injured patients: A psychiatric clinical description.* Scand J Rehabil Med 10:7, 1978.
14. Lishman, WA: *Brain damage in relation to psychiatric disability after head injury.* Br J Psychol 114:373, 1968.

15. SWEET, WH, ERVIN, F, MARK, VH: *The relationship of violent behavior to focal cerebral disease.* In GARUTTINI, S AND SIGG, EB (EDS): *Aggressive Behavior.* Proceedings of International Symposium on the Biology of Aggressive Behavior, Milan, May 1968.
16. KRETSCHMER, E: *Cerebral orbital and diencephalic syndromes following fractures of the brain and skull.* Archives of Psychiatry 182:452, 1949.
17. JENNETT, B: *Assessment and prediction of outcome after head injury.* Presented at the International Symposium on the Brain Injured Adult and Child, Boston, 1981.
18. BOND, MR: *Psychosocial effects of head injury.* Presented at the fourth Annual Post-Graduate Course on the Rehabilitation of the Traumatic Brain Injured Adult, Williamsburg, Va, 1980.
19. LEZAK, MD, ET AL: *Relationships between personality disorders, social disturbances, and physical disability following traumatic head injury.* Presented at the International Neuropsychological Society Meeting, San Francisco, 1975.
20. LEVIN, HA, ET AL: *Long-term neuropsychological outcome of closed head injury.* J Neurosurg 50:412, 1979.
21. ROBERTS, AH: *Severe Accidental Head Injury.* Macmillan, London, 1979.
22. OTA, Y: *Psychiatric studies on civilian head injuries.* In CAVENESS, WF AND WALKER, AE (EDS): *Head Injury.* JB Lippincott, Philadelphia, 1966, p 110.
23. TAYLOR, AR AND BELL, TU: *Slowing of cerebral circulation after concussional head injury.* Lancet 2:178, 1966.
24. HARRISON, MS: *Notes on the clinical features and pathology of post-concussional vertigo, with especial reference to positional nystagmus.* Brain 79:474, 1956.
25. MILLER, H: *Problems of medicolegal practice.* In WALKER, AE, CAVENESS, WF, AND CRITCHLEY, M (EDS): *The Late Effects of Head Injury.* Charles C Thomas, Springfield, Ill, 1969, p 429.
26. ALEXANDER, MP: *Traumatic brain injury.* In BENSON, DF AND BLUMER, D (EDS): *Psychiatric Aspects of Neurologic Disease,* Vol 2. Grune & Stratton, New York, in press.

Chapter 15

EFFECTS ON THE FAMILY SYSTEM

Michael R. Bond, M.D., Ph.D.

Sudden serious head injury to a member of any family causes psychologic and social changes within the family. The nature and extent of the changes depend on several factors, including the composition of the family group, its place in the fabric of society, the role formerly played by the injured person, and the ability of each member of the family to cope with the stress that develops. The main burdens for relatives are caused by the injured person's residual physical and emotional deficits, especially the latter, and by secondary alterations of interpersonal relations, family income, work patterns, and social activities. Recovery from injury is a drawn-out, continuous process that has clearly defined stages, each of which throws different kinds of stresses on the victim and family, over a period of many months or even years.[1] Until very recently, little systematic work had been carried out on the psychosocial consequences of head injury for patients and their families, but sufficient information exists to permit consideration of the following issues:

1. The general social characteristics of head-injured persons and their families
2. The physical and mental consequences of head injury reported by family members
3. The psychosocial consequences of the injured person's deficits for the family.

THE HEAD-INJURED PATIENT AND THE FAMILY

Jennett and MacMillan[2] reported that the incidence of head injuries is highest among males between the ages of 15 and 35; therefore, many are on the threshold of adult life, and about half are married or in the early stages of establishing their families. In addition to being young, head-injured persons tend to come from lower social and economic groups, and there is evidence that a higher proportion of them have had a previous head injury (see Chapter 2) and a history of antisocial behavior than uninjured individuals from the same social background; for example, Fahy and coworkers[3] noted that 46 percent of patients had evidence of social maladjustment in a study carried out in Britain. Most injured persons come from a group of physically active and emotionally immature men who are socially unsettled or only newly established in an adult role; although they have had a high degree of spending power, their levels of responsibility tend to be low, and many are heavy drinkers. For example 72 percent of head-injured patients in a recent study in the United States had alcohol in their blood on admission to hospital, and 52 percent were intoxicated by legal definition (see Chapter 2). Therefore, within their own social group, young men who have head injuries are among the most vulnerable psychologically and in terms of frequency with which their social supports are found to be impoverished.

There is a second peak in the incidence of head injuries among persons over age 70. However, the emphasis in this chapter will be on those in the larger and younger group of victims, toward whom most effort in rehabilitation is directed.

PHYSICAL AND MENTAL CONSEQUENCES OF INJURY

Several ways of defining the outcome of head injury have been developed and are described in Chapter 7. To recapitulate briefly, the results of studies using various measures, whether from those dealing with overall disability (e.g., Glasgow Outcome Scale—see Chapter 7) or specific psychologic and physical deficits, reveal that the greater part of recovery occurs within 6 to 12 months after injury, mostly within the first 6 months. Moreover, although further recovery of basic physical and mental abilities *does* occur in the second half of the first year after injury and later, *the rate and degree of change are small.*[4] A considerable part of the process of recovery in its later stages—that is, from 6 months onward—seems to involve the development of successful strategies for coping with the physical, emotional, and social consequences of injury by the injured person and family. However, there is evidence that many injured persons do not reach their full potential for recovery for reasons related both to their own failure to develop adequate means of coping with deficits and to the failure of family members to give the injured person the help needed for full recovery; in fact, they may even prevent the person's full recovery.[5]

There is general agreement that mental rather than physical deficits give rise to the most taxing problems for the victim of a head injury and the family, and that disorders of personality and behavior are the source of most of their difficulties. However, this is not to say that residual physical disabilities, which are usually neurologic or orthopedic, are of little or no consequence because they are known to be of great concern to the injured person during the early stages of recovery.[6] If severe and multiple, or of a certain type (e.g., incontinence), physical deficits may well place a very considerable burden on the sufferer's family.

The mental and behavioral consequences of injury to the brain may be divided into *those attributable chiefly to brain damage,* and *those that are reactions to the primary deficits* caused by injury and their consequences. The former consist of changes in volition, cognition, and emotion; the latter are usually a mixture of emotional and behavioral changes, which often have a further deleterious effect on basic intellectual activities. For example, impairment of memory is the most common of all basic changes attributable directly to brain injury and yet may show considerable variation as a result of depression of mood or poor motivation. Frequently, moderately to severely injured persons also exhibit slowness in thinking, distractability, and reduced powers of concentration. Changes in personality, especially in the early stages of recovery, include evidence of irritability, aggressiveness, impatience, and restlessness. Although these changes tend to lessen with time, apathy and euphoria, if they occur, appear to be permanent. In a review spanning the years 1959 to 1978, Lezak[7] commented on the basic changes of personality and behavior reported as most likely to cause problems to the families of head-injured persons, and constructed five broad and at times overlapping categories of change, as shown in Table 15-1.

The emotional responses of injured persons to their deficits show considerable variation. In almost all but the very severely handicapped, where apathy, aggressiveness, irresponsibility, or euphoria occurs, elements of the pretraumatic personality remain, often in an accentuated way. For example, the character traits of proneness to anxiety, hypochondriasis, or aggressiveness often become more marked. In addition, the secondary development of depression is common, especially where the person retains insight into the nature and consequences of

TABLE 15-1. Effects of Head Injury Upon Personality and Behavior

Personality or Behaviorial Construct	Changes Caused by Head Injury
Capacity for social perceptiveness	Self-centered behavior Diminution or total loss of self-criticisms Loss of ability to show empathy
Capacity for self-control	Random restlessness Impatience and impulsivity
Learned social behavior	Diminution in or loss of initiative; power to make judgments, plan, and organize Increased social dependency
Ability to learn	Mental slowness and rigidity of thought Reduced learning capacity
Emotion	Irritability, silliness, lability of mood, apathy, and increased or diminished sexual drive

the deficits. Some persons may develop an anxiety neurosis, an important feature of which may be agoraphobia or a social phobia; whereas others have an obsessional disorder that, on further examination, seems to be based on underlying slowness of thought processing and impaired powers of decision-making. A very small proportion develops conversion syndromes with hysterical symptoms, especially loss of motor power and sensation. However, these symptoms generally occur among those with mild injuries. On occasions, such patients have a combination of symptoms reflecting the presence of brain injury, secondary conversion symptoms, and additional and consciously added deficits, making a difficult diagnostic problem and one that is very resistant to treatment. Often, this particular combination of symptoms is linked to claims for financial compensation for injury.

The comments made so far depend chiefly on objective assessments of brain-damaged people by physicians, nurses, and other professional groups involved in their care. However, such studies do not reach the heart of a very important problem, namely, the effects of sudden changes in the health and behavior of the victim of injury on the structure and functions of the family as seen from their point of view. To examine the problems experienced by families, it is necessary to analyze the feelings, attitudes, and reactions of those directly involved, and it is only comparatively recently that work has been carried out with close relatives of injured persons. There are few accounts of their perceptions as "lay people" of the changes that occur to them and their ways of life. Although we have been aware for some time of the disturbing effects on families of high levels of behavioral and emotional disturbances among survivors of severe head injury, the first major family study was not carried out until 1976 by Rosenbaum and Najenson.[8] They studied head-injured victims of the Israeli/Arab War of Yom Kippur and the consequences of their injuries for their wives in personal and social terms. Their observations on the head-injured group were compared with their findings among families of men rendered paraplegic by the same war, and they found that those with head injury were reported as more selfish, childish, demanding, and dependent. Head-injured persons took a smaller share in running the household and, in particular, in caring for their children. The effects of head injury led to a reduction in family leisure time and time spent in contact with relatives. The frequency with which meetings with old friends took place lessened, and this was regarded by the families as a significant loss in their social lives. The wives of both injured groups reported a marked reduction in, or in some cases complete absence of, sexual activity. This was reported most often by the wives of paraplegics, some of whom found the prospect of physical contact with their disabled husbands most disagreeable and unwelcome.

In 1978, Oddy and colleagues[6] in Britain reported the results of an investigation of the residual deficits of men with head injuries that were mostly moderately severe. Six months after the injuries occurred, 20 percent of the men were symptom-free. One third (35 percent) had six or more symptoms, and two thirds (65 percent) suffered from one of the most frequent triads of symptoms encountered—namely, poor memory, loss of temper control, and fatigue. The authors commented that both patients and relatives reported intellectual and personality changes as the most common post-traumatic deficit (Table 15-2). Work by the Glasgow group has revealed that severe head injuries result in residual changes in personality in as many as two thirds of those injured and may be the only mental deficit in about one third,[9] and also that changes in personality are almost invariable in patients with marked cognitive or physical deficits. The relationship of changes to outcome as measured by the Glasgow Outcome Scale and described elsewhere (see Chapter 7, Table 7-8) shows that even one third of the Glasgow patients who made a good recovery had mild changes in personality, observed by family members, and that this proportion increased to two thirds among those with moderate disability. Almost 20 percent of the severely disabled had severe personality changes. Therefore, those involved in rehabilitation will encounter problems produced by personality changes after injuries of all grades of severity, but especially those that are severe. In some cases, an individual's character actually improves, usually by alteration to a less tense person with a more ready sense of humor. For the most part, however, the changes pose personal and interpersonal difficulties of various kinds, generated by the appearance of irritability, temper outbursts, emotional lability, loss of social restraint, and childishness.

McKinlay and others[10] in Glasgow carried out a careful prospective study in which they examined the difficulties most often reported by close relatives of 55 men with severe brain injury 3, 6, and 12 months after the injuries occurred. They examined seven categories of change, both physical and mental (Table 15-3). As in other studies, mental changes were the most common; irritability, tiredness, slowness, and poor memory were reported as the most frequent early changes. McKinlay and colleagues also observed that reports of changes in personality (irritability, impatience, and bad temper) increased during the year following injury (Table 15-4), whereas reports of impairment of memory, tiredness, and slowness fell, and reports of tension, anxiety, and depression in the injured person did not alter. The category designated in Table 15-3 as "disturbed behavior" was characterized by bizarre or puzzling conduct, and violent and inappropriate behavior. These behaviors were reported in less than 20 percent of cases, but where such changes did occur, having been absent before injury, they were of the greatest concern to relatives. The most frequent changes reported in this category were excessive talking, which lessened dramatically after 3 months, and childishness, which increased. Many other items in this category increased or fluctuated, but very few declined.

TABLE 15-2. Symptoms of Head Injury Most Frequently Reported by Injured Persons and Their Close Relatives 6 Months After Injury

Symptoms Reported by Head-Injured Persons (N = 48)	Symptoms of Head-Injured Persons Reported by Close Relatives (N = 48)
Trouble remembering things (18)	Trouble remembering things (21)
Frequent loss of temper (17)	Tiring very easily (18)
Tiring easily (16)	Often impatient (17)
Poor concentration when reading (14)	Frequent loss of temper (16)
Often irritable (14)	Often irritable (15)
Often impatient (13)	Difficulty with eyes (12)
Often restless with difficulty in developing interests (10)	Bumping into things (10)

From Oddy, Humphrey, and Uttley,[12] with permission.

TABLE 15-3. Mean Number of Residual Difficulties in Each of Seven Categories Reported by Relatives of Head-Injured Men*

Category	3 Months	6 Months	12 Months
Physical	1.8	1.6	1.5
Subjective	4.5	4.3	4.5
Language	2.4	2.2	2.1
Emotional	4.6	5.1	5.4
Dependence	1.8	1.5	1.4
Disturbed behavior	1.4	1.6	1.9
Memory	2.7	2.3	2.7

*Total score for each category was 10.
From McKinlay, et al,[10] with permission.

The number of physical problems initially reported by relatives was small at 3 months and even smaller at the end of the first year after injury.

The investigators examined the extent to which injured persons could care for themselves and the degree of supervision they required. It was discovered that between 20 percent and 25 percent could not be left in charge of the household 1 year after injury; but, in contrast, only 17 percent needed help with washing and dressing after 3 months, a figure that was reduced to 9 percent by 12 months. Thus it must be obvious that when comments are made about "dependency," a precise definition should be given.

The conclusions from the three studies quoted confirm earlier reports that mental problems caused by head injury are more common and longer lasting than physical ones. These studies give more information about the way in which the pattern of symptoms changes during the first year after injury. The extent to which relatives find the deficits described stressful to them remains to be discussed, to determine whether the pattern of stress changes with the passage of time, and to survey the ways in which patients' families cope with burdens placed on them.

PSYCHOSOCIAL CONSEQUENCES OF THE SYMPTOMS OF SEVERE HEAD INJURY FOR FAMILIES OF INJURED PERSONS

The families' problems may be divided into those that affect all members to some extent; those that arise in the main caring relatives, usually the wife or mother; and those that afflict

TABLE 15-4. Ten Most Frequent Symptoms Reported as Problems by Relatives of Head-Injured Men (Percent Reporting)

Problem Symptoms	3 Months	6 Months	12 Months
Slowness	86	69	67
Tiredness	82	69	69
Irritability	63	69	71
Poor memory	73	59	69
Impatience	60	64	71
Tension/anxiety	57	66	58
Bad temper	48	56	67
Personality change	49	58	60
Depression	57	52	57
Headaches	54	46	53

From McKinlay, et al,[10] with permission.

others in the family but which arise out of the main caretaker's own reactions to the injured person. Minor changes in personality are usually well tolerated, but changes beyond this level affect family life considerably. For example, the presence of an irritable, mentally slow, demanding, and perhaps aggressive person who cannot be left alone except for short periods curbs freedom drastically; as a result, family members feel trapped in the home and socially isolated. For example, they cannot get out as often as before the injury occurred and therefore tend to lose contact with friends and social interests. Naturally, relatives at times feel hostile toward the injured person because of the limitations placed on them, especially if the patient is abusive, or accuses the family of rejection or the spouse of unfaithfulness. However, as might be expected, relatives also experience guilt at having such feelings about someone who is disabled. Relatives outside the immediate family often give help in the early stages of recovery; but as time passes and the injured person's recovery slows, they may withdraw their support. In addition, more distant relatives may become critical of attempts by those who are very close to rehabilitate the disabled person; this tendency is particularly obvious among parents of the injured person—usually a man. Thus, a mother may become very critical of her daughter-in-law and make matters worse rather than better by increasing the wife's sense of frustration, anger, guilt, and perhaps failure.

Relatively little work has been carried out on the early reactions and expectations of the relatives of head-injured persons. Often, relatives seem overoptimistic about the extent to which the injured person will recover. This is to be expected for several reasons. First, if the patient is going to survive after a severe injury, the patient will improve quite rapidly within the first few weeks from a state that initially seemed, to the relatives at least, quite hopeless. Next, the views of surgeons and nurses about recovery may be interpreted in an overoptimistic way by relatives; in part, this may be due to natural reluctance of medical and nursing staff to be specific about long-term outcome once survival is assured. Lastly, relatives' high hopes for a good recovery may also be due to the mental mechanism of *denial*, which operates very strongly in these circumstances: in other words, relatives tend to repress the worst possibilities of the immediate and late outcome of the injury.[11] This process, which is a common and natural response to the threat of death or disability occurring to one's self or others who are close, continues to operate to a variable extent for many months into the process of recovery, and is shown by the way in which subtle changes in personality are glossed over and excuses are made for antisocial or aggressive behavior that would not have occurred or been tolerated previously. Relatives may, for example, tell the patient he or she is lazy and should try harder, may expect more self-control than is possible, and may feel anger when it does not materialize. Their expectations of patient's capacity for work outside the home and social activity are often far too ambitious, especially among more educated persons, and a period of deep gloom and despondency occurs when the realities of the victim's limitations are appreciated eventually. In simple terms, for the most part, "people see and expect what they most wish to see." One practical consequence of family denial is an imbalance in expectations about the injured person's speed and degree of recovery between medical and paramedical staff on the one hand and the family members on the other, a situation that may provoke hostility toward the former groups.

After severe injuries where mental changes are prominent and permanent, the family members slowly begin to appreciate the true extent of the changes and to react to them. They are bewildered initially but are anxious and yet hopeful about the outcome. Depression and despair may develop at any time, and attempts to mourn are thwarted because the "mourners" have "the body" with them. Eventually, in my experience, most members of the family will separate emotionally from the disabled person between 1 and 2 years from injury, to such an extent that they have a realistic view of the person's level of disability and develop appropriate social and emotional coping strategies.

The general reactions described are common to all adult family members, especially the main caretaker. For a wife, the injury to her husband means loss of her partner whom she cannot mourn properly; her affectional and sexual needs cannot be fulfilled; and her husband has a role in which he is childlike and dependent. The study of the wives of Israeli soldiers[8] revealed something of the nature of the crisis wives go through in the first year after injury. A very high proportion of them become depressed. This appears to be caused by several factors, including a sense of isolation and loneliness; increased responsibility for household affairs; complete responsibility for childrearing; tensions in the relationships between wife and husband and between herself and her husband's parents, who perhaps take a critical and overprotective attitude to their son's care; and perhaps also loss of her main confiding relationship—known to be a "predisposing factor" for the development of depression. Therefore, the wife experiences little enjoyment in her life, and she loses her main confiding relationship (i.e., with her husband). Her efforts in caring for her husband and children, if she has any, are not positively reinforced. From studies of psychiatric patients, it is known that she is exposed to factors that make individuals very vulnerable to depression.

In a detailed study in England, Oddy and associates[12] found that depression among wives was commonest during the first month after injury and that although its incidence fell thereafter, the numbers of depressed wives did not change between 6 months and 1 year. They also found that the presence of depression was chiefly related to adverse personality changes in the injured person and to his having a high number of symptoms—physical, mental, or both. However, depression was not related to whether or not the husband was back at work or to his number of social contacts. Apart from depression, it seems that illnesses of other kinds increase in incidence as a result of the stresses; examination of all relatives in the study 6 to 12 months after the injury revealed that 25 percent had some form of illness in the previous 6 months and that half were expressions of stress, being either psychosomatic or purely emotional. A study by Panting and Merry[13] of relatives attending a rehabilitation center several years after injury had occurred revealed that 61 percent of relatives were under stress. It should be appreciated that this group was carefully selected because of the problems being experienced, but the findings have obvious implications for those providing rehabilitation sought voluntarily at a late stage after injury.

The changes described in wives could well become the basis for separation of wife and husband, and for divorce; for example, Panting and Merry[13] observed a 40 percent divorce rate. However, in my experience, the figure is smaller than this, and Walker[14] in a 25-year follow-up gave a figure of only 11 percent among World War II veterans compared with 25 percent for the male population of the United States at that time. In contrast to the reported frailty of marriages exposed to the consequences of head injuries to husbands, there is a belief that mother-and-son relationships are much more durable.

In a more recent study of stress among the wives and mothers of seriously head-injured men in Glasgow, McKinlay and others[10] revealed that although in the first 3 months after injury there is a significant correlation between the severity of injuries, as assessed in terms of the duration of post-traumatic amnesia, and levels of stress experienced, this relationship is barely present after 6 months and absent after 1 year (Table 15-5). Therefore, stress in families does *not* simply appear to be a reflection of the initial severity of a person's injury—it is a reflection, or the consequence, of certain specific types of problem. Furthermore, although overall levels of stress reported by relatives did not alter appreciably during the first year, the nature of the problems giving rise to stress did change. Emotional and behavioral changes, subjective symptoms, and impairment of memory were all significantly related to the burden of relatives 3 months after injury occurred. By 12 months, memory impairment had ceased to be significant in this respect; but from 6 months onward, the overall dependency of the patient emerged as a source of burden, while emotional, behavioral, and subjective changes

TABLE 12-5. Comparison by Means of One-Way Analysis of Variance (ANOVA) of the Duration of PTA in Patients Whose Relatives Experience Low, Medium, or High Stress

	Mean PTA		
	3 Months	6 Months	12 Months
Group 1 (SB = 1 or 2) Low	13.3	14.4	17.7
Group 2 (SB = 3 or 4) Med	24.0	33.9	31.2
Group 3 (SB = 5–7) High	49.7	38.9	37.7
One-way ANOVA: probability of F	.0002	.0359	.1013

NOTE: The changes that occur over time are due only to changes in burden reported by relatives (SB) and consequent changes in the composition of the three SB groups. Only one value of PTA was used for each case.

remained significantly stressful. In fact, reports of bad temper (48 percent at 3 months, 67 percent at 12 months) and mood swings (33 percent at 3 months, 62 percent at 12 months) increased as the year progressed, suggesting the patients were responding emotionally to appreciation of their handicaps and loss of ability to resume a normal life. Therefore, the close relatives have a secondary and very difficult form of stress with which to cope when these changes emerge in the later stages of recovery.

CONCLUSION

To conclude, it is clear that the problems families encounter as a result of one of their relatives being severely brain-damaged begin from the moment injury occurs. However, the pattern of stresses they encounter changes with time, and probably the most significant points for them in the recovery process are in the first days, at the time of discharge from hospital, and when they finally realize and accept the full extent of the victim's deficits. The first stage is significant for the very obvious mixture of denial and hope; the next, because of the mixture of depression, despair, and denial it causes; and the last, for the return of some degree of emotional equilibrium brought about by acceptance of the reality of the problems in the family and of ways of solving them. Each stage demands a different approach from those involved in rehabilitation, and the increasing detail accumulating about them makes it possible to begin to *design and test* techniques of rehabilitation to meet relatives' various needs.

REFERENCES

1. Bond, MR and Brooks, DN: *Understanding the process of recovery as a basis for the investigation of rehabilitation for the brain-injured.* Scand J Rehabil Med 8:127, 1976.
2. Jennett, B and MacMillan, R: *Epidemiology of head injury.* Br Med J 282:101, 1981.
3. Fahy, TJ, Irving, MH, and Millac, P: *Severe head injuries: A six-year follow-up.* Lancet 2:475, 1967.
4. Bond, MR: *Stages of recovery from severe head injury with special reference to late outcome.* Int Rehabil Med 1:155, 1979.
5. Humphrey, M and Oddy, M: *Return to work after head injury: A review of post-war studies.* Injury 12:107, 1980.
6. Oddy, M, Humphrey, M, and Uttley, D: *Subjective impairment and social recovery after closed head injury.* J Neurol Neurosurg Psychiatry 41:611, 1978.

7. LEZAK, MD: *Living with the characterologically altered brain-injured patient.* Journal of Clinical Psychiatry 39:592, 1978.
8. ROSENBAUM, M AND NAJENSON, T: *Changes in life patterns and symptoms of low mood as reported by wives of severely brain-injured soldiers.* J Consult Clin Psychol 44:881, 1976.
9. JENNETT, B, ET AL: *Disability after severe head injury.* J Neurol Neurosurg Psychiatry 44:285, 1981.
10. MCKINLAY, WW, ET AL: *The short-term outcome of severe blunt head injury as reported by relatives of the injured person.* J Neurol Neurosurg Psychiatry 44:527, 1981.
11. ROMANO, MD: *Family response to traumatic head injury.* Scand J Rehabil Med 6:1, 1974.
12. ODDY, M, HUMPHREY, M, AND UTTLEY, D: *Stresses upon relatives of head-injured patients.* Br J Psychiatry 133:507, 1978.
13. PANTING, A AND MERRY, PH: *The long-term rehabilitation of severe head injuries with particular reference to need for social and medical support for the patient's family.* Rehabilitation 38:33, 1972.
14. WALKER, AE: *Long-term evaluation of the social and family adjustment of head injures.* Scand J Rehabil Med 4:5, 1972.

Chapter 16

EDUCATIONAL AND VOCATIONAL DEFICITS

John P. Bolger, M.S.

The head-injured adult must overcome a multitude of barriers to succeed in independent living. As our society places demands of educational achievement and vocational productivity on all individuals, these become two key areas in which the head-injured client must gain to live independently. The goal of this chapter is to examine some of the specific deficits that are outcomes of head injury. These deficits ultimately prevent the client from entering society and attaining independent function.

Emphasis will be placed on personal reflections from head-injured individuals, along with observations from professional staff members who have come in contact with these clients in comprehensive rehabilitation settings. Factors that must be considered in facilitating the successful return of the adult to a vocational setting in which effective learning may occur include:

1. Behavioral adjustment to disability—interpersonal skills
2. Physical status of recovery—activities of daily living functioning
3. Mental status—memory and cognition, communication.

These factors are most frequently cited as handicaps to successful return to gainful employment.[1]

The theoretical network and function of the brain will be correlated with the many individualized deficits the head-injured adult may possess, to provide the reader with a potential scheme for assessing deficits and initiating specific therapy.

BRAIN FUNCTION

Human beings are unique in their ability to fully adapt to the environment. The brain is able to receive and interpret numerous and complex bits of information simultaneously. Using past experiences and new learning, humans can alter their condition to adapt to any stimulus. The brain is capable of adapting and compensating, not only to the environment but also for most individual deficits. A simple example of this process is wearing glasses to improve vision or using tools to perform a task that would otherwise be impossible.

In the case of head-injured clients, these individuals have partially lost this ability.[2] Indications are that they may not be as aware of the need to adapt or compensate. Another problem is found in the ability to properly design, through the use of past experience, a specific plan to adapt or compensate. Finally, these individuals may not be able to receive the necessary feedback from the environment to indicate that they have performed an adequate compensation technique. Head-injured clients constantly mention these problems as a rationale for their inability to succeed. These individuals tend to state that they often perceive themselves as being wrong or making the wrong choice. They explain that they feel different but can't define how they are different or what they can do to change. Some discuss how they seem to have lost some control or ability to concentrate on something long or hard enough to achieve success. All these problems are indicative of their inability to compensate and adapt to changes in their environment. Often, there appear to be certain selective inabilities to learn new information. These learning disabilities may be due to deficits in particular functional systems, which prevent the proper conceptualization of new information.[3] These individuals are incapable of designing new strategies to compensate for their present deficits. The result is an increase in frustration while attempting to achieve success in specific learning situations.

PRE-INJURY STRENGTHS AND WEAKNESSES

The importance of assessing pre-injury conditions cannot be stressed strongly enough in designing the rehabilitation program of the head-injured client. In most cases, any pre-injury educational or vocational problem becomes more apparent after the onset of a traumatic head injury.[4] This relationship is apparent in personality, intelligence, and behavior. The assertive individual usually becomes more assertive, often to the point of being labeled aggressive. The client who was unmotivated to work prior to injury would probably be even less motivated in this area. Successful manipulators may spend all of their mental energy trying again to manipulate. The structured organizer may become compulsively fastidious in nature.

Pre-injury problems have a decided bearing on the design and success of the rehabilitation program. It becomes necessary to address these disturbances to secure an independent placement for the individual. These problems often slow or prevent a placement. Pre-injury learning disabilities are devastating to re-education endeavors. The adult who had a pre-injury reading disorder such as dyslexia has a much lower chance of regaining reading ability than the client who was a competent reader. Correlation of premorbid education levels and successful job placements indicates that clients with a stronger educational background are more successful in being vocationally placed.[5] Also, one of the greatest pre-injury disabilities occurs when someone has never experienced the world of work. The ability to learn proper work skills and accept orders and criticism from an employer may need additional attention. Finally, a problem may be created by an inability to lower one's standards for a successful job placement. A third-year medical student may totally reject a vocational goal of becoming a nurse's aide. The inability to fully assess one's own strengths and weaknesses reduces the ability to set appropriate vocational goals.

EFFECTS OF UNIVERSAL DEFICITS

The results of a traumatic injury to the brain can be basically separated into two broad areas, following current neuropsychologic theory. Certain deficits appear to be universal, as they exist in all head-trauma victims regardless of the specific areas of the brain that may have been injured. Following equipotential theory, it appears that the greater the total damage to the brain, the greater the occurrence and severity of the behavioral manifestations.[6]

Some of the universal problems that occur in all head-injured clients include self-centered behavior, impulsivity, poor planning skills, and rigidity.[7] Additional deficits include an inability to abstract, perseveration, loss of internal feedback, and a shortened attention span. All of these cognitive processes and personality functions become essential when applied to performing vocational or educational tasks.

Cognitive processing can be simply defined as the ability to perform a task while thinking about something else. In other words, this means the ability to do more than one mental operation at the same time.[8] In the case of the head-injured client, depending on the severity of the injury, the ability to process huge amounts of information simultaneously is lost. The behavioral results of this loss are quite devastating.

If someone is unable to perform numerous processes simultaneously, one can see how individuals would become very impulsive in nature. They might not be capable of delaying gratification, responding instead to stimulation in a typical stimulus-response format. Obviously, attention span and on-task behavior would be affected. Individuals would be highly distractable and would be unable to concentrate or attend to a task unless there were no distractions. These clients are unable to perform in any educational or vocational setting where they might become bombarded with too much stimulation. Telephones ringing or peers conversing would be enough of a distraction to end productive work on even the simplest task.

Through a loss in cognitive ability, head-injured persons might become very rigid or incapable of correcting errors. Their awareness of failure may be affected by an inability to internally process feedback from the environment. The inability to process information can result in the individual returning to a previous mental set, which would then be initiated in a variety of situations. Rigid and perseverative behavior is one of the most devastating of the maladaptive behaviors the head-injured client can possess. For all who come in contact with these clients, only frustration can result, owing to clients' inability to learn from their errors or accept different ways of performing tasks. This behavior cannot be tolerated by the instructor or employer. These students or employees refuse to accept instruction on the proper way to perform their jobs. Eventually, the employer, although attempting to educate the individual on meeting the rules established by the organization, becomes frustrated by the employee's inability to change. This ultimately results in the termination of the employee.

The inability to perform numerous cognitive processes at the same time results in inadequate abstract reasoning. Tasks need to be clearly structured, defined, and organized for the individual to achieve success. Deviations from this structure are met with confusion, as the individual is incapable of solving new problems alone. Very few employers could accept an individual who, because of an inability to abstract information or effectively deal with the unexpected, would need a totally structured, closely supervised environment. Assembly line workers who perform an identical task each day must be able to make quick decisions in the case of errors. Students and workers must be able to organize, planning the best use of their time to meet their needs. This involves performing numerous cognitive processes simultaneously.

When head-injured clients are concentrating on performing a task to the best of their ability, they often exceed their mental capacity to perform all the aspects of the tasks.[9] In other words, they exceed their intellectual limit. In response to the drive to succeed, they usually perform the task but sacrifice the process of remembering the information. Memory loss is the most common manifestation of the universal deficits of head-injured persons. The vocational and educational prognosis for a client with memory deficits is poor.

EFFECTS OF SPECIFIC DEFICITS

Adults who have suffered focal or penetrating head wounds may exhibit specific learning disabilities, perceptual disturbances, or motor deficits.[11] Localization theory states that certain functions of the brain can be correlated to specific cortical areas. It does appear that when specific areas of the brain are injured, predictable deficits are observed.

Hemiplegia is possibly one of the most readily understood disabilities brought on by damage to a specific area of the brain. Paralysis on the right side of the body usually indicates damage to the left hemisphere of the brain. Although rehabilitation engineering can provide these patients with a multitude of adaptive devices, some vocations require full use of all extremities. The ability to write may also be limited, further impairing academic abilities.

Language and speech disturbances present a multitude of barriers to successful understanding and application of educational principles. Also, the ability to return to an occupational position requiring any amount of communication skill is impaired.[12] Usually in the case of the right-handed individual, damage to the left hemisphere of the brain will result in language deficits. Receptive aphasia will prevent the employee from being able to follow through with specific directions. Often, employers attribute this lack of follow-through to poor motivation and noncompliance and release the employee from the job. Comprehending any communication, either spoken or written, becomes increasingly difficult, thus preventing the student from quickly learning new material. A more severe hearing disorder due to brain stem damage may prevent the client from returning to a noisy work environment. The ability to distinguish important and relevant auditory information within a field of background noise is impaired; thus the client becomes increasingly confused as the noise level is raised. Yet another disorder, auditory asymbolia, might prevent the individual from recognizing the different sounds of a telephone or door bell. Expressive difficulties have a similar effect both in the classroom and on the job. The ability to write complete sentences and spell correctly may be lost, and often workers' inabilities to express themselves not only prevent them from returning to positions requiring communication with the public, but also from returning to positions where they must defend their actions or decisions. Mathematical skills may be lost due to dysgraphia and dyscalculia. These deficits include an inability to recognize or write numbers or to perform basic mathematical concepts.

In the right-handed individual, the right hemisphere is associated with spatial abilities. Visual-spatial deficits can create severe handicaps.[13] Vocations involving any form of assembly work, or following blueprints and diagrams, may become impossible to perform. Awareness of extrapersonal space may be altered, preventing the individual from fully comprehending the surroundings. This client may not be able to recognize familiar objects. Hemianopsia and other visual field deficits might endanger the employee's ability to perceive unsafe conditions in a factory situation. Additional problems are associated with reading, due to neglecting half of the presented material and trying to make sense with only half the information.[14] Oculomotor deficits can lead to further problems in route finding, locating objects, eye-hand coordination, and reading.[15]

Specific behavioral manifestations include lability (an inability to control emotions and mood swings) and altered affect. Often, employers view workers with flat affect as unmotivated and uninterested in performing their jobs. Adults with this syndrome lose assertive skills, thus reducing their ability to sell themselves in employment interviews or to work well with fellow employees. The labile adult is met with complete misunderstanding. It is obvious that periods of hysterical laughter and/or uncontrollable crying would prevent an individual from successfully completing an educational or vocational program.

Other specific deficits may occur in head-injured adults. In many cases, through compensation and remediation, these individuals can return to active and productive lives. A problem develops, however, since as the number of problems increases, the ability to compensate and make special allowances is diminished.

REMEDIATION

Because many chapters in this book deal with the various techniques used to remediate the deficits of the head-injured adult, emphasis here will be placed on specific programs designed to increase the individual's ability to return to the educational or vocational setting. Above all else, the individual needs to be educated as to the nature of the disability and its consequences. Appropriate feedback must be given as soon and as often as possible. A recent technique (originally used to improve the bedside manner of physicians) is known as Interpersonal Process Recall.[17] Videotaping is employed to provide accurate and immediate feedback of interpersonal, social, and communication skills. The technique has been found to be beneficial in modifying these skills in the head-injured client.[18]

Perceptual and cognitive retraining involves the appropriate shaping of skills through the use of cues or prompts that are gradually faded.[19] Attention span, visual scanning, visual-spatial abilities, auditory perception, simultaneous problem solving, and other abilities can be relearned through these techniques.[20] Results have been very promising, though conclusive findings based on controlled research have not yet been reported.

Prevocational work adjustment programs are designed to improve work-related behaviors. These programs need to be specifically molded to meet the needs of head-injured persons. Placing these clients in the same surroundings as the mentally retarded can be devastating.[21] Workshop experiences need to be challenging, since head-injured clients state that they do not want to be treated as if they were retarded. Often, book material may be substituted for the less intellectually based instruction more common to this environment. Sessions on job interviewing, application forms, and providing feedback on job-related strengths and weaknesses need to be stressed. Through the use of a stimulating environment, work adjustment experiences are more successful.

Individualized behavioral and academic instruction is required to provide specifically tailored programs to meet each individual's needs. Academically, a client might be performing at a third-grade level for months and then miraculously advance to a sixth- or seventh-grade ability in 1 week. Without close supervision (one-to-one), this advancement might go unnoticed, raising the frustration of the client. Individualized cognitive behavior modification programs may need to be established. These programs allow the client to be responsible for modifying inappropriate behavior by providing internal satisfaction and gratification as reinforcers.[22] This technique has been shown to be very effective in anger control.[23]

Later in the rehabilitation process, psychosocial counseling provides a base for the client to express frustrations, fears, and anxieties that may prevent a complete return to independent living. Assertiveness training, social skills development, and rational emotive therapy are excellent educational and psychosocial techniques that have been adapted to meet the needs of head-injured persons.[24]

A very recent vocational development program is receiving some recognition. In this program, vocational evaluation, vocational training, and resources from the home community are combined to develop an appropriate and feasible vocational goal for the client. The evaluation assesses specific job-related strengths and weaknesses, and this information is transferred to the rehabilitation counselor in the community. A task analysis produces a possible job, which is tailored to meet the strengths of the client. A prescriptive training program is then initiated, training students in specific job tasks in which they possess basically adequate skills. In this approach, the client is better prepared for the transition from the institutional training experience to the on-the-job situation.

Thus, remediation needs to be highly specific, tailored to meet each individual's needs. Unlike many other disability groups, too few generalizations can be made about the head-injured population, thus necessitating specificity and individuality in programming.

CONCLUSION

Each year, the public is becoming more aware of the devastating consequences of head trauma. The number of people receiving head injuries is steadily growing each year.[25] Modern medical discoveries are saving more of these individuals every year. This is placing a greater demand on providing rehabilitation services for the head-injured client.

There is a great need for more community education on head injury and the effects of rehabilitation. Education for the families of the head-injured patient needs to begin in the acute phase of treatment. Neurologists and neurosurgeons should be encouraged to learn more of the long-term, 5-year post-trauma effects of head injury. There needs to be a more structured process of rehabilitation through the stages of acute hospitalization, to intermediate care, through vocational rehabilitation, and on to transitional living before independence. Community-based mental health settings should provide more services to this growing population. A nationally based advocacy system needs to be established to coordinate services, provide information to facilities on new techniques, and initiate community educational programs.

It is apparent that the process of educational and vocational rehabilitation of the head-injured adult is in its infancy. Little is known about the relative efficacy of various techniques of cognitive remediation and their eventual outcome in terms of job placement. Specialized programs need to be developed that address the unique educational and vocational needs of this population.

REFERENCES

1. DuBose, L: *Vocational Planning.* Presented at the Third Annual Post-Graduate Course on the Rehabilitation of the Traumatic Brain-Injured Adult, Williamsburg, Va, 1979.
2. Gross, Y: *Cognitive Re-training.* Presented at the JFK Medical Center, Edison, NJ, 1979.
3. Knights, R and Bakker, D: *The Neuropsychology of Learning Disorders.* University Park Press, Baltimore, 1976.
4. Smolkin, C and Cohen, S: *Socioeconomic factors affecting the vocational success of stroke patients.* Arch Phys Med Rehabil 55:269, 1974.
5. Najenson, T, et al: *Rehabilitation outcome of brain damaged patients after severe head injury.* Int Rehabil Med 2:17, 1980.
6. Lashley, KS: *Brain Mechanisms and Intelligence.* University of Chicago Press, Chicago, 1929.
7. Lezak, M: *Living with the characterologically altered brain injured patient.* Journal of Clinical Psychiatry 39, 1978.
8. Case, R: *Validation of a neo-Piagetian capacity construct.* J Exp Child Psychol 14:287, 1972.
9. Case, R: *Mental strategies, mental capacity, and instruction.* J Exp Child Psychol 18:382, 1974.
10. Golden, CJ: *Diagnosis and Rehabilitation in Clinical Neuropsychology.* Charles C Thomas, Springfield, Ill, 1978.
11. Luria, AR: *The Working Brain.* Basic Books, New York, 1973.
12. Najenson, T, et al: *Rehabilitation outcome of brain damaged patients after severe head injury.* Int Rehabil Med 2:17, 1980.
13. Benton, AL: *Disorders of Spatial Orientation.* In Vinken, JP and Pam Bruyn, GN (eds): Handbook of Clinical Neurology, Vol 3. North Holland Publishing, Amsterdam, 1969, p 212.
14. Diller, L, et al: *Methods for the Evaluation and Treatment of the Visual Perceptual Difficulties of Right Brain Damaged Individuals.* Supplement to the 8th Annual Workshop for Rehabilitation Professionals, NYU Medical Center, 1980.
15. Weinberg, J, et al: *Visual scanning training effect on reading related tasks in acquired right brain damage.* Arch Phys Med Rehabil 58:479, 1977.
16. DuBose, L: *Vocational Implications for Brain Damaged Individuals.* Presented at the Second Annual Post-Graduate Course on the Rehabilitation of the Traumatic Brain-Injured Adult, Richmond, Va, 1978.

17. KAJAN, N: *Studies in Human Interaction: Interpersonal Process Recall Stimulated by Video Tape.* Educational Publications Services, College of Education, East Lansing, Mich, 1967.
18. HELFFENSTEIN, D: *The effects of interpersonal process recall on the interpersonal and communication skills of the newly brain injured.* Doctoral dissertation, University of Virginia, 1981.
19. BEN-YISHAY, Y, ET AL: *Working Approaches to Remediation of Cognitive Deficits in Brain Damaged.* Supplement to the 6th Annual Workshop for Rehabilitation Professionals, NYU Medical Center, 1978.
20. DILLER, L, ET AL: *Studies in Cognitive and Rehabilitation in Hemiplegia.* Rehabilitation Monograph No. 5, Institute of Rehabilitative Medicine, NYU Medical Center, New York, 1974.
21. HENDRIX, R: Personal communication, 1980.
22. MEICHENBAUM, D: *Cognitive Behavior Modification.* Plenum Press, New York, 1977.
23. THORESON, C AND MAHONEY, M: *Behavioral Self-Control.* Holt, Rinehart, & Winston, New York, 1974.
24. TUMBARELLO, R AND MCDONALD, L: *Group Therapy for Head Trauma Rehabilitation Clients.* Presented at the Second Annual Conference, Head Trauma Rehabilitation—Coma to Community, San Jose, Calif, 1979.
25. RIMEL, R: *Epidemiology and Recovery Following Head Injury.* Presented at Brain Injury '80—Accent on Treatment, Fishersville, Va, 1980.

CONCLUSION

Mitchell Rosenthal, Ph.D.

The uniqueness of head injury is well illustrated in the diversity of mental and physical sequelae described in this section. By the time these problems are fully manifest, the patient has likely entered the subacute phase of recovery, sometimes known as early rehabilitation. Taken individually, any of these problems (e.g., epilepsy or communication deficit) would pose significant obstacles for a patient with a "good" recovery, as defined by the criteria used in the Glasgow scales. In combination, as is so often the rule rather than the exception, one cannot avoid being awed by the tremendous challenge that confronts physicians and therapists alike who endeavor to restore lost function or develop remedial strategies to re-educate or compensate for these deficits. It is therefore small wonder, as Bond suggests, that the families of head-injured persons often feel overwhelmed and greatly stressed by the burden inherent in the long-term management of their relatives.

To paraphrase Brooks in his chapter on memory deficits, one may ask several pertinent questions about the nature of deficits secondary to brain injury: (1) How much do we know about these deficits?, (2) What is their natural course of recovery?, and (3) Which deficits can be ameliorated, and by what means? It is within this context that we shall review the major themes of this section.

A major long-term medical complication of brain injury is the risk of late epilepsy. Though the percentage of patients (5 percent) developing epilepsy is relatively small, the effects of living with a potential or actual seizure disorder are considerable. Because of the prophylactic seizure medication often prescribed, victims of head trauma are often restricted for several years in important life activities, for example, operating an automobile and returning to certain occupational endeavors. These limitations create frustrations for head-injured persons and their relatives. Yet advanced methods of predicting those patients likely to develop late epilepsy and the level of risk involved have greatly assisted those responsible for regulating the anticonvulsant program for the patient. If appropriate management protocols are followed, it is now less likely that late uncontrolled epilepsy will develop and create even greater neurologic insult, resulting in more severe disability.

Because of the often rapid, dramatic recovery of motor function in head injury, motor deficits are often downgraded in their importance in the total, long-term management plan for head-injured patients. As Griffith describes, however, spasticity can create major problems, resulting in loss of balance, decreased self-care skills, impaired mobility skills, and unacceptable cosmesis. The techniques of spasticity management have been well documented in other disability categories (e.g., cerebral palsy, stroke) but rarely addressed in the literature on head trauma. Some useful guidelines for the clinician are presented, which address the diversity of educational, pharmacologic, and surgical techniques that may be used singly or in combination to alleviate spasticity in this patient population.

For the clinician concerned with the long-term treatment of head-injured patients, the complex of cognitive, behavioral, and communicative impairments secondary to trauma is perhaps of greatest concern. Taken as a whole, this represents the "invisible" disabling consequences of the injury. Though basic expressive and receptive language skills usually return to a functional level within 6 months, Groher highlights the recent research that has documented the presence of lingering subtle, high-level language deficits in the processing, organization, and structure of both oral and written language. The process of communication cannot be isolated from the cognitive impairments found in head trauma. Brooks provides ample documentation to support the notion that memory disorders are the most pervasive and debilitating of all the cognitive deficits accompanying head injury. In a description of their model of cognitive deficits, Ben-Yishay and Diller address the complex array of discrete problems that inhibit the patient from attending to stimuli, retaining and processing information, responding to complex and novel stimuli, and engaging in practical problem-solving behavior.

Another category of sequelae known as behavioral dysfunction has been described by Bond as the most difficult for family members to understand, accept, and cope with. Rosenthal discusses the classic syndromes of emotional and personality change that accompany head injury. Apathy, lethargy, aspontaneity, impaired affect, poor emotional control, low frustration tolerance, impulsivity, rigidity, depression, and the like are major obstacles in the restoration of the patient to a suitable role within the family and community. Whether these deficits originate from the specific lesion itself or from the process of living with brain damage is certainly of academic import, but makes little difference for the family who are at a loss to comprehend and effectively interact with their loved one. The manner in which cognitive, communicative, and behavioral deficits affect practical living skills has been well described by McNeny. Though head-injured persons often have the capability of performing most basic activities of daily living (e.g., dressing, feeding, bathing, driving), the aforementioned problems are great limiting factors in the therapist's attempt to restore the patient to a level of functional independence. Bond's description of the stresses on the family underscores the importance of helping the family, as well as the patient, adjust to the trauma and find adequate methods of assisting and caring for their loved ones.

Perhaps the disabling effects of head injury are best exemplified in the process of educational and vocational rehabilitation. The goal of any rehabilitation program is to return injured persons to a level compatible with their premorbid level of function. Often, this would imply some measure or recovery of the ability to live independently, continue in an educational program, or return to work. Unfortunately, as Bolger points out, the rehabilitation community is currently lacking in the specialized programs that can meet the unique needs of this population. Too often, the result is prolonged dependence on family and government resources for financial and social support.

To return to the theme presented earlier, our understanding of the deficits following head trauma has greatly advanced within the last decade. We now can specify the nature of many physical and mental sequelae of head injury and can make some predictions about their severity and duration. This is certainly clearer for the physical sequelae. Our understanding of the unique cognitive and behavioral deficits has greatly improved, but our power of prediction of duration is not yet refined. Even less developed is our ability to definitively prescribe specific interventions that are likely to remediate these deficits and restore head-injured persons to an adequate role within the family and community.

Section 4

SPECIALIZED METHODS OF ASSESSMENT

Chapter 17

MEDICAL ASSESSMENT

Sheldon Berrol, M.D.

Assessment of rehabilitation potential begins with the initial determination of the neurologic status of the patient at the scene of the injury. Ongoing re-evaluation by emergency personnel and the neurotrauma team adds substantial information relative to potential outcome. The current use of the Glasgow Coma Scale permits rapid anticipation of rehabilitation potential, and brain evoked potential studies may add significant data regarding prognosis. Thus, we may now identify earlier patients who might benefit maximally from a rehabilitation program.

It is important to understand the mechanism of injury in each case, so that we may better anticipate the consequences of terms of dysfunction as the patient evolves from coma. Coma itself does not necessarily imply conclusive evidence of brain stem damage, since coma may result from purely cortical disruption. It is, therefore, necessary that skull x-ray films, computed tomography (CT) scans, neurologic assessment forms, and so forth be evaluated by the physiatrist in charge of the head-injury rehabilitation unit to determine the most effective treatment approaches. Rotational forces, occurring in the majority of head-trauma cases, produce diffuse and extensive tissue damage, setting the stage for further ischemia, hemorrhage, edema, metabolic changes, and raised intracranial pressure. Evidence of blood in the ventricular system may presage the later development of hydrocephalus. Thorough recording should be made of prognostic factors, such as presence of a lucid interval, eye signs, length of coma, and blood pressure. Only through a careful analysis of both positive and negative factors can a realistic use of the limited resources for head-injury rehabilitation be accomplished.

Patients should ideally be considered for admission to head-injury rehabilitation programs at a level of 7 to 9 on the Glasgow Coma Scale. This allows for early introduction of comprehensive rehabilitation management, which would include a multimodality stimulation program, positioning programs to prevent contractures, and earlier removal of nasogastric tubes, tracheostomy tubes, and catheters. Maintenance of such foreign bodies during the evolution from coma contributes to patient discomfort and adds to their overall level of confusion. The presence of these auxiliary measures is sometimes considered as suggesting medical instability when, in fact, the patient is frequently sufficiently stable to allow their discontinuation. The majority of patients admitted to our center with tracheostomy tubes are able to have them removed within the first week after admission to the rehabilitation unit.

CRITERIA FOR REHABILITATION

EVIDENCE OF NEUROLOGIC IMPROVEMENT

Improvement in the level of coma, as reflected by the Glasgow Coma Scale, provides the early basis for assessment. The patient must also demonstrate some degree of contact with the environment and some ability to react with it. The rehabilitation process is a learning process; thus, the patient must have the potential to establish some basic communication system. The visual system is a prime route of information access, so the ability to fix and focus should be present. Information should be presented to all quadrants of the visual field, for the field of vision may be quite contracted. The presence of visual tracking is yet a higher level of function. One must recognize that the stimulus should be appropriate, and, since visual acuity may be severely impaired, the intensity of the stimulus may have to be increased to evoke a response.

Appreciation of auditory stimuli should be evaluated. It is not necessary that a patient be able to respond to commands. The ability of the patient to localize to sound is frequently the first stage of auditory sensory reintegration and can be used to develop higher-level responses to auditory information.

Vocalization at this early phase is generally quite limited, if present at all. Though the rating of early vocalization on the coma scale may be important prognostically, it appears to be of less value for evaluation of rehabilitation potential.[1] More importantly, it is the patient's capability to integrate sensory stimuli into symbolic information of *any* kind that establishes a basis for continued learning. A comprehensive evaluation of each sensory modality must be made to assess the potential for appropriate responses.

Appropriate motor responses may be inhibited as a result of pathologic reflex activity; thus, inhibiting postures and facilitation techniques must be used in an attempt to establish a baseline for potential function.

MEDICAL STABILITY

Patients are frequently not transferred to rehabilitation wards until their acute medical problems have resolved. This may produce unnecessary delay in instituting appropriate nursing and therapy regimens.

The patient should be transferred to the acute rehabilitation program when there is sufficient stabilization so that the major emphasis of patient care is rehabilitation. It is thus not uncommon that patients still maintain tracheostomies, nasogastric tubes, and so forth. The confusion accompanying the recovery from coma leads to significant behavioral problems that interfere with the individual's recovery. The failure to understand the origin of the patient's agitation and to deal with it effectively leads to the excessive and often inappropriate use of multiple restraints and tranquilizers. The former only increases agitation, and the latter intensifies the clouding of the sensorium. Most tranquilizers additionally interfere with memory and learning, the fundamental prerequisites for recovery. Early admission to a rehabilitation program allows for more effective institution of orienting and behavior modification programs, while proceeding with continued assessment of response to stimuli and the shaping of motor responses. The early institution of a program of mobilization combats the catabolic effects of prolonged bed rest, more effectively prevents and treats contracture formation, and facilitates orientation to one's body. Balance, equilibrium, and righting reflexes are more rapidly established, and bowel and bladder training initiated. A study within our own program suggests that early rehabilitation admission for patients in coma of 8 to 14 days shortens total hospitalization by an average of 2 months.

POST-TRAUMATIC AMNESIA

The duration of post-traumatic amnesia (PTA) is felt to be related to the extent of brain damage and, therefore, to possess prognostic significance. It marks that point in time when the patient has recall of the previous day's events and thus is the foundation for functional memory. Because the patient's return of speech is frequently delayed, the assessment of that moment when PTA has ended is frequently overrated. It is not uncommon to have an individual initiate a previously learned motor task, such as activities of daily living, without the visual, auditory, or tactile cues that were previously provided. It is this point in time that may be considered the end of PTA. Thus, we may determine this important milestone in aphasic or severely dysarthric patients who have not as yet developed nonoral communication systems.

CRANIAL NERVE DEFICITS

The persistence of altered sensory input contributes significantly to the confused state of the patient. Anosmia is a common consequence of severe head trauma that is frequently not recognized until the post-hospital period. Patients who have sustained fractures of the frontal bone or the sinus areas have a higher incidence of olfactory nerve impairment. Anosmia will occur in about 50 percent of the patients with cerebrospinal fluid rhinorrhea.[2] Even without gross fracture, a rotational injury may shear the terminal fibers of the olfactory nerve as it passes through the fine, sieve-like, cribriform plate. Stimulation and testing of olfactory function should be repeated throughout the rehabilitation phase using a series of strong, moderate, then mild odors. (Strong odors, however, may stimulate cranial nerve V as well as I.) It is essential to continue to evaluate and stimulate because recovery of function may occur either partially or completely.

Visual function should be evaluated early for light perception. The stimulus must be presented to each quadrant of the visual field. The time of visual fixation should be recorded as a baseline, and visual function should continue to be reassessed. Spontaneous nystagmus is a principal sign of peripheral or central disturbance. Spontaneous vertical nystagmus, however, is generally a sign of a midbrain lesion.[3] The visual stimulus should be novel enough (intensity, form, and so forth) to elicit a response; simply requesting attention to a finger or pencil may be inadequate. The optokinetic drum may provide such a novel stimulus and, in addition, may provide the earliest appraisal of visual acuity. If the patient does respond to the drum, then acuity must be at least 20/200. The optokinetic drum further allows us to suspect cortical blindness, for in that case the patient may see movement but not a stationary object. An assessment of visual fields should be made to determine how visual information should be presented to maximize the treatment program. Recording of dysconjugate gaze enables the clinician to develop treatment approaches, including orthoptic training, and to determine when and if strabismus surgery is indicated. In third-nerve palsies, most muscle function will return, but frequently there is a residual superior rectus weakness, which may persist. It is important to assess extraocular muscle function, since diplopia may also result from orbital fractures rather than from cranial nerve impairment. Visual acuity may be estimated, as stated above, by the use of the optokinetic drum, but more detailed assessment is essential to determine the ability of the patient to accurately perceive visual information.

The facial nerve is more often damaged than any other motor nerve as a result of its long course in a bony canal. The only cranial nerve more commonly injured is the olfactory nerve. Transverse fractures of the temporal bone produce facial nerve palsy in 30 to 50 percent of patients and are a result of severe frontal or occipital blows. Since the entire height of the petrous bone is frequently involved, both branches of the eighth nerve may be severely impaired in up to 50 percent of patients. Longitudinal fractures are more common, occurring in 70 to 80 percent of temporal bone fractures. Facial nerve injury in these cases is usually delayed in onset and has a better prognosis for recovery. Some sign of recovery is usually present within 8 weeks, if recovery is to occur. Early nerve conduction and electromyographic studies frequently provide a basis for prognostic estimation. Longitudinal fracture may produce dislocation and disruption of the ossicles as a cause for conductive hearing loss; thus, a potential exists for surgical repair. Early assessment of vestibular nerve function can be made while the patient is still in coma by oculovestibular and caloric stimulation tests. When the patient is alert, more detailed information may be provided by the electronystagmogram. The lacrimal branch of the facial nerve may be evaluated at this stage by the Schirmer tearing test.[4,5]

The patient who demonstrates an insensitive cornea, as demonstrated by an absent corneal reflex, combined with facial nerve paralysis (especially if the lacrimal branch is involved) is greatly at risk to develop neurotropic ulcers of the cornea. These patients should be considered for a tarsorrhaphy to protect the cornea. Corneal lubricants should be used liberally.

When the patient is sufficiently alert, audiologic testing should be performed to define any hearing impairment. Brain stem evoked potentials can determine the integrity of the auditory nerve and the cochlear nucleus.[6] Dichotic listening tests may provide additional information regarding auditory perception problems.

LATE EFFECTS OF FACIAL BONE FRACTURES

When loss of continuity of the facial nerve has occurred, permanent paralysis results. The development of microvascular surgical techniques now offers a variety of approaches for the re-establishment of facial nerve function. Once it has been determined that normal function will not return, such surgical procedures may be explored. The best rehabilitation of the face occurs with re-establishment of nerve continuity with the ipsilateral or contralateral nerve. If this is not possible, then a nerve-muscle-pedicle graft from the ansa hypoglossi may be considered. Tonus and some motion may be expected a few weeks after such a procedure, rather than in 6 months as in nerve crossovers. If the fifth cranial nerve has not been damaged, then a regional muscle-nerve transposition using the temporalis or masseter muscle may be performed. If the fifth cranial nerve is also damaged, then the sternocleidomastoid can be used as the donor, or a free nerve-muscle graft from a distant part of the body may be done.[7]

The most common sign of displaced fracture of the facial bones, except for the nose, is malocclusion of the teeth. The single most valuable x-ray view for the diagnosis of facial fracture is the Water view, but it does not visualize the mandible well. Management of such fractures is generally well established prior to transfer to the rehabilitation unit. Some facial fractures, however, produce late effects that must be assessed and managed in the rehabilitation facility. A blowout fracture of the orbit is a result of a fracture of the floor of the orbit. Such a lesion commonly traps the inferior rectus muscle and, occasionally, the inferior oblique. This results in a vertical diplopia with limitation on upward and downward gaze. Additionally, enophthalmos may be associated and may present as a pseudoptosis. Even with early repair of the fracture, excessive scar tissue may form and bind the extraocular muscles. Surgical implants must be used to cover the defect in the orbital floor. If diplopia persists after release of the excessive scar tissue, at least 6 months should elapse before doing strabismus surgery.

An occasional patient may sustain a chronic, recurring dislocation of the temporomandibular joint if the ligaments have become too relaxed. The patient will have trouble chewing and closing the mouth, and the condyle of the mandible will be readily palpated. This can be easily reduced (sometimes requiring local anesthetic injection into the capsule to relax spasm) and is best held in place with wires.[8]

EPILEPSY

Epilepsy after the first week of injury occurs in 5 percent of severely head-injured patients. Incidence is significantly increased if there has been an acute hematoma, a depressed skull fracture, dural penetration, or the occurrence of seizure within the first week of injury. Patients at low risk who are admitted to the rehabilitation center without seizure prophylaxis are generally not given antiseizure medication unless a seizure occurs. Our rule, however, is to initiate seizure prophylaxis if the patient has one or more of the factors that increase risk. The risk of developing late seizures decreases significantly after the first year but remains a potential for some patients even after 4 years.[9,10] (See Chapter 8 for further discussion of post-traumatic epilepsy.)

INFECTIONS

Prevention of infection is primary in the management of penetrating craniocerebral trauma. Retained bone fragments are a common cause of infection and should be sought radiographically when indicated. If postoperative x-ray films reveal even a single bone fragment, reoperation is indicated. Closure of a dural defect is essential to prevent intracerebral infection. All penetrating wounds require radical debridement and primary closure.

Meningitis as a late sequel to skull fracture usually involves a fracture of the floor of the middle cranial fossa. Even when signs of cerebrospinal fluid leakage, such as otorrhea or rhinorrhea, dictate the early administration of antibiotics, late meningitis may develop and should be aggressively treated.

Post-traumatic brain abscess may occur beneath, or in association with, a traumatic wound, generally by direct extension. This complication occurs in penetrating wounds rather than in closed head injury. Its presence may be heralded by the onset of convulsions, and focal signs may or may not be present. A positive CT scan requires surgical evacuation and drainage.

Fever may occur as a result of hypothalamic injury, but a search for infection must always be made. The most common source of such infection is the respiratory tract; the second most common, the urinary tract. Early removal of the indwelling catheter is necessary to eliminate this as an ongoing potential for infection. An intermittent catheterization program may delay the patient's ability to appreciate the sensation of bladder filling, so this should be used with caution.

Other sources of fever include wound infections, thrombophlebitis, and pulmonary embolism. The patient who has severe spasticity may become febrile from the increased metabolic rate associated with such movement. Temperature elevations in such individuals may be controlled by the judicious use of antispasticity medication.

Blood cultures should be obtained with temperature spikes, and a lumbar tap for cerebrospinal fluid culture, if indicated, should be done.

POST-TRAUMATIC HYDROCEPHALUS

Three mechanisms may be responsible for ventricular enlargement. The first may be a result of blood in the ventricular system, which causes increased osmolarity and subsequent adhesions. Hydrocephalus ex vacuo results from replacement of atrophic brain tissue by an expansion of the ventricles. The third form, normal-pressure hydrocephalus resulting from decreased reabsorption of cerebrospinal fluid, may be suggested by a deterioration of the patient's condition, resulting in incontinence, a decrease in the sensorium, and unexplained loss of motor function. If the ventricular system is under high pressure, then shunting frequently improves function. Normal-pressure hydrocephalus, however, responds to surgery in only 25 percent of the cases. The CT scan can identify the presence of ventricular enlargement, but not the type. Radioisotope serum albumin (RISA) scans are essential to identify the etiology.[1]

CRANIOPLASTY

The indications for cranioplasty are to provide the brain with adequate protection and to improve cosmetic appearance. Contrary to some early reports, there is no relationship between seizure activity and skull defects. Though many cranioplasty materials are available, autogenous bone and methyl methacrylate are the most commonly favored. Large cranial defects in children are best repaired with split rib grafts. If the periosteum is left, regeneration is rapid. In closed head injuries without evidence of infection, repair of the defect may be made relatively early; but penetrating injuries must be considered as potentially contaminated, and repair should be delayed a minimum of 1 year. Immediate postoperative management requires constant observation for signs of elevated intracranial pressure, which result from intracranial bleeding or massive edema, or both. This would be heralded by a change in the level of consciousness or the advent of abnormal eye signs. These signs, of course, can be obscured by the concomitant administration of narcotics (pupillary constriction) or sedatives (altered awareness). Postoperative complications include infection, osteomyelitis, and, more commonly, subgaleal fluid accumulations. The latter can be managed quite readily with elastic bandage compression.[11,12]

ORAL-FEEDING STATUS

Bulbar symptoms are almost universal in severe head injuries. An assessment of oral-feeding status is necessary to determine an approach to nutrition and to establish a basis for motor impairment of the peripheral speech mechanisms. If the patient has a poor prognosis for early feeding, then alternate approaches for nutrition must be considered. Patients with severe head injury generally lose between 10 and 40 percent of their body weight, and recovery of this loss may take up to a year. Oropharyngeal response to cutaneous stimulation should be noted, as well as the presence or absence of pursuit responses, cough reflex (and its degree of effectiveness), mobility of tongue and cheek muscles, and the quality of movement. A constant moist quality to respirations or voice suggests poor pharyngeal control. Adequate lip closure is an essential feature of controlled feeding. If oral feeding does not appear imminent after 2 weeks of oral bulbar training, then one should consider a gastrostomy or esophagostomy, rather than long-term maintenance of a nasogastric tube. The presence of a nasogastric tube produces significant irritation, leading to granulomatous tissue formation and stenosis, maintenance of a flexion posture, pain, and chronic blood loss. Gastrostomies should ordinarily be considered as a temporary feeding system; thus, the Janeway permanent gastrostomy should not be performed unless there are strong indications of permanent dysphagia. The tube should be placed as lateral to the midline as possible, so as not to interfere with the early mat program in therapy. In children, esophagostomies are preferred by some. This procedure should not be used when significant torticollis or a strong asymmetric tonic neck reflex is present.

HETEROTOPIC OSSIFICATION

Heterotopic ossification occurs with greater frequency than is commonly appreciated in head injury. Its presence may first be suspected by an elevated alkaline phosphatase level. One must recognize, however, that elevations may occur in the presence of bone fractures and as a natural consequence of growth in a teenager. Heterotopic ossification may also be suspected when limited ranges of motion are encountered in a stretching program. The most common sites for heterotopic ossification in head injury are the hips, axillae, shoulders, and elbows. As in spinal-cord-injured patients, thrombophlebitis must be ruled out in the differential diagnosis. A bone scan frequently demonstrates areas of increased uptake, even in the presence of negative x-ray views. Diphosphonates may be used to prevent bony ankylosis, but their efficacy in head injury has not yet been clearly established. The maintenance of passive range of motion may prevent further ankylosis, and the previously held views that passive range of motion should be restricted are not valid. If the ossification threatens joint motion, then serial bone scans with computerized ratios should be obtained to determine when activity has ceased, signaling the potential time for surgery.[13,14]

AIRWAY OBSTRUCTION

The patient with respiratory difficulty should be considered early for a tracheostomy. If an endotracheal tube is left in place for 5 to 7 days, there is an increased risk of laryngeal stenosis. Any patient who has maintained an endotracheal tube for a week or more prior to tracheostomy should have indirect or direct laryngoscopy to evaluate vocal cord function, the status of the pyriform fossa, and the patency of the larynx. The late development of labored respiration or tachypnea should suggest laryngeal stenosis. An attempt should be made to remove the tracheostomy tube as early as the patient's respiratory status indicates. Once the pulmonary problems have resolved, the patient's ability to breathe adequately with the tracheostomy tube plugged should be monitored by blood gas studies. Healing of the stoma after tube removal is rapid and rarely requires surgical closure. The tracheostomy tube, while in place, should receive aseptic care. Suctioning should be preceded by oxygen administration for a few minutes. Constant use of a humidifier when the patient is in bed decreases crust formation and increases the liquefication of the sputum.[15]

SKELETAL TRAUMA

Almost 50 percent of our cases of severe head injury sustain some associated skeletal trauma. Although a search for associated trauma is made in the acute neurotrauma unit, undiagnosed osseous trauma frequently becomes evident during the rehabilitation phase. As the patient becomes more alert, attention should be paid to any complaint of pain that may be osseous in nature, and the complaint should be evaluated both functionally and with x-ray studies. Casting of bony trauma generally should not be done in flexion because of the element of spasticity and its role in contracture formation. Patients must be treated as if they will fully recover from head trauma, even when trauma involves a densely hemiplegic extremity. Any teenaged child who is immobilized for long periods is a candidate for the development of hypercalcemia. Routine serum calcium levels should be obtained on all teenagers and young adults; if calcium is elevated, parathormone levels should be obtained to distinguish immobilization hypercalcemia from primary hyperparathyroidism. The onset of serum calcium elevations usually occurs 6 to 15 weeks after trauma and frequently returns to normal with the onset of full mobilization. Occasional cases may require aggressive medical treatment. The presence of this syndrome may be undetected because the usual clinical symptoms of nausea, vomiting, constipation, weakness, and emotional lability may not be present in the head-injured patient.[16]

HYPOTHALAMIC FUNCTIONS

Diabetes insipidus occurs after severe head injury with an incidence of 1 in 200. Symptoms are frequently transient, usually lasting several weeks. Diabetes insipidus may be suspected on the basis of polyuria and polydipsia with a consistently low urinary specific gravity that cannot be raised above 1.010. Occasionally, patients may require intranasal vasopressin to control the symptoms. In two of our cases, the control of these symptoms was accompanied by improved memory function, as suggested by DeWeid.[17] Hyperphagia, which may result from hypothalamic damage, has not responded to any drug therapy.[18]

A listing of some of the general medical complications that may be encountered at various times before or during the hospital rehabilitation program is presented in Chapter 3, Types of Disability.

CONCLUSION

The potential for medical problems can ofttimes be suspected or anticipated from evaluation of the records of the neurotrauma center. The establishment of uniform terminology and reporting systems, such as the Glasgow Coma Scale, provides the physiatrist with an increased ability to deal with the rehabilitation needs of the head-injured patient.

The patient with severe head injury must be assessed to determine the potential for functional improvement in the rehabilitation program. There are no concrete minimal established criteria for admission to such a program. Instead, one must determine the access to the environment that the patient has and then, based on the unique residuals of each patient, determine the sensory avenues open for enlarging that access. Assessment must be an ongoing continuum throughout the rehabilitation process, and an integral part of the treatment program. Plateaus are rarely achieved. Instead, the rate of change may slow to a level that does not match the level required by the program for cost effectiveness. Because change continues, patient assessment must continue long after discharge from the rehabilitation center. Evidence suggests that neurophysiologic return parallels normal developmental milestones, reflex patterns, and maturational behaviors in evaluating response to treatment. Since response to treatment is essential to determine a head-injured patient's potential, we can rarely begin to determine that potential in less than 2 weeks.

REFERENCES

1. YEN, JK, ET AL: *Numerical grading of clinical neurological status after serious head injury.* J Neurol Neurosurg Psychiatry 41:1125, 1978.
2. JENNETT, B AND TEASDALE, G: *Management of Head Injuries.* FA Davis, Philadelphia, 1981.
3. GAY, AJ, ET AL: *Eye Movement Disorders.* CV Mosby, St Louis, 1974.
4. NELSON, JR: *Neuro-otologic aspects of head injury.* In THOMPSON, RA AND GREEN, JR (EDS): *Advances in Neurology,* Vol 22. Raven Press, New York, 1979, p 107.
5. MCHUGH, HE: *Auditory and vestibular disorders in head injury.* In CAVENESS, WF AND WALKER, AE (EDS): *Head Injury: Conference Proceedings.* JB Lippincott, Philadelphia, 1966, p 97.
6. RAPPAPORT, M, ET AL: *Evoked brain potentials and disability in brain-damaged patients.* Arch Phys Med Rehabil 58:333, 1977.
7. BAKER, C (ED): *Clinics in Plastic Surgery: Facial Paralysis.* WB Saunders, Philadelphia, 1979.
8. NATVIG, P AND DORTIZBACH, RK: *Facial bone fractures.* In GRABB, C AND SMITH, JW (EDS): *Plastic Surgery.* Little, Brown & Co, Boston, 1979, p 242.
9. JENNETT, B: *Epilepsy after Non-missile Head Injuries,* ed 2. Heinemann, London, 1975.
10. JENNETT, B: *Posttraumatic epilepsy.* In THOMPSON, RA AND GREEN, JR (EDS): *Advances in Neurology,* Vol 22. Raven Press, New York, 1979, p 137.
11. RISH, BL, ET AL: *Cranioplasty: A review of 1030 cases of penetrating head injury.* Neurosurgery 4:381, 1979.

12. SMITH, J AND GEIST, BL: *Evaluation and care of the acute craniotomy patient.* Journal of Neurosurgical Nursing 10:102, 1978.
13. GARLAND, DE: *Heterotopic ossification: Incidence, location and management.* In *Rehabilitation of the Head Injured Adult.* Rancho Los Amigos Hospital, Downey, Calif, 1980.
14. ROBERTS, JB AND PANKRATZ, DG: *The surgical treatment of heterotopic ossification at the elbow following long-term coma.* J Bone Joint Surg 61-A:760, 1979.
15. *Stenosis following tracheostomy.* JAMA 216:1984, 1971.
16. CRISTOFARO, RL AND BRINK, JD: *Hypercalcemia of immobilization in neurologically injured children: A prospective study.* Orthopedics 2:486, 1979.
17. DEWEID, D: *Hormonal influences on motivation, learning, and memory process.* Hospital Practice January 1976:123.
18. MOSES, AM: *Diabetes insipidus and ADH regulation.* In KRIEGER, DT AND HUGHES, JC (EDS).: *Neuroendocrinology.* Sinauer Associates, Sunderland, Mass, 1980, p 141.

Chapter 18

MOTOR ASSESSMENT

Arthur J. Nelson, Ph.D., R.P.T.

Motor activity is developed as a result of harmonious action of many portions of the brain, spinal cord, and peripheral nervous system. Abnormalities of movement resulting from head injuries are most commonly involved in the cortical regions and their connecting pathways.[1] The disorders of movement resulting from head injury may be loosely classified into two major categories. First are movement deficiencies, or lack of function, such as loss of motor power, agility, coordination, and control. Second are movement abnormalities such as spasticity, dystonia, and/or unwanted movement patterns.[2]

The purpose of this chapter is to formulate a clinical method of assessing movement in head-injured adults that can lead to an inventory of deficiencies and problem areas which can be used by the therapist for treatment planning and for assessing outcome of that treatment. Some important variables should be kept in mind in any evaluative procedure and especially in estimating motor function. The subject being examined should ideally be alert and capable of following directions and remembering commands. Furthermore, the individual should understand the procedures involved and be willing to perform them. Therefore, the purpose and method should be explained to the subject in simple terms so that the subject may comprehend the procedures. Pain, discomfort of any type, sedatives or other narcotics, apprehension, anxiety, fatigue, and other factors may all interfere with the consistent observation of the behaviors. If the patient is in an obtunded or lowered state of consciousness, or if intelligence is impaired and the patient fails to understand the examiner's directions, the procedures need to be even further simplified. If the person does not persist in the activity, the examination should be repeated at least twice and preferably five times to determine consistency of performance.

The patient should be suitably clothed for examining the limbs and, if possible, for visualization of the trunk, hips, and shoulders. At the same time, the patient should be reasonably warm and comfortable and not be distressed (needing to void or feeling embarrassed by not being properly covered). The accuracy and consistency of motor assessment are influenced by a number of variables, the foremost of which is the patient's sense of need to move.

Other important variables are the ability to attend and the length of time for the individual to hear a command and respond. People have different reasons for attending to different matters; quite obviously, what the therapist considers to be an important matter may not be considered so by the patient. Among the head-injured population, there may be complicating factors such as multiple injuries to other parts and other compromises of internal organ function; therefore, the person's state of health in general must be taken into consideration.

MOTOR PROBLEMS OF THE HEAD-INJURED ADULT

The motor problems of the head-injured adult fall into three major categories: (1) the loss of power or ability to exert tension in the muscles sufficiently; (2) the loss of balance, in both sitting and standing; and (3) the disorders of muscle tone or spasticity of varying degrees. Loss of motor power may be quite diffuse, involving all limbs, or may be focal, leading to changes such as weakness of grasp and/or extension of the fingers of a single limb. Loss of motor power is evidenced not only by inability to exert tension but also by fatigability or variation in output on repeated testing. Of importance also is the range at which that movement is occurring.

In this same regard, it is important to consider the pattern with which the movement is executed. Is it clumsy? Does it involve a whole limb mass being moved? Or is a portion of the limb active and the other portion of the limb somewhat frail and limp? Conversely, when the movement is attempted, does the individual tighten up abnormally and become somewhat rigid in attempting the pattern of motion?

The loss of motor power may be in various types of distribution such as a monoplegia, paralysis of one extremity; a diplegia, paralysis of two sides of the body; hemiplegia, paralysis of one half of the body; paraplegia, paralysis of the legs; quadriplegia, paralysis of all four extremities; or hemiplegia alternans, paralysis of one part of one side of the body and another part of the opposite side of the body. There may be a bilateral hemiplegia such as decorticate hemiplegia of one side with flexion of the upper extremity predominating and extension of the lower extremity, while on the opposite side there may be a decerebrate configuration consisting of extension of the upper extremity as well as extension of the lower extremity.

When muscles have been left in positions of shortening for considerable periods of time, contracture or connective tissue restrictions of the joint-muscle complex may take place. Therefore, even though a muscle may be capable of contraction and relaxation, if the joint is restricted and/or the muscle is inflexible, obviously the muscle cannot be carried through its normal excursion. This may reflect unfairly on the production of motor output in the opposing muscles that must pull against this restriction and tightness, and should be carefully noted in the recording of the problem. In the head-injured adult, who may have considerable trauma of multiple body parts, it should be noted that the joint changes might be related to a primary musculoskeletal disorder and should not always be ascribed to the central nervous system motor disorder. However, the orthopedic problem may considerably complicate matters in assessing motor performance.

OBSERVATIONAL PHASE OF ASSESSMENT

The initial encounter of the physical therapist with the patient is a significant one. The adage "first impressions are lasting ones" is no less significant for patient assessment. A head-injured patient who is rolled into the physical therapy department in a wheelchair, slouched to one side, drooling, and seemingly unresponsive to verbal commands may create an unfavorable impression within a very short time of observation. Hence, it might be suggested that motor behavior assessment not be immediately started while the patient is in this compromised position. Rather, the testing should be done in a systematic fashion with maximal patient readiness.

MOTOR EXAMINATION

With the patient reclining in a comfortable position with the limbs suitably exposed so that one can observe them easily, the first consideration would be to look at the general pattern of the individual's posture. Is one limb more extended and/or flexed than the other? Is one side of the body in generally a different pattern than the other? Does the person seem to prefer to rotate the neck to one side? Care should be exercised in this regard to be sure that the rotation is not caused by being stimulated more from one side of the treatment table or bed than the other. Therefore, the examiner should move from one side of the bed or table to the other to assure that this is not the case.

The next observation should be made for any spontaneous movements that occur without provocation, noting their extent, duration, and intensity. The limbs should be examined also for any wasting, thinness, or abnormal distribution of muscle bulk that may be noted on a lined diagram that the examiner may use.

The next part of this observational phase would include giving verbal commands to the patient, should the patient have language capability, and determining what response there is to those commands and how long it takes. If the patient is aphasic or appears not to comprehend verbal commands, an attempt should be made to gesture and have the person follow that gesturing. The first muscle groups to be examined would be the lower extremity, since these patients would be more likely to be able to move it earlier than the upper extremity. An emphasis should be on succeeding rather than making the individual's examination involve the most difficult part first.

Asking or demonstrating to the person to lift one leg off the surface of the bed or table would be the first action looked for. The knee would be expected to bend slightly, and the head would flex. This might involve ankle dorsiflexion. Therefore, one would note deficiencies in components of the movement that would normally be encountered when the individual would actively lift one leg off the surface of the table. The inventory form should have a recording of the arc, the intensity of the movement, and the ability of the individual to repeat the activity five times. For example, does the person initiate the movement after a considerable delay? Does the individual persist in carrying out all five of the movements with equal intensity, range, and fervor? Or does the individual wax and wane in carrying out the movement pattern?

The next movement assessment would be the distal portion of the limb, which might be considerably more difficult to attain. In this next pattern, the patient would be asked to dorsiflex or bring the foot and ankle toward himself or herself and push the foot away. The movement that ensues should be one of extending or lifting the toes and dorsiflexing the ankle, keeping the foot neutral with respect to the plane of movement; the counterpart of plantarflexion coupled with flexion of the toes should be present. This should be repeated with equal intensity and range five times to be classified within the normal range.

It might be anticipated that patients with cortical lesions may experience difficulty in executing distal movements, so there may be attempts to produce the ankle movement by substituting inversion and/or supination of the foot rather than dorsiflexion with the foot held in a neutral position. Similarly, there may be more power exercised in plantarflexion that may not be easily reversed when the repeated dorsiflexion is attempted. It should be underscored that these movements are done without assistance by the therapist; if they are unsuccessful, the therapist should not assist at this particular stage of the assessment.

The next movement to be tested is the asymmetric tonic neck reflex. The patient is asked to rotate the head from side to side. Notation should be taken of the ability to pass the midline, and of the range, extent, and persistence of the movement. While this rotation from side to side is occurring, the therapist should also be observing the arms and legs for any influence that this neck movement may have on the limbs. Do the limbs on the side toward which the chin is rotating tend to extend or remain in an extension pattern for prolonged periods after the head rotates away from that side? Some head-injured patients in the early phases are able to rotate the head and face to one side but are not able to cross the midline and rotate to the other side. This should be noted carefully. (See Appendix 1 at the end of the chapter for Motor Behavior Inventory.)

The next test is the symmetric tonic neck reflex. One asks the individual to flex the head and neck forward, lifting the head and neck off the pillow or support. Is this accomplished with symmetry and adequate range, or is it difficult? Does it elicit pain? Or is it simply not accomplished? Similarly, can the person push the head and neck back into the pillow (or towel roll) behind the patient? Can the patient then reverse this readily and easily to move toward flexion? Again, the range, rate, and persistence of the activity are noted.

Finally, the upper extremity is tested by asking or gesturing to the patient to elevate the arm, flexing at the shoulder with the elbow extended, forearm in pronation, and the hand and fingers extended, neutral, or slightly fisted. If the movement is different from this pattern, that is, the elbow flexes and the forearm remains in pronation, and there is some flexion of the shoulder or the elbow flexes with the forearm supinating, these should be noted and recorded on the inventory form. The movement should be performed throughout the arc that is available to the person, bringing the arm up near the side of the head if possible and then returning it to the side of the body using again the same pattern of elbow extension and forearm pronation. The movement is repeated five times, and one observes the rest of the body during the performance of this activity to determine whether it either is influenced by other parts or is influencing other parts of the body, especially rotation of the head and neck.

The distal muscles of the wrist, forearm, and hand would be assessed next by asking the person to attempt a paraprehensile pattern of pinching the thumb and second and third fingers together and releasing the same, separating the fingers by a short distance, repeating the pinch, releasing and pinching five times. The extent of the movement, the accuracy of the placement, and the ability to rapidly release the pinch would all be noted on the inventory.

MUSCLE TONUS AND MYOTATIC REFLEXES

While the patient is in the supine position, muscle tone should be observed. Tone has been defined as the tension produced by muscles when they are relaxed or their resistance to passive movement when voluntary control is absent. From a functional viewpoint, this means how much resistance to passive stretch the muscles offer when being lengthened. If one taps on the tendon of the muscle, do the muscles respond with a stretch response?

Assessment of muscle tone or the response of muscles to stretch or the inability of a muscle to relax readily is very difficult because it demands the utmost in cooperation by the patient as well as a good deal of clinical skill on the part of the examiner. (See Appendix 2 at the end of the chapter for Sensory Inventory.) For instance, normal muscle shows some slight resistance to passive movement in spite of voluntary relaxation. While abnormal increase in tone may be a slight increase in this resistance to passive movement, it is simply a matter of judgment, therefore, and can be learned by the therapist only through repeated investigations of many normal subjects and many patients with abnormalities in tone. Palpation of the muscles to note their consistency, firmness, or turgor is helpful, but is certainly not the only factor that needs to be tested in assessing this phenomenon of tone. For example, a person may have very loose muscles in the resting state, while having hyperresponsiveness to stretch when the muscle is tapped. Inconsistencies found between palpation and response to tapping of the muscle should be noted.

The testing of tone should be done with the individual in a relaxed, passive state because any slight active contraction of muscles will mask the responses of the stretch system. The specific tests that may be applied at this time are to test the biceps, brachioradialis, and triceps tendons with a tendon tap applied either with the tips of the fingers or with a tendon hammer. Should the person assume a dystonic or fixed position of a limb during the testing, this should be noted on the inventory form. A standard operating procedure should be used in testing the muscle stretch response in the arms. That is, the elbow should be flexed passively to 90 degrees and cradled by the examiner's arm; the forearm should be in midposition for testing the brachioradialis; and when the triceps are tested, the arms should be rotated 45 degrees from the vertical to permit access to the triceps area (but the elbow should be kept again at 90 degrees of flexion). The head and neck should remain in the same position and not be moving during the testing.

The elbow flexors and extensors are then tested for resistance to passive stretch simply by bending and straightening the limbs at a fairly rapid pace, and the resistance that is offered by the muscles is estimated. Landau[2] defines spasticity as the progressive and consistent increase in resistance to passive elongation of the muscle that builds to a peak. Then suddenly that tension is released or relaxed in what is called the "knife-clasp" phenomenon. The examiner may shake the forearm to and fro while holding the elbow region to see how relaxed the hand and wrist remain during this movement. The normal muscle stretch response would be that the hand remains loose and limp. Similarly, if the arm is passively lifted and suddenly released, the arm will be lowered slowly by the individual if the individual has active control; if the arm is weak, it will suddenly drop. The resistance of the lower extremities to passive stretch would then be done in similar fashion, that is, the knee-jerk response should be tested with the knees at a right angle and the ankle-jerk response also should be tested with the ankle at a right angle. Passive movement of the knee and ankle should similarly be tested to determine resistance to passive elongation of those muscles. While in this area, the plantar stimulation may be carried out by stimulating with a blunt instrument along the inferior lateral surface of the foot; in the normal person, this results in plantarflexion of all the toes, whereas in the head-injured person, it may result in either extension of the great toe or fanning of the lateral four toes, or both.

HEAD-DROPPING TEST

The patient should be supine without a pillow and completely relaxed with the eyes closed and the attention diverted. The examiner places a hand under the patient's occiput, and with the other hand briskly raises the head and then allows it to drop rather suddenly into the other hand. Normally, the head drops rapidly into the examiner's hand, but in the patient with increased tone, there is a delayed, slow, and gentle dropping of the head. Should the patient have meningeal irritation and/or pressure on the structures in the neck, this movement might be painful during flexion and should be noted accordingly.

ASSESSMENT OF SENSORY RESPONSIVENESS

In assessing motor behavior, the matter of sensation takes on importance, and one must be aware of the gross sensory responsiveness of the patient. During sensory testing, it is frequently necessary to occlude the person's vision. It is better to block the vision with a card, piece of paper, or blindfold rather than to ask the person to close the eyes. When one has to keep the eyes closed, attention must be diverted from other factors, and the sensory evaluation might be somewhat distorted as a result. Similarly, communication problems will provide an extreme frustration to the examiner as well as to the patient. Therefore, whenever possible, replacement of the naming of objects with the identification of similar sets of objects can be an advantage.

The recognition of crude sensations of pinprick, temperature, and touch should be used at the outset to determine whether there is gross damage to sensory discrimination. Pinprick is tested by touching the skin with a sharp pin. The therapist may, for example, determine whether it is perceived as sharp or dull by reversing the pin from the sharp to the dull end, over the regions of the limbs affected. Temperature may be tested by using two test tubes, one filled with cold water and the other filled with hot water. The individual is given the test in such a fashion that sufficient time is permitted for the temperature to be mediated to the part. Care should be exercised that the temperature does not change in the course of the examination to the point that discrimination is rather minimal. Light touch may be tested by use of the finger or a piece of cotton or cloth. This test might be made more quantitative by the use of tactile hairs that have specific pressure gradients.

All of the major affected parts should be tested, though it may be instructive to also test in a hemiplegic patient, for instance, the unaffected side to determine if there is sensory impairment. During the testing of touch, the therapist observes for signs of tactile defensiveness. This phenomenon is a withdrawal on contact that leads to the patient being apprehensive or, in fact, fearful of touch stimuli. In the early phases of care, the head-injured adult may indeed demonstrate tactile defensiveness.

The sensory examination may next move to proprioceptive sensibilities such as the position of joints in space, and may be done at the more distal arm joints and the distal leg joints. The standard procedure is to test the distal joints first, such as the great toe, the lateral four toes, the foot, the ankle, and then the thumb and fingers of the hand. When testing the joints, it is important to hold the patient's joint laterally on each side of the segment, not on the top and bottom.

STEREOGNOSIS

Stereognosis is the tactile and proprioceptive recognition of common objects held in the hand and the recognition of textures of different objects. The absence of this ability is termed astereognosis. Difficulty in determining these sensations is termed dystereognosis.

The test is usually done in two ways. The subject is offered an object with vision obstructed and asked to name it. These may be common objects such as a paper clip, a coin, a ballpoint pen, a small golf ball, and so forth. The object is placed in the hand and the patient can manipulate it, but the patient must not use the other hand for assistance. The patient then should be able to identify the comparable object in another set of similar objects using the other hand. In the second part of the test, the subject may be offered a selection of different textures to identify, for example, a piece of velvet, sandpaper, or carpet. The patient is then asked to identify a similar texture with the other hand while the vision is still occluded.

TWO-POINT DISCRIMINATION

This is the ability for the individual to perceive as dual tactile stimuli small distances of separation between two points. A caliper that can be set for specific distances should be available, and when its points are placed at a distance as close as 5 mm, they should be distinguishable at the tips of the fingers. A separation of 1.5 to 2 cm on the dorsal surface of the hand may be required before a double stimulus is sensed. In the trunk and abdomen, the calipers may need to be separated 6 to 8 cm before the individual can discriminate two points of contact. This test is usually applied in the hand, for this is where discriminations may be most significant for function.

BILATERAL SIMULTANEOUS STIMULATION

After the patient has been tested for tactile sensibility and can localize unilateral and single touch, the simultaneous presentation of two stimuli will be assessed. For instance, with the patient's vision obstructed, the examiner touches the patient lightly on the ends of the toes with the eraser end of a pencil held in each hand. The patient then points to the spot touched, if capable of doing so, or responds verbally if that is possible. The same would be done at the knees, the fingertips, and finally the elbows. The patient with tactile inattention will not recognize the stimulus from the affected part of the body or may displace that stimulus proximally. For example, presentation of double and simultaneous stimulation of the toes may result in displacement of the affected side response to the level of the lower leg or may extinguish that response so that the person may perceive only the stimulation on the unaffected side. It should be stressed that this inattention to tactile stimulation may also apply to vision and hearing. It should be determined if a person can respond to visual stimuli when presented to one side but extinguishes that sensibility when presented with stimuli from both sides of the visual field. This can have an extremely important impact on how a patient functions and therefore on how one designs a training program.

BODY SCHEMA

The way in which a patient may see the body parts or may be able to identify body parts when asked to do so by the examiner is a crude way of determining if the person actually has the sense of those parts being present. A method of determining this would be to ask patients to draw a picture of themselves in a crude line drawing. Although many interpretations of this can be made, it will be evident if the patient does not conceptualize major portions of the body. It is extremely difficult to have patients engage in movement patterns with body parts that are not present in their minds. An illustration of this obtained from a hemiplegic patient may be seen in Figure 18-1.

Related to this problem of sensory inattention is a difficulty with right/left discrimination. It should not be confused with unilateral neglect. Quite simply, the way this is determined is to ask the person to point to the right hand or left hand, right foot or left foot, right ear or left ear, and so forth. An important factor in this observation is the difficulty that the person

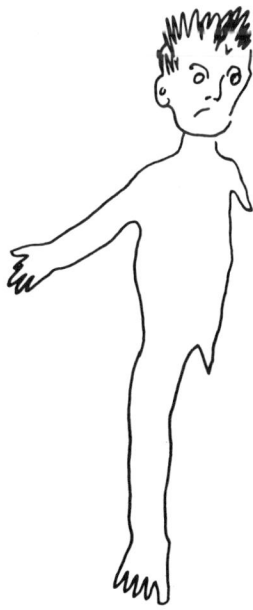

FIGURE 18-1. Self-portrait of a head-injured patient. A male patient with right hemisphere brain injury was asked to draw a simple picture of himself. This patient demonstrated left-sided neglect on clinical examination.

may have with pointing across the midline of the body versus being able to point to things on the same side of the body. The ability to recognize right and left should not be confused with an inability to cross the midline.

VISUAL FUNCTION

The head-injured adult may have an unusual variety of visual impairments, involving the retina, optic nerves, or any portion of the optic radiation, including the visual cortex where the visual signals are interpreted or appreciated. Therefore, a crude assessment of these functions should be made. If a patient normally wears glasses, they should be worn during the assessment. Such field defects as homonymous hemianopsia (blindness in half of the field of vision), visual extinction, and more limited visual field defects should be noted. Special problems relating to the discrimination of figure-ground or the recognition of common visual portrayals such as faces, numbers, and other common communication symbols should be noted. The tendency to extinguish when presented with bilateral and simultaneous visual stimuli should be noted.

TONIC REFLEXES

The next aspect of evaluation includes a rating of the primitive tonic reflexes. The primitive responses such as the tonic neck, tonic labyrinthine, and rotational responses can be rated on a scale from 0 to 4 according to the method described by Capute.[3] The subject is examined in the supine position, and the neck is either passively or actively rotated to one side. When this is done, either the tone or position of the limbs is noted. The rating scale for the asymmetric reflex is indicated below. (See Appendix 2 at the end of this chapter.)

When the asymmetric tonic neck reflex is tested, the patient remains in the supine position, and the flexion of the neck should be accomplished from a neutral position. That is, the patient should not have a pillow propping the head into ventral flexion during the testing because the relative position change of the neck would be minimal.

TONIC LABYRINTHINE REFLEX

The labyrinthine responses would be tested with the person in the supine position and the neck in a neutral position and not moving. The limbs would be assessed in terms of either tone change or resistance to passive stretch of the limbs when the individual is supine, as opposed to when the patient is rolled from one side to the other and then rolled to the prone position. The rating used would follow the one proposed by Capute.

The asymmetric labyrinthine responses are those mediated in the side-lying position. Care should be exercised that the neck does not change its alignment but stays in a neutral position during the testing of these responses. Some have advocated the use of a cervical collar to retard excessive neck movement during this procedure.

In summary, the major influences of these tonic reflexes would be to determine whether or not the responses were obligatory or if they had significant impact on the performance of movement, tending to impair or hamper the person's movement of the limbs.

TRIGGERED RESPONSES

The righting reflexes or responses can best be assessed with the patient in the supine position by rotating the head and neck passively and determining the amount of response that occurs in the trunk and limbs as a result of that rotation. The most primitive response is one in which the whole trunk rolls as a kind of "log-rolling" response to that of a minimal one of segmental movement of the upper trunk in response to the rotation of the neck to one side.

The opposite pattern of distal to proximal would be assessed by rotating the legs and pelvis and determining the amount of rotation that occurred in the head and neck in response to this rotation. Again, the Capute rating scale would be used.

EQUILIBRIUM REACTION

The placing, hopping, and/or equilibrium reactions may be tested in the supine position by placing the subject on a tilting surface. When that tilting surface is suddenly moved to one side, the limbs tend to spread in abduction and give the appearance of an attempt to balance oneself and prevent oneself from falling or, in other words, to increase the base of support for the body. Tilting would be repeated five times to each side, and any asymmetry of response would be noted. This would complete the assessment of the person in the supine position.

SEATED POSITION

The next position to be tested would be that of the sitting position. The examiner may perform a shoulder-shaking test with a seated patient. The patient's back should not be supported. The hands should be dropping down by the sides of the body in a relaxed fashion during the examination. The examiner places the hands on the person's shoulders, and shakes the patient briskly in forward and backward directions and also in a rotary direction. With significant increases in tone, the arm swinging on the affected side will be rather restricted. With hypotonicity, or reduction in tone, the affected side will lead to greater than normal arcs of movement or a pendular type of response.

THE ARM-DROPPING TEST

The patient's forearm may be briskly raised and suddenly dropped. With increase in tone, there is a delay in the downward movement of the arm, while with hypotonicity, the dropping is abrupt. A similar maneuver can be engaged in for the legs that are draped over the edge of the table, whereby the leg is brought up briskly and let go suddenly. Rate of fall toward the surface should be observed.

PRONATION AND SUPINATION OF FOREARMS

With hypertonicity, the patient may experience difficulty in performing full supination of the forearm. The patient will have an asymmetry when asked to perform both movements symmetrically. In the presence of hypotonicity, there is a tendency for the hands to assume a position of pronation, which is continued even when the arms are outstretched horizontally but is exaggerated when lifted above the head. On forward elevation, there is a characteristic position of the hands, flexion of the wrists, hyperextension of the proximal and terminal phalanges, and some overpronation of the forearms. When the arms are continued above the head, there is increased pronation of the forearms with internal rotation of the shoulders, and as a result, the palms are turned outward. When assessing movement progress, one should note whether or not there are missing portions of the movement or whether there are abnormal aspects within the performance. Secondly, how does the individual maintain upright or excessive amounts of activity? And, finally, does the function produce increased tone or involuntary movement or instill tremor or other abnormal components? An important movement of the arms when the patient is seated would be to reach forward to grasp objects, bring them to the head and mouth region, and return them to the same position.

SITTING BALANCE WHEN DISTURBED

With the patient seated on the edge of a treatment platform, feet on the floor, the patient is suddenly shifted from one side to the other. Observations of movement of the arm are then made to determine whether or not the limbs extend to support the individual in the direction of the shift. The upper trunk should shift away from the side being tilted to for a proper equilibrium reaction. Care should be exercised so as not to overstimulate the individual so that it would be impossible or difficult to accomplish the movement. As in previous evaluations, it is important to note whether the individual rotates the neck toward one side or the other, and if this has an influence on the movement when shifted.

The next movement assessed would be shifting the patient to the side and rotating so that both hands are placed on one side of the leg. For instance, the left and right hands are

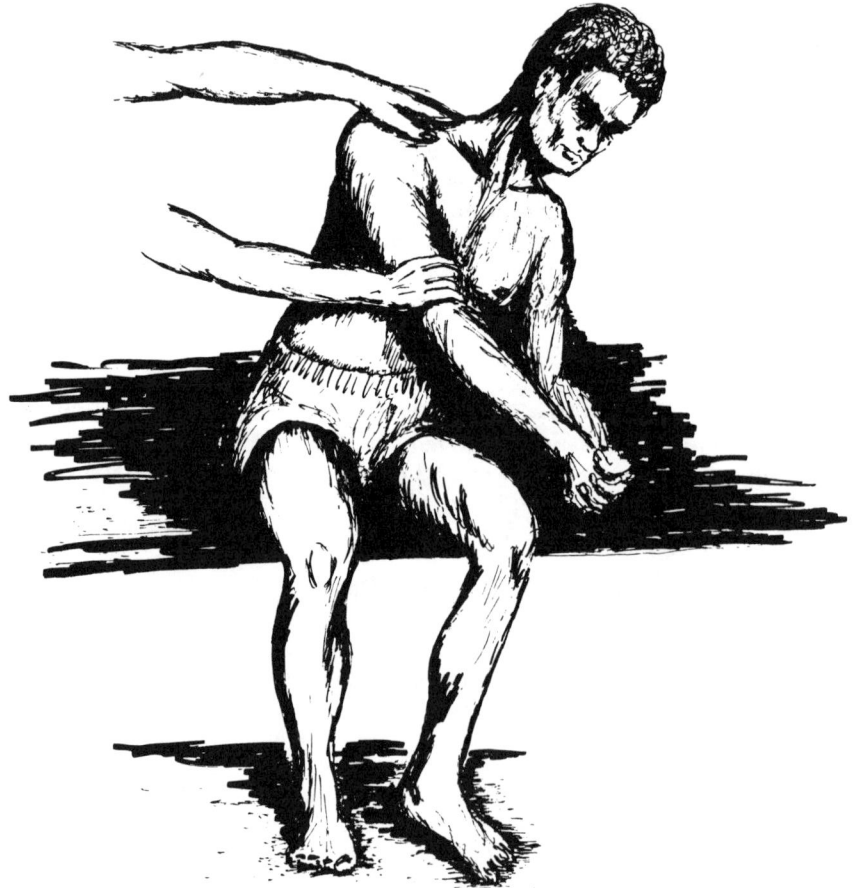

FIGURE 18-2. Weight shifting in seated position. The patient with a left hemiparesis in this illustration is tilted to the left and, with hands folded, attempts to prop himself for support. The therapist shifts the trunk by lifting under the right buttock and left axilla. The goal is to distribute weight to the left buttock.

placed on the left hip region, and weight is shifted to that side. The reverse is also tested. The relative participation of each of the arms would then be recorded (Fig. 18-2).

SITTING TO STANDING

The patient then demonstrates the ability to slip forward and sit nearer the edge of the table and/or frame. Particular attention is paid to the ability to place weight on both sides equally and to keep weight on the heels of both feet during the process of shifting forward. Any tendency to use abnormal movements or to function with unilateral weight shift to one side would be noted in the inventory (Fig. 18-3).

Similarly, in observing the rate of movement from the seated position to standing, the examiner would note whether the individual, when finally assuming the upright position, puts weight on both feet equally or tends to keep weight to one side preferentially.

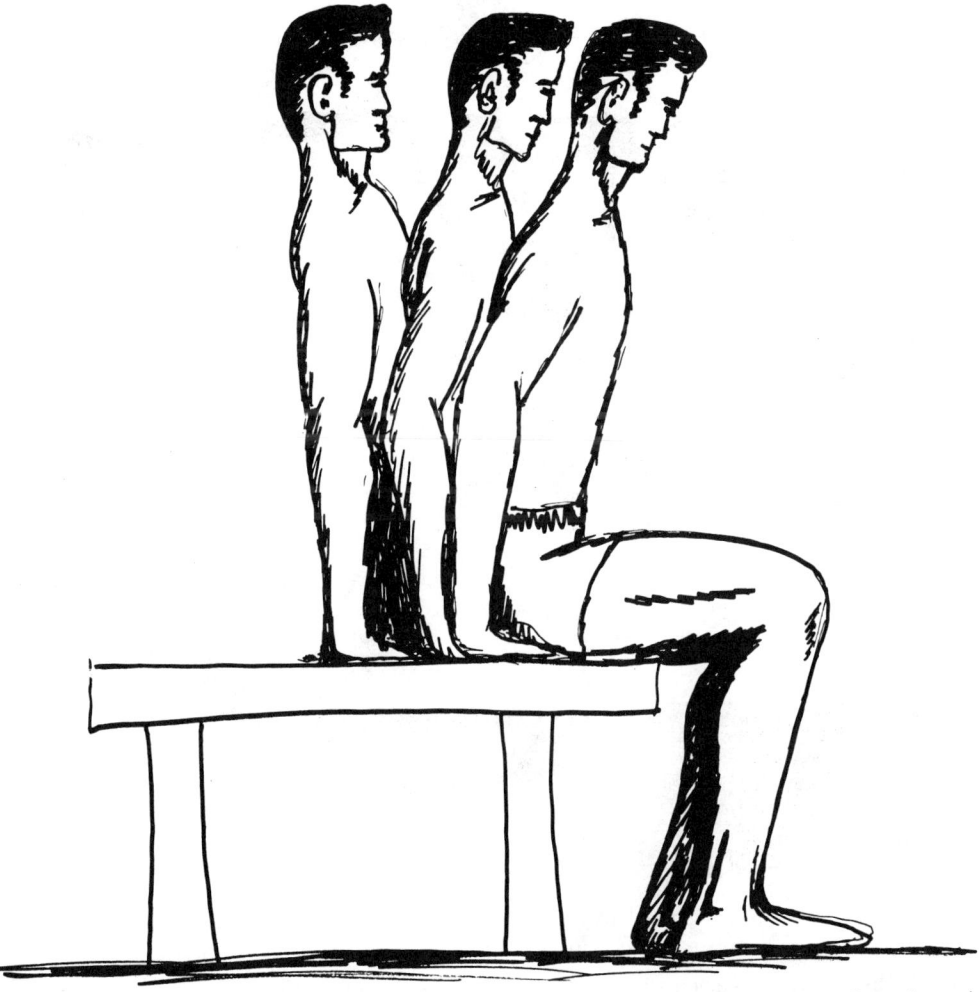

FIGURE 18-3. Forward weight-shift in seated position. Can the seated patient flex sufficiently at the hips and slide forward to place weight evenly on both feet in preparation for moving from the seated to the standing position?

THE STANDING POSITION

In the upright position, the assessment of balance is of utmost importance. The balance reactions are tested while standing by shifting the person from side to side. Observations of the limbs are made to determine if they move appropriately and symmetrically from one side to the other. It is particularly noteworthy to determine if lateral flexion of the head and trunk occurs. Attention should be directed toward the movement of the pelvis and shoulder to see whether or not the person is capable of depressing the shoulder and elevating the pelvis.

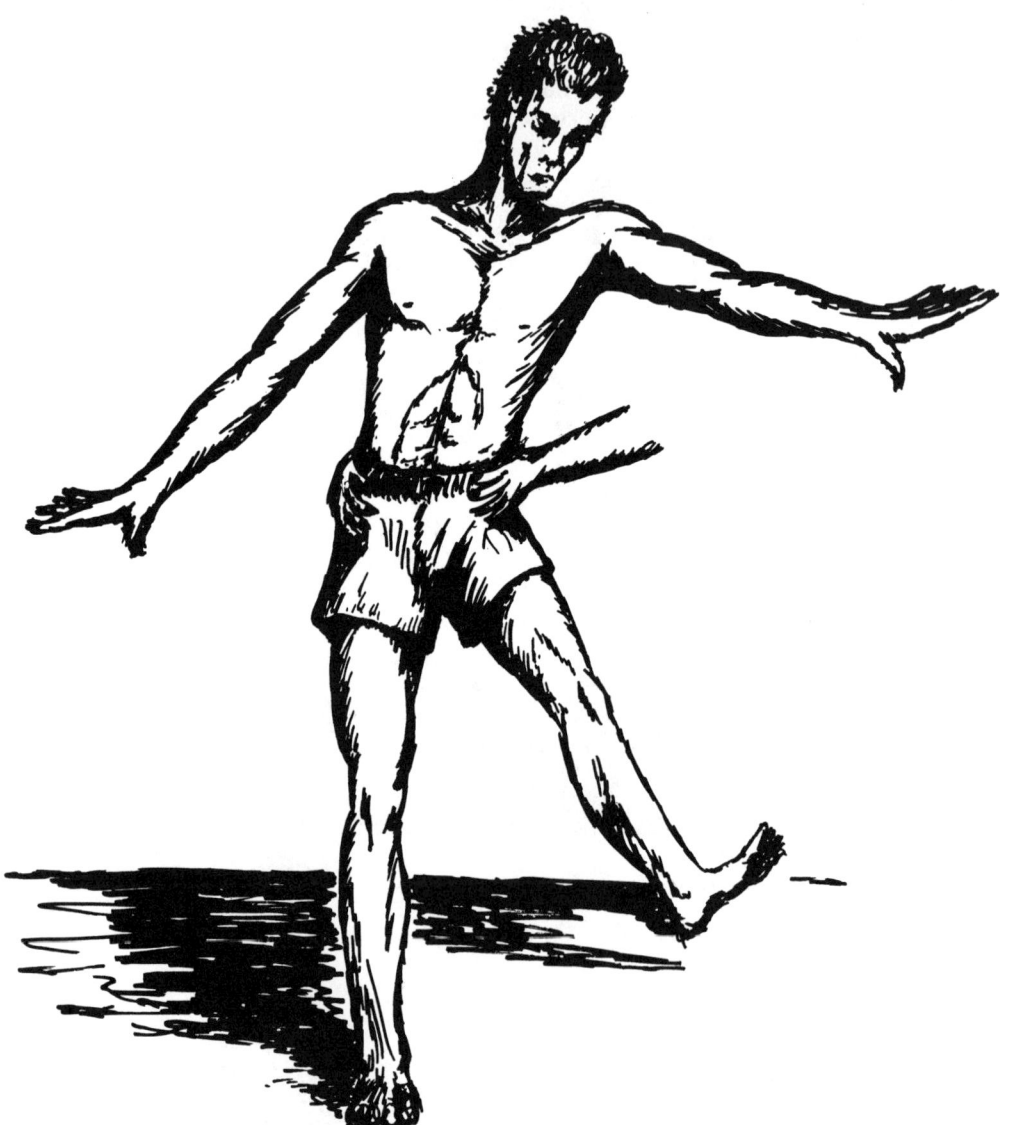

FIGURE 18-4. Balance reactions in standing position. During upright stance, the patient is suddenly shifted from side to side, and the adjustments of the limbs are observed. A normal response of upper and lower limbs is illustrated; however, a head-injured patient may make inappropriate adjustments by narrowing the base of support.

These are important components of lateral flexion. The presence of abnormal movements and/or increases in tone should be noted during the movements laterally as well. After side-to-side equilibrium responses, oblique, forward, and backward shifts may be performed to observe for rotational and lateral movements of the pelvis and thorax. These movements are crucial as precursors to locomotor behavior (Fig. 18-4).

AUTOMATIC BEHAVIORS

LOCOMOTION (FORWARD)

The first aspect for assessment of locomotion would be to determine the mechanism used by the patient in initiating locomotion. As Cooke and Cousins have identified, forward locomotion is initiated by a reduction in tension of the calf muscles; therefore, it would be looked for in the patient as an indication of normal initiation of locomotion. One would not direct the patient as to which foot to start with, but certainly this would be noted in recording the initiation of locomotion. Locomotion may be scored by the test devised and modified by Nelson. It provides for a relative score or ratios of performance.[4]

FUNCTIONAL AMBULATION SCORE

The Functional Ambulation Score (FAS) is shown in Figure 18-5. The ambulation test is conducted over a smooth surface with a recording mat or carbon paper on which the patient walks. The distance used has been 10 ft (approximately 3 m). The patient is instructed to walk at the preferred rate, neither rapidly nor slowly, but at a comfortable, customary rate of speed. The equipment necessary for the test includes a stopwatch or timing device that records in tenths of a second, a steel ruler or tape measure, and some means of producing marks on the floor from the feet or a type of substance that will produce a change that can be recorded for footfalls. The Krusen gait mat is an excellent device for this purpose. An automated microprocessor ambulation scoring device, under development by Nelson and Tucker, will employ footswitches for contact and release of the foot from the surface. Gait analysis can be performed by conventional methods, and may be augmented by audiovisual recordings and feedback or by photography for further analysis. (For further discussion of gait analysis using the FAS, refer to Nelson.[4])

ASSESSMENT OF HAND FUNCTION

While hand function may take many forms, the intent of this section is to limit discussion to the major forms of grasp and release. The test is conducted by having the patient sit at a table in a chair that is the appropriate height for the patient. Distractions should be minimal, and the patient's position should be as symmetric as possible. The therapist should note how the hands are when in the resting state. Are any tremors or coarse movements present without commands to move?

The most commonly employed form of grasp appears to be that of palmar prehensile grasp between the thumb and the second and third fingers. This would be evaluated first by the use of either a pinch meter or simply a qualitative assessment of the movement pattern. As essential feature of that grasp is to determine whether or not the individual can release or inhibit the grasp response. The inhibition of the grasp response should be differentiated from the active release of the grasp. Inhibition of the grasp is simply the relaxation of the flexor muscles involved, while the active release is the active extension of the muscles opposing the

FUNCTIONAL AMBULATION
PERFORMANCE SCORE

Name _____

Location _____

Age _____ Sex _____

Disability _____

Left Leg Length (cm) _____)   Gr. Troch. to Floor
Right Leg Length (cm) _____)   Below the Lateral Malleolus

Instructions: Subject to walk at preferred rate a distance of 3 meters, two times. The average is then taken for data to be recorded below.

FUNCTIONAL AMBULATION DATA	Test no. 1 Date	Test no. 2 Date	Test no. 3 Date	Test no. 4 Date	Test no. 5 Date	Test no. 6 Date	Test no. 7 Date
Three meter test Number of steps							
Time (for 3 meters— in seconds)							
Velocity (cm/sec)							
Cadence (Steps per min) No. of steps per sec X 60							
Left step length (cm) (Left heel to right heel)							
Right step length (cm) (Right heel to left heel)							
Difference: Larger/Smaller (cm)							
Ratio: Left step/leg length							
Ratio: Right step/leg length							
Time: Left step time (sec) (R step length ÷ velocity)							
Time: Left step time (sec) (R step length ÷ velocity)							
Subtract amount taken Table No. 1							
Subtract: Step/ext vs time (left) Table No. 2							
Subtract: Step/ext vs time (right) Table No. 2							
AMBULATION PERFORMANCE SCORE							

Deduct additional five (5) points for any of the following (put total in adjusted score)
SUPPLEMENTAL INFORMATION: Indicate orthotics, devices, or assistance below

Orthoses/Prothesis							
Walking Aid (Cane, crutches, parallel bars)							
Personal assistance – dependent							
Requires guarding*							
Adjusted ambulation score							

*Requires verbal guidance but no physical contact.   Copyright: Nelson, A. J. & Tucker, J.

FIGURE 18-5. Functional ambulation performance score.

flexors. Ability to inhibit grasp is a higher-level function than an opposing action such as extension of the fingers. Should the patient have difficulty releasing the grasp, this should be noted and the degree of difficulty in releasing things should be indicated.

A whole range of objects may be used for the testing of grasp so that the range of type of grasp might be assessed such as radial and ulnar grasp, pincer grasp, and whole-hand grasp. It is important, however, to determine whether the grasp is sufficient to carry on many of the usual activities of daily living. When this is determined, items such as a glass, a pen or pencil, toothbrush, and other similar objects may be used to determine the degree of functional grasp that may be present. The grasp and release should also be tested in a variety of postures of the arm, for example, with forearm pronated and supinated, and with the elbow flexed and extended. The purpose of the latter would be to determine whether there is some indication of relative independence of action from mass synergy patterns. Other quantitative tests of hand function may be used, such as those described by Jebsen and coworkers[6] and Chyatte and Birdsong.[7]

RECORDING OF MOTOR BEHAVIOR

The patient's movements may be recorded in a standardized fashion by the use of home movie film or in a more professional manner with 16-mm film. Other options include use of a tape recording with a video player and recorder, and still more elaborately, one might employ a three-dimensional film analysis technique. For clinical purposes, it seems appropriate to use some videotaping of characteristic movements in postures that can be accomplished in a relatively short period of time with a minimum of equipment. One approach has been the use of a single video camera to record the patient performing some characteristic movements in the supine, seated, and standing positions as previously described. Included in the filming is some measurement of distance and time so that movement may be analyzed at a future time.

DYNAMOMETRY

A clinical dynamometer known as the Cybex II Isokinetic Dynamometer is available. The Cybex II Dynamometer is an instrument that is capable of keeping the velocity of a limb segment moving at a constant rate, while the resistance offered by the limb is developed as a result of the individual attempting to exceed the speed that is set by the unit. The device is an electromechanical and hydraulic system that works on a servo-driven, electrical motor gear reduction mechanism, which serves to convert any speed in excess of the one set on the unit into resistance offered through the gear reduction system of the device. Hence, the resistance that is produced is known as an accommodating resistance (Fig. 18-6).

The speed settings can vary from 0 degrees per second velocity to 300 degrees per second in a continuous fashion. The range in torque that may be created will be from 0 to 448 Newton meters. An illustration of the device is provided as it would be set for determining shoulder flexion and extension. Other movements are possible, ranging from a wide variation in the upper extremity to movements of the lower extremity, including inversion and rotatory movements. A sample tracing is provided in Figure 18-7.

The Cybex makes possible a recording of torque derived from the flexors and from the extensors in a reciprocating fashion, as well as a range-of-motion indicator that describes the arc through which the segment is moving. By calculating from the beginning of the movement to the attainment of its peak output, one could develop the rate at which tension is being developed. The latter rate of tension development is somewhat masked or distorted by the

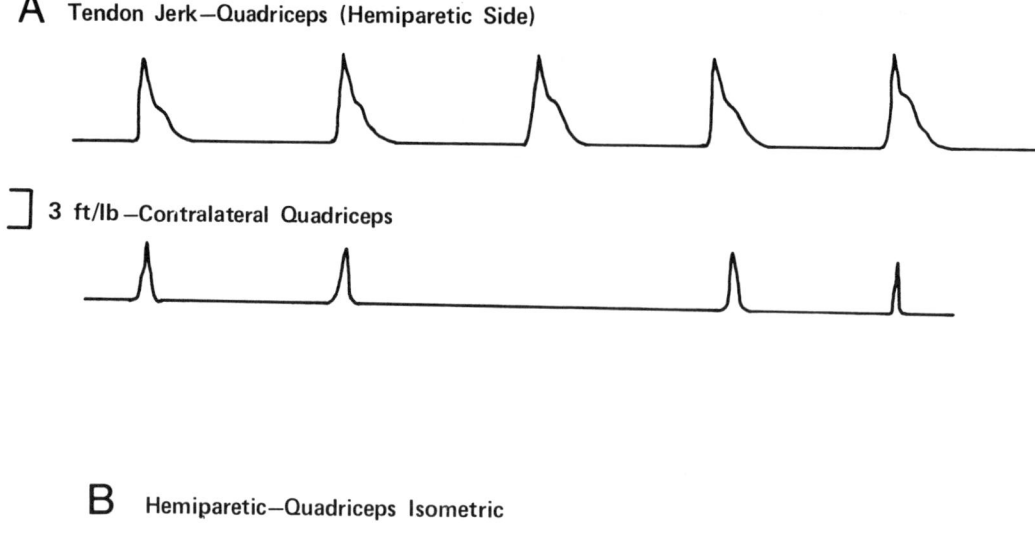
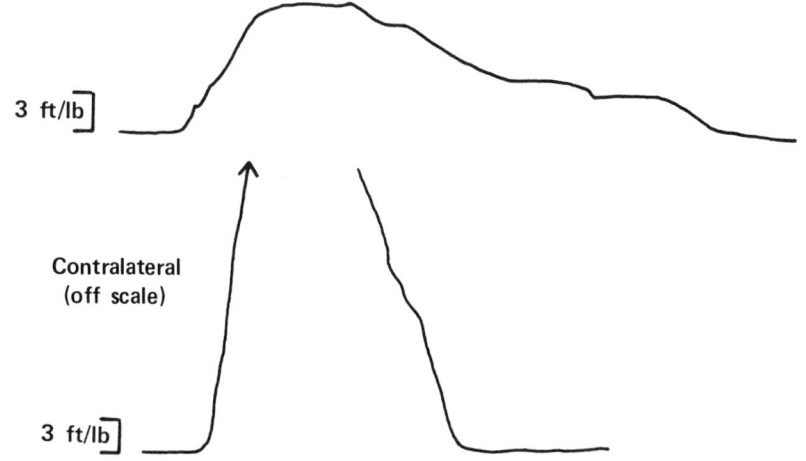

FIGURE 18-6. Isokinetic dynamometer recordings of a head-injured hemiparetic. (A) Tracing of patellar tendon jerk response on each limb illustrates the increased amplitude and prolongation of the response of the paretic side, as contrasted with that of the unaffected side. (B) Tracing of the isometric tension developed by the paretic side as opposed to that of the opposite quadriceps shows that the greater tension of the unaffected limb develops at a much further rate than the tension of the involved side.

hydraulic mechanism within the system. However, it may give a relative indication of quickness of movement.

Similarly, because the range of motion is indicated, one can determine at what point in the range of movement a particular force is being developed, so that one might determine what is known as specific strength or the specific torque that is developed in a given point in the range of movement (Fig. 18-8).

Another measure that can be determined from these tracings when comparing the plegic extremity with the contralateral extremity is the ratio of one muscle group to another. That of the hamstrings to quadriceps is normally a two to three output. In the hemiparetic patient, one can observe that the hamstrings' output is roughly one third to one fourth the output of

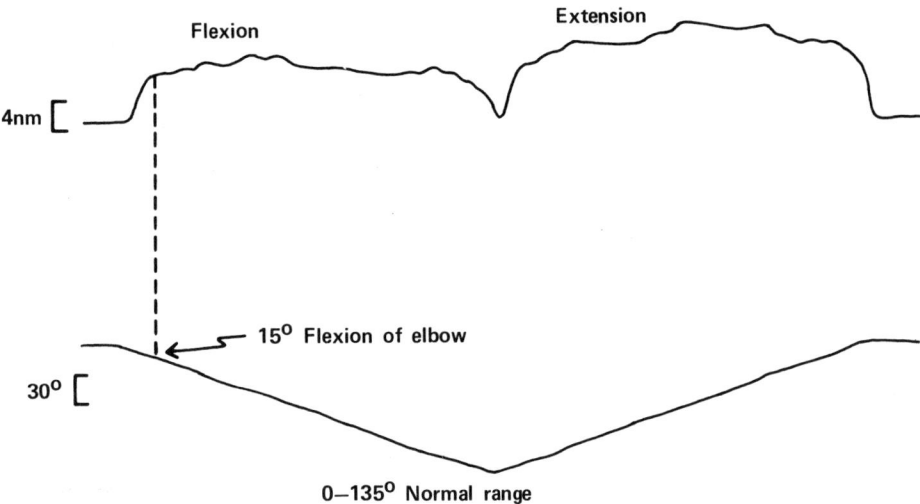

FIGURE 18-7. Hemiparetic performing elbow flexion and extension. Arrow on range-of-motion tracing indicates a 3-Nm torque at 15 degrees of flexion. Specific strength may be determined at any given point in the motion. The torque was recorded by the Cybex II isokinetic dynamometer.

the quadriceps. Furthermore, there appears to be very poor ability to determine the contraction of one muscle group before the other muscle group takes over so that reciprocal activation is poorly processed by the patient. An additional measurement of control of force output may be rendered by simply asking the patient to contract to the same level in a series of pulls at any given speed. To determine that the contractions came to the same level, a target zone would be placed on the recorder, and the patient would observe where that target was and try to meet that consistently throughout the tracing (Fig. 18-8). Another method would require

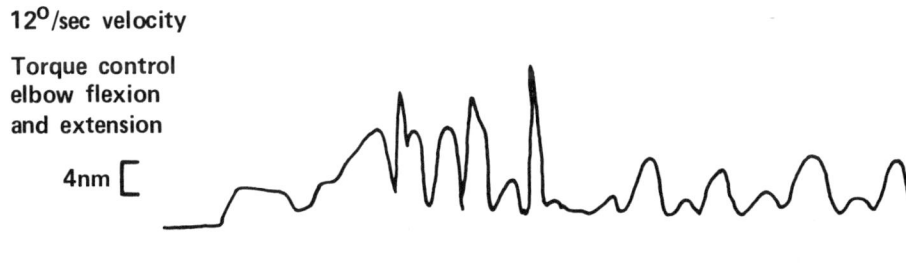

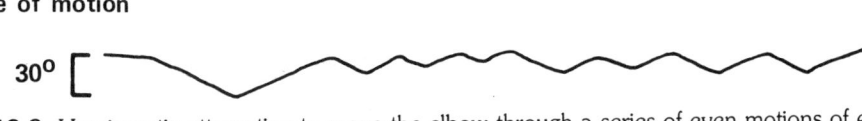

FIGURE 18-8. Hemiparetic attempting to move the elbow through a series of even motions of equal torque. Note the uneven performance initially, followed by more regular movements of elbow flexion and extension at isokinetic velocity of 12 degrees per second.

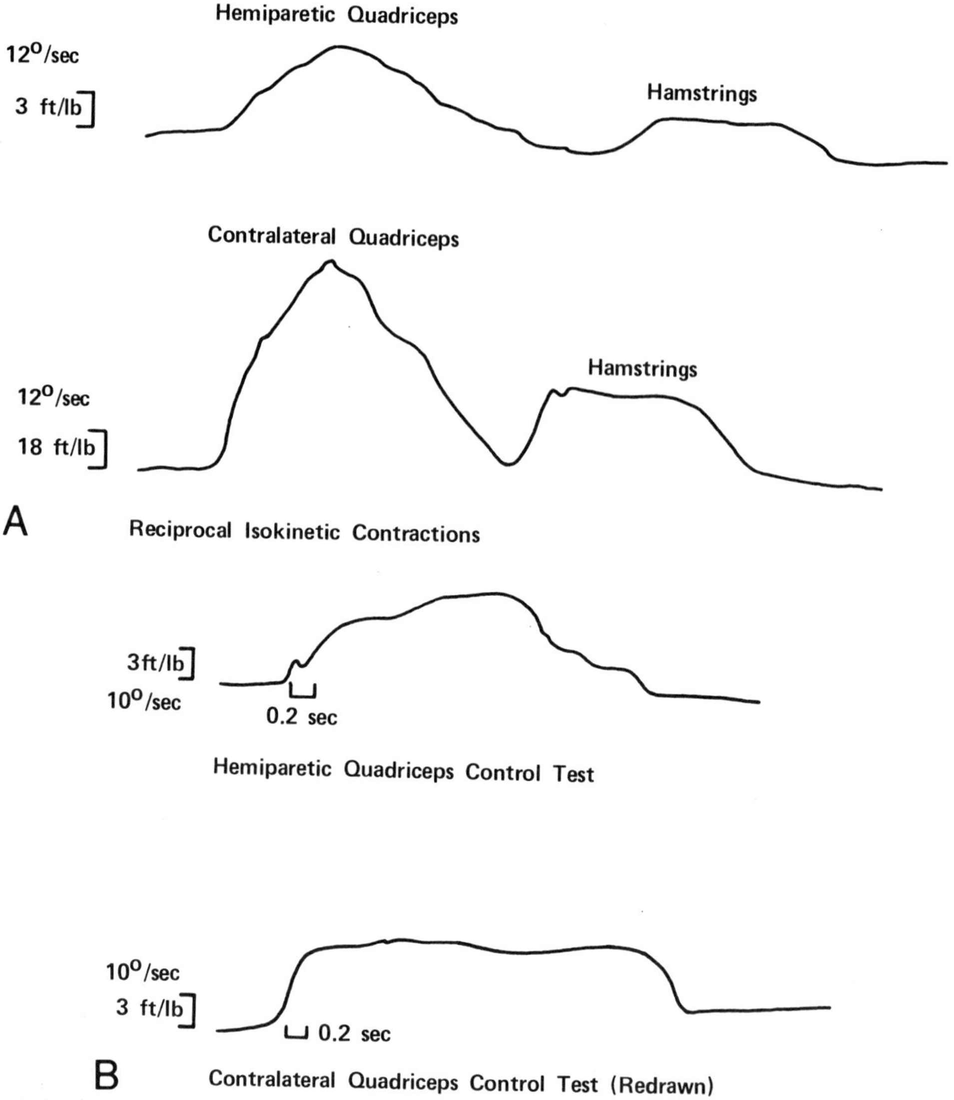

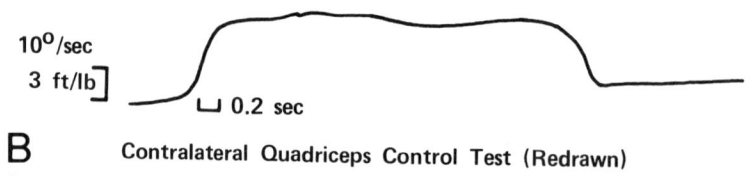

FIGURE 18-9. Isokinetic (Cybex II) Dynamometer recordings of a head-injured man with left hemiparesis. (A) Illustration of reciprocal isokinetic torque production of quadriceps and hamstrings of the involved and uninvolved limbs. On the involved side, there is a loss of torque development with prolongation of relaxation, resulting in poor reciprocation that is disproportionately below the expected 2:3 ratio of normal hamstring-quadriceps torque productions. (B) Illustration of the attempts of the patient to draw a rectangular pattern with the recording pen of the isokinetic dynamometer set at a 10 degrees per second velocity. It is evident that the paretic quadriceps is incapable of providing a smooth, continuous line.

the patient to trace a horizontal line or a box-like configuration and to see how level the patient can maintain this. The amount of deviation provides an indication of the degree that a hemiparetic patient during the acute phase of recovery moved when attempting to maintain this horizontal line. It is clear that this line was not maintained by the patient, while the contralateral extremity did considerably better (Fig. 18-9).

Finally, by taking a series of velocities, the force-velocity relationship may be plotted to determine how adequate the person's force development is at any given velocity. Quite typically, the patient with a cerebrovascular accident lesion has difficulty developing sufficient force even at slow velocities, but this becomes progressively more apparent as the velocities increase. It is quite common for patients to be unable to develop tension at velocities above 70 or 80 degrees per second. This assumes added significance when one considers that movements like locomotion require a movement of the shank on the knee at a minimum speed of 100 degrees per second when walking at average rates of locomotion. These data may be compiled and reported in several different ways or may even be reduced and printed directly through a microcomputer, which may process the signal in a series of torque productions automatically.

VALIDITY AND RELIABILITY OF THE DYNAMOMETER

The calibration and face validity of the instrument may be established by hanging known weights on the end of the dynamometer and recording the torque that is developed on the device.

It may be noted that although the relationship is a linear one, the torques at the lower speeds tend to record at a higher level, whereas the torques at the higher speeds for the same weight will be recorded at a lower level. This would suggest that as a patient improves and can move to the higher speed level, the recording at higher speed is not as recognizable or tends to be somewhat masked by this mechanism. Furthermore, it is important to underscore the changes in recordings that occur as a result of providing different damping settings on the dynamometer. The optimal damping settings appear to be either 0 or 1, and the others tend to lose a good deal of information, especially at the higher velocities of testing.

The measurements recorded with this instrument have a high degree of reliability. However, the dynamometer does provide a permanent record of the person and an individual may indeed be compared against himself or herself for performance change.

As was suggested in previous discussion of testing of motor power, either individual segments may be tested or whole limb components may be evaluated. For instance, the elbow flexors and extensors may be isolated so that motion of one may position the patient in such a fashion that the patient may engage in a flexion and extension synergy to produce a movement pattern. Similarly, the leg may be engaged in a total hip, knee, and ankle flexion and extension movement, or it may involve a simple ankle flexion and extension movement, or it may involve a simple ankle dorsiflexion and plantarflexion. This provides one with the opportunity of comparing the magnitude and intensity of one type of movement over the other, if such a difference exists. Some recordings taken from patients and normal subjects have been included for review.

The major problem of data reduction is a considerable one unless one seeks to automate the procedures with microprocessors or minicomputers. In this instance, one would then look at the rate of tension development, the ability of the individual to let that tension disappear rapidly, the ability to start the opposite muscle group action quickly, and the appropriateness or balance between the two muscle groups, as well as whether the individual can control torque production to a given level and maintain that consistently through a reasonable series of actions.

SUMMARY AND CONCLUSIONS

The evaluation of central nervous system motor deficits may involve the use of objective dynamometer determination with scales of performance, such as the functional ambulation performance score, and other indices of functional performance, such as timing one's performance of standard activities of daily living. Or it may simply be a subjective observational analysis of the quality of movement that may be subsequently studied more definitively through filming and analysis of those films on a frame-to-frame basis.

From a clinical standpoint, it seems evident that limitation in clinical resources would warrant the development of tests that can be conducted with a minimum of equipment and instrumentation. The assessment of motor behavior should provide insight into substitutions or behavioral "tricks," as well as an indication of the relative ease with which the movement is accomplished and whether it is accompanied by other deviations from those normally encountered.

There should be some clear indication as to whether the overall pattern was primitive or more advanced. Also, an assessment of tone should be determined at a variety of intervals and circumstances during the testing procedures. Most of the impact of primitive reflexes may be identified through the rating scale described, and the relative dominance of those movements may be seen to relate to other performance tests. Thus, the assessment must take into account the reflex basis, the turning responses of the neck and labyrinthine systems, the imposition of the more dynamic righting responses, and finally, the ability to engage in equilibrium reactions.

All of these categories are incorporated in the process we refer to as willed acts, or voluntary movement. Many of these voluntary acts, including ambulation, are quite automatic. The functional ambulation performance score is a useful tool to assess the general level of performance of subjects while also accumulating specific data that may be referred to for future comparisons.

REFERENCES

1. JENNETT, B AND TEASDALE, G: *Management of Head Injuries.* FA Davis, Philadelphia, 1981.
2. LANDAU, WM: *The upper motor neuron syndrome.* In ELIASSON, SG, PRENSKY, AL, AND HARDIN, WB (EDS): *Neurological Pathophysiology.* Oxford University Press, London, 1974.
3. CAPUTE, AJ, ET AL: *Primitive Reflex Profile; Monographs in Developmental Pediatrics.* University Park Press, Baltimore, 1978.
4. NELSON, AJ: *The functional ambulation profile.* Physical Therapy 54(10):1059, 1974.
5. DEJONG, RN: *The Neurological Examination,* ed 4. Harper & Row, New York, 1979.
6. JEBSEN, RH, ET AL: *An objective and standardized test of hand function.* Arch Phys Med Rehabil 50:311, 1969.
7. CHYATTE, SB AND BIRDSONG, JH: *Methods-time measurement in the assessment of motor performance.* Arch Phys Med Rehabil 53:38, 1972.

APPENDIX 1. MOTOR BEHAVIOR INVENTORY

INSTRUCTIONS FOR ASSESSMENT AND RATING OF MOTOR BEHAVIOR

The measurement of deep tendon jerk responses may be derived through use of a tendon hammer or the tips of the third and fourth fingers but should be consistently performed with standard postures described in the text.

When moving the limb for determination of passive resistance, efforts should be toward even, steady lengthening to avoid accelerations. The exaggerated and sustained classifications exhibit increasing resistance as the elongation progresses with the sudden release of tension determining the sustained (4) rating. Testing for clonus should, however, involve an acceleration of the stretch to the calf muscles.

Stimulation of the plantar surface of the foot should be performed with a blunt instrument, with the stroke moving from the lateral border of the heel to the lateral metatarsal area and thence across the foot to the base of the great toe.

The Hoffman response is determined by "flicking" the nail bed of the third finger and observing if the thumb and forefinger flex following the stroke.

Distinguishing between the primitive grasp and true grasp involves the response to a distal moving stimulus in the former and pressure in the palmar area in the latter. If the grasp cannot be released, it is rated as sustained (4).

Primitive responses such as the flexor withdrawal, extensor thrust, and crossed extension reflexes are most readily tested in the supine position with consistent stimuli as described in the text. Each response is tested five (5) times and rated on the basis of at least three of the five trials. Sufficient time (30 seconds) should be permitted for the response to be manifested. Whenever possible, the stimulus (i.e., neck rotation) should be provided through active motion, but it should be equal in effort and range of motion from one side to the other.

Righting responses are stimulated with relatively rapid movements of the patient's head and neck or legs and pelvis, or by tipping the person from side to side, or by shifting a vertically oriented frame in front of the patient, or by sudden release of the head from an elevated position. As these are "triggered" by the stimulus, the response is expected to be in proportion to it. It is virtually impossible to delimit responses to one particular stimulus, and only an estimation of the response may be made.

Balance reactions to a shifting surface are most readily determined by using a surface that permits shifting or tilting in the supine, sitting, and standing positions. The three levels of weight shifting, weight bearing, and then protective response involve progressively increased degrees of shift. Ratings are made as designated in the key, and procedures are described in the text.

The testing of voluntary movement is intended only to provide a crude assessment of selected movements that represent difficult motions for those with CNS lesion. The quality of the motion is distinguished by its relative independence from mass action (stereotyped pattern). All motions are repeated five (5) times, and successful completion of three out of five is used as the basis for the rating.

A summary score may be determined by adding each component. The higher the score, the more primitive or deficient is the motor behavior of the patient.

CHART A.   Motor Behavior Inventory

Pt. Name: _____ Location: _____

I.D. No. or S.S. No.: _____ Age: _____ Sex: _____ Diagnosis: _____

_____ Complications: _____

INSTRUCTIONS: ALL RESPONSES ARE RECORDED AS THE AVERAGE OF FIVE (5) TRIALS; STANDARDIZED POSTURES AND ENVIRONMENT ARE USED; THE STIMULI ARE APPLIED CONSISTENTLY.

REFLEX KEY: 0—Normal; 1—Decreased; 2—Absent; 3—Exaggerated; 4—Sustained

I. REFLEXES	No. 1 Date:		No. 2 Date:		No. 3 Date:		No. 4 Date:		No. 5 Date:		No. 6 Date:	
	R	L	R	L	R	L	R	L	R	L	R	L
A. Deep Tendon Jerk												
Ankle (PF)												
Knee (Bx)												
Elbow (FL)												
Elbow (Ex)												
Wrist (FL)												
DTR Summary Score:												
B. Passive Resistance Stretch												
Ankle (PF)												
Knee (Ext)												
Elbow (FL)												
Elbow (Ext)												
Wrist (FL)												
Passive Resistance Summary Score:												
C. Clonus Ankle (PF)												
Wrist (FL)												
Clonus Summary Score:												
D. Plantar Stimulation												
(Babinski) Plantar (FL)												
Extensor												
Babinski Summary Score:												
E. Hoffman Response												
(Hand and Fingers)												
F. Grasp Response												
Traction												
Primitive												
True												
Grasp Response Summary Score:												
Reflex Summary Score:												

MOTOR ASSESSMENT

CHART B. Motor Behavior Inventory

Pt. Name: _____ Location: _____

I.D. No. or S.S. No.: _____ Age: _____ Sex: _____ Diagnosis: _____

_____ Complications: _____

INSTRUCTIONS: ALL RESPONSES ARE RECORDED AS THE AVERAGE OF FIVE (5) TRIALS: STANDARDIZED POSTURES AND ENVIRONMENT ARE USED; THE STIMULI ARE APPLIED CONSISTENTLY.

KEY: 0—Absent; 1—Tone change in extremity; 2—Visible movement of extremity; 3—Full movement of extremities; 4—Obligatory and sustained movement

II. PRIMITIVE RESPONSES	No. 1 Date:		No. 2 Date:		No. 3 Date:		No. 4 Date:		No. 5 Date:		No. 6 Date:	
A. Spinal	R	L	R	L	R	L	R	L	R	L	R	L
Flexor withdrawal												
Extensor thrust												
Crossed extension												
Spinal Summary Score:												
B. Tuning Responses (Brain Stem)												
Asymmetric tonic neck R/L												
Symmetric tonic neck VF/DF												
Asymmetric tonic labyrinthine R/L												
Symmetric tonic labyrinthine												
Associated arm												
Leg												
Tuning Response Summary Score:												

III. RIGHTING RESPONSES

KEY: 0—Present with complete motion; 1—Moves with incomplete motion; 2—Moves with inconsistent mass pattern; 3—Moves always with mass pattern

A. Derotational												
Neck on trunk												
Legs on trunk												
B. Labyrinthine												
Sitting (side to side)												
Sitting (forward and back)												
D. Moro												
Sitting (side to side)												
Sitting (forward and back)												
C. Optical												
Sudden extension of head												
Righting Responses Summary Score:												

CHART C.   Motor Behavior Inventory

Pt. Name: _____ Location: _____

I.D. No. or S.S. No.: _____ Age: _____ Sex: _____ Diagnosis: _____

_____ Complications: _____

IV. BALANCE REACTIONS

KEY: 0—Present with all components; 1—Pattern lacking some component; 2—Pattern lacking all components; 3—Patterns opposite to normal

	No. 1 Date:	No. 2 Date:	No. 3 Date:	No. 4 Date:	No. 5 Date:	No. 6 Date:
A. Prone on Forearms						
Weight transfer (side to side) _____						
Weight bearing _____						
Protective response						
Prone Summary:						
B. Sitting (feet unsupported)						
Weight transfer (side to side) _____						
Weight bearing _____						
Protective response						
Sitting Summary:						
C. Standing (feet parallel)						
Weight transfer _____						
Weight bearing _____						
Protective response						
D. Standing on Left Leg						
Protective response						
E. Standing on Right Leg						
Protective response						
Standing Summary:						
Balance Reaction Summary Score:						

MOTOR ASSESSMENT 265

CHART D.   Motor Behavior Inventory

Pt. Name: _____ Location: _____

I.D. No. or S.S. No.: _____ Age: _____ Sex: _____ Diagnosis: _____
_____ Complications: _____

V. VOLUNTARY MOVEMENTS

KEY: 0—Present with all components; 1—Present with insufficient motion or speed; 2—Present with partial mass patterns (synergy); 3—Present only in mass pattern (synergy); 4—No movement possible

	R	L	R	L	R	L	R	L	R	L	R	L
A. Supine Position												
1. Hip extension with knee flexion _____												
2. Ankle dorsiflexion with knee extended _____												
3. Knee flexion with hip extended _____												
4. Hold extended arm in elevated position when placed there _____												
5. Flexion of elbow _____												
6. Extension of elbow _____												
7. Flexion of wrist _____												
8. Flex and extended wrist _____												
9. Supination of forearm (elbow flexed at 90°) _____												
10. Pronation of forearm (elbow flexed at 90°) _____												
11. Rolling to left side _____												
12. Rolling to right side _____												
B. Sitting Position												
1. Abduct arm to side (with elbow extended) _____												
2. Supinate forearm (elbow flexed trunk fixed) _____												
3. Pronate forearm (without adduction) _____												
4. Externally rotate (extended arm) _____												
5. Flex elbow and touch shoulder same side _____												
6. Extend elbow (return from same shoulder) _____												
7. Flex elbow to opposite shoulder _____												
8. Extend (or return) to original position _____												
9. Extend wrist with fingers flexed _____												
10. Extend wrist with fingers extended _____												
11. Perform palmar prehension _____												
C. Standing Position												
1. Stand on both legs (30 sec) _____												
2. Stand on left leg (30 sec) _____												
3. Stand on right leg (30 sec) _____												
4. Alternating stepping in place (record seconds for 8 steps or 4 cycles) _____												
5. Stand on left leg and lift toes _____												
6. Stand on right leg and lift toes _____												
Voluntary Summary Score:												
Total Motor Inventory Summary Score:												

APPENDIX 2. SENSORY INVENTORY

INSTRUCTIONS FOR SENSORY INVENTORY

All questions asked of patients presume ability to comprehend speech; if the patient cannot, an asterisk should indicate gestures or other forms of communication used (notation on bottom of form). The testing is done with patient in supine position (or seated, which is noted) in a quiet, uncluttered area.

Background data are mainly observationally determined or derived from simple questioning. Cues or prodding is prohibited, and the procedure should be standardized.

Joint motion is determined passively on patient by the therapist as a gross estimation using a goniometer for compilation of the average estimation of percentage from normal that is lost.

Muscle flexibility is assessed by passively lengthening the muscle groups noted and rating them as (a) partially restricted if the terminal 10% to 20% of motion can be completed, only with stretching; (b) moderately restricted if the terminal motion (10%–20%) cannot be completed even with stretching; (c) contracture when fixed muscular (not joint primarily) restriction does not give way to passive stretching or inhibition.

Somatic sensation is rated according to the key with the patient in a seated position (or supine if necessary). Whenever possible, the patient should point to the stimulus as well as verbalize its location and quality. Difficulty with communication should be noted, and the best estimate made of the patient's response. See text for specific test directions.

MOTOR ASSESSMENT

CHART A. Sensory Inventory

Pt. Name: _____ Location: _____

Age: _____ Sex: _____ Diagnosis: _____

I. BACKGROUND INFORMATION	No. 1 Date:	No. 2 Date:	No. 3 Date:	No. 4 Date:	No. 5 Date:	No. 6 Date:
A. Consciousness Level						
Key: 0—alert						
1—lethargic						
2—somnolent						
3—stuporous						
4—comatose						
B. Affective Level						
Key: 0—cooperative						
1—indifferent						
2—anxious						
3—agitated						
4—hostile						
C. Orientation Level						
Key: 0—yes; 1—partially;						
2—disoriented						
TIME: _____						
PLACE: _____						
PERSON:						
D. Memory Level						
Key: 0—present/complete						
1—partial/concrete						
2—partial/abstract						
3—absent for all						
RECENT: _____						
REMOTE:						
E. Calculation Level						
Key: 0—correct; 1—partial;						
2—incorrect						
HOW MANY QUARTERS IN A DOLLAR?						
HOW MANY NICKELS IN A QUARTER?						

F. Joint Range of Motion		R	L	R	L	R	L	R	L	R	L	R	L
	1. Neck (% loss) _____												
Rating	2. Shoulder (% loss) _____												
0 = Zero	3. Elbow (% loss) _____												
2 = 5-25%	4. Wrist (% loss) _____												
3 = 25-50%	5. Fingers (% loss) _____												
4 = 50-100%	6. Hip (% loss) _____												
	7. Knee (% loss) _____												
	8. Ankle (% loss)												
G. Muscle Flexibility													
0—Flexible	1. Hamstrings _____												
1—Partial loss	2. Adductors _____												
2—Moderate loss	3. Calf _____												
3—Contracture	4. Flexors of arm _____												
	5. Wrist and finger flexors												

CHART B.   Sensory Inventory

Pt. Name: _____ Location: _____

Age: _____ Sex: _____ Diagnosis: _____

Key: 0—Intact; 1—Poor localization; 2—Long latency; 3—Absent

II. SOMATIC SENSATIONS	No. 1 Test:		No. 2 Test:		No. 3 Test:		No. 4 Test:		No. 5 Test:		No. 6 Test:	
	R	L	R	L	R	L	R	L	R	L	R	L
A. Touch												
Face _____												
Neck _____												
Upper arm _____												
Forearm _____												
Hand _____												
Thigh _____												
Calf _____												
Foot _____												
Touch: Summary Score												
B. Pain												
Face _____												
Neck _____												
Upper arm _____												
Forearm _____												
Hand _____												
Thigh _____												
Calf _____												
Foot _____												
Pain: Summary Score												
C. Joint Position												
Shoulder _____												
Elbow _____												
Wrist _____												
Fingers _____												
Hips _____												
Knee _____												
Ankle _____												
Toes _____												
Joint Position: Summary Score												
D. Cortical Integration												
Key: 0—present; 1—partial/displaces; 2—absent												
1. Stereognosis _____												
2. Graphesthesia _____												
3. Tactile; simultaneous _____												
4. Two-point discrimination _____												
5. Gnosis for fingers _____												
6. Figure-ground discrimination _____												
7. Praxis: Ideational _____												
Ideomotor _____												
Limb-kinetic _____												
8. Right-left orientation _____												
9. Body schema (illustrate) _____												
Cortical Integration: Summary Score												
OVERALL SENSORY SCORE:												

MOTOR ASSESSMENT

CHART C.   Sensory Inventory

E. Other: Narrative Summary

Test no. 1, date: _____
_____

Test no. 2, date: _____
_____

Test no. 3, date: _____
_____

Test no. 4, date: _____
_____

Test no. 5, date: _____
_____

Test no. 6, date: _____
_____

Chapter 19

OCCUPATIONAL THERAPY EVALUATION

Paula E. Wahlstrom, O.T.R.

Assessing the patient with a head injury requires the modification of traditional evaluation techniques. The patient's level of cognition often limits the ability to cooperate with evaluation requests and may prevent an initial interview with the patient to gather accurate background information. An adequate assessment includes a thorough chart review, followed by multiple short evaluation sessions. Before the evaluation is begun, a general assessment of the patient's cognitive abilities must be made. The environment and evaluation can then be structured to support the best performance according to the cognitive level. Careful observation and ingenuity in evoking the response appropriate to that aspect of the assessment makes the head-injury evaluation a challenge.

The occupational therapy evaluation presented in this chapter is useful for assessing patients who are past the acute stage of head injury. They may still have nasogastric tubes in place, catheters, and/or gastrostomies, and may be at a low cognitive level. The primary purpose of the evaluation is to assess the influence of physical, perceptual, or cognitive impairments on the patient's ability to perform purposeful or functional tasks. Modifications of commonly used evaluation techniques that are effective with severely cognitively impaired patients will be discussed.

REVIEW OF MEDICAL HISTORY

The review of the medical chart can provide information regarding the extent of injury. Prognosis and goal setting can be determined by other findings. Since the head-injured patient is often an unreliable historian, information regarding premorbid psychosocial history should also be gathered from the chart or family members, or both.

Factors to note include the patient's age, length of time since onset of injury, duration of the comatose state if applicable, and the patient's score on the Glasgow Coma Scale.[1] The duration of coma and the coma scale score combined with other factors are used as predictors of recovery in many facilities. For example, the young patient who is relatively close to onset of injury and who is noted to have had a brief duration of coma and a high score on the coma scale is predicted to have a fairly successful rehabilitation outcome.

Etiology of injury and injury site are equally important in attempting to determine prognosis of the patient. Blunt versus penetrating blows to the head or multiple sites of injury that may produce concomitant involvement must be considered. For example, a patient may fall from a ladder, landing on head and shoulder. Impact to the head produces brain injury, and torsion to the neck may produce brachial plexus injury. Frontal lobe involvement produces different behaviors than does parietal lobe injury.

If the patient has a history of early decerebrate or decorticate posturing, the therapist should be alerted to the possibility of joint-range limitations. Range-of-motion limitations can also be caused by fractures, which can cause peripheral nerve damage. Typically involved are the ulnar and peroneal nerves.

Medications should be noted, since antiseizure drugs, tranquilizers, and so forth can produce extreme lethargy in many patients.

Previous therapy assessments should be reviewed, as they can provide a basis for comparison with the patient's current status. Finally, if possible, the extent of family involvement with the patient should be determined so that early discharge planning can be initiated.

GENERAL EVALUATION PROCEDURES

Observation of the patient is the next step in the evaluation. The examiner should observe the patient at rest without stimulation from staff intervention. The position of the patient lying quietly in bed can provide clues to location of areas of the body with increased muscle tone, that is, neck flexed to either side, extremities held in extremes of flexion or extension, or trunk laterally flexed. Any motion that the patient initiates spontaneously should be noted; if possible, an attempt should be made to determine if the motion observed is selective or synergistic in quality.[2] Observation may be the only means available to the therapist to determine approximate muscle strength with a patient who is in a very agitated state. Such patients are frequently unable to cooperate with standard muscle testing, but observation of functional performances reveals their ability to use available motor control.

The next step in the evaluation is to determine the patient's ability to orient to time and place. It is not uncommon for a patient to be unable to tell the examiner the name of the hospital or the day of the week. In that case, the therapist can give the patient this information at the beginning of a short session and ask the patient to repeat it at the end. This method can be used to grossly determine immediate recall or short-term memory. It is also important to determine the patient's ability to follow one-step or multi-step commands. The instruction should be kept simple and related to body parts, for example, "open your eyes, raise your arm off the bed, or take my hand." Observe for general decrease in awareness, agitation, or brevity of attention span. This information will allow the therapist to structure the remaining evaluation procedure and choose the environment that supports the patient's most appropriate responses.

Generally, minimally responsive patients require a nondistracting setting where the therapist can stimulate and arouse the patient using firm commands and tactile input. The agitated patient requires an evaluation setting that does not increase agitation. It may be necessary to seek out the least distracting environment for each patient prior to continuing the evaluation. The therapist's manner should be calm and soothing, and all commands brief and concrete. The length of treatment sessions for both of these patient groups should be brief, possibly 10 to 15 minutes, several times per day. As the cognitive level rises, less modification and structure of the evaluation process and setting are required. Patients at a higher cognitive level may need only performance checks of self-care abilities at the appropriate times of day and in the appropriate environment, that is, dressing evaluations in the morning when they awaken, followed by feeding evaluations at the ensuing breakfast meal.

MOTOR CONTROL

Assessment of motor control is the next step in the evaluation. Passive range of motion, muscle tone and strength, sensation, and motor planning will be discussed as components of motor control, since smooth, coordinated motions are dependent on these factors.

RANGE OF MOTION

If the physical examination is started with the range-of-motion measurement, the therapist has an opportunity to observe the patient's reaction to passive movement, to get a general feel for the patient's muscle tone, and to get an objective measure of motion available at each joint. The range may be limited by soft tissue contracture or muscle fiber shortening secondary to increased tone. Another reason for reduced range of motion may be heterotopic ossification. Diagnosis of this problem may require serial bone scans, alkaline phosphatase determinations, x-ray studies, or temporary nerve blocks to reduce the effects of spasticity.[3] Painful reactions to range of motion should alert the therapist to the possibilities of occult fractures. Frequently, however, patients are more sensitive to tactile stimulation and tend to overreact to ranging. Once x-ray studies have assured the absence of fractures or dislocations, the therapist must help the patient "work through" this pain.

The therapist may require assistance from another person when evaluating the agitated patient's passive upper extremity motion to prevent interference with the measurement.

MUSCLE TONE

The most common finding during this assessment is the presence of increased muscle tone. Muscle tone is most efficiently tested by applying a quick stretch to a muscle or muscle group to see if an exaggerated stretch response is elicited. It is unusual to find a head-injured patient with decreased muscle tone. If this condition is discovered, a lower motor neuron lesion should be suspected. That complication will be discussed later in this chapter. The usual finding is spasticity or rigidity in muscle groups such as flexors of the upper extremity or antagonistic muscle groups. This patient group frequently lacks the ability to relax the extremities, so that frequently the standard quick-stretch evaluation techniques cannot be used. Under these circumstances, the therapist may have to resort to observation of general body posture or any available voluntary motion, as previously discussed, to identify areas of increased tone. In either case, the differences in muscle tone with the patient in the supine, prone, and sitting positions should be noted, as well as any changes at different times of day or during periods of wakefulness or sleep. These variations in tone have implications for treatment. For example, the limb with variable tone that can be easily ranged to its maximum limit may be managed by vigorous daily range of motion, whereas the limb with spasticity that prevents full ranging may benefit from a serial casting program.[3] (See Chapter 9 for further information on spasticity.)

MUSCLE STRENGTH

Identification of selective muscle control must be completed before manual muscle testing can be initiated. This technique of grading muscle strength is not appropriate for use on a muscle that is working in synergy. For the patient who is unable to consistently follow instructions, observation is the therapist's best tool. Note any spontaneous motion for selectivity and ability to move against gravity. The agitated patient may not be able to consistently respond to commands, but observation of an extremely agitated patient destroying casts or mattresses indicates good to normal muscle strength. The confused patient responds best to concrete commands such as "comb your hair," and "wash your face." Again, the therapist must observe for apparent muscle strength.

SENSATION

The validity of a specific sensory evaluation depends on establishing a consistent form of communication with the person to be tested. For this reason, patients at a very low cognitive level are frequently only grossly evaluated for their response to pain stimuli. This is really more of an indication of their cognition rather than their sensation, but it is a relevant test in that it requires a certain amount of cognition to put higher-level sensory systems to use.

The confused patient often becomes agitated by attempts to complete the entire sensory examination at one time. The examination can be divided and presented to the patient in several sessions. Generally, attending skills are inadequate for testing responses to sharp-dull discrimination, two-point discrimination, and stereognosis in the standard manner.

Patients who are confused, but not agitated, can be successfully tested for sensory responses if instructions are very simple and concrete. The common areas tested are position sense, sharp-dull discrimination, and light touch. The test for two-point discrimination correlates with return of hand function after a peripheral nerve injury. This test has not been found to be as reliable with head-injured patients because of their inability to attend to the test.[4]

Test of stereognosis is a controversial issue as some feel that verbal identification of an object with vision occluded is a skill that is too language/cognitive-oriented to be a pure sensory-motor test. At the Rehabilitation Institute of Chicago, a test consisting of the presentation of unfamiliar objects is being developed.[5] The patient responds by pointing to a choice of objects on a card that pictures all the objects presented. This test eliminates the preverbal and memory components of the more commonly used familiar object stereognosis test.

PERCEPTUAL-MOTOR

Indications of sensory-motor deficits can be noted by observing the patient's voluntary motions and approach to functional tasks. In order for these skills to be smooth, coordinated, and functional, the patient must receive adequate input from all sensory systems. The input from all systems must be integrated at the brain stem and at higher levels.[6] Many head-injured patients have primary cortical injuries or secondary brain stem damage, resulting from edema, that interfere with sensory integration. During specific testing procedures, note ability to cross the midline of the body, and tendency to avoid a visual field or neglect an extremity or entire body half. The areas that will be discussed for specific testing are visual perception, somatosensory functions, perception of form and space, and motor functions.

VISUAL AWARENESS

Visual field deficits are common in this patient group. The low-level patient can be tested by noting responses of eye movements to threat of a rapidly approaching therapist's hand toward the periphery of either eye. A normal response would be a rapid eye blink. Although the normal response may be slowed in the low-level patient, complete absence of a response indicates visual field dysfunction. The patient's ability to track an object vertically and horizontally in all visual fields should be noted. In order to get a low-level patient to track, a photograph of a loved one or pet may be used. A frequent complaint of the awakening patient

OCCUPATIONAL THERAPY EVALUATION

is double vision, and the therapist should have eye patches on hand to treat this problem. As the patient progresses in recovery, the patient usually learns to compensate for the double vision so that it remains a limiting factor only for close hand work and driving.

Cortical blindness may be caused by direct insult to the occipital cortex or, more frequently, by arterial compression to the vessels serving this area. The quality of the ensuing ischemia can determine the prognosis for the patient's vision. Ischemia of sudden onset produces irreversible damage. Gradual ischemia, possibly associated with secondary brain edema, does not lead to tissue destruction; therefore, the visual function can return after days, weeks, or months.

Recovery occurs in the fields of vision whose representative cortical areas are nearest to functioning blood vessels. For example, in basilar artery insufficiency, the occipital poles suffer least as they can receive some blood from the middle cerebral arteries. In this case, blindness may reverse, with central vision returning first.[7] Clinically, this problem should be suspected in patients with intact optic nerves who complain of blindness. It may not be complete blindness but instead may be limited to parts of the visual fields.

Evaluation of vision should proceed over a period of time, with the examiner being alert to changes in visual acuity that indicate improvement.

If the patient is cognitively able to learn new tasks, some training in self-care techniques for the visually impaired may be used. The patient who is confused rarely benefits from this training and needs considerable assistance in functional activities.

SOMATOSENSORY FUNCTIONS

Awareness of light touch, stereognosis, executing anticipatory motor acts, and initiating motor acts are all somatosensory functions.[8,9] The identification of body parts and knowledge of their relationship to each other and the position of the body in space can be affected by deficits in this area. Right-left discrimination and the perception of double simultaneous tactile stimuli may also be impaired.

In the low-level patient, observe abnormal or inappropriate responses to tactile input. Notice if the patient displays tactile defensiveness or increased restlessness from tactile input. This may be the only evaluation of this system possible with the patient who is unable to cooperate with paper-and-pencil tests or who is unable to consistently follow commands.

Body image (Draw-A-Person) tests, puzzles of people, and the simultaneous presentation of two tactile stimuli can be administered to the highest-level patient. Observe the patient in familiar activities such as "catch." Frequently, people with deficits in this area are unable to produce the "postural set" to prepare to catch a ball until it almost strikes them. They may also have difficulty with functional activities such as preparing to perform a transfer from bed to wheelchair or assuming the appropriate position to dress themselves.

FORM AND SPACE

Form and space perception includes the ability to recognize consistencies in shapes and colors, body image, and ability to move the body through space and perceive objects against a background.[4] Also included are the abilities to perceive the position of objects in space and in relationship to each other. These perceptual skills underlie self-care tasks such as dressing, feeding, and hygiene-grooming.

Design copying, spatial relations, and figure-ground evaluations (Ayers or Frostig) can be used to assess the higher-level patient. More concrete tasks such as solving simple puzzles, copying block designs, and shape and color form-sorting activities can be used with the low-level patient. Further indication of abilities or deficits in this area can be obtained through observation of minimal self-care skills. Notice if the patient has difficulty selecting toiletries from a cluttered drawer, choosing the requested color of garments, and putting clothes on correctly.

MOTOR PLANNING

The patient's ability to properly initiate, sequence, and complete motor acts can be assessed by asking the patient to imitate postures or touch the therapist's finger at different points in space. Reciprocal motions can also be used to assess difficulties in motor planning in this patient group, as patients typically initiate motions by first co-contracting antagonistic muscle groups. Instruct the patient to flex and extend the elbow as rapidly as possible. Gestures can be used to help eliminate difficulties created by any language disorders. Performance as a result of verbal or manual assistance is an indication of a probable deficit in the area of motor planning.

ACTIVITIES OF DAILY LIVING (ADL)

This cluster of skills can be divided into self-care, home, and community skills. The patient's ability to perform in these areas can be limited by deficits in any or all of the previously discussed areas. The therapist must determine if inability to perform these tasks is secondary to cognitive, physical, or perceptual dysfunction or a combination of all three. Treatment approaches will vary according to the reasons for performance problems.

SELF-CARE SKILLS

Self-care skills are those personal care tasks such as feeding, dressing, hygiene, grooming, bed mobility, transfers, bathing, toileting, handwriting, and telephone use. The minimally responsive patient is dependent in all these activities, but performance can be still challenged by presenting pre-"self-care" tasks such as handing patients a wet washcloth, a foam tooth cleaner, or a comb and brush in an attempt to elicit purposeful activity. Goals for treatment can be established based on responses to these items.

An early morning self-care program works well for evaluating the confused patient. More than one evaluation session is needed to compensate for inconsistent behaviors. Evaluating the patient on the unit in the early morning allows the patient to see others preparing for the day and helps to eliminate some disorientation for the patient. A complete self-care regimen can be instituted that can be carried over into treatment.

HOME SKILLS

Home skills include bed making, clothing organization, laundry, meal preparation, and housework. Assessment of these skills is not accomplished immediately with the low-level patient. If the patient does not surpass the physically assisted level in performance of self-care skills, it is not practical to proceed with further ADL evaluation. However, patients at a higher cognitive and physical level may be evaluated for home skills immediately after a self-care program is established and implemented. Ability to organize materials and methodic approaches to tasks are observed during activities such as bed making or folding laundry.

Kitchen experiences should not be delayed until the patient is ready for discharge. Experience in some rehabilitation programs has shown that even confused patients, if their behavior is appropriate, can benefit from minimal kitchen exposure early in the treatment process. All the home activities can be graded for the patient's level by increasing or decreasing complexity over a period of time. The factors most limiting to performance are impaired cognition and ataxic motor disturbances.

COMMUNITY SKILLS

Community skills include shopping; eating out; managing street crossings, lights, and curbs; driving; and vocational skills. A prerequisite performance of "verbally assisted" should be reached before a community evaluation is considered. If the patient cannot attain this level owing to cognitive impairment, the patient will not perform in the community.

Like home skills assessment, evaluation of community skills should occur early enough in the program to allow ample training prior to discharge. The extent of the community skills evaluation and training program for any given patient depends on the ultimate discharge setting.

Driving and vocational assessments are frequently instituted after discharge. The driving program at Rancho Los Amigos Hospital requires that patients be seizure-free on controlled medication for 1 year postinjury before referral for driving assessment. Judgment, memory, and visual problems are the factors that most often limit successful driving.[10] Patients can be taught to drive with adapted equipment even with severe, nonataxic motor problems.

Prevocational assessment is indicated, as many head-injured patients are young and have not held regular jobs. The therapist can contribute such information as ability to keep appointments and organize work materials, approach tasks, standing tolerance, and a general clinical picture of the patient in the vocational counselor's evaluation.

GOAL SETTING

In setting goals, the examiner must realize that the physical findings constitute only part of the equation that adds up to a final discharge plan. The interplay of cognition and motor control is the important consideration in predicting a patient's functional status. Recovery of cognition and motor control may not be parallel. Prognosis for recovery of cognition will influence how the patient is ultimately able to use available motor control to compensate for sensory or motor deficits.

A patient who is minimally responsive will be limited by a short attention span and ability to concentrate on tasks. This will preclude functional use of available motor control. The individual who is confused, with or without agitation, will be unable to spontaneously compensate or learn to compensate for deficiencies in sensory motor systems. The patient lacks judgment and requires assistance with functional activities for safety. The patient who is demonstrating appropriate behavior but has decreased money management and problem-solving skills is able to learn to compensate in overlearned activities (self-care) through much repetition but will not have carryover for new situations. This patient will require supervision (verbal cueing) for activities of daily living. Very minimal cognitive problems with memory or problem-solving may not interfere with the patient's ability to learn to compensate for motor or sensory deficits, but the patient may require supervision for activities in the home and community.

SUMMARY

The evaluation process includes the chart review, careful observation of patient behavior, modification of evaluation techniques, and structuring of the environment. Goal setting must take into account all available information that will assist the therapist in determining the patient's final discharge placement.

Observation, as an evaluation tool, is necessary when assessing all patients. With the head-injured patient, it is invaluable. The patient's decreased cognitive functioning may make it impossible to use traditional evaluation techniques. Observation of the patient's behaviors provides a basis for the modification of these procedures to gather the most accurate information. Along with modifying the evaluation techniques, structuring the environment to support the patient's best response increases the amount of information that can be gathered during the assessment. Modifying the environment includes choosing the time of day, the length of the evaluation session, and people present, as well as avoiding background distractions.

When setting treatment goals, the therapist must be aware of all available information. A thorough chart review is in order to gather data on medical status, premorbid social functioning, and family involvement. This information, in addition to current assessments by the rehabilitation team, provides the basis for determining functional goals that lead to the final discharge placement goal.

REFERENCES

1. JENNETT, B, ET AL: *Prognosis of patients with severe head injury.* Neurosurgery 4(4), 1979.
2. BOBATH, B: *Adult Hemiplegia: Evaluation and Treatment.* William Heinemann, London, 1970.
3. GARLAND, DE, BOOTH, BJ, AND DOYLE, M: *Early Management of Spasticity.* Presented at the conference of the Rehabilitation of the Head Injured Adult: Comprehensive Physical Management, Professional Staff Association of Rancho Los Amigos Hospital, Downey, Calif, 1979.
4. GARLAND, EE AND WATERS, R: *Orthopedic evaluation in hemiplegic stroke.* Orthop Clin North Am 9:291, 1978.
5. CHAPPARO, C AND RANKA, J: *Application of sensory integrative treatment principles to adult hemiplegics.* Presented at AOTA Conference, 1980.
6. AYERS, AJ: *Sensory Integration and Learning Disorders.* Western Psychological Services, California, 1972.
7. LENDENBERG, R, WALSH, F, AND SACKS, J: *Neuropathology of Vision.* Lea & Febiger, Philadelphia, 1973, p 460.
8. KORNHUBERS, HH (ED): *The Somatosensory System,* ed 3. Publishing Sciences Group, 1975.
9. WALL, PD: *The sensory and motor role of impulses traveling in the dorsal columns toward the cerebral cortex.* Brain 93:505, 1970.
10. LANGRAN, S: *Handbook for the Establishment of a Driving Program for the Physically Handicapped.* Occupational Therapy Department, Rancho Los Amigos Hospital, Downey, Calif, 1975.

Chapter 20

SPEECH AND LANGUAGE ASSESSMENT

Robert M. Smith, M.Ed.

The speech and language assessment of any head-injured patient involves the review of pertinent medical and biographical information, formation of a speech and language diagnosis, and determination of the prognosis for speech and language improvement. This assessment should include an analysis of motor speech ability, receptive and expressive language skills, cognitive ability, and the patient's physical and psychologic recovery processes. A comprehensive assessment is needed because many head injuries cause a multiplicity of problems.

This chapter will discuss assessment of speech and language problems and how the head-injured patient's cognitive problems affect this assessment. It will also include a discussion of the natural recovery process and the prediction of recovery from severe head injury. These factors greatly influence the speech and language assessment as well as the subsequent therapeutic program.

ASSESSMENT OF LANGUAGE AND COGNITIVE FUNCTION

Assessment of head-injured adults is often a challenge. Dysfunction of language and cognitive skills may cause considerable difficulty in formal testing. At times, formal testing will have to be delayed until cognitive behavior improves.

Assessment of language and cognitive skills should provide information to the head-trauma team as to how well the patient is able to process language and whether a problem is due to a specific neurologic lesion or generalized cerebral dysfunction. The cognitive assessment will include tests of attention, memory, and thought processing. The language assessment also involves these skills but includes the higher cognitive processes of reading, writing, and speaking.

COGNITIVE EVALUATION

Cognitive functions are usually diminished by head injury regardless of the site of lesion.[1] These functions include the ability to remember learned material, process thought, translate thought into verbal behavior, and control verbal behavior through an intact feedback system. Therefore, reduction of cognitive function will be directly reflected in reduction of speech and language skills.

The cognitive aspect of the speech and language evaluation should include tests of attention, memory, and thought processing. Although these aspects of cognition theoretically can be treated differently, in practice they are difficult to separate. These cognitive skills may be evaluated with such standardized tests as Digit Span, Wechsler Memory Scale, Rey Auditory-Verbal Learning Test, and the Peabody Individual Achievement Test.

The Digit Span is a test for assessing attention and immediate auditory memory. The Digit Span subtest on the Wechsler Adult Intelligence Scale is probably the most widely known standardized version of this test.[2] A series of digits is presented in increasing number to the patient to repeat orally. One series is presented, followed by another series for the patient to repeat in reverse order. An adult should be able to repeat six digits forward and five in reverse order.

The Wechsler Memory Scale[3] is a widely used test that surveys memory and short-term learning. This scale includes seven areas that relate to memory: (1) personal and current information, (2) orientation, (3) mental control, (4) logical memory, (5) digit memory, (6) visual memory, and (7) learning of associated word pairs.

The Rey Auditory-Verbal Learning Test evaluates immediate memory span, provides a learning curve, and elicits retroactive and proactive interference tendencies, as well as tendencies to word confusion or confabulation on memory tasks.[4] This test consists of six oral presentations of a list of 15 words with a seventh recall trial. (See Chapter 13 for further discussion of memory).

The Peabody Individual Achievement Test (PIAT)[5] can be useful tool for evaluating general knowledge and thought processing. There are five subtests in the battery: mathematics, reading recognition, reading comprehension, spelling, and general information. The reading comprehension subtest is, in essence, a word association test that is especially vulnerable to problems in thought processing, immediate memory, and difficulty with flexibility of thinking.

Another way of evaluating cognitive function is by use of a functional performance scale. The Rancho Los Amigos Scale[6] is a hierarchic behavior scale that systematically describes and categorizes the patient's level of function. The levels of cognitive function as described by the Head Trauma Service of the Rancho Los Amigos Hospital are:

1. No response
2. Generalized response to stimulation
3. Localized response to stimuli
4. Confused and agitated behavior
5. Confused with inappropriate behavior (nonagitated)
6. Confused but appropriate behavior
7. Automatic and appropriate behavior
8. Purposeful and appropriate behavior

The patient's behavior is compared with this scale to determine what level of cognitive function the patient is exhibiting. Those who are functioning at a *confused level* or lower can be expected to exhibit confused language behavior because of generalized cerebral dysfunction. Those patients exhibiting appropriate behavior on the scale should not exhibit language dysfunction purely because of cognitive difficulty. Therapy for aphasic and dysarthric conditions may be provided for patients at a *confused but appropriate behavior* level or higher, whereas those functioning at a lower level will benefit most from cognitive retraining. Cognitive retraining is needed as a prerequisite to many speech and language therapeutic procedures.

Additional testing of such cognitive skills as conceptual flexibility and nonverbal reasoning may be indicated for some patients. Tests such as the Proverbs Test[7] and the Raven's Progressive Matrices Test[8] may be used to evaluate these skills. Other tests of cognitive ability, including tests of intellectual ability, are discussed in psychologic texts.[9,10]

LANGUAGE EVALUATION

Some patients with head trauma will have language problems caused by specific lesions to language centers in the brain rather than generalized cognitive dysfunction. In most cases, the language problems found will be due to a combination of specific lesion and cognitive dysfunction. In a differential assessment of a patient, the cause should be determined so that proper treatment can be provided.

The evaluation of language skills may be accomplished with a comprehensive aphasia battery or a group of formal and informal tests. To provide a comprehensive assessment of aphasia, a test battery should be used that will evaluate all modalities of language, and one that is broad enough to be used with patients with a wide range of difficulty. There are a number of comprehensive test batteries available for the evaluation of aphasia. These include the Boston Diagnostic Aphasia Examination,[11] Minnesota Test of Differential Diagnosis of Aphasia,[12] Porch Index of Communicative Abilities,[13] and the Neurosensory Center Comprehensive Examination of Aphasia.[14]

Many tests of aphasia are only diagnostic in nature and are not useful for prognosis or planning a comprehensive therapeutic program.[15] Only the Porch Index of Communicative Ability has a numerically based prognostic scale. All test authors discuss therapeutic programming, but most do not provide a program based on the test results.

Prognosis for improvement of language skills can be made when the aphasic patient is given a comprehensive evaluation with a test built on a linguistic hierarchy such as those developed by Porch and Schuell. The prognosis is based on the difference between the linguistic level at which the patient can perform normally (diagnostic level) and the maximum level at which the patient can perform inconsistently. The reliability of this prediction will vary depending on the etiology and time after insult.[16-18]

Head-injured patients frequently exhibit aphasia during the early stages of recovery. This aphasia is usually due to cognitive dysfunction rather than to a specific neurologic lesion in one of the language centers. When the problem is due to cognitive dysfunction, it should be labeled "transient" aphasia, because the language skills improve as the patient's cognitive abilities improve. Aphasia test batteries can be used with such patients only to obtain a baseline of linguistic function. Improvement from "transient" aphasia comes about as part of the natural recovery and is due to improved brain function.

At times, an aphasia test battery is not appropriate for assessing language skills of head-injured patients. Other tests are available that can be used to evaluate various aspects of language. A comprehensive assessment will include tests of auditory reception, visual reception, graphic expression, and oral expressive skills. Severe head trauma often results in reduction in all of these modalities.

Auditory Receptive Evaluation

The ability to perceive, process, retain, and use auditory information is vital to human communication. The aphasia batteries mentioned above evaluate these abilities in some detail. Additional auditory receptive evaluative tools include the Token Test[19] and the Peabody Picture Vocabulary Test.[20]

At some time during the course of recovery, an audiometric assessment should be provided. This includes the evaluation of hearing acuity for both speech and pure tones, as well as a test of auditory discrimination of words.

Visual Receptive Evaluation

Head injury may result in a number of visual problems, including visual field deficits, dyslexia, reduced reading level, and reduced reading comprehension. Several aspects of reading should be evaluated, including word recognition, word comprehension, sentence comprehension, paragraph comprehension, and reading rate. The following tests can be used to evaluate these reading skills: Wide Range Achievement Test,[21] Gray Oral Reading Test,[22] Woodcock Reading Mastery Test,[23] and the Gates-MacGinitie Reading Test.[24]

Included in the visual receptive evaluation should be an evaluation of the patient's visual field and general visual acuity.

Graphic Expressive Skill Evaluation

Writing is the most complex of the linguistic skills.[16] Writing requires high-level perceptual ability, motor control, understanding of spatial relationships, and linguistic processing ability. Graphic expressive tests include tasks of copying, word writing, sentence construction, paragraph construction, use of syntax, spelling, and writing fluency.

Copying tasks should include items such as geometric shapes, letters of the alphabet, and printed words. Word writing and spelling can be evaluated with a test such as the Wide Range Achievement Test.[21]

Writing fluency can be evaluated with the Thurstone Primary Mental Abilities Test.[25] On this test, the subject is instructed to write as many words beginning with the letter "S" as the subject can in 5 minutes, followed by writing as many four-letter words beginning with "C" as the subject can in 4 minutes. The average 18-year-old can produce 64 words within the 9-minute total time period.

Writing skills of sequential organization, syntax, punctuation, and graphomotor ability can be evaluated by asking the patient to write a paragraph. The Picture Story Language Test[26] is an example of this type of evaluation.

Verbal Expression Evaluation

Evaluation of verbal expressive skills may include many formal and informal tests. Aspects of speech evaluated should include fluency, rate, repeating abilities, naming abilities, vocal quality, articulation, syntax, and logical expressive thinking.

After head injury, many patients experience changes in the speed and fluency of verbal production. Impaired verbal fluency is often associated with a frontal lobe lesion.[27] The Word Naming subtest on the Stanford Binet test is an example of an evaluation of word fluency.[28] The subject is required to say as many words as possible in 1 minute, but not in a sentence or number series. On Form L-M, a 10-year-old should be able to produce a minimum of 28 words. A similar test is the Controlled Word Association Test, which consists of three word-naming trials, using the letters F, A, and S, respectively.[29] The subject is directed to name as many words as possible which begin with the given letter, excluding proper nouns and numbers. Norms have been established in relation to age, sex, and education.

Content, grammar, vocal quality, and logical thinking can be evaluated by asking the subject to give biographical information orally. Questions that elicit such responses are "What is your". . . address, age, reason for the evaluation, hobbies, work history, and school history. There are no formal tests for this area of the evaluation, but the experienced evaluator should have an understanding of normal behavior and should keep notes on abnormal aspects of the patient's conversation.

An evaluation of ability to repeat is important to rule out conduction aphasia and gross memory problems. Repeating numbers from 1 to 10 in sequence is one of the simplest verbal tasks. Repetition of monosyllabic words beginning with various phonemes can serve as a test of articulatory ability as well as a test of ability to repeat. Auditory memory can also be evaluated by repeating polysyllabic words, three-word phrases, and sentences. The average adult can repeat sentences of 24 to 25 syllables.[30] Memory for Unrelated Sentences test is a structured test of this type.[31]

ASSESSMENT OF THE NEUROMUSCULAR SPEECH SYSTEM

Head-injured patients frequently have neuromuscular problems that cause difficulty in the motor production of speech. The two major motor speech problems are dysarthria and apraxia of speech.

DYSARTHRIA

Dysarthria can be defined as difficulty in speech production owing to insult to a motor speech nerve tract. Usually the problem is due to insult to the pyramidal or extrapyramidal motor tracts in the central nervous system but may also be due to a peripheral nerve lesion. Such lesions result in compromised speech production affecting respiration, phonation, resonance, articulation, and/or prosody.

Darley[32] has described five types of central dysarthria based on site of lesion and dysfunction of speech: flaccid, spastic, ataxic, hypokinetic, and hyperkinetic. Head-injured patients frequently exhibit a mixed spastic and flaccid dysarthria.

Insult to the brain stem frequently results in reduced function of one or more of the cranial nerves. During the motor speech evaluation, detailed assessment of the motor and sensory aspects of the cranial nerves should be provided. Those nerves involved in speech production are trigeminal, facial, glossopharyngeal, vagus, accessory, and hypoglossal.

The prognosis for complete recovery from dysarthria is often poor. Only if the nervous system returns to normal will the speech return to normal. Therefore, the therapeutic goal for severe dysarthria is usually to improve speech intelligibility rather than to achieve normal speech. Improvement is based on the patient's ability to compensate for impaired neurologic control of the speech musculature.

APRAXIA OF SPEECH

Persons suffering head injury may exhibit apraxia of many kinds as a result of general cerebral dysfunction. Apraxia for any motor activity may be observed, including apraxia of speech and apraxia of oral movements. When the problem is due to transient cognitive dysfunction, the apraxia will dissipate as thinking processes improve. Apraxia of speech due to permanent cortical lesions will require therapeutic intervention for maximum return of speaking skills.

Apraxia of speech is caused by neurologic impairment of articulatory programming. The site of lesion is believed to be in the motor association area of the left hemisphere.[16,17] There is no significant weakness of the oral musculature in the apraxic patient. Even in severe cases, automatic movements for coughing, chewing, and swallowing are performed normally. Only the voluntary oral movements are impaired.

Patients with mild apraxia of speech will exhibit inconsistent articulatory problems or have difficulty pronouncing polysyllabic words. Severely apraxic patients may be completely mute.

MOTOR SPEECH EVALUATION

Evaluation of the neuromuscular speech system includes (1) testing the strength of muscles involved in speaking, (2) testing coordination of muscle groups during speaking and nonspeaking activities, (3) evaluating respiration as the basic aspect of speech production, and (4) evaluating the motor aspects of phonation, resonance, articulation, and prosody of speech. The examiner will listen to the patient's speech, observe the various muscle groups during speech and nonspeech activities, and frequently manipulate the muscles. Results of electromyography and spirometry can be useful in making a diagnosis and prognosis.

One systematic approach to assessing motor speech function is to evaluate the speech systems of respiration, phonation, resonance, articulation, and prosody of speech. Each muscle and muscle group involved in these aspects of speech production should be assessed for strength, movement, and coordination. A determination of the patient's ability to monitor speech as well as the patient's motivation to improve should also be included in the evaluation.

Respiration

Head-injured patients frequently have difficulty coordinating respiration, causing reduced breath support for speech. Any problem in strength, control, or coordination of respiration will cause difficulty in loudness of speech and/or dysfunction in prosody. Respiration is evaluated by observing the patient during conversation and during requests to inhale, hold the breath, prolong vowel sounds, and speak. Lung capacity can be measured on a spirometer or other respiratory volume device.

The vagus nerve innervates much of the musculature involved in breathing. An evaluation of both sensory and motor aspects of this complicated nerve should be made during the motor speech evaluation.

Phonation

Weakness and reduced tone of the laryngeal muscles often result in breathiness and hoarseness. Spasticity of these muscles may result in a strained-strangled voice. Listening to the patient converse and go through a series of word and sentence production requests is a necessary part of the assessment of phonation.

Phonation is controlled by branches of the vagus nerve. When there is dysfunction of the vagus caused by impairment of the brain stem, all motor functions of this nerve should be evaluated.

Resonance

Speech resonance is the result of vibrating air passing up from the lungs, through the pharynx, and out through the nasal cavity and/or the mouth. Flaccidity or spasticity of any muscles in these areas will alter the resonance quality of speech. The facial, glossopharyngeal, vagus, and accessory cranial nerves are involved in control of the musculature in these areas.

A common speech resonance problem in head-injured patients is hypernasality. Patients with lower brain stem trauma may exhibit this problem as a symptom of flaccid dysarthria. Listening to the patient's spontaneous speech should alert the examiner to significant resonance problems. Formal tests of velopharyngeal function and observation of soft palate movement are essential parts of the motor speech evaluation.

Articulation

Articulatory speech impairments are found in most dysarthric patients. Such problems cause reduction of speech intelligibility. Articulation of speech should be evaluated by observing static muscles and movement during conversation. Some problems occur from poor coordination during running speech and not in single word utterances. Soft voice associated with reduced openness of the mouth is common in head injury and should be evaluated.

Oral movements needed for the articulation of speech are dependent on adequate innervation from the trigeminal, facial, glossopharyngeal, and hypoglossal nerves. Motor aspects of these nerves are evaluated by having the patient attempt various activities that mobilize the different parts of the tongue, lips, jaw, face, palate, and throat.

Prosody

Prosody refers to the changes in loudness, pitch, timing of articulation, and pause time that give speech its tonal quality, stress, and rhythm. These features of the patient's speech should be assessed during conversation and during specific speech tasks such as repeating words and sentences and reading orally.

Prosody is the result of the motor activity of speech production. Deficiency of muscular strength or control will be reflected in the prosody of the speech. Incoordination of the various cranial nerves or lack of monitoring one's speech will affect prosody.

The assessment of motor speech problems has been astutely discussed by such researchers as Darley[32] and Johns.[33] Persons desiring detailed procedures should refer to the literature.

NATURAL RECOVERY PROCESS

To understand any disease or physical disability, one must know the natural recovery process of that condition. When this is known, prediction can be made as to future outcome of individual cases. Making a prognosis for improvement of speech and language skills is an integral aspect of the assessment.

Head-injured patients who improve are observed to do so in an orderly way.[34] Coma is usually followed by return of basic psychophysical, motor, psychologic, and social skills. The length of time for a patient to go through this process may vary from 1 to 10 years. Table 20-1 is an outline of the severe head-injury recovery process. Many do not recover completely but plateau at some level in the process.[12]

The length of coma is often indicative of the severity of the head injury.[35] After the patient awakens from coma and starts to interact with the environment, a number of behaviors can be observed. These early manifestations are basic psychophysical skills. They include a period of stupor followed by regaining ability to nod the head (indicating understanding), swallowing, and then speaking words aloud. The speed at which the patient passes through

Table 20-1. Outline of the Recovery Process From Severe Head Injury

Early Recovery Skills (basic vegetative abilities)
1. Stupor
2. Nod head for understanding
3. Swallow
4. Speak words aloud

Motor Skills
1. Feed self
2. Perform manual tasks
3. Sitting balance
4. Standing
5. Transfer by self from chair to bed
6. Walking
7. Independent activities of daily living
8. Bimanual coordination

Psychologic Skills
1. Attention span
2. Memory
3. Cognitive skills
4. Emotional stability

Social-Economic Skills
1. Social and family competency
2. Vocational and financial security

these early stages is indicative of the brain's ability to function and may be used as an indicator of future recovery from the head trauma.[36]

The recovery of these basic psychophysical skills is followed by the recovery of higher-level motor skills. These include self-feeding, performing manual tasks, maintaining balance for sitting in a chair, standing without the support of another person, transferring from a wheelchair to another seat independently, walking independently with or without an appliance, performing activities of daily living independently, and finally, performing rapid bimanual activities. Depending on the severity and location of the cerebral damage, a few or all of these motor tasks may be achieved. Patients with severe motor lesions may not be able to perform the higher-level motor skills.

Throughout the period of recovery of basic physical skills, psychologic skills improve. The return of psychologic skills can be observed in a hierarchic pattern. The first level is the recovery of attending skills. These include an awareness of the environment, and achievement of an adequate auditory and visual attention span.

The next psychologic skill that can be evaluated is memory. Short-term and long-term memory skills may take months to return to normal limits. Residual deficits may always remain for some patients. Visual, auditory, and verbal memory skills should be evaluated during this phase of the recovery process.

Cognitive dysfunction is the most obvious and difficult problem to overcome for most head-injured patients. Cognitive skills include ability to retain, analyze, compare, integrate, and form ideas from information. Cognition requires high-level integrity of the brain. This integrity is beyond the functional ability of many head-injured patients, especially in the early stages of recovery.

The final psychologic skill level is emotional stability, which is defined as behavior that is within normal acceptable limits. It includes rational thinking and an adequate self-concept.

Regaining social and economic skills is frequently a major problem for individuals whose head injury has required an interruption in gainful employment. Achievement of these goals often depends on the professional help that the patient receives during the rehabilitation process. Social and family competencies must also be regained for the patient to have a rewarding social life and a secure family role. The need for economic security will cause some persons to seek employment, whereas others will rely on public assistance programs. Full-time employment is a goal achieved by only a minority of severely head-injured adults and only after a long period of professional help.

BRAIN TRAUMA RECOVERY LEVELS

During the past 15 years, a number of scales of recovery from traumatic head injury have been published.[37–40] Most of these scales are limited to only a few levels. This limits their value to the rehabilitation specialist who works with patients over a long period of time. Progress is often too slow for these scales to exhibit functional change from one level to the next. Smith[36] published a scale of recovery from severe head trauma that has 10 levels (Table 20-2). The Functional Scale of Recovery From Severe Head Trauma has two levels of death and a level for complete recovery. This leaves seven levels that can be used to document recovery over time during the rehabilitation process. A scale of this type can be used not only to describe how a patient functions but also to predict the level of recovery.

Prediction of recovery has been based on length of coma by researchers.[35,41–43] Recovery potential can also be based on the speed of recovery of other functions. Smith and associates[44] examined the relationship between early recovery patterns and recovery. They found that swift reinstatement of swallowing, nodding the head, and verbal responses, after the patient regains consciousness, is characteristic of patients who eventually return to pre-

Table 20-2. A Functional Scale of Recovery From Severe Head Injury

1. DEATH: Within 48 hours of trauma.
2. LINGERING DEATH: Occurring more than 48 hours after trauma.
3. PERSISTENT VEGETATIVE STATE: Unresponsive and speechless.
4. SEVERE HELPLESSNESS: Conscious but severely disabled. Functional movements with some communication and intellectual responses. May be able to swallow and speak some words. Unable to perform ADL. Dependent on others for all daily needs.
5. SEVERE PHYSICAL DISABILITY: Severe physical limitations. Nonambulatory with fair communication and intellectual responses. Considerable nursing care needed. Able to sit upright and feed self.
6. SEVERE MENTAL DISABILITY: Mentally incapacitated. Usually ambulatory but with severe psychologic and/or intellectual problems. Needs supervised living environment.
7. MODERATE DISABILITY: Disabled but independent. Independent ambulation with or without equipment. Has one or more of the following disabilities: (a) requires assistance in ADL, (b) has reduced communication skills, (c) needs ongoing psychologic support.
8. MODERATE TO MILD DISABILITY: Independent in ADL and has good communication skills. Mild to moderate physical, psychologic, and/or intellectual impairment. Usually able to live outside institution with family/social support. May require a modified work or living environment.
9. GOOD RECOVERY: Return to normal life style. Minimal physical, intellectual, or psychologic impairments but completely independent.
10. COMPLETE RECOVERY: Full functional recovery to pre-injury level. Able to return to employment or other pretrauma activities. Patient is emotionally stable and has regained pretraumatic intellectual facilities.

traumatic functional ability. Head-injured patients who exhibit slow reinstatement of these basic skills have a poor prognosis.

CONCLUSION

The speech and language assessment of head-injured patients should include an analysis of speaking, reading, writing, understanding, cognitive ability, and recovery process. This information is needed to formulate a diagnosis of any speech and language problem and to develop a prognosis for improvement. These two clinical judgments will determine the subsequent therapeutic program.

A detailed speech and language evaluation should use sophisticated psychometric tools and clinical judgment. The evaluation should include tests of auditory and visual receptive skills, tests of graphic and verbal expressive skills, and tests of motor speech function.

Cognitive dysfunction is often the most debilitating problem patients exhibit subsequent to severe head injury. It significantly interferes with speech and language processing. The assessment determines whether the impairment of speech and language skills is due to cognitive dysfunction, a specific neurologic lesion, or a combination of these two causes.

Developing a prognosis for improvement of speech and language skills is an integral aspect of the assessment. Knowledge of the natural recovery can be helpful in predicting future improvement. Patients with potential for recovery only to a severe disability level may need considerably more speech and language rehabilitation than the patients whose prognosis is for complete recovery.

REFERENCES

1. YACORZYNSKI, GK: *Organic mental disorders.* In WOLMAN, BB (ED): *Handbook of Clinical Psychology.* McGraw-Hill, New York, 1965.
2. WECHSLER, D: *Wechsler Adult Intelligence Scale Manual.* The Psychological Corp, New York, 1955.

3. WECHSLER, D: *Wechsler Memory Scale.* The Psychological Corp, New York, 1972.
4. TAYLOR, EM: *Psychological Appraisal of Children with Cerebral Defects.* Harvard University Press, Cambridge, Mass, 1959.
5. DUNN, LM AND MARKWARDT, FC: *Peabody Individual Achievement Test.* American Guidance Service, Circle Pines, Minn, 1970.
6. HAGEN, C, MALKMUS, D, AND DURHAM, P: *Levels of cognitive functioning.* Head Trauma Rehabilitation Seminar, Rancho Los Amigos Hospital, Los Angeles, 1977.
7. GORHAM, DR: *Proverbs test for clinical and experimental use.* Psychological Reports, Monograph Supplement 1:1, 1956.
8. RAVEN, JC: *Guide to the Standard Progressive Matrices.* HK Lewis, London, 1960.
9. GOLDEN, CJ: *Diagnosis and Rehabilitation in Clinical Neuropsychology.* Charles C Thomas, Springfield, Ill, 1978.
10. LEZAK, MD: *Neuropsychological Assessment.* Oxford University Press, New York, 1976.
11. GOODGLASS, H AND KAPLAN, E: *The Assessment of Aphasia and Related Disorders.* Lea & Febiger, Philadelphia, 1973.
12. SCHUELL, H: *Differential Diagnosis of Aphasia with the Minnesota Test.* University of Minnesota Press, Minneapolis, 1965.
13. PORCH, BE: *Porch Index of Communicative Ability.* Consulting Psychologists Press, Palo Alto, 1967.
14. SPREEN, O AND BENTON, AL: *Neurosensory Center Comprehensive Examination for Aphasia.* University of Victoria Press, Victoria, British Columbia, 1969.
15. DISIMONI, FG: *Assessment factors in effective treatment of aphasic patients.* Journal of Pennsylvania Speech and Hearing Association 8:2, 1980.
16. CRITCHLEY, M: *Aphasiology.* Edward Arnold, London, 1970.
17. EISENSON, J: *Adult Aphasia.* Prentice-Hall, Englewood Cliffs, NJ, 1973.
18. SMITH, RM: *Prognosis of aphasia: Etiology, time and linguistic factors.* Proceedings of International Association of Logopedics, Washington, DC, 1981.
19. DERENZI, E AND VIGNOLO, LA: *The token test: A sensitive test to detect receptive disturbances in aphasics.* Brain 85:665, 1962.
20. DUNN, LM: *Revised Peabody Picture Vocabulary Test.* American Guidance Service, Circle Pines, Minn, 1980.
21. JASTAK, JE AND JASTAK, SR: *The Wide Range Achievement Test.* Guidance Associates, Wilmington, 1965.
22. GRAY, WS: *Gray Oral Reading Tests.* Bobbs-Merrill, Indianapolis, 1967.
23. WOODCOCK, RW: *Woodcock Reading Mastery Tests.* American Guidance Service, Circle Pines, Minn, 1973.
24. GATES, AI AND MACGINITIE, WH: *Gates-MacGinitie Reading Tests.* Teachers College Press, New York, 1969.
25. THURSTONE, LL: *Primary Mental Abilities.* University of Chicago Press, Chicago, 1962.
26. MYKLEBUST, HR: *Development and Disorders of Written Language.* Grune & Stratton, New York, 1965.
27. GREEN, E: *On the contribution of studies in aphasia to psycholinguistics.* Cortex 6:216, 1970.
28. TERMAN, LM AND MERRILL, MA: *The Stanford-Binet Intelligence Scale* (1972 norms edition). Houghton Mifflin, Boston, 1973.
29. BORKOWSKI, IG, BENTON, AL, AND SPREEN, O: *Word fluency and brain damage.* Neuropsychologia 5:135, 1957.
30. WILLIAMS, M: *Mental Testing in Clinical Testing.* Pergamon Press, Oxford, 1965.
31. OSTREICHER, H: *Memory for unrelated sentences.* In LEZAK, MD: *Neuropsychological Assessment.* Oxford University Press, New York, 1976, p 360.

32. DARLEY, FL, ARONSON, AE, AND BROWN, JR: *Motor Speech Disorders.* WB Saunders, Philadelphia, 1975.
33. JOHNS, DF (ED): *Clinical Management of Neurogenic Communicative Disorders.* Little, Brown & Co, Boston, 1978.
34. BECKER, DP, ET AL: *The outcome from severe head injury with early diagnosis and intensive management.* J Neurosurg 47:491, 1977.
35. JENNETT, B AND BOND, M: *Assessment of outcome after severe brain damage.* Lancet 3:480, 1975.
36. SMITH, RM, ET AL: *A functional scale of recovery from severe head trauma.* Clin Neuropsychol 1:48, 1979.
37. HEISKANEN, O AND SIPPONEN, P: *Prognosis of severe brain injury.* Acta Neurol Scand 46:343, 1970.
38. JENNETT, B: *Prognosis after severe head injury.* Clin Neurosurg 19:200, 1972.
39. STOVER, SL AND ZIEGLER, HE: *Head injury in children and teenagers: Functional recovery correlated with the duration of coma.* Arch Phys Med Rehabil 57:201, 1976.
40. VAPALAHTI, M AND TROUPP, H: *Prognosis for patients with severe brain injuries.* Br Med J 3:404, 1971.
41. CARLSON, CA, VONESSEN, C, AND LOFGREN, J: *Factors affecting clinical course of patients with severe head injuries.* J Neurosurg 29:242, 1968.
42. GILCHRIST, E AND WILKINSON, M: *Some factors determining prognosis in young people with severe head injuries.* Arch Neurol 36:355, 1979.
43. PAZZAGLIA, P, ET AL: *Clinical course and prognosis of acute post-traumatic coma.* J Neurol Neurosurg Psychiatry 38:149, 1975.
44. SMITH, RM, ET AL: *Prognosis after severe head trauma.* Presented at the Fourth Annual Post-Graduate Course on the Rehabilitation of the Traumatic Brain-Injured Adult, Williamsburg, Va, 1980.

BIBLIOGRAPHY

HEIMBURGER, RF AND REITAN, RM: *Easily administered written test for lateralizing brain lesions.* J Neurosurg 18:301, 1961.

Chapter 21

NEUROPSYCHOLOGIC ASSESSMENT

William J. Lynch, Ph.D.

DEFINITION AND BACKGROUND

Clinical neuropsychologic assessment involves the evaluation of human brain-behavior relationships by means of standard testing methods.[1] While there are certain similarities between the clinical neurologic examination and the typical neuropsychologic evaluation, the two should be considered complementary, rather than redundant or interchangeable. The neuropsychologic evaluation provides an extensive assessment of higher cortical functions in addition to a limited evaluation of more basic sensory-motor processes, whereas the reverse may be said of the traditional clinical neurologic examination.

Another distinction between the two approaches lies in their general purpose. The clinical neuropsychologic assessment is designed to identify specific and general cognitive and perceptual-motor abilities and deficits with an eye toward defining functional, impaired, and nonfunctional cortical areas. Beyond an attempt to localize the hemisphere and lobe(s) that are maximally involved, clinical neuropsychologic assessment seeks to articulate the cortical functions that require rehabilitative attention, as well as those that are essentially intact. The tests are such that they provide an objective baseline for future comparison during various stages of recovery.

The clinical neurologic examination, on the other hand, is designed to thoroughly evaluate the central nervous system, at all levels, in order to detect the presence of dysfunction. There is no intent to provide a comprehensive objective baseline for serial evaluations, and rehabilitative prescriptions tend to be based on general impressions and clinical experience rather than on specific findings from a given examination.

While both the clinical neurologic assessment and the clinical neuropsychologic examination evaluate cognitive functions, the procedures used by the former are much more detailed than those of the latter. For example, the neuropsychologist may use a formal mental status examination, intelligence scale, and comprehensive memory evaluation. The neurologist frequently determines "mental status" by evaluating temporal and spatial orientation. The neurologist may typically assess intelligence in a global fashion by presenting informational or proverb interpretation items (perhaps along with an impression gained by noting the patient's vocabulary level). Memory is typically tested by such tasks as digit recall, retention of three words, or naming of prominent cities or political figures. The difference between the two approaches is more quantitative than qualitative, and the relative merit of each depends on how the data obtained are to be used. Briefly, if the question is one of *presence* or *absence* of cognitive dysfunction, either approach would suffice. However, if the need is for more detailed analysis, such that the specific *type* and *degree* of deficit can be defined, then a more comprehensive cognitive evaluation is required. This brings to mind a truism that applies to assessment of all types but especially to neuropsychologic assessment, namely, that specific and detailed interpretations require specific and detailed testing procedures.

In an effort to expand the evaluation of higher cortical functions as carried out in the traditional neurologic examination, Halstead[2] and later Reitan[1] developed a neuropsychologic test battery known today as the Halstead-Reitan Battery. More recently, Christensen[3,4,5] has published a version of Luria's neuropsychologic procedures[6] under the title *Luria's Neuropsychological Investigation*. Golden and colleagues[7] have published a standardized version of the Luria Neuropsychological Investigation that revises, restructures, and eliminates many of the procedures outlined by Christensen. This standardized version is entitled *The Luria-Nebraska Neuropsychological Battery*.

In the following section, these three general approaches to neuropsychologic assessment (Halstead-Reitan, Christensen-Luria, Golden-Luria) will be described so that the reader will become aware that there are a number of methodologies available, each of which has particular strengths and weaknesses in given situations.

DESCRIPTION OF THE PROMINENT TEST BATTERIES

HALSTEAD-REITAN BATTERY

Halstead[2] developed a set of standard procedures that he felt were sensitive to frontal lobe functions. These procedures emphasized problem solving, abstraction, logical analysis, motor speed, attention, and incidental memory. His introduction and popularization of the test battery approach to assessment and his use of cut-off scores for evaluating individual patients' performances were among his significant contributions to the field of clinical neuropsychology. Further, he introduced the use of a numerical index of deficit (the Impairment Index), which depended on the patient's level of performance on 10 (later reduced to 7) separate measures of cognitive and perceptual-motor ability.

Halstead's work was carried on, expanded, and popularized by Reitan, who for the past 30 years has carried out numerous research studies using Halstead's tests and others from various sources.[8]

Reitan added measures of psychometric intelligence (the age-appropriate Wechsler Intelligence Scale), academic achievement (the Wide Range Achievement Test by Jastak and Jastak[9]), a standardized cortical sensory evaluation (the Sensory-Perceptual Examination), a measure of manual strength (Strength of Grip), and a test of rapid visual-motor integration and problem solving (Trail Making Test). Reitan also added a measurement of nondominant index-finger-tapping speed (Halstead used only the dominant finger). In addition to these extensions and modifications, Reitan eliminated two of the original 10 tests employed by Halstead (the Time-Sense and Critical Flicker Frequency Tests) because of their inferior discriminative power in comparing subjects with brain lesions with normal subjects.[1] The resulting set of tests, along with a brief description of each, is provided in Table 21-1.

Reitan[8] describes four methods of inference for dealing with neuropsychologic data:

1. *Level of performance:* The traditional application of cut-off scores in order to divide test scores into a normal and abnormal range.
2. *Pattern of performance:* The analysis of *differences* in scores within the battery as they reflect strengths, weaknesses, and performance variability.
3. *Specific behavioral deficits or pathognomonic signs:* Pathognomonic signs are behaviors that occur only in pathologic conditions. This approach to data interpretation is illustrated by attendance to such phenomena as hemiparesis, hemianopsia, or anomia, none of which occurs in non-brain-damaged persons.

4. *Comparison of performance of the two sides of the body:* The analysis of performance on unilateral and bilateral motor and sensory measures can provide useful data as to the relative efficiency of each side of the body (and presumably the brain).

A more detailed description of the interpretation of Halstead-Reitan tests can be found elsewhere.[10]

LURIA'S NEUROPSYCHOLOGICAL INVESTIGATION

Although Luria's work had been well publicized for nearly 20 years, it was not until the publication of Christensen's test[3,4,5] that his assessment techniques were presented in an organized format. Luria's method rests on his theory of functional systems, which characterizes psychologic processes as being the result of complex interactions among brain regions. Processes such as reading, writing, and speaking are viewed as being multidetermined. An inability to perform such behaviors does not implicate a problem in a specific brain area, but rather a problem somewhere in the particular system in question. Thus, an inability to read aloud may result from a failure in vision or visual recognition (input) as well as in speaking (output).

Luria expresses the premise that if a particular system is affected by a brain lesion, all other functions that use that system should be affected. Likewise, functions that do *not* include that system should be unaffected.

Luria's Neuropsychological Investigation consists of 11 principal segments, each of which has two or more subsections. These principal segments and subsections are listed in Table 21-2.

Scoring of Luria's Neuropsychological Investigation is impressionistic, although a three-point system (none, slight, or severe) of rating disturbances is provided on the test forms.[4] A sheet containing five brain diagrams (left and right hemispheres, lateral and sagittal views, and a basal view) is provided for the indication of the specific site of damage deduced from the examination.

Christensen[3] describes three main stages of the investigation. The first stage consists of the administration of numerous brief tests that evaluate the status of the principal systems ("analyzers" in Luria's terminology) that mediate basic visual, auditory, kinesthetic, and motor functions. The second stage deals with more specific tests suggested by the patient's performance during the first stage. Testing at this stage is "strictly individualized," according to Christensen. The emphasis here is on qualitative, rather than quantitative, observations. Stimuli may, for example, be presented at varying rates as one way of assessing the critical factors operating in the performance of a task. The third stage is described as the formulation of a conclusion based on the results obtained. The clinician must attempt to identify the etiology of the deficit and to describe the ways in which the deficit intrudes on the patient's cognitive and/or perceptual-motor activity. A detailed analysis of the results will lead to an identification of one or more "syndromes" or "symptom complexes," which will point the way to the locus of the lesion. An evaluation of Luria's Neuropsychological Investigation as an assessment tool in rehabilitation settings will follow the discussion of the third and final neuropsychologic battery, the Luria-Nebraska Neuropsychological Battery.

LURIA-NEBRASKA NEUROPSYCHOLOGICAL BATTERY

Golden and colleagues[11] recently published initial data on a test battery based on Luria's Neuropsychological Investigation. The intent was to provide a standardized and objectively scored version of the Luria investigation. This, it was felt, would allow implementation of more meaningful validity and reliability studies and would permit the accumulation of data on various types of neurologic disorders. Subsequent papers[12-14] have addressed the problems of validity and localization of dysfunction.

TABLE 21-1. Halstead-Reitan Battery (Adults 15 and Older)

Test Name	Brief Description	What the Test Measures
Halstead's Tests		
1. Category Test	208 slides divided into 7 subtests are presented on a rear projection screen. Patient must discern a consistent organizing principle or concept for each subtest in trial-and-error fashion, with immediate feedback provided by a bell (correct) or buzzer (incorrect). Score is given as the number of errors.	Attention, concentration, visual problem solving, ability to generate and test hypotheses, abstract reasoning, ability to attend to and make constructive use of feedback, ability to generalize from familiar to new-but-similar situations.
2. Tactual Performance Test	A modified Seguin-Goddard form board is employed. Patient is blindfolded; empty board and loose blocks are placed before patient. Patient must replace as many blocks as possible with a time limit (10 to 15 min). Dominant, nondominant, and both-hand trials are obtained consecutively. After board and blocks are hidden, blindfold is removed and patient must draw a picture of the board, correctly depicting as *many* of the shapes as possible in their proper relative *locations*. Score is given as total time, blocks correctly recalled (memory), and blocks correctly located (localization).	Motor problem solving, stamina, transfer of training from one trial to the next, tactile-motor-spatial integration, spatial and tactile memories, incidental learning.
3. Rhythm Test	Presented on audio tape, the test items consist of 30 pairs of monotonic rhythmic patterns. Patient must indicate "same" or "different" for each pair (15 are same; 15 are different). Score is again given as either a scaled score (1 to 10) or as number of errors.	Attention, concentration, nonverbal auditory discrimination, nonverbal memory.
4. Speech Sounds Perception Test	Presented on audio tape, 60 nonsense words in sets of 10. Patient must underline on an answer sheet the correct choice among four alternatives for each item. Score given as number of errors.	Attention and concentration, verbal auditory discrimination, visual discrimination, high-frequency sound perception.
5. Finger Tapping Test	Using a mechanical counter affixed to a 9 × 9.5 inch board, patient taps as rapidly as possible with index finger for 10 sec. Preferred and nonpreferred hands are used alternately until five trials are obtained	Motor speed (although there is a small visual-proprioceptive component). The ability to establish and sustain a regular rhythm of tapping is required,

	which vary by less than five taps from one another. Score is given as the mean number of taps for five trials with the preferred hand. (Although not contributing to the Impairment Index, the nonpreferred hand's performance is recorded for comparison.)	and therefore basal ganglia or cerebellar dysfunction may impair performance.
Additional Measures:		
6. Grip Strength	Using a hand dynamometer calibrated in kilograms, the relative strength of each hand grip is measured (two trials per hand). Score is given as the mean number of kilograms, across two trials, with each hand.	Strength of the upper extremities.
7. Trail Making Test	Using a pen or pencil, patient must rapidly draw a line sequentially connecting 25 circles scattered on an 8½ × 11 inch sheet of paper. On Part A, the circles contain only numbers (1 to 25); on Part B, the circles contain both numbers (1 to 13) and letters (A to L). On Part B, the patient connects the circles in a number-letter-number-letter sequence. Score is given as the number of seconds required to complete each part. Errors (incorrect sequences) are also recorded.	Visual-motor speed; scanning and searching; ability to deal with numeric and linguistic symbols; ability to execute a sequential sensory-motor activity; ability to maintain and alternate smoothly between parallel mental sets.
8. Aphasia Screening Test	32 items, dealing with aspects of language, constructional skill, articulation, right-left orientation are presented either verbally or by means of a booklet of small stimuli cards. Scoring is of a plus-minus or pass-fail variety. No total score is used, although some researchers have attached weight to the items.	Communicative abilities (naming, reading, writing, spelling), auditory comprehension, calculating, drawing ability, recognition of body parts, clarity of speech, ability to imagine and carry out a motor set.
9. Sensory Perceptual Examination	Basic tactile, auditory, and visual signal detection are evaluated. Bilateral simultaneous stimulation is also carried out in each modality. Finger localization, number writing perception, and tactile object recognition are evaluated. Visual fields are approximated by confrontation.	Cortical sensory functions. The presence of sensory "neglect" (suppression or inattention) is measured, along with the ability to locate one's fingers, graphesthesia, stereognosis, and integrity of visual fields.

TABLE 21-2. Principal Segments and Subsections of Luria's Neuropsychological Investigation*

Segment	Subsections
1. Preliminary conversation	a. State of patient's consciousness b. Principal complaints
2. Motor functions	a. Functions of the hands b. Functions of the mouth (oral praxis) c. Speech regulation of the motor act
3. Acousticomotor organization	a. Perception and reproduction of pitch b. Perception and reproduction of rhythm
4. Higher cutaneous and kinesthetic functions	a. Cutaneous sensation b. Muscle and joint sensation
5. Higher visual functions	a. Visual perception b. Spatial orientation c. Intellectual operations in space
6. Impressive speech	a. Phonemic learning b. Word comprehension c. Understanding simple sentences d. Understanding logical grammatical structures
7. Expressive speech	a. Articulation of speech sounds b. Repetition of speech sounds c. Naming d. Narrative speech and fluency
8. Writing and reading	a. Phonetic analysis of words b. Writing c. Reading
9. Arithmetic skill	a. Comprehension of number structure b. Arithmetic operations
10. Mnestic processes (Memory)	a. Learning b. Retention and retrieval c. Logical memorizing
11. Intellectual processes	a. Understanding pictures and texts b. Concept formation c. Discursive intellectual activity

*From Christensen.[3]

The Luria-Nebraska Battery consists of 269 items divided among 14 scales.[15] The scales are listed in Table 21-3.

Each item is assigned a numerical score of 0 (best), 1 (borderline), or 2 (impaired) based on criteria provided in the manual.[7] Methods for adjusting raw score totals for both age and education and for transcribing raw scores onto a T-score profile are also presented. The resulting profile may be interpreted much as one would an MMPI profile in which T-score elevations over 60 or 70 are felt to be significant. Golden[15] asserts that while *two* scales over a T-score of 60 are strongly suggestive of brain damage, *three* scales over 60 are associated with brain damage in normal populations about 90 percent of the time.

TABLE 21-3. Brief Summary of 14 Scales of the Luria-Nebraska Neuropsychological Battery

Scale Name	Number of Items	What the Scale Evaluates
1. Motor functions	51	Basic and complex motor functions (including fingers, hands, tongue, mouth; drawing).
2. Rhythm or acousticomotor organization	12	Rhythm and pitch abilities
3. Tactile or higher cutaneous and kinesthetic functions	22	Kinesthetic and cortical sensory skills
4. Visual functions	14	Visual and spatial skills
5. Receptive (impressive) speech	33	Ability to understand spoken speech
6. Expressive speech	42	Ability to express speech orally
7. Writing	13	Writing and spelling skills
8. Reading skills	13	Basic and complex reading skills
9. Arithmetic skills	22	Simple math skills from number identification to simple algebra
10. Memory	13	Verbal and nonverbal memory skills, along with effects of proactive and retroactive interference
11. Intellectual processes	34	Patient's general intellectual level
12. Pathognomonic	32*	The 32 items found to be most discriminating in initial validation study[11] indicate overall impairment a patient is showing.
13. Right hemisphere	34*	Items dealing with motor and sensory functions that evaluate the functioning of the left side of the body.
14. Left hemisphere	37*	Items dealing with motor and sensory functions that evaluate the functioning of the right side of the body.

*Items are special subsets of the basic 269-item pool. See Golden, Purisch, and Hammeke[7] for precise item composition.

ADDITIONAL TECHNIQUES

A number of additional assessment techniques, although not part of the aforementioned batteries, may be useful in a number of situations. Two key areas of interest in neuropsychologic assessment—language and memory assessment—are more ably evaluated by special tests that are often used in conjunction with a standard neuropsychologic battery.

LANGUAGE FUNCTIONS

In most rehabilitation settings, speech pathologists are available for performing detailed evaluation of the patient's language functions. Typically, the principal measurement tool employed will be one of the following:

1. *Boston Diagnostic Aphasia Examination* (BDAE)[16] evaluates the major components of language in an effort to determine qualitative and quantitative aspects of the patient's communications system. Impaired patients are classified into categories such as Broca, Wernicke, conduction, or global aphasia. Performances are scored on a rating scale and are plotted on an elaborate Z-score profile for quick reference.
2. *Minnesota Test for the Differential Diagnosis of Aphasia*[17] is a very detailed language evaluation procedure that seeks to methodically determine the precise problem by systematically examining each principal facet of speaking, comprehending, and writing. Here, as in the BDAE, the scoring system is based on ratings of "pass-fail" considerations.
3. *Porch Index of Communicative Ability* (PICA)[18] is a relatively brief (45 to 90 minute) procedure consisting of 18 subtests divided among graphic (6), verbal (4), and gestural (8) response requirements. The PICA uses a complex 16-point multidimensional scoring system that translates clinical behavior into a numeric value. The PICA is not designed to diagnose or label a patient's communication problem, but rather to quantify the patient's abilities in a variety of situations. The PICA is useful in initial assessment, treatment planning, and outcome measurement.

In addition to these measures, there are a number of excellent procedures that can be employed in special situations. The Token Test[19] is a measure of verbal comprehension that enjoys the advantages of highly flexible input complexity and consistently uncomplicated output requirements (touch or pick up). Briefly, the patient is confronted with 10 variously shaped and colored plastic tokens and is asked to touch or point to one or more of them, either singly or in a prescribed sequence. The Token Test is an excellent technique for evaluating auditory comprehension because of its de-emphasis upon complex verbal, graphic, or gestural output as an indicator of understanding. Recently, Holland[20] published the Communicative Activities of Daily Living (CADL) technique, which was designed to assess practical "real-life" communicative skills, such as filling out simple forms, reading product labels, understanding common signs, or expressing emotional states. Although the CADL is relatively new, it is quite promising and certainly points out the need to evaluate speech and language in more natural and realistic contexts.

The *Neurosensory Center Comprehensive Examination for Aphasia*[21] is an aphasia assessment technique that has been gaining in popularity in recent years. It consists of 20 subtests that evaluate language (expression and comprehension), repetition, reading, and writing. Norms are available for aphasic patients, as well as for right-hemisphere-damaged persons and normal persons. (See Chapter 20 for further discussion.)

MEMORY FUNCTIONS

The evaluation of memory functions is typically accomplished by two types of assessment procedures. The first involves determination of auditory verbal memory. The most popular method for measuring various forms of auditory verbal memory is the Wechsler Memory Scale (WMS).[22] The WMS consists of eight subtests measuring such abilities as orientation, mental control, logical memory, digit span, and associate learning. Raw scores are converted to a Memory Quotient, which is roughly equivalent to a deviation IQ. In recent years, age-weighted standard scores for each subtest have been provided,[23] and norms for a 30-minute delay format for two of the WMS subtests have been published.[24]

Visual memory is typically evaluated by a memory for geometric designs. The Revised Benton Visual Retention Test[25] is one of the most widely used visual memory assessment techniques. This test consists of 10 designs, most of which consist of two major figures and one minor figure that is peripheral to these. There are three parallel forms and norms for various age and intellectual levels.

NEUROPSYCHOLOGIC ASSESSMENT IN REHABILITATION SETTINGS

Neuropsychologic assessment has a number of applications in rehabilitation settings. The following discussion will highlight the principal ways in which such testing can assist in the diagnostic and treatment process.

BASELINE DETERMINATIONS

Neuropsychologic assessment can be helpful in determining the patient's initial status with regard to cognitive and perceptual-motor abilities. By comparing the patient's performance with that of an appropriate normative group, the clinician can establish a pattern of deficits and preserved abilities for the patient for comparison with future evaluations. Progress in general, as well as in specific areas, can be documented by comparing periodic assessments with the baseline data.

IDENTIFICATION OF STRENGTHS AND WEAKNESS

Aside from the determination of a baseline reference point for future comparison, neuropsychologic data can be useful in articulating the patient's problems and strengths. This can be done directly by transforming the raw scores obtained to age-weighted scores, which are then plotted on T-score profiles. Scores that fall below T-score of 40 or 30 can be considered impaired for the purposes of identifying liabilities, while scores in the average range (or higher) can be considered to reflect strengths or assets. Figure 21-1 illustrates a portion of such a profile.

It should be emphasized that the clinician does not consider test performances per se as weaknesses or strengths. Rather, the behavior represented by the test performance is the focus of attention in rehabilitation.

The specific problems that are identified may be stated in various forms, although it is preferable to employ standard terminology. A fairly comprehensive list of problems for use in head-injury rehabilitation has been published recently.[26] Some examples of these standard problems are presented in Table 21-4.

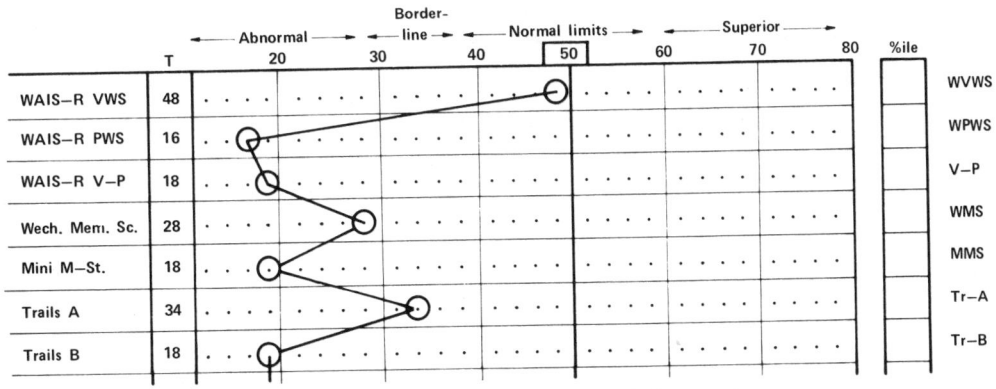

FIGURE 21-1. Portion of T-score profile for plotting neuropsychologic test scores.

TABLE 21-4. Portion of Standard Problem List for Patients With Brain Dysfunction

1. COGNITIVE
   A. Memory difficulty
      1. Auditory
      2. Visual
      3. Spatial
      4. Temporal disorientation
   B. Impaired receptive language in
      1. Reading comprehension
      2. Word recognition
      3. Auditory comprehension
   C. Impaired expressive language in
      1. Writing
      2. Word finding
      3. Fluency
      4. Spelling
   D. Math difficulty

Adapted from Lynch and Mauss.[26]

PRESCRIPTIONS FOR TREATMENT

Once the patient's problems have been identified, the next step in the process is deciding on specific treatment strategies. Generally, this is accomplished by selecting tasks that either retrain impaired abilities or substitute new techniques or strategies for carrying out a motor or cognitive activity. Neuropsychologic tests provide useful information in this regard. By analyzing the patterns of performance on these tests, the clinician is able to identify functions that are maintained, as well as those that are partially or totally "lost." By skillful use of the preserved function, the impaired abilities can often be retrained or replaced by alternative methods.

It is most helpful to consider the more basic functions—such as alertness, attention, and concentration—as fundamental to the acquisition of the more complex abilities such as sequential memory, mathematical computation, or abstract reasoning. Neuropsychologic measures that evaluate mental status, reaction time, and simple memory functions would thus be given greater emphasis initially.

Qualitative aspects of neuropsychologic test performance are also of great importance in prescribing specific treatments for the head-injured patient. By observing the patient on a variety of test procedures, one can gain insight into the patient's strategies of problem solving, recognition of and response to failure, capacity for abstract reasoning, and ability to persist at a task that is mentally or physically demanding. Such information can be invaluable in determining not only *what* treatments are to be employed, but *how* and *when* they are to be instituted into the patient's rehabilitation program.

The reader is referred to papers by Diller and Gordon,[27] Gudeman and Craine,[28] and Luria and colleagues[29] for a more thorough presentation of specific treatment prescriptions that can be gleaned from careful neuropsychologic assessment.

PREDICTION AND DETERMINATION OF OUTCOME

The reliable prediction of specific outcomes from early neuropsychologic assessment has not yet been accomplished. Recently, studies from other fields have demonstrated that certain predictions of outcome are possible. Jennett and Teasdale[30] describe their system of predicting broad categories of outcome by using a combination of variables, such as the patient's age, duration of impaired consciousness, and presence of abnormal eye movements. These authors claim a "hit-rate" of more than 0.90 when predicting whether a patient will eventually recover with moderate or minimal disability, or will either die or remain comatose.

Roberts[31] presents a detailed system for predicting long-term outcome after head injury. He states that the three crucial variables in determining prediction of outcome are (1) the *degree of neurologic dysfunction* during the acute stage, (2) the *rate* at which recovery of neurophysical disability takes place, and (3) the patient's *age* at time of injury. Roberts presents a series of "predictive procedures" in the form of decision trees, which use various combinations of variables in a sequential fashion. Aside from predicting neurophysical (neurologic) and mental (cognitive-emotional) disability, Roberts presents data that relate to the prediction of when a head-injured patient will return to work.

From the field of speech pathology, Porch and colleagues[32] have shown that in stroke patients, communicative status at various points in time can be fairly well predicted by a combination of test data (from the Porch Index of Communicative Ability) and age. The authors conclude that the most accurate predictions are those which are made beyond the first month postonset, and which predict for a fairly brief time span, that is, from the first to the twelfth month.

Unfortunately, no such studies have been published using standardized neuropsychologic tests. This is not to say that clinicians do not make inferences about the test data. Rather, it seems that certain traditions have evolved that seem to be borne out clinically but lack firm experimental foundation. Examples of such traditional "rules of thumb" would be the feeling that poor performance on the Trail Making Test, Part B, with normal performance on the Category Test is a sign of recovery, whereas poor performance on both measures is an unfavorable sign.

Likewise, it is generally accepted that wide variation or scatter within or among test performances is suggestive of a potential for improvement, while a flat, invariant level of performance across subtests is consistent with a stable or static state that is less apt to respond to treatment.

It seems clear that studies that examine the predictive strength of neuropsychologic test variables are needed. Such studies have been carried out on neurologic and demographic variables using stepwise multiple regression procedures.

The determination of outcome is accomplished by using one of a number of excellent outcome measures that are in use in a number of centers. The Glasgow Outcome Scale (GOS)[33] is a popular measure of general levels of outcome: good recovery, moderate disability, severe disability, persistent vegetative state, and death.

Roberts[31] presents two separate schemes for grading both central neural and mental disability in head-injured patients. Each scale ranges from "no disability" (scored 0) to "decerebrate dementia" (scored 5). Roberts' scales have the advantage of being more precise than the GOS, thus permitting more accurate description of the patient's current level of disability in two principal areas (neurologic and mental). The use of numeric weights for each grade lends itself more readily to statistical recording or calculations. And finally, the use of clear inclusion/exclusion criteria tends to improve the interrater reliability of the scales.

Recently, Rappaport and others[34] at Santa Clara Valley Medical Center devised the Disability Rating Scale (DRS). The DRS consists of eight categories of potential disability, each of which is assigned a numerical value according to a set of simple objective criteria. Table 21-5 presents the principal scoring categories of the DRS. Although it is as yet not thoroughly validated across a number of centers, the DRS has shown a great deal of promise as a reliable, clear, and yet comprehensive tool for describing levels of disability, both at the outset and conclusion of treatment.

TABLE 21-5. Principal Scoring Categories of the Disability Rating Scale

I. Arousability, awareness, and responsivity
Items: eye opening, verbalization, and best motor response

II. Cognitive ability for self-care activities
Items: feeding, toileting, and grooming

III. Dependence on others
Item: level of functioning

IV. Psychosocial adaptability
Item: employability

Adapted from Disability Rating Scale by Rappaport et al.[34]

It seems clear that whatever outcome measure the clinician chooses, it should be one that will be meaningful, not only to the clinician but to those in other centers who may wish to evaluate or compare data.

ORGANIZATION AND PRESENTATION OF NEUROPSYCHOLOGIC DATA

The utility of neuropsychologic test data is dependent in large part on the manner in which the data are organized and represented. Originally, Halstead-Reitan test data were presented in raw score form on a complex raw score summary sheet. Eventually, clinicians began to question the efficiency and legitimacy of analyzing raw score data on patients of various age groups. The logical solution, for many at least, was to attempt to portray the data in a more concise, easily interpreted fashion by employing standard score profiles. An example of such a profile was presented above (see Fig. 21-1). Typically, in order to construct a standard score profile, the raw scores obtained from testing are transformed to T-scores (having a mean of 50 and a standard deviation of 10), which are then plotted on a profile form.

Most neuropsychologic test batteries have adopted the convention of arranging the profile so that low T-scores (<50) represent poorer-than-average performance, whereas high T-scores (>50) represent greater-than-average performance. An exception to this convention is the profile employed by the Luria-Nebraska battery, which is plotted so that higher scores represent increasing levels of pathology.

In order to provide for a standard interpretation of T-score data, the clinician can employ the following strategies: (1) to calculate the average T-score for all tests, and (2) to calculate the percentage of T-scores that fall at or below a certain cut-off point (usually a T-score of 30). Both the average T-score technique[35] and the percentage of impaired scores[36] have been shown to be effective techniques in certain circumstances. At the Brain Injury Rehabilitation Unit in Palo Alto, we employ a combination of the two methods. Figure 21-2 illustrates the decision model that is used in order to standardize interpretation of the patient's general level of performance.

It should be emphasized that, although it is important, level of performance is only one of several ways in which neuropsychologic data can be interpreted. The following case will illustrate how neuropsychologic tests can be helpful in determining the deficits sustained by a patient following a head injury.

NEUROPSYCHOLOGIC ASSESSMENT

NEW CRITERIA FOR EVALUATING NEUROPSYCHOLOGIC T-SCORE PROFILES
(July 1980)

I. **Data Required:**

   A. **Deficit Index:** (DI) i.e. the percentage of T-scores falling at or below T-score of 30.

   B. **Average T-score:** (AT) i.e. the average or mean of all T-scores obtained.

II. **Decision Tree**

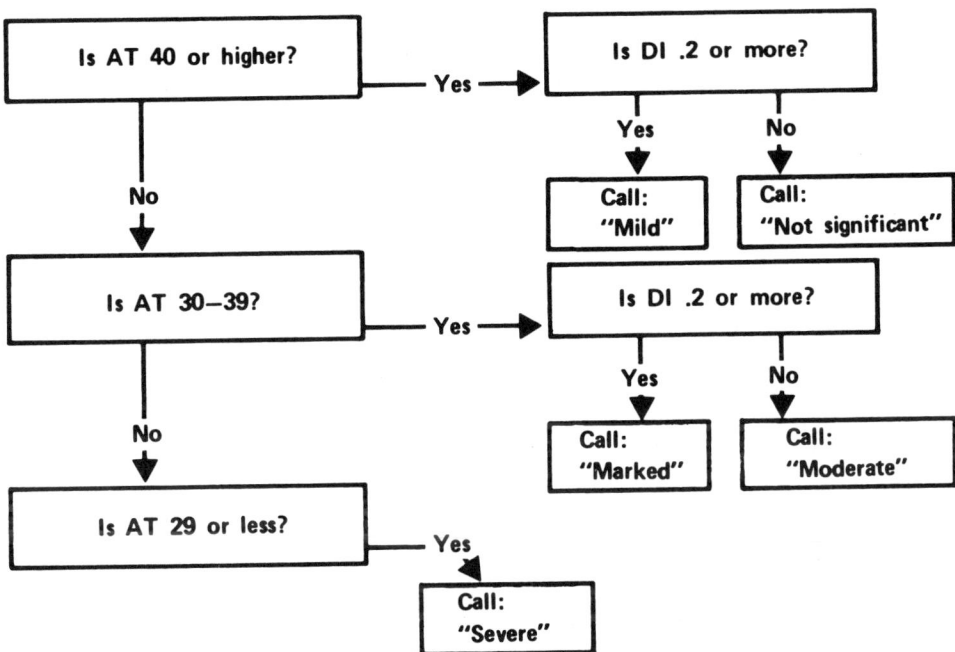

FIGURE 21-2. Decision model for determining level of performance from T-score profiles.

Illustrative Case, Case #2522

The patient was a 32-year-old single man with 13.5 years of formal education. Six months prior to admission to the Brain Injury Rehabilitation Unit, he sustained a closed head injury to the left cerebral hemisphere, resulting in an epidural hematoma. He had a prior seizure disorder, and it appeared that he had a seizure, fell, and struck his head on the street. He was unresponsive to voice or pain when brought in to the emergency room at a nearby hospital. Initially, his pupils were roughly equal and reactive, and the disks were "sharp." However, the patient soon became apneic, and it was noted that his left pupil had become dilated and nonreactive. An emergency left temporal-parietal craniotomy revealed an epidural hematoma (about 200 cc). Over the next several days, his neurologic status improved, and he appeared to be more alert and awake, although his expressive speech was described as incoherent. He stabilized with a mild right hemiparesis and ptosis of the left eyelid.

He was transferred to the rehabilitation department where he spent approximately 3 months before being admitted to the Palo Alto VA Brain Injury Rehabilitation Unit.

TABLE 21-6. Raw Scores on Baseline Neuropsychologic Measures for Case #2522

Trail Making Test
Part A 63 sec
Part B 275 sec

Grip Strength
R = 26 kg
L = 31 kg

Purdue Pegboard
R = 9
L = 12
B = 8
T = 29

Porch Index of Communicative Ability
Overall average 12.26
Gestural   13.36
Verbal   13.68
Graphic   9.87

Wide Range Achievement Test

	Grade	Std Score
Reading	13.0	132
Spelling	8.7	101
Arithmetic	3.9	80

Wechsler Adult Intelligence Scale
Verbal IQ = 94
Performance IQ = 67
Full Scale IQ = 81
Verbal weighted score = 42
Performance weighted score = 24
Difference VWS − PWS = +18

Subtests:

Verbal:
INF = 14
COM = 7
ARI = 4
SIM = 10
DSP = 7
VOC = 13

Performance:
DSY = 2
PCO = 7
BLD = 7
PAR = 4
OAS = 4

Halstead's Tests
Category (errors) 67

Tactual Performance Test (min):
Right 17.3
Left   9.7
Both   9.1
Total 36.1
Memory   8
Localization 1
Rhythm (errors)   1
Speech (errors)   8
Finger tapping: R 42
                L 45
Impairment Index = .7

Sensory Errors:
R = 23
L = 0

TABLE 21-7. General Problem Areas and Total Treatment Hours for Case #2522

Impairment	Treatment Hours
1. Memory difficulty (auditory and visual)	34
2. Impaired expressive language (writing; fluency)	5
3. Math difficulty	26
4. Fine motor dyscoordination (right hand)	28
5. Motor weakness (right side)	36
6. Depression	45
7. Nonassertion	20
8. Impaired independent living (finances; housing)	—

Diagnostic Studies: Computed tomographic scans at the time of the injury and 6 months later indicated focal damage in the left temporal lobe. No atrophy or dilation of the cerebral ventricles was noted. An electroencephalogram that employed nasopharyngeal leads was performed while the patient was sleep-deprived. Aside from the expected slowing over the craniotomy site, no abnormalities were noted.

Results of Neuropsychologic Assessment: Table 21-6 contains the raw scores obtained by the patient on the admission evaluation.

The baseline evaluation indicated greater impairment on the Wechsler Adult Intelligence Scale (WAIS) performance subtests than on the verbal subtests, despite the definite presence of a left hemisphere lesion. The general level of performance reflected marked impairment of higher cortical functions, although certain abilities were quite well maintained. The Porch Index of Communicative Ability (PICA) indicated moderate impairment of language abilities. Tests of motor functions evidenced mild right-sided weakness and slowness. The problems that were identified as a result of this battery of tests (including personality assessment), as well as a listing of the total number of treatments for each problem, are summarized in Table 21-7.

The outcome of treatment was determined by readministering the majority of the neuropsychologic battery after the 6-month period of treatment. Table 21-8 contains the follow-up data on the neuropsychologic tests for Case #2522.

It can be seen that the patient improved dramatically in a number of areas, most notably in general psychometric intelligence, memory, language abilities, and mathematics skills. While a number of other variables are taken into consideration in determining treatment strategies and outcome, it is clear that neuropsychologic tests are quite helpful in documenting the presence and extent of deficits and strengths, as well as the outcome of treatment in head-injured patients.

SUMMARY

This chapter has attempted to present a brief review of the three principal neuropsychologic test batteries in use in the majority of rehabilitation settings. Each of these batteries (Luria, Luria-Nebraska, and Halstead-Reitan) has particular strengths and weaknesses that can limit its effectiveness in certain circumstances. However, each has proven useful in defining and measuring extent of deficits both before and after treatment.

Although it is fairly expensive and time-consuming, neuropsychologic assessment can be invaluable in rehabilitation. When skillfully administered and carefully interpreted, these test batteries can provide critical information regarding both the quantitative and qualitative effects of brain injury on each patient. Such knowledge will assist the clinician in devising a treatment program that makes maximum use of the patient's retained skills while aggressively seeking to retrain skills that are temporarily impaired.

TABLE 21-8. Raw Scores on Follow-up (6 Months Later) Neuropsychologic Measures for Case #2522

Trail Making Test
Part A: 56 sec
Part B: 113 sec

Grip Strength
R = 25 kg
L = 34 kg

Purdue Pegboard
R = 9
L = 12
B = 8
T = 29

Porch Index of Communicative Ability
Overall average 14.44
Gestural 14.64
Verbal 14.18
Graphic 14.37

Wide Range Achievement Test

	Grade	Std Score
Arithmetic	5.9	92

Wechsler Adult Intelligence Scale
Verbal IQ = 123
Performance IQ = 86
Full Scale IQ = 113
Verbal Weighted Score = 65
Performance Weighted Score = 39
Difference VWS − PWS = +26

Subtests:

Verbal:
INF = 14
COM = 10
ARI = 11
SIM = 16
DSP = 14
VOC = 19

Performance:
DSY = 5
PCO = 9
BLD = 11
PAR = 5

Halstead Tests
Category (errors) 29

Tactual Performance Test (min):
Right: 15.2
Left: 7.8
Both: 5.9
Total: 28.9
Memory 8
Localization 3
Rhythm (errors) 1
Speech (errors) 1
Finger tapping: R. 40
L. 50

Impairment Index = .37

Wechsler Memory Quotient 101

REFERENCES

1. REITAN, R: *An investigation of the validity of Halstead's measures of biological intelligence.* Archives of Neurology and Psychiatry 73:28, 1955.
2. HALSTEAD, W: *Brain and Intelligence: A Quantitative Study of the Frontal Lobes.* University of Chicago Press, Chicago, 1947.
3. CHRISTENSEN, A-L: *Luria's Neuropsychological Investigation* (text), ed 1. Spectrum Publications, New York, 1975.
4. CHRISTENSEN, A-L: *Luria's Neuropsychological Investigation* (manual), ed 1. Spectrum Publications, New York, 1975.
5. CHRISTENSEN, A-L: *Luria's Neuropsychological Investigation,* ed 2. Munksgaard, Copenhagen, 1980.
6. LURIA, A: *Higher Cortical Function in Man.* Basic Science Books, New York, 1966.
7. GOLDEN, C, PURISCH, A, AND HAMMEKE, T: *The Luria-Nebraska Neuropsychological Battery.* University of Nebraska Press, Lincoln, 1979.
8. REITAN, R: *A research program on the psychological effects of brain lesions in human beings.* In ELLIS, N (ED): *International Review of Research in Mental Retardation.* Academic Press, New York, 1966, p 153.
9. JASTAK, J AND JASTAK, S: *The Wide Range Achievement Test Manual of Instructions,* ed 3. Jastak Associates, Wilmington, 1978.
10. BOLL, T: *The Halstead-Reitan neuropsychological test battery.* In FILSKOV, S AND BOLL, T (EDS): *Handbook of Clinical Neuropsychology.* John Wiley & Sons, New York, 1981, p 577.
11. GOLDEN, C, HAMMEKE, T, AND PURISCH, A: *Diagnostic validity of a neuropsychological battery derived from Luria's neuropsychological tests.* J Consult Clin Psychol 46:1258, 1978.
12. HAMMEKE, T, GOLDEN, C, AND PURISCH, A: *A standardized, short and comprehensive neuropsychological test battery based on the Luria neuropsychological evaluation.* Int J Neurosci 8:135, 1978.
13. LEWIS, G, ET AL.: *Localization of cerebral dysfunction by a standardized version of Luria's neuropsychological battery.* J Consult Clin Psychol 47:1003, 1979.
14. OSMON, D, ET AL: *The use of a standardized battery of Luria's tests in the diagnosis of lateralized cerebral dysfunction.* Int J Neurosci 9:1, 1979.
15. GOLDEN, C: *A standardized version of Luria's neuropsychological tests: A quantitative and qualitative approach to neuropsychological evaluation.* In FILSKOV, S AND BOLL, T (EDS): *Handbook of Clinical Neuropsychology.* John Wiley & Sons, New York, 1981, p 608.
16. GOODGLASS, H AND KAPLAN, E: *The Assessment of Aphasia and Related Disorders.* Lea & Febiger, Philadelphia, 1972.
17. SCHUELL, H: *The Minnesota Test for the Differential Diagnosis of Aphasia.* University of Minnesota Press, Minneapolis, 1965.
18. PORCH, B: *The Porch Index of Communicative Ability.* Consulting Psychologists Press, Palo Alto, 1967.
19. DERENZI, E AND VIGNOLO, L: *The Token Test: A sensitive test to detect disturbances in aphasics.* Brain 85:665, 1962.
20. HOLLAND, A: *Communicative Abilities in Daily Living.* University Park Press, Baltimore, 1980.
21. SPREEN, O AND BENTON, A: *Neurosensory Center Comprehensive Examination for Aphasia.* Neuropsychology Laboratory, Victoria, BC, 1969.
22. WECHSLER, D AND STONE, C: *A standardized memory scale for clinical use.* J Psychol 19:87, 1945.
23. OSBORNE, D AND DAVIS, L: *Standard scores for Wechsler Memory Scale subtests.* J Clin Psychol 34:115, 1978.
24. RUSSELL, E.: *A multiple scoring method for the assessment of complex memory functions.* J Consult Clin Psychol 43:800, 1975.
25. BENTON, A: *Revised Visual Retention Test,* ed 4. Psychological Corp, New York, 1974.

26. LYNCH, W AND MAUSS, N: *Brain injury rehabilitation: Standard problem lists.* Arch Phys Med Rehabil 62:223, 1981.
27. DILLER, L AND GORDON, W: *Rehabilitation in clinical neuropsychology.* In FILSKOV, S AND BOLL, T (EDS): *Handbook of Clinical Neuropsychology.* John Wiley & Sons, New York, 1981, p 702.
28. GUDEMAN, H AND CRAINE, J: Unpublished data, 1976.
29. LURIA, A, ET AL: *Restoration of higher cortical function following local brain damage.* In VINKEN, P AND BRUYN, G (EDS): *Handbook of Clinical Neurology, Vol 3.* North Holland, Amsterdam, 1969, p 368.
30. JENNETT, B AND TEASDALE, G: *Management of Severe Head Injuries.* FA Davis, Philadelphia, 1981.
31. ROBERTS, A: *Severe Accidental Head Injury.* Macmillan, New York, 1979.
32. PORCH, B, ET AL: *Statistical prediction of change in aphasia.* J. Speech Hear Res 23:312, 1980.
33. JENNETT, B AND BOND, M: *Assessment of outcome after severe brain damage: A practical scale.* Lancet 1:480, 1975.
34. RAPPAPORT, M, ET AL: *Disability rating scale for severe head trauma patients: Coma to community.* Arch Phys Med Rehabil 63:118, 1982.
35. KIERNAN, R AND MATTHEWS, C: *Impairment index versus T-score averaging in neuropsychological assessment.* J Consult Clin Psychol 44:951, 1976.
36. KNIGHTS, R AND WATSON, P: *The use of computerized test profiles in neuropsychological assessment.* Journal of Learning Disability 1:696, 1968.

CONCLUSION

Ernest R. Griffith, M.D.

There are a number of commonalities to consider in conceptualizing the medical, physical, communications, and mental assessments of head-injured patients. Traditional methodology of evaluating these spheres of function must be modified so as to adapt to the circumstances and the needs of individuals with this complex disability. The earliest attempts at assessment may be greatly restricted by the mental status of the patient. Very limited or no information may be obtained from the subject, who is either unable or unwilling to cooperate or communicate with the evaluator. The availability of background information on the premorbid medical and functional status of the patient becomes critical. Additionally, the evaluator must have access to information concerning the management of the patient from the time of injury until the moment of assessment. The major sources of this information include family, medical records, previous health-care professionals treating the patient, and various community resources such as educational institutions and previous employers. Thus, any specialized assessment must start with a baseline of detailed levels of premorbid physical, psychosocial, communications, and vocational-educational functions.

With head-injured persons, the substrate of all evaluations is the mental assessment. Mental function will determine what techniques of assessment should be used, how complete the assessment can be, what degree of limitations in functions are directly attributable to mental dysfunctions, and what treatment strategies are possible within the learning capabilities of the patient.

The assessment by each discipline is a dynamic process, often yielding cumulative information as the patient becomes gradually more awake and cooperative. In addition to serving as a means of ascertaining premorbid functions, the assessment discloses current function against which periodic reassessments will be compared. Hence, the assessment serves the primary purpose of establishing a plan of management, which will be modified as indicated by the results of later assessments. Furthermore, assessment is a major tool in the prognostication of ultimate functional outcomes. Such prognostication is becoming less anecdotal, global, and intuitive, and increasingly systematic, specific, and quantitative in scientific terms. Within each discipline, the evaluation becomes a combination of the employment of clinical skills of observation and the utilization of sophisticated instruments of measurement. We are no longer content with the mere identification of specific deficiencies within a functional area. Rather, we have become concerned with the detailed description of the nature and degree of each deficiency. Moreover, we are equally attentive to the nature and degree of proficiencies within each functional area.

Instruments of measurement are often well standardized, and methods of recording allow precise comparisons with subsequent assessment results. The methods of clinical observation and the instruments of testing are not the exclusive domain of any one specialty. Physician, occupational and physical therapist, speech pathologist, and psychologist share many clinical skills, and there is a certain amount of duplication in their evaluative techniques. Well-coordinated rehabilitation teams managing head-injured patients should be able to avoid some of this duplication by establishing protocols of evaluation that still permit the necessary flexibility of individual assessments. However, a certain amount of duplication of evaluation methods is essential to corroborate vital information that may be based on constantly fluctuating patient behavior and outputs. Moreover, there may be major variations in interpretation of common data which require interdisciplinary discussion before effective treatment can be established. One of the arts common to these various forms of assessment is the ability to observe the patient's reactions to the assessment itself. An astute observer will constantly modify the evaluation, based on the reactions of the patient, in order to derive maximum information. Ofttimes, the very portions of the evaluation showing specific dysfunctions are the bases for the therapies that ensue. Indeed, the instruments of testing may become the instruments of treatment.

As our experience and expertise in assessment grow, an increasing standardization of methodology is expected, which will allow legitimate comparisons of both spontaneous changes in function and treatment outcomes among institutions. Only then will the assessment of the head-injured patient have reached its full maturity as a science.

Section 5

TREATMENT APPROACHES

Chapter 22

STRATEGIES FOR IMPROVING MOTOR CONTROL

Arthur J. Nelson, Ph.D., R.P.T.

The major objectives of this chapter are to identify several mechanisms involved in recovery from central nervous system (CNS) injury and to formulate some conceptual models for physical therapy that form the bases for strategies to improve motor control in the head-injured adult. Some techniques that derive from the conceptual models are presented.

MECHANISMS OF RECOVERY FROM CENTRAL NERVOUS SYSTEM LESIONS

In a comprehensive review of major concepts of recovery from CNS lesions, Johnson and Almi[1] identify eight major mechanisms: (1) diaschisis (shock), (2) equipotentiality, (3) vicarious function, (4) behavioral substitution, (5) functional reorganization, (6) denervation supersensitivity, (7) collateral sprouting, and (8) regeneration of damaged neurons.

DIASCHISIS OR CEREBRAL SHOCK

The profound attenuation of function that accompanies trauma to the brain may, at times, completely resolve spontaneously. Recovery following diaschisis, then, is simply the re-emergence of temporarily attentuated function. Treatment effects should not be attributed to recovery that occurs spontaneously. However, it seems appropriate to maintain joint and muscle flexibility and the integrity of the patient's skin while awaiting this phase of spontaneous recovery.

EQUIPOTENTIALITY

The mechanism of equipotentiality has been attributed to Lashley,[2] who postulated that deficits from lesions of the cerebral cortex are mostly influenced by the size of the lesion and not its location. He believed there was considerable redundancy of cortical tissue and therefore when a lesion destroyed some tissue, remaining tissue was capable of assuming its function. Whereas Lashley postulated that there was no localized function, Myers[3] demonstrated that cats showed interhemispheric transfer of learning when the corpus callosum was intact, but transfer learning did not occur when it was sectioned. Therefore, focal lesions on the cortex may not eliminate a behavior, as there may be engrams of the learning impressed on the opposite side or in diverse areas of the cortex.

VICARIOUS FUNCTION

Removal of the left hemisphere in children who have not attained speech is an illustration of vicarious function whereby they subsequently attain speech. It is evident that they are "speaking" with the remaining right cortex. However, more comprehensive and detailed analysis of their speech reveals subtle deficits. Furthermore, such functions as space and depth perception, motor planning, and other attributes of the right hemisphere are deficient. Apparently, "taking on" the function of speech must sacrifice the proficiency of other functions already housed in the right hemisphere.

BEHAVIORAL SUBSTITUTION

Behavioral substitution or "tricks" are quite similar to vicarious function but require careful analysis to delineate when a substitute behavior is taking place. Gazzinaga[4] notes that the right cerebrovascular accident (CVA) victims who appear capable of form discrimination (e.g., cubes, spheres, circles) are no longer capable of these discriminations when confronted with shapes formulated by twisting wire into a particular configuration. He explains that the wire configurations cannot be verbalized or reduced to calculations, whereas the familiar shapes can; therefore, the left cortex only appears to produce form discrimination and is actually engaging in a type of "trick" or behavioral substitution.

Another example of behavioral substitution offered by Goldberger[5] is the phenomenon of recovery from forced grasping resulting from premotor (area 6) lesions in Rhesus monkeys. He notes that it appears as though the monkey is able to inhibit the grasping, but the animal is actually using active extension of the fingers (avoidance reaction) because a second lesion to the parietal region (areas 5 and 7) produces a return of forced grasping that is never eliminated. In functional terms, extension of the fingers produces a reciprocal inhibition of the flexors, which is a substitution (or trick) for inhibition of the grasp per se.

FUNCTIONAL REORGANIZATION

For many years it was believed that the CNS in mammals was incapable of regeneration. There is recent evidence of collateral sprouting from one pathway to the septal muscles of rats when the other pathway is interrupted.[6]

Another example of neuronal plasticity is demonstrated by Bechterew's nystagmus. Acute labyrinthectomy results in nystagmus (among other symptoms) for several weeks, which finally disappears. Damage to the second labyrinth produces nystagmus opposite to that of the previous damage. A bilateral labyrinthectomy produces no nystagmus; therefore, one must assume the single-stage operation results in functional reorganization.[7]

SUPERSENSITIVITY OF DENERVATION

A form of transmitter supersensitivity has been recognized in peripheral nerve injuries as acetylcholine administered to denervated skeletal muscle results in contraction or fibrillation. Eccles and McIntyre[8] found post-tetanic potentiation lasting several hours in chronically deafferented animals. It has been suggested that the postsynaptic membrane becomes hypersensitive to the transmitters usually liberated there, which results in hyperactivity of the pathway distal to the postsynaptic area. This might explain some of the increased responsiveness to stretch in some spastic persons who do not also have increased activity in the fusimotor efferents to the muscle spindles.

COLLATERAL SPROUTING

Hypersensitivity of denervated skeletal muscle to acetylcholine is usually followed by the attraction of sprouts from adjacent intact axons. It appears that the hypersensitivity may actually be an attractant for this collateral sprouting, and spontaneous fibrillation typically decreases with reinnervation.[9]

REGENERATION

The formulation of permanent memory storage in the CNS has been attributed by some[10,11] to be the result of structural change involving the interaction of oligodendroglial cells, neural cells, and ribonucleic acid (RNA) molecules derived from deoxyribonucleic acid (DNA) coding. Initially, the potentiation of synaptic transmission by repeated stimuli results in eventual dendritic growth and new formation of axonic boutons terminaux in posterior root axons in the segments below a spinal transection.[7] This would imply that if a motor behavior is to become part of a person's long-term memory storage system, it would require not hundreds but thousands and thousands of repetitions. Kottke[12] notes in the motor restoration of persons with CNS lesions that hundreds of repetitions of a behavior are relatively meaningless and the only meaningful number of repetitions would be in the millions. Nevertheless, Schneider[13] has demonstrated neural growth in brain-injured hamsters, but the regrowth frequently resulted in abnormal behavior patterns.

PRINCIPLES OF IMPROVING MOTOR CONTROL

The principles of physical therapy for head-injured patients may be applied to those with severe injuries during the early, acute phase of care and to head-injured patients after the comatose stage when greatest recovery of function may be expected.

MANAGEMENT DURING THE ACUTE PHASE

Bed Positioning

The acute, "comatose" patient with severe head injury must be positioned appropriately to provide for optimal joint and muscle function should recovery of movement take place. Passive range of motion should be rendered as a source of maintaining flexibility as well as a source of central stimulation. Respiratory care is an essential for continued improvement. Sensory stimulation is one component of care for the semicomatose patient that may have some benefit, but there is only subjective evidence in its support.

Positioning becomes an important consideration in the obtunded or comatose patient. The alterations in position may be varied from side-to-side to supine. The knees should not be propped on a pillow so that knee flexion contractures do not develop, and the foot and ankle may be kept in a posterior splint to preserve ankle dorsiflexion. The splints should be removed at frequent intervals for observation of skin changes. The use of a foot board is not advocated as the patient is frequently moved away from the foot board during nursing care and the foot would drop into plantar flexion position as a result. The side-lying position requires placement of a pillow between the knees to prevent ulceration at bony prominences. A functional position of the hand can be maintained by simply placing a rolled-up face cloth between the thumb and second fingers much as a handle might be placed in the palm of the hand. A small tab of tape or a loop of Velcro might be applied on either end to assure that it stays in place.

Passive Range of Movement

While the patient is unresponsive to commands and may only respond minimally to painful stimuli, passive range of movement is mandatory to preserve continuity of joint surfaces and flexibility of tendons and muscles. Ruch and Patton[7] indicate that passive movement in primates is a significant input source for stimulation of pyramidal tract neurons and is rated as equal to that of spontaneous conditioned responses in those neurons. Similarly, Brodal[14] indicated that the separation of mind and body following a cerebrovascular accident at age 63 was considerably relieved through the passive range-of-movement exercises given by the physical therapist. The impact that passive range of movement may have in a semicomatose patient may be only speculated on; however, logic would dictate that one should make an attempt to provide some input to the system.

Respiratory Function

As the head-injured patient may have considerable difficulty with adequate respiratory activity, passive assistance of rib movement may be of some value; positioning the patient so that gravity assists postural drainage of the bronchial tree may also prove of some limited value. Should the patient be capable of following commands, teaching the patient to cough with some depth would obviously be of some help. As Jennett and Teasdale[15] indicate, the accumulation of secretions and the subsequently decreased ventilation are significant problems in the head-injured patient. This may be particularly compounded if the patient had sustained a chest injury with the head injury, further compromising ventilation.

Sensory Stimulation

The obtunded patient may derive some benefit from specific patterns of sensory stimulation. The application of rough toweling and/or brushing, or the application of ice to various surfaces in the patterns is advocated by Rood.[16] No controlled studies to date have attested to the validity of this procedure. However, on the premise that it is impossible to evoke a voluntary response, the only available resource appears to be that of applying sensory stimuli to the organism. A fine brush may be applied over areas such as the extensors at the elbow, the extensors of the wrist and fingers, and the dorsiflexors and evertors of the foot and ankle, as these areas tend to suffer the greatest deficit of motor activity. Further response may be obtained by tapping over the muscle or its tendon to elicit a muscle stretch response.

As noted previously, it would be quite probable that movement would be initially discerned in response to pain. The next response one might encounter would be the response to proprioceptive stimulation such as muscle stretch response. Following the cutaneous stimulation with brushing, or the use of ice stroking, one would apply a brisk muscle stretch and attempt to elicit active movement.

Axial Rotation of the Trunk

During the positioning of the patient in the side-lying posture, some attempts should be made to rotate the thorax on the pelvis during these sessions to bring about a breaking up of the "log-rolling" effect of trunk movement. The rotatory movement of the thorax on the pelvis is associated with more highly elaborated movements and indeed may assist in later training of the patient should more recovery occur. Once the patient can be moved more readily, gentle rocking side-to-side with pivoting of the thorax on the trunk or pivoting of the neck on the thorax followed by pivoting of the leg and pelvis on the thorax could be employed to attempt to stimulate some movement of the limbs in response to the truncal rotation patterns.

SUBACUTE PHASE (POSTCOMATOSE PATIENT)

The subacute phase may commence at a variable length of time following the acute episode and is usually characterized as the emergence from cerebral shock (diaschisis). The first manifestation of emergence from this shock-like state is the appearance of some deep tendon-jerk responses, usually in flexors of the arm and the extensor muscles of the leg.

These deep tendon-jerk responses may be used to facilitate voluntary response if the patient is capable of responding to commands. However, it should be underscored that proprioceptive stimulation is usually the result of motor behavior and not the cause of that behavior. To be more specific, when one steps forward with one leg during walking, the quadriceps muscle contracts and the muscle stretch response increases. Not only is the load anticipated, but also the particular length of the muscle is established. Should the individual step instead into a hole, the load will be considerably increased, owing to the increase in momentum and distance that the person has traveled. Consequently, the muscle will undergo a stretch, activating spindle afferents that facilitate the anterior horn cells to "catch up" by producing muscular contraction proportional to the "error." In this vein, the receptor functioning can be seen as a type of error detector that responds to deviation from an expected activity pattern. Thus, proprioceptive stimulation would be more appropriate to apply during activity, not to initiate the activity if the therapeutic session is to duplicate the usual mode of CNS function.

Another mode of sensory input would come from cutaneous input. It may be noted that touch applied to the dorsum of the foot during flexion typically enhances flexion of the patient's extremity. Conversely, touch applied to the dorsum of the foot during the extension phase decreases the extension. Touching the patient on the foot during the appropriate movement would serve to facilitate the action, but one must consider the practical limitation of this form of stimulation not being available except during formal therapeutic sessions.

As noted by Landau,[17] the patient with a CNS lesion develops two major categories of difficulties. The first may be termed the negative one, in which there is a deficiency of output recognized in the motor system as weakness or loss of motor power. The second would be positive symptoms such as increased muscle stretch response and/or adventitious movements or other involuntary movements such as dystonic posturing.

In patients with cortical lesions, one might anticipate three deficits: (1) the loss of power, that is, inability to develop tension rapidly; (2) difficulty in attaining the right degree of power; and (3) the inability to release that tension rapidly so that the opposite muscle group may take over (Fig. 22-1). As voluntary movement is the most difficult type of movement for a head-injured patient, it is unlikely that training can overcome all three of these deficiencies. As an alternative, movement is elicited through rapid vestibular stimulation, since it permits fairly rapid action that more closely resembles voluntary movement in rate of tension development.

The vestibular system has two major components, a so-called "static" component and a more dynamic component. The static one is most explicitly demonstrated by the tonic labyrinthine responses, which are largely postural in nature. The dynamic component is evident in the righting responses that require movement of the head through space, with its

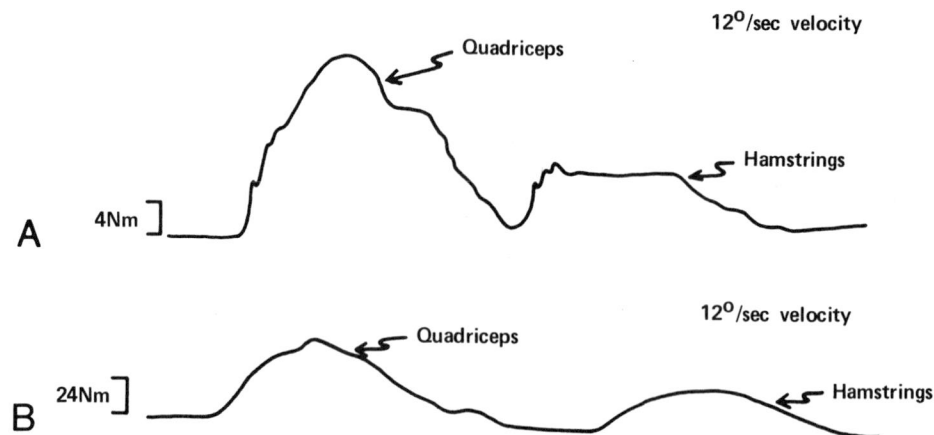

FIGURE 22-1. The isokinetic torque developed in reciprocation at 12 degrees per second velocity. The first curve is the torque developed by the quadriceps, while the second is developed by the hamstrings. (A) Isokinetic torque curves of acute hemiparetic. (B) Isokinetic torque curves of chronic hemiparetic.

subsequent acceleration and deceleration, which results in fairly rapid limb adjustments known as righting responses.

Because many head-injured patients demonstrate a loss of dynamic action, it would seem more appropriate to use this form of vestibular stimulation as the major input. Dynamic vestibular stimulation is most readily applied in younger patients by the use of a large ball over which the patient is suspended. Two persons attend and rock the patient to and fro, side to side, and in an oblique and circular fashion in increasing arcs to increase the patient's rate of movement response. Should the use of a beach ball be too complex or present a risk to the patient, a rocking chair or simply sitting on the edge of a plinth or table in which both feet can be placed on the floor could also serve the purpose for stimulating the patient by shifting the patient to and fro and from side to side (Fig. 22-2).

Weight-shifting may also be done with a patient in an all-fours position or an on-knees position if other injuries or disabilities do not interfere. A stimulation should be intense enough to initiate a response that is appropriate to the needs of preserving the individual's alignment in space. Should it be too strong and overcome the patient, the response becomes maladaptive. Therefore, the stimulus should be brought back to the level at which an appropriate limb motion was obtained. This should then be repeated until the person can expand to a further range at a later time. By pairing the unconditioned righting response with either verbal or cutaneous cues, it may eventually be possible to elicit responses without the vestibular stimulus.

Linking Vestibular Stimulation to Voluntary Movement

Once movement has been initiated by vestibular stimulation, it should be immediately linked to the person's conscious perception of that movement and an attempt made to duplicate the action or at least to participate in voluntary activity that stimulates it. For instance, if shifting the patient sideways on a plinth results in extension of the arm and a propping-type reaction, the patient may then be asked to discern whether he or she feels the movement or not and, if so, if the patient can now push on the arm and duplicate the extension pattern. It is important not to ask the patient to initiate the activity voluntarily. The patient may do so in a laborious fashion or invoke the more primitive mechanisms, which are often readily avail-

STRATEGIES FOR IMPROVING MOTOR CONTROL

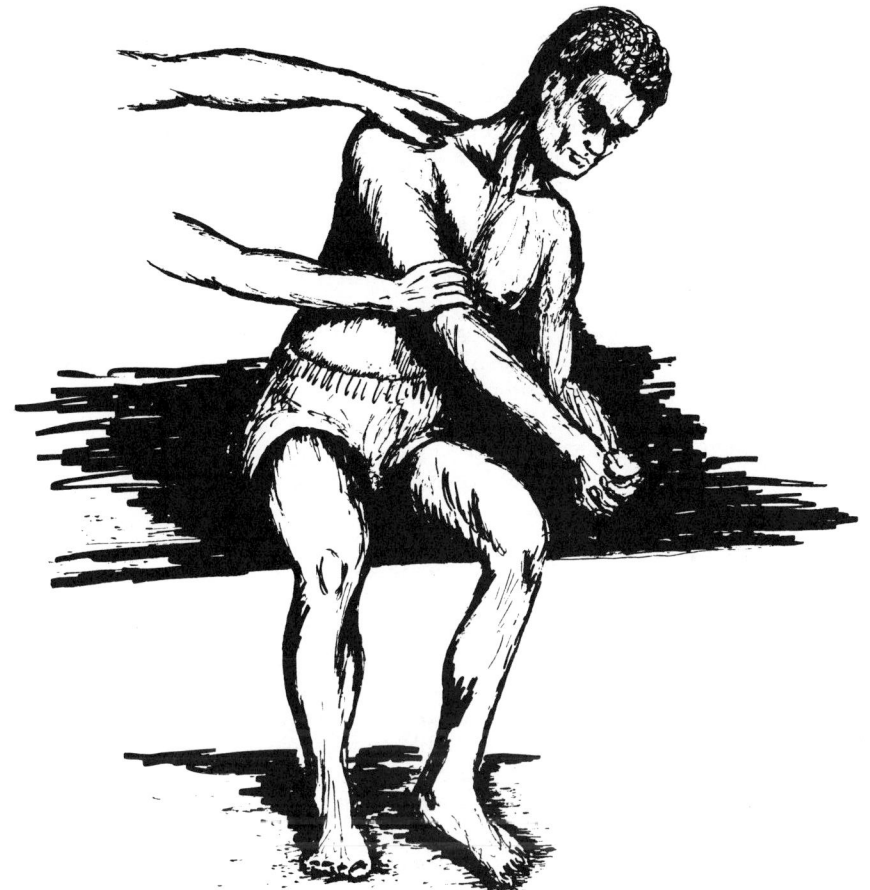

FIGURE 22-2. Weight-shifting in seated position. The patient with a left hemiparesis in this illustration is tilted to the left and, with hands folded, attempts to prop himself for support. The therapist shifts the trunk by lifting under the right buttock and left axilla. The goal is to distribute weight to the left buttock.

able. The speed and range of movement may be gradually increased, as a sudden imposition of movement may be overwhelming, resulting in excessive muscle activity that may actually produce a dystonia or spastic fixation.

The sequence of developing transition from stimulated movement or triggered responses to voluntary ones should progress from neck and trunk rotation, to propping responses of the upper extremity, and then to movements of the legs in response to weight shifting in the seated and standing positions. The first pattern of rotating the head and neck, controlling the trunk, and subsequent limb movements can begin in the supine position. Then the patient moves to the prone position for propping reactions or pushing off and rotating to each side, progresses to the all-fours position to perform the same head and neck rotations, flex one arm, and extend the other, and then reverses the movement. Finally, the pattern is done in the seated position on the edge of a treatment table or mat, at which point the person would rotate to one side, placing both hands on the side of the opposite leg, and reverse again to the opposite side, placing both hands on the one side (see Fig. 22-2).

The next group of training procedures would involve placing the feet flat on the floor and shifting the weight forward. The patient attempts to move toward the standing position, distributing equal weight on both feet, standing with the heels pressing firmly into the floor while the knees are in the process of extending. If the patient tends to place more weight on one side and extend both at the ankle and knee, the weight should be replaced over that extremity and the movement should involve extension of the knee with the ankle remaining in a dorsiflexed position, that is, the heels pressing against the surface.

To be more explicit, the simulation of weight shift and balance might begin with the subject seated, with legs over the edge of the bed. The therapist lifts under the shoulders or axilla, and also under the unaffected hip. This allows the patient to feel weight shift to the opposite side should the patient be loading equal weight on both sides. As the person shifts forward, this shift should be maintained over the affected limb in preparation for standing. Some head-injured patients have a tendency to extend excessively at the hips and therefore are not able to assume an erect seated posture. If this is the case, it might be desirable to have the patient lean on the forearms with a table or tray placed under the forearms to support the trunk, while the patient extends the neck. If, however, the tension remains excessive or there are muscle contractures, this would not be feasible. Work must then be directed toward stretching the contractures and developing an adequate range of hip flexion to permit an erect seated position. It is desirable to eventually have the person assume a 90-degree position of thighs on trunk so that the semireclining posture is avoided.

Stimulation of Weight Shift and Standing Balance

The beginning of standing balance takes place when the patient is seated on the edge of the table or chair. Both feet should rest squarely on the floor; if one limb is affected more than the other, it should be placed further back than the other. Next, the person should be encouraged to shift weight forward with the therapist assisting by lifting up and forward under the axilla on the affected side. The patient should shift forward actively as much as possible while continued pressure is applied against the entire surface of the foot; the heel should not lift, especially during the early phase of gait training (Fig. 22-3).

Stimulation of Weight Bearing in the Upright Position

Once the patient is capable of moving from the seated position, the emphasis should be placed on the ability to shift weight from side to side while standing. It has been observed that normal individuals initiate locomotion by decreasing stiffness in the calf muscles, thereby allowing the trunk and legs to shift forward. Because the stiffness in the calf muscles is somewhat asymmetric, the shift occurs to one side more than the other. Training patients to be able to release calf tension might be facilitated by use of electromyographic (EMG) feedback instrumentation. The emphasis in this instance would be placed on the ability to decrease the EMG discharge in calf msucles as rapidly as possible. Furthermore, one might emphasize a differential release of calf tension by having the individual release one calf faster and to a greater degree than the other, thereby assuring the oblique shift of body weight to the opposite side.

The EMG feedback may be done with the person in the supine position, using resistance against the therapist's hands; as the EMG output decreases, the patient could note the sensation associated with this decreased output. By substituting the supine for the upright position, the patient is not initially concerned about factors such as aligning the body in space while attempting to control the tension in the calf muscles. Once the patient has assumed the standing position, the EMG feedback could continue as a means of testing the transfer of this ability from the more secure position to the standing position. Eventually, it is hoped that the patient could accomplish this relaxation by use of conscious proprioceptive sensibilities within the muscles themselves. With the reduction in tension in the calf muscles, the individual is

STRATEGIES FOR IMPROVING MOTOR CONTROL

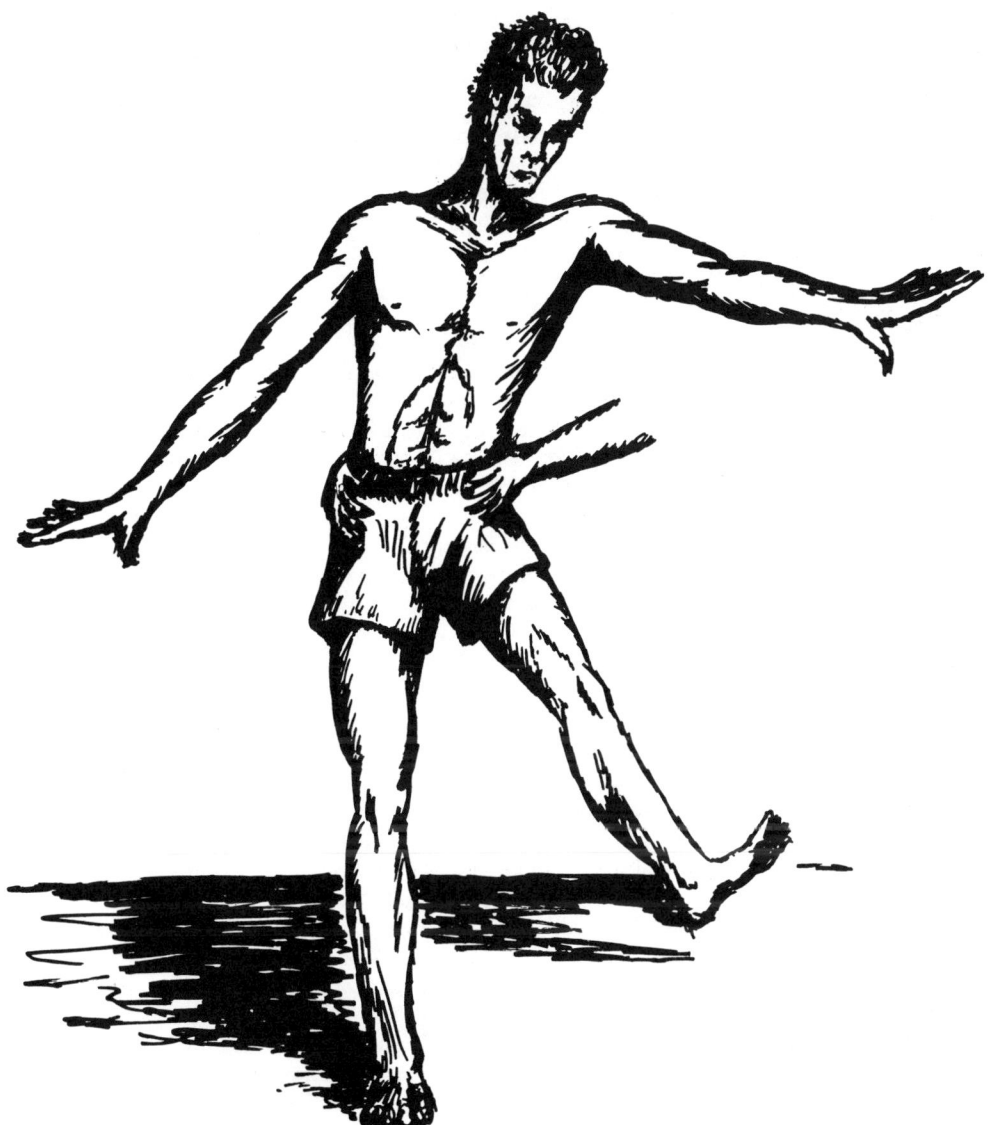

FIGURE 22-3. Balance reactions in the standing position. During upright stance, the patient may be suddenly shifted from side to side and the adjustments of the limbs observed. A normal response of upper and lower limbs is illustrated; however, a head-injured patient may make inappropriate adjustments by narrowing the base of support.

expected to shift forward and obliquely to one side, at which point the leg should swing up underneath the pelvis to move into position to accept weight. At that point, the heel should come in contact with the floor, and the person should accept the weight on the leg mainly by using hip extensors and not permitting the knee to go into full extension.

As the normal individual demonstrates an ability to shift weight and initiate locomotor patterns rapidly, it is desirable to attain as rapid a weight shift and movement of the patient as possible so that one may invoke patterns similar to those previously engaged in by the patient. For practical purposes, this means the person should be able to attain a set speed, that is, to be able to go through one cycle in approximately 1 to 1.5 seconds by the second step. As this rapid movement of the legs might pose some threat to a patient, it is desirable to practice these rapid, alternating movements of the legs in a secure, controlled environment.

The isokinetic device known as the Kinetron is designed with two pedal-like arrangements that can be set for a range of speeds that correspond to those used in locomotion (ranging from rather slow to fairly rapid movements). There is also a seat whose height and depth are modifiable depending on the degree of trunk control the patient has. The seat also has a belt to hold the person in place and arm rests to provide additional support, if necessary (Fig. 22-4). The use of the Kinetron is described below.

Bilateral Reciprocal Training Program

The training of the patient should proceed by increasing the rate of limb movements while the rhythm is maintained. The amount of force the legs expend is deliberately restricted. The dials that indicate pressure on the pedals should be set so that the individual does not exceed 100 pounds per square inch. The purpose of restricting the force exerted is to place the emphasis on quickness of leg movement. If the individual stresses force, there may be a tendency to decrease rather than increase the velocity of movement. The isokinetic device develops what is termed an accommodating resistance; that is, resistance is not offered until the individual matches and starts to exceed the speed of the setting on the device. In the early stages, it may be necessary to set the speed quite slow so that the individual will develop some resistance to the movement and therefore have a sense of pressure developed in response to the movement.

The use of the limb load monitor developed by the Krusen Rehabilitation Research Center is useful at this stage for augmenting the sensory responses of pressure on the feet. Should the person have one side unaffected more than the other, it is obvious that the unaffected or less affected side would be capable of higher velocities of movement. Therefore, one must stress increased velocities on the affected side and decreased velocities on the unaffected side.

The emphasis in early training should be on symmetry of performance and the development of a good rhythmic exchange between the extremities during this activity. As the affected part is capable of attaining greater velocity, which would be indicated by attaining the maximum allowed of 100 pounds per square inch on each dial, the speed may then be advanced from a setting of 3 to 4. This progression takes place as soon as the patient is capable of responding with symmetry of movement in terms of speed, arc of movement, and the amount of pressure exerted on each extremity. The symmetry of rhythm might be further enhanced by the use of a metronome or other sources of constant rhythm.

The goal of this particular training would be to develop reciprocal movements that approximate the normal 1-second cycle time from heel-strike to heel-strike of one extremity. Therefore, one may test the device using a stop watch, simply timing the individual moving from the foot-down position on one side to the foot-down position on the same side; when this approaches 1 second, it would be considered to be an appropriate rate. Obviously, both limbs should be moving at the same rate. Simultaneous with the progression of rate of movement would be the continual elevation of the seat to the point that the individual is practically standing in the device. As early as possible, the patient should be stimulated to rotate the pelvis forward and back during the bilateral reciprocating movement of the leg. This may be stimulated by stretch and/or pressure applied by the therapist's hands to the pelvic brim during the reciprocating movements of the legs by the patient.

In the early phase, the flaccid patient may have difficulty developing sufficient output on the affected side. Therefore, one may employ counterweights on the opposite lever arm. This counterweight would assist the affected limb moving downward by pressing the pedal

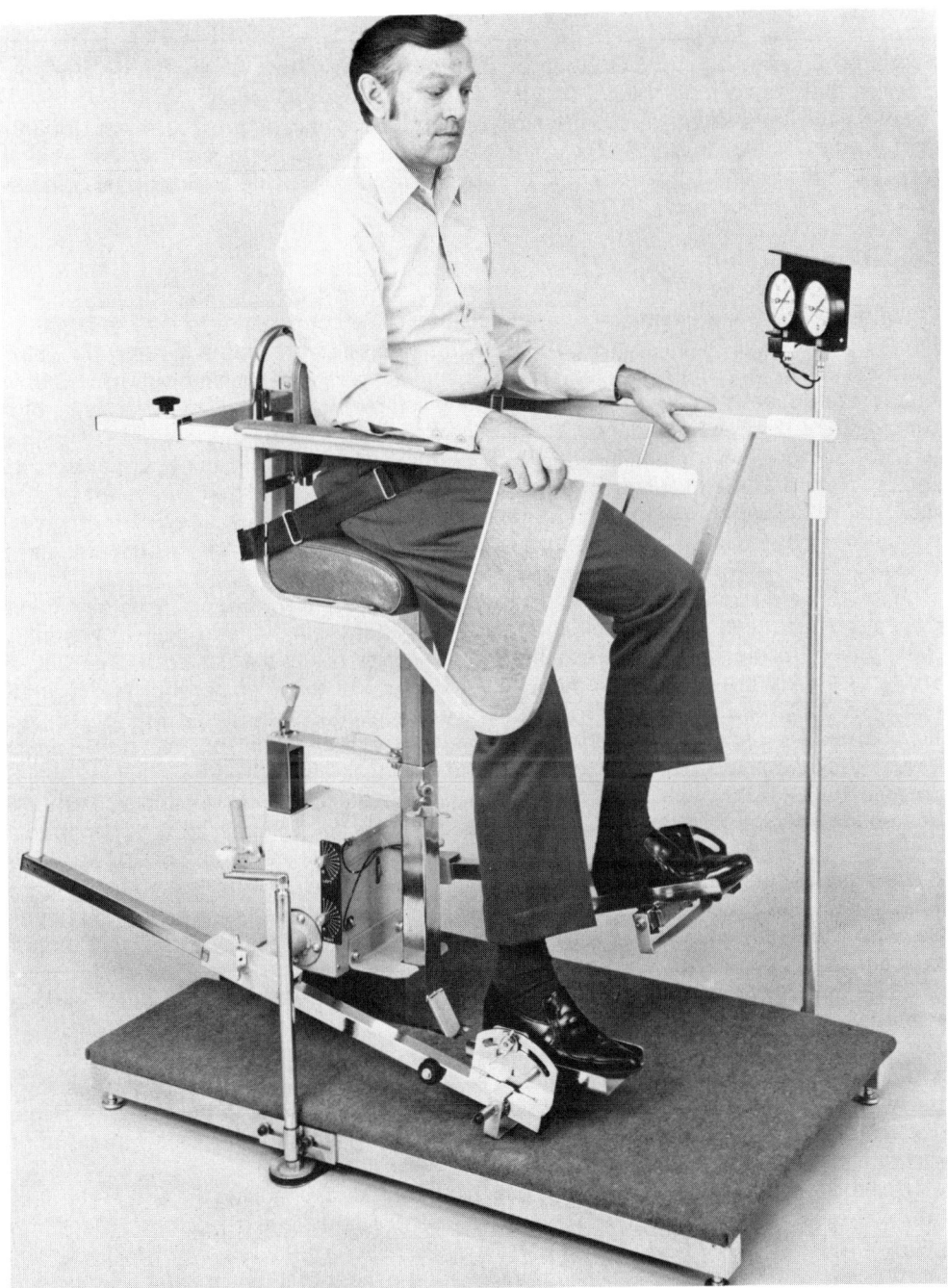

FIGURE 22-4. The Kinetron is an isokinetic device to permit training in bilateral movements that simulate lower extremity action during ambulation. The velocity of each foot lever may be set at the same speed or at a different speed.

on the opposite side in an upward direction. As improvement takes place, obviously less weight may be placed in counterbalancing this effect. The emphasis is always toward development of symmetry in speed and the amount of force exerted by each of the limbs during the reciprocating movement. It is preferred that the patient's arms not be on the arm rest of the device, but rather hang relaxed on each side during the movements. While this may not be possible in some patients due to insecurity, it should become the goal, as placing too much weight on the unaffected side would disrupt the symmetry of the movement. For later ambulation, use of the arms during locomotor movements may provide an additional confounding factor.

Ambulation Training

Once a patient has attained a rate of movement that corresponds to the 1-second cycle time, gait training out of the Kinetron may commence. It is preferable to start this training without the use of a cane or parallel bars. The major reason for training without the use of parallel bars or cane is to keep the weight shifting symmetric and to keep movements of the lower extremities in correspondence with those of the upper extremity. Should the patient's balance be so poor that the patient cannot support himself or herself without upper extremity propping, there is some question as to whether the training program should revert to developing balance before progressing to gait training. If it is elected that gait training progress at this time, emphasis should be placed upon maximum weight bearing on both sides in an alternating, even fashion.

Should the patient's reciprocating movements be sufficiently rapid and their vertical alignment be adequate, it is desirable to require the patient to move as rapidly as possible so that the patient may approach the usual rate of progression that the patient had prior to the injury. This usually means an attainment of velocity of less than 1.6 seconds per cycle: the time it takes to go from heel-strike of one foot to heel-strike of the same foot during locomotion. Should a patient be capable of this velocity of movement on one side only, the emphasis should again be placed upon symmetry of movement, not on rapidity per se. It has been my experience that hemiparetic patients, when achieving this velocity, appear to improve dramatically and lose many of the characteristic gait deviations associated with hemiparesis. There may be other adaptations as well, but it becomes obvious that a normal subject walking at a slow rate of progression invokes many adaptations in gait that in many evaluations of locomotion are classified as abnormalities of gait. Should a patient with a CNS lesion invoke these adaptations, it does not seem warranted to classify them as abnormalities. Therefore, in slow ambulation, one should anticipate encountering these adaptations, but other changes such as asymmetry or loss of rhythm should be underscored and training instituted to eliminate the loss of symmetry.

As soon as feasible, the rate of progression should be increased, but rate should not take precedence over rhythm and symmetry of movement. Thus the patient should not be instructed to "walk as fast as possible," but rather the rate should be progressively increased by the therapist when it is apparent that the patient can tolerate the increase without undue loss of rhythm and symmetry.

This may be effected by holding the patient about the waist, taking the arm and running it around the therapist's waist, and holding the patient's hand in a position of extension of the fingers, external rotation of the shoulder, and supination of the forearm.[18] While walking in this position, the therapist should attempt to get the patient to track on him or her, and the therapist should be careful not to assume the abnormal rhythm of the patient. This is especially true if patients are being ambulated by aides in maintenance or endurance gait training programs.

Frequently patients will dramatically improve their locomotion during this "training program." It appears that the motion is improving as a result of eliciting patterns that were already present in the undamaged nervous system and simply had to be stimulated. The principal aspect of training would be to develop in the individual the capacity to elicit this motor program at will. Once the ambulation pattern is rapidly formed, another requirement would be to rapidly terminate this pattern. Head-injured patients may have difficulty terminating the walking behavior. This may be looked upon as a type of perseveration. Thus, the therapist may practice the initiation, the proper execution, and the termination of locomotion on command or on the presentation of a certain stimulus to place the pattern in an operant conditioning format. More research is needed to determine what factors may be involved in triggering the normal subject to terminate movement. Is it the active contraction of opposing muscles or simply the inhibition of the active muscles that leads to cessation of the activity pattern?

In the group of patients that may not attain rapid locomotion, certain key factors should be considered. First, the emphasis in training should be on good dynamic alignment and control, the maintenance of good rhythm and rate of movement, and balanced output from each side of the body. Particular attention should be paid to movements of the pelvis, as the leg will move in synchrony with it. For example, the speed of leg movement cannot be increased without increasing the rate of pelvic rotation. If the pelvis remains retracted, the leg will tend to externally rotate. Similarly, the pelvis should not remain advanced, as this would lead to an internally rotated leg and possibly "scissoring." Emphasis should therefore be placed on the rotation of the pelvis that corresponds with the movement of the advancing and supporting limb. It may be necessary to perform this movement manually for the patient in the early phases, but the ultimate goal would be to have the person attain this rotation actively without assistance.

In addition to training in forward locomotion, the patient should be instructed on methods of sidestepping to each side, and also should be able to step backward. It is necessary to step to one side to avoid oncoming people or objects. In addition, it may be necessary to step backward, for instance, when opening a door. It has been my experience that these movements are considerably more difficult to evoke in a patient with a CNS lesion than is forward locomotion.

Effectiveness of Bilateral Reciprocal Isokinetic Exercise

The effectiveness of bilateral reciprocal isokinetic (Kinetron) versus conventional programs of training hemiparetics was investigated in a study of 34 hemiparetic patients at three health-care facilities (Kessler's Institute for Rehabilitation, Mercer Hospital, and Eger Nursing Home).

Hemiparetic patients were randomly assigned either to conventional physical therapy or to bilateral reciprocal isokinetic (BRI) training. The BRI group received training on the Kinetron with the objective of attaining a velocity close to that found in preferred locomotion in normal subjects (i.e., cycle time of 1.5 seconds or less), whereas the conventional treatment group received reciprocal exercise to both legs applied with manual contact by the therapists. Both groups received gait training in addition to the specialized training noted, and each subject was given 20 training sessions.

On the basis of pretreatment and post-treatment scores for balance, ambulation, velocity, and dynamic weight shifting (in place), the BRI group revealed significant increase in unilateral stance (both limbs), velocity of ambulation, and ability to rapidly shift weight and step from one foot to the other (Fig. 22-5).

In a retrospective study of 12 head-injured hemiparetic patients in an active rehabilitation program using the Kinetron for training, it was found that the five left hemiparetics had a

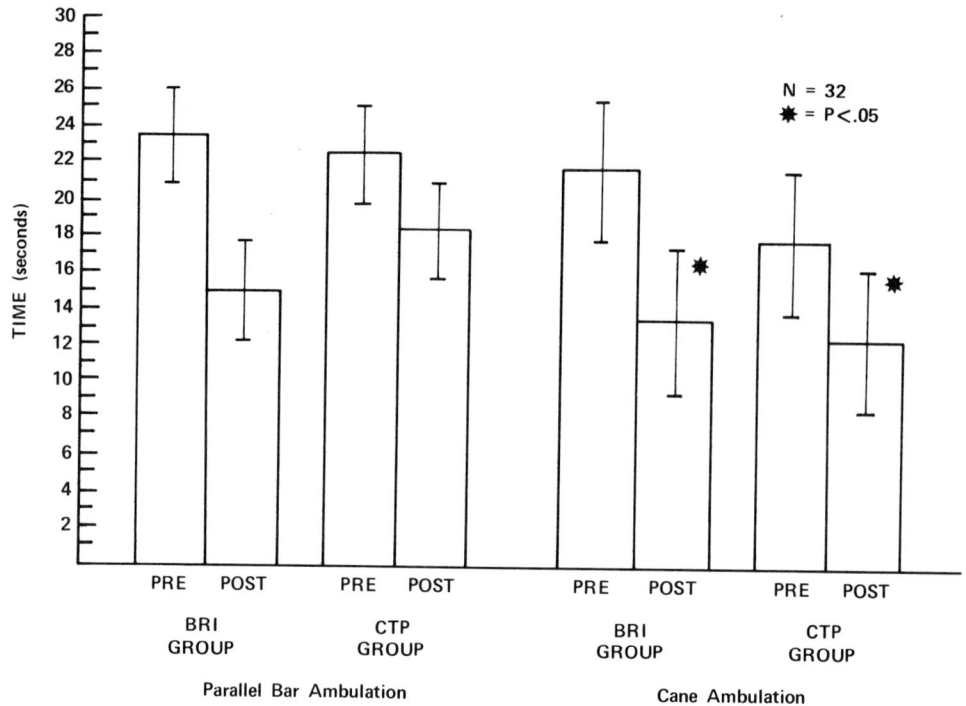

FIGURE 22-5. Comparison of ambulation velocity of 32 hemiparetic patients after two training approaches: bilateral reciprocal isokinetic (BRI) training of 4 weeks (20 sessions) and conventional training program (CTP) of same duration and number of sessions. Both groups revealed improved velocity, but the BRI improvement was significant at the .05 level of confidence.

lower average initial functional ambulation profile (FAP)[19] score and a lower discharge score than the seven right hemiparetics (Tables 22-1, 22-2).

Closer analysis revealed that those patients with low FAP scores also had higher ratings for primitive motor behaviors on the motor inventory and had poorer motor planning and body schema than those with higher scores. The small numbers in the study precluded statistical analysis. The goal of future training would be directed toward further improvement of motor power, especially extension to increase the thrust and step length bilaterally, without producing a distortion of the symmetry already present.

By closer analysis of the components of the FAP score, it may be possible to uncover the source of deficient locomotion and establish a training program to meet that need. Lack of muscular power would be evident to the physical therapist when the linear attainment (step length) is deficient.

Motor Control of the Upper Limb

Bobath[18] suggests that control of the upper limb starts with rotation about the midline whereby the pelvis rotates on the thorax and vice versa. Nashner[20] indicates that movements of the upper extremity, responding to perturbations, result in electromyographic (EMG) actions in the trunk and lower extremities prior to those found in the upper extremities. Therefore, in the supine position, the patient should be positioned in such a way that the pelvis and

TABLE 22-1. Traumatic Left Hemiparetic Functional Ambulation Profile Scores.
(Five left hemiparetics revealed an average initial FAP score of 33 and a discharge FAP score of 47.8. The average number of days of care was 70.)

Subject	Age	Sex	Race	Onset to Admit	Length of Stay	Initial FAP*	Discharge FAP*	Change FAP*
8	25	M	W	63	35	71	88	+17
9	22	F	W	250	95	0	3	+3
10	54	M	B	92	55	37.5	78.5	+41
11	19	F	W	108	107	1	41.5	+40.5
12	26	M	W	408	59	56	28	−28
$\bar{X}$	29.2	—	—	184	70.2	33.1	47.8	+14
$SE_{\bar{x}}$	6.31	—	—	64.58	13.35	14.32	15.80	7.24

*FAP = Functional Ambulation Profile Score (100 maximum)

thorax are asymmetric and then asked to attempt to realign them. It is important to determine the position from which the patient can initiate axial rotation. Emphasis should be placed on strengthening those movements that are the weakest so as to match the more effective ones.

Once the patient can roll over from supine to prone forearm rest position, a bolster or several large pillows may be placed under the chest of the patient to support some of the weight, permitting the elbows and upper arm to form a right-angle position. Movements of the arms may be stimulated by shifting the person diagonally or from side to side, to attain active movement as previously described. Once the person attains movement in one position of the arm, its position may be altered to a different angle with the thorax. The person should

TABLE 22-2. Traumatic Right Hemiparetic Functional Ambulation Profile Scores.
(Seven right hemiparetics revealed an initial FAP score of 61.5 and a discharge FAP score of 68.7. The average number of days of care was 64.)

Subject	Age	Sex	Race	Onset to Admit	Length of Stay	Initial FAP*	Discharge FAP*	Change FAP*
1	23	M	W	70	92	70	84	+14
2	51	M	W	886	70	24.5	15.8	−8.7
3	18	M	W	178	72	78.5	71.5	−7.0
4	36	M	W	63	62	77	91	+14
5	17	F	W	78	30	75	78	+3
6	36	M	B	98	49	70	83	+13
7	41	M	W	32	71	36	57.5	+21.5
$\bar{X}$	31.71	—	—	200.7	63.7	61.57	68.68	+7.11
$SE_{\bar{x}}$	4.81	—	—	115.5	7.43	8.27	9.70	2.26

*FAP = Functional Ambulation Profile Score (100 maximum)

attempt to restabilize himself or herself with the arm in the new position. The patient is questioned as to the ability to "feel" that position and subsequently duplicate it.

This forearm rest position may also contribute to the production of conjugate eye movements.[16] The placement of a book or picture in the patient's line of view may facilitate reading while so positioned.

Stability of the forearm rest position may be enhanced through movement by pushing the patient's shoulders to either side, then forward and back. Oblique shifts are added later. When any movement is elicited, it should be followed up by the suggestion that the patient sense the movement and at the next occasion attempt to count while performing the movement. This would invoke the method suggested by Peto (see Clarke and Evans,[21] Carr and Shepherd,[22] and Cotton and Parnwell[23]), which is called the *rhythmic intention method*. For example, the therapist and patient verbalize together the movement taking place (i.e., "I am shifting weight to my right arm"); then counting is linked to the activity and continued until completed. If the whole movement is completed in association with verbalizing the intended pattern, counting need not be added. The components of a complex act are identified, and the person practices each component until mastered and then adds the next until the several components can be fitted together. An example would be the grasping of a glass of water, bringing it to the mouth, drinking, swallowing, and returning the glass to the original location. Each unit of movement would be broken down to its simplest components and each of these practiced separately until mastery is attained. Subsequently, all are fitted together in the total activity. Stability of the shoulder girdle and shoulders would be an important component involved in reaching for a glass.

With the patient in the side-lying position, the patient's arm is draped over the therapist's shoulder (near the neck), and the therapist has the patient slide the arm forward while mobilizing the scapula on the rib cage. Many patients may move only at the glenohumeral joint and not at the scapulothoracic junction because the scapular muscles may be in spasm. If the arm is forced into flexion without increasing scapular movement, the shoulder joint (glenohumeral) may become hypermobile. This may eventually result in further subluxation and pain.

Progression to elbow flexion and extension of raising and lowering the opened hand to the patient's forehead would be practiced next with the same simultaneous verbalization and rhythmic pattern. Once the patient holds the limb in a variety of alterations of posture, the limb is now ready for drill and many repetitions to perhaps effect an engram.[12] This aspect of training involves placing the arm or hand in many different positions and determining if the patient can hold that posture for several alterations.

The stability of the upper extremity may be further stimulated by weight shifting in the seated position. Here the patient is shifted from side to side while keeping head and neck aligned (not turning from side to side). The intention is to elicit arm movement that would lead to a propping or supporting action. The initial response may result in merely landing on the flexed arm, but the shifting should continue with the goal of extension of the elbow. The patient may verbally repeat along with the therapist and perform the action in a rhythmic fashion until the movement becomes a conditioned one.

Placing the patient's limb in a given posture, usually at 90 degrees of flexion or abduction to start with, and withdrawing support as advocated by Bobath[18] can be practiced repeatedly until a series of movements are attained for the major components of upper extremity actions. Producing action in the patient's limb is interrupting the process of learning not to use the arm on the affected side. The notion that the patient actively learns not to use the extremity has been tested by Yu,[24] who has restrained the unaffected extremity and simply placed the demand for action on the affected extremity. Lifting the arm forward and returning it were employed in a standard conditioned response format with the intrinsic reward of movement success as a reinforcement. He found that hemiparetic patients had increased movement as a result of this "forced" activity of the involved extremity.

Hand Activities

The pessimistic outlook for hand function frequently prevents the full expression of treatment effectiveness. This lack of hand function is especially evident in the hemiparetic patient, for this patient has one hand functioning and tends not to strive to regain function in the affected limb.[25]

Short of restraint of the functioning arm, therapy might be directed to bilateral tasks that accomplish a functional goal. For example, holding a large ball with two hands and rotating the ball can assist hand and arm function, especially as it progresses to smaller and smaller objects (still requiring bimanual manipulations). Much later, opening a sock to place on the foot would require both hands.

As many activities of the hand require palmar prehension, thumb and forefinger opposition and apposition should be practiced by the therapist, by holding the patient's hand and requesting duplication by the patient. This may be expanded to holding an object between thumb and forefingers and moving the wrist in extension and flexion while maintaining pinch. A substitute movement of crude grasp (with all fingers in hook-like pattern) should not be confused with the palmar prehension involved with pads of thumb and second and third fingers pinching together. In specific lesions of the motor cortex, Goldberger[26] suggests pincer grasp may not return and only a substitute pattern of gross grasp will be possible.

Forced grasping is another hand function disorder encountered in head-injured patients, especially in the early phase. Forced grasping or the inability to inhibit the finger and thumb flexors has been attributed to lesions in area 6 of Brodman by Goldberger. He notes Rhesus monkeys appear to recover the ability to release the grasp but do so by the substitute motion of actively extending the fingers and abducting the thumb. He finds that a second lesion in area 5 in the monkey voids the ability to release the grasp and the dual-lesioned animal never gains inhibition of the forced grasping. If this same substitution holds true for humans, it would appear that therapists should employ electromyographic feedback (EMG, FB) to the flexors to augment the sensory changes associated with relaxation of those flexors. This would be using the EMG, FB as an assist in training for inhibition of grasping. Should the patient not attain inhibitory control of the flexors, one might employ facilitation of the extensors to thereby effect reciprocal inhibition of the flexors. This might be accomplished via EMG, FB or through facilitation of the extensors by vibration, tapping, or electric stimulation.

Foot Control

While forced grasping is well established for the hand, it is not well understood in the foot. However, there is evidence to suggest that plantar stimulation and the excessively supinated foot (usually accompanied by an extended great toe) are correlated. Again, the use of EMG, FB during cutaneous stimulation of the plantar skin of the foot should prove helpful. The training goal would be to decrease EMG discharge with continued presentation of plantar stimuli. Should the patient not develop inhibition in 2 to 3 weeks, EMG, FB for the purpose of increasing activity in the evertors and pronators of the foot would be the substitute training goal (i.e., to reciprocally inhibit supination).

SUPPLEMENTAL TREATMENT

Many treatment supplements are available such as ice, vibration, or electric stimulation. A study of the beneficial effects of electric stimulation to extensors of the fingers has recently been reported. While this study employed low voltage, it is not possible to use high-voltage stimulation. I used the EGS High-Voltage Stimulator to assist in training of wrist and finger extension. A smaller, portable unit has been employed for more consistent application that employs a switch that stimulates the wrist and finger extensors when the elbow is extended.

A similar application has been made to electrically stimulate the dorsiflexors during gait to simulate the normal pattern of activity. The reports from Emory Rehabilitation Center suggest that there is carryover to increased activity (e.g., the person moves even though the current has been interrupted). To date, the high-voltage units have not been employed for this purpose, but it seems probable that they can provide a greater stimulus to activity than low-voltage generators.

I have also used high-voltage galvanism (EGS High-Voltage Galvanic Generator) in a pilot project as a cutaneous stimulation during training on the Kinetron. Ruch and Patton[7] note that cutaneous stimulation on the dorsum of the foot during flexion will enhance the flexion, while stimulation of the dorsum of the foot during extension will result in decreased extension. Conversely, stimulation on the plantar surface or even on the sural nerve (a cutaneous nerve) will increase the extensor movement. The key factor in this application is to provide an interruptor for current flow that is sequenced at the correct time in the limb movement cycle. This has been accomplished through the use of a mercury switch at the knee or a foot pressure switch in the heel of the opposite shoe. When the pressure is released on the opposite foot (with a switch), it turns the stimulus on, thereby synchronizing it with the extension movement.

Cryotherapy

The use of cold can be separated into two major categories: the brief application of ice and ice packs applied for longer periods of time.

BRIEF APPLICATION OF ICE. Application of an ice cube or ice pop to the surface of a limb has been advocated by Rood[16] and described more fully by Stockmeyer[27] (Fig. 22-6). It is obviously a strong stimulus to the skin and is purported to facilitate fusimotor discharge to the spindles when applied to the dermatome of the muscle in question. Unfortunately, although this has been clinically observed, it has not been documented in a controlled investigation to date. Rood indicates that ice applied to the radial extensor surface can be effective in improving grasp by increasing the spindle "bias" in those same muscles. She maintains that pinching an ice cube will improve grasp as well as release; however, she adds that quick ice application to the palm of the hand will increase spasticity. Clearly, those observations require further verification.

ICE PACKING. The application of crushed ice packs for spasticity has been advocated for many years,[28] as it has been associated with subjective evidence of relief of pain and spasticity according to Chambers.[29] However, Urbscheit and Bishop[30] reported an increase in motoneuron discharge, and Knutsson[31] reported no decrease in hypertonicity.

Ice packs have been applied to the spastic muscle by Turkish toweling covering the part. Generally it is advocated that the ice be applied for 20 to 30 minutes. Initially, the ice brings discomfort but later leads to progressive relaxation (Fig. 22-7).

Total Contact Casting

Dystonic postures of the lower extremity have been reported by Hayes and Burns[32] to be alleviated by the application of total contact plaster-of-Paris casting. The foot and ankle posture is passively moved to a position of maximum correction and a plaster cast applied. A rubber pad is placed in the plaster on the plantar surface to permit ambulation and weight bearing. The cast may be removed in 4 to 7 days for inspection of the skin and for further correction of the deformity. Care should be exercised to pad bony prominences and to provide a relief at the region of the common peroneal nerve. The toes are exposed on the dorsal

STRATEGIES FOR IMPROVING MOTOR CONTROL

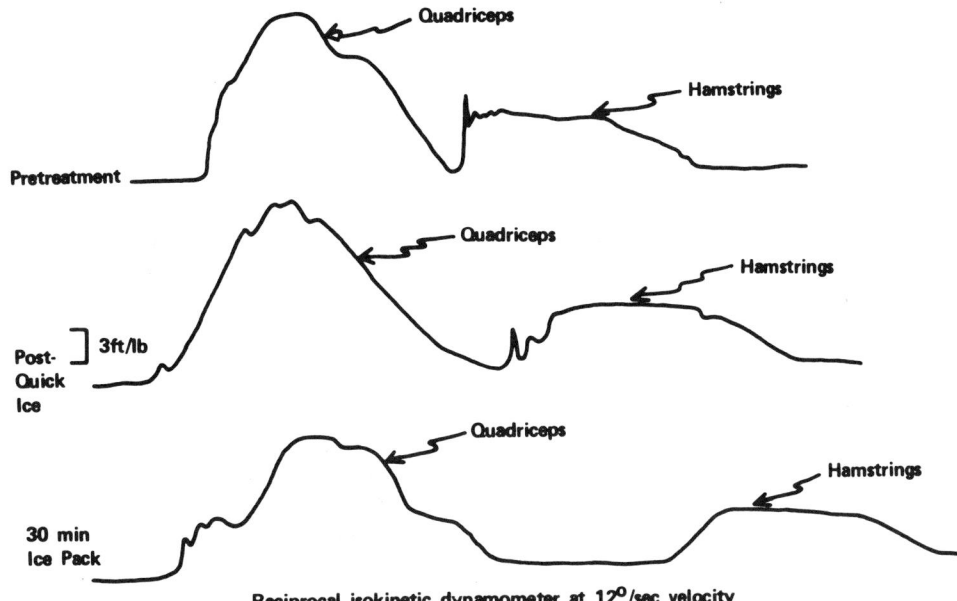

FIGURE 22-6. The effects of cryotherapy (cold) on a traumatic head-injured patient. The effect of quick ice application to the anterior thigh (post-quick-ice) and the application of an ice pack to the same area for 30 minutes are shown on reciprocal isokinetic contractions recorded by the Cybex isokinetic dynamometer.

surface but are supported on the plantar surface in slight extension. Generally, the cast is worn for 3 weeks, but it may require several more weeks in some cases. A series of applications may be required.

Although casting of the upper extremity has been more limited, it has been used for patients with dystonic configuration of the arm. More recently, casting has been used in the early management of spasticity states in head-injured patients (see Chapter 9).

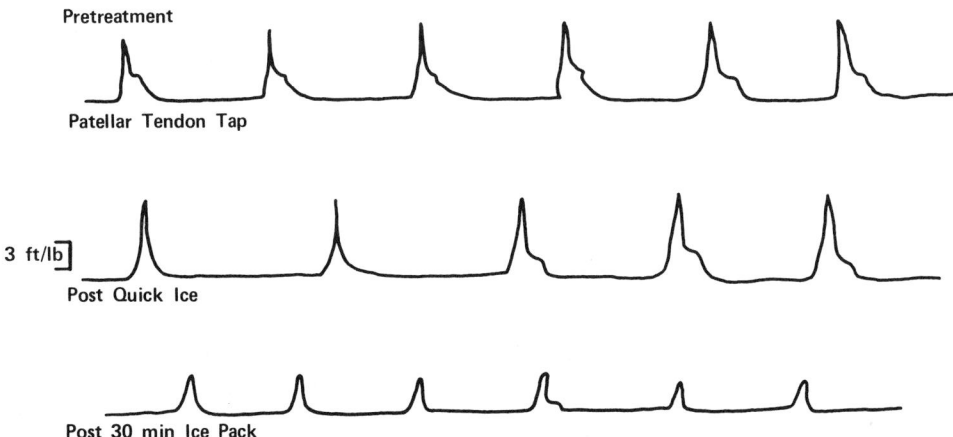

FIGURE 22-7. The effects of ice application (quick and long duration) to the anterior thigh of a traumatic hemiparetic patient on the deep tendon jerk response of the quadriceps. The recording was made on a Cybex dynamometer at a damping of zero, using an electromagnetically driven tendon hammer.

Electronic Feedback

The most widely recognized source of feedback is electromyographic feedback. It has been applied to patients with spasmodic torticollis by Brudny, Grynbaum, and Korein[33]; and Basmajian and coworkers[34] reported on its effectiveness in training stroke victims in ambulation. Basmajian indicates the augmented information provides the patient and the therapist with an immediate knowledge of results.

Amato, Hermsmeyer, and Kleinman[35] used EMG feedback to increase inhibitory control of spastic plantar flexors so as to increase dorsiflexion. In a controlled experimental design for foot drop associated with hemiparesis, Basmajian and coworkers[34] reported a beneficial effect for the EMG feedback group. However, the duration from time of stroke was different in the control group.

In a long-term (3-year) follow-up of 39 hemiplegic patients, Brudny and coworkers[33] found 20 had significant functional gains and had been weaned from the EMG feedback. Another controlled experiment by Lee and colleagues[36] failed to note significant increases in upper extremity function of hemiparetic patients as compared with placebo techniques. I have studied visual, mirror-image, EMG, and no feedback and have found EMG feedback only slightly superior to visual and mirror-image feedback in training intrinsic foot musculature not under voluntary control.

Exteroceptive Feedback for Coordination

Harris[37] contends that "inapproprioception" may be the basis for impaired postural stability and poor control in cerebral palsy. Using electronic position transducers and electronically generated visual and auditory displays, he was able to demonstrate effective functional gains in all but 1 of 18 cerebral palsied subjects tested. The instrumentation was reported as quite costly and therefore not feasible for the average clinical setting.

Vibratory Stimulation

Small-amplitude (1 to 2 mm) high-frequency (100 to 200 Hz) vibration applied to a tendon or a muscle typically results in a sustained low-grade state of contraction.[38] This response is termed the tonic vibratory reflex. In the intact person, this reflex is readily inhibited within a half dozen trials. However, patients with CNS lesions do not appear capable of inhibiting the response. For example, a normal person can easily extend the elbow when the biceps brachii muscle has been vibrated, but a hemiparetic patient cannot accomplish extension against the tonic vibratory reflex (TVR).

The clinical application of this technique appears to be in the stimulation of the antagonistic muscle of a spastic pair. A TVR established in the triceps when the biceps is spastic should effect a reciprocal inhibition of the biceps because of the facilitation of the triceps. As a facilitatory measure, the TVR may be employed to reinforce motor unit discharge in weakened states. This is particularly true if there is an associated loss of muscle stretch response (hypotonia).

The TVR applied to an intact person has been reported[39] to result in a distorted spatial orientation. It is suggested that it might serve to improve perception of spatial orientation in the head-injured patients. The maximum effect of the TVR is obtained when the muscle is not allowed to shorten. Hagbarth and Eklund reported that subjects receiving an isometric TVR felt as though the limb was slowly moving in a shortening direction.

Eklund and Steen[40] found TVR to be effective in the care of cerebral palsied children for improvement of motor control. Patients reported greater awareness of the state of relaxation in muscles previously vibrated. Bishop[41] cautions that the exact mode of TVR, muscles selected, duration, and pattern should be worked out carefully by the therapist. Furthermore,

CONCLUSION

Through careful analysis of movement behavior and assurance that the spontaneous recovery from diaschisis is not misinterpreted as relearning of movement, an estimation of the effectiveness of training may be made.

The extent of the head injury, age and sex of the victim, associated extracranial injuries and disorders, the duration from time of injury and extent of care rendered, the premorbid conditioned motor behavior, and the motivation of the individual are all important qualifying influences on motor recovery.

The major problems of lack of motor power, loss of balance, agility, and discrete movements, as well as spasticity or rigidity, are identified, and procedures have been recommended for their amelioration.

Training principles include those advocated by Bobath,[18] Knott and Voss,[28] and Brunnstrom,[42] which incorporate various approaches to the activation of CNS patients. The isokinetic training I describe places emphasis on increasing the velocity of the movements with rapid alternation of muscle groups and symmetric activity. Body balance is integrated with the development of limb control, and specific conditioning routines are suggested. Bilateral reciprocating isokinetic movements are used in a training format in preparation for locomotion. With proper rate of limb control, the automatic locomotor behavior may be elicited, leading to resumption of an efficient gait.

An experimental design comparing two methods of ambulation training has been presented; superior results were obtained with bilateral reciprocal isokinetic training. Retrospective analysis of head-injured hemiparetic patients revealed better overall performance by right hemiparetics, but the left hemiparetics made greater gains from training.

REFERENCES

1. JOHNSON, D AND ALMI, CR: *Age, brain damage, and performance.* In FINGER, S (ED): *Recovery from Brain Damage.* Plenum Press, New York, 1978, p 115.
2. LASHLEY, KS: *Functional determinant of cerebral localization.* Archives of Neurology and Psychiatry 38:371, 1937.
3. MYERS, RE: *Corpus callosum and grosis.* In DELAFRESNAYE, J (ED): *Brain Mechanisms and Learning.* Blackwell Scientific Publications, Oxford, 1961.
4. GAZZINAGA, MS: *Is seeing believing: Notes on clinical recovery.* In FINGER, S (ED): *Recovery From Brain Damage.* Plenum Press, New York, 1978, p 409.
5. GOLDBERGER, ME: *Restitution of function in the CNS: The pathologic grasp in Macaca mulatta.* Exp Brain Res 15:29096, 1972.
6. RAISMAN, G AND FIELD, P: *A quantitative investigation of the development of collateral reinnervation after partial deafferentation of the septal nuclei.* Brain Res 50:241, 1973.
7. RUCH, T AND PATTON, HD: *Physiology and Biophysics,* ed 20. WB Saunders, Philadelphia, 1979, p 643.
8. ECCLES, JC AND MCINTYRE, AK: *The effects of disuse and of activity on mammalian spinal reflexes.* J Physiol (Lond) 121:492, 1953.
9. LIVESON, JA AND SPILEHOLZ, NI: *Peripheral Neurology.* FA Davis, Philadelphia, 1979, p 5.
10. HEBB, DO: *The Organization of Behavior.* John Wiley & Sons, New York, 1949.
11. GALAMBOS, R: *A glia-neural theory of brain function.* Proc Natl Acad Sci USA 47:129, 1961.
12. KOTTKE, F: *Training of coordination.* Arch Phys Med Rehabil 61:551, 1980.

13. SCHNEIDER, GE: *Early lesion of the superior colliculus: Factors affecting the formation of abnormal retinal projections.* Brain Behav Evol 8:73, 1973.
14. BRODAL, A: *Self observations and neuroanatomical considerations after a stroke.* Brain 96:675, 1973.
15. JENNETT, B AND TEASDALE, G: *Management of Head Injuries.* FA Davis, Philadelphia, 1981.
16. ROOD, M: Unpublished material, 1963.
17. LANDAU, WM: *The upper motor neuron syndrome.* In ELIASSON, SG, PRENSKY, AL, AND HARDIN, WB (ED): *Neurological Pathophysiology.* Oxford University Press, London, 1974.
18. BOBATH, B: *Adult Hemiplegia: Evaluation and Treatment.* Heinemann, London, 1978.
19. NELSON, AJ: *Functional ambulation profile.* Phys Ther 54:1059, 1974.
20. NASHNER, L: *Fixed patterns of rapid postural responses among leg muscles during stance.* Exp Brain Res 30:13, 1977.
21. CLARKE, J AND EVANS, E: *Rhythmic intention as a method of treatment for cerebral palsy.* Australian Journal of Physical Therapy 19(2):57, 1973.
22. CARR, JH AND SHEPHERD, R: *Physiotherapy in Disorders of the Brain.* Heinemann, London, 1980.
23. COTTON, E AND PARNWELL, T: *The Peto method.* Special Education 56(4):7, 1967.
24. YU, J: *Neuromuscular recovery with training after CNS lesions.* In INCE, LP (ED): *Behavioral Psychology in Rehabilitation Medicine.* Williams & Wilkins, Baltimore, 1980, p 402.
25. TAUB, E: *Somatosensory deafferentation implications for rehabilitation medicine.* In INCE, LP (ED): *Behavioral Psychology in Rehabilitation Medicine.* Williams & Wilkins, Baltimore, 1980, p 371.
26. GOLDBERGER, ME: *Motor recovery after lesions.* Trends in Neural Sciences 3(11):288, 1980.
27. STOCKMEYER, S: *A sensorimotor approach to treatment.* In PEARSON, P AND WILLIAMS, C (EDS): *Physical Therapy Services in the Developmental Disabilities.* Charles C Thomas, Springfield, Ill, 1972, p 223.
28. KNOTT, M AND VOSS, DE: *Proprioceptive Neuromuscular Facilitation.* Harper & Row, New York, 1968.
29. CHAMBERS, R: *Clinical uses of cryotherapy.* Phys Ther 49:3, 1969.
30. URBSCHEIT, N AND BISHOP, B: *Effects of cooling on the ankle jerk and H response.* Phys Ther 50:1041, 1970.
31. KNUTTSON, E: *Topical cryotherapy in spasticity.* Scand J Rehabil Med 2:159, 1970.
32. HAYES, NK AND BURNS, YR: *Discussion on the use of weight-bearing plasters in the reduction of hypertonicity.* Australian Journal of Physiotherapy 16(3):108, 1970.
33. BRUDNY, JB, GRYNBAUM, BL, AND KOREIN, J: *Spasmodic torticollis: Treatment by feedback display of EMG.* Arch Phys Med Rehabil 55:403, 1974.
34. BASMAJIAN, JV, ET AL: *Biofeedback treatment of foot drop after stroke.* Arch Phys Med Rehabil 56:231, 1975.
35. AMATO, A, HERMSMEYRE, CA, AND KLEINMAN, KM: *Use of EMG feedback to increase inhibitory control of spastic muscles.* Phys Ther 53:1063, 1973.
36. LEE, K, ET AL: *Myofeedback for muscle training in hemiparetic patients.* Arch Phys Med Rehabil 57:588, 1976.
37. HARRIS, FA: *Inapproprioception: A possible sensory basis for athetoid movements.* Phys Ther 51:761, 1971.
38. EKLUND, G AND HAGBARTH, KE: *Normal variability of tonic vibration reflexes in muscle.* Exp Neurol 16:80, 1966.
39. HAGBARTH, KE AND EKLUND, G: *The muscle vibrator: A useful tool in neurological therapeutic work.* Scand J Rehabil Med 1:26, 1969.
40. EKLUND, G AND STEEN, M: *Muscle vibration therapy in children with cerebral palsy.* Scand J Rehabil Med 1:35, 1969.
41. BISHOP, B: *Vibratory stimulation, Part 3.* Phys Ther 55(2):139, 1975.
42. BRUNNSTROM, S: *Movement Therapy in Hemiplegia.* Harper & Row, New York, 1970.

Chapter 23

REMEDIATION OF PERCEPTUAL DYSFUNCTION

Paula E. Wahlstrom, O.T.R.

Perceptual dysfunction, in combination with cognitive limitation, has a devastating effect on the brain-damaged person. Limited cognition may prevent the individual from taking advantage of compensatory training, and impaired perception may lead to impaired processing of information from the environment into the cognitive system.

Perception is also influenced by physical disabilities (sensory dysfunction, tone impairments, poor motor control) that prevent the patient from exploring and receiving valid sensory information from the environment. This information forms the basis of motor activity. If based on information from a damaged sensory-motor system, motor activity will be impaired. Damage to the central nervous system can prevent the integration of sensory input. Therefore, there are many levels on which the sensory integrative process can be interrupted: distally through damaged sensory receptors; at brain-stem level where tactile, vestibular, and proprioceptive input is integrated and forms the basis for visual perception; and at the cortical level where it forms the basis for movement.[1]

The characteristic pattern of diffuse injury makes the head-injured patient likely to have involvement at all levels. Sensory-integrative deficits have been considered to be the basis of higher-level perceptual deficits. This forms the basis for beginning treatment at the most elementary level: tactile, vestibular, and proprioceptive. The patient may not have the physical mobility to independently provide the neurologic system with this input; this becomes the job of the therapist. The environment must be structured to provide stimulation to these basic systems as well as to challenge the higher-level systems.

The evaluation of perception begins with the observation of the patient's body posturing and movements. Patients at the lowest cognitive levels can be assessed by this method. Movements of the extremities should be observed for ability to cross the midline. The posture of the head and neck should be in midline. Flexion of the neck to either side indicates influence of tone on the body and will affect the integration of sensory input and the patient's ability to act on it. The patient is presented with a brightly colored object or familiar photograph and requested to follow as the object is moved throughout the visual field. The eye excursions are observed for smooth movements to extreme corners of both eyes and crossing the midline.

The patient's capability to learn new material or to remember the remote, recent, or immediate past can be determined from the psychology or speech evaluation, or both. The speech therapist provides data concerning language and communication capabilities. Either evaluation may contribute information regarding premorbid learning and intellectual abilities that can affect the patient's ability to participate in the rehabilitation program.

(For the specific evaluation of perceptual deficits, refer to chapters 19 and 21.)

TREATMENT APPROACHES

Cognitive, motor, or functional skills levels can be used as a frame of reference from which to evaluate and treat the head-injured person. I will use the cognitive levels model established at Rancho Los Amigos Head Trauma Service for this purpose.[2]

Generally, the eight levels in the scale can be summarized into three categories for purposes of treatment: (1) The low-level patient who is minimally responsive may respond to stimuli in a generalized or specific manner but displays little spontaneous activity and only inconsistent responses to command. The patient requires a program of stimulation. (2) The level of functioning in which confusion or agitation or both are present requires a very structured and concrete approach. (3) Finally, the higher-level individual who is generally appropriate but may be functioning in a very automatic mode requires varied and challenging experiences.

Areas of integration to be considered for treatment will be clustered into the following areas:

1. *Visual perception* includes depth perception, visual field neglect, and figure-ground and spatial relations. Functionally, the patient may overreach for objects and may have difficulty finding objects in a cluttered drawer or distinguishing buttons on clothing. The patient may also ignore one field of vision or objects in that field.
2. *Somatosensory* includes body concept, image, and scheme; body neglect; right/left discrimination; body part localization; and the ability to initiate motor activity.
3. *Form and space* includes some overlap with the visual area as well as body in space, shape and color discrimination, and relationship of objects in space. Patient may have difficulty maneuvering a wheelchair, especially through crowded spaces. Dressing and hygiene/grooming skills may be disorganized. The patient may have difficulty orienting self to clothing—front, back, right side from wrong.
4. *Praxis* includes the planning and control of movement, and the ability to initiate, sequence, and complete motor acts in a smooth fashion. Patients with apraxia may demonstrate difficulty imitating motor acts. This interferes with learning new skills such as transfers, one-handed dressing techniques, or ambulation with adaptive equipment. Activities to tap into each of these areas will be discussed.
5. *Visual activities* include any activity that requires the use of sight. Many incorporate motor skills. Tracking an object into all visual fields is one that requires only oculomotor skills. It is appropriate for the minimally responsive patient who is able to focus but does not spontaneously look in all visual fields. With some physical assistance, many are able to attempt color-matching activities with cards or blocks.

    The patient requiring structure who has visual field neglect may be required to do puzzles starting at midline and gradually moving into the neglected visual field. Both groups of patients will require assistance or close supervision to complete the task. Short periods of treatment, 10 to 15 minutes, are most effective.

    The higher-level patient will be able to do paper-and-pencil tasks with minimal supervision. Eye-hand coordination work sheets and mazes can be used. Those visual tasks of a more motoric nature include games such as ring toss, horseshoes, and catch. These are particularly helpful for training those patients with depth perception problems.
6. *Somatosensory* activities for the low-level patient can be very basic. The patient can be given brisk tactile stimulation to body parts and encouraged to initiate motion. Very simple commands such as "straighten your arm" or "raise your leg" may be used.

    The patient who is confused will benefit from a functional approach. The self-care training program can be used to help structure input. As it is a familiar task, it provides a feedback system to help the person monitor performance.

    Completing human figure puzzles is also helpful. Having the patient dig small objects out of a sand box gives tactile stimulation. Stereognosis can be challenged if the high-level patient is required to do this task with vision occluded and name the objects as the patient discovers them (Fig. 23-1).

REMEDIATION OF PERCEPTUAL DYSFUNCTION

7. *Form and space* activities can be easily graded for all levels of patient ability. The low-level patient will be able to attempt shape, size, and color-sorting activities (Fig. 23-2). The patient may require some physical assistance to complete the task.

    Gross motor activities that tap into form and space and provide vestibular, tactile, or proprioceptive input are particularly useful with the agitated patient. These include ring toss, beanbag throwing, and jousting.

    Tasks of directionality challenge the high-level patient. The patient may be required to get to and from therapy alone and with the use of a map. Paper-and-pencil tasks can be used; design copying, form constancy, spatial relations, and figure-ground work sheets from Frostig workbooks can be used.

8. *Motor activities* include those that provide vestibular, proprioceptive, and tactile input. These may be graded from the low-level patient who is able to raise the head from being flexed on the chest to the ability to imitate intricate postures. Gross motor games such as "Simon says," catch with a large ball, or maneuvering through obstacle courses may be used. The higher-level patients respond to light sports such as Velcro dartboard, tether ball, and shuffleboard.

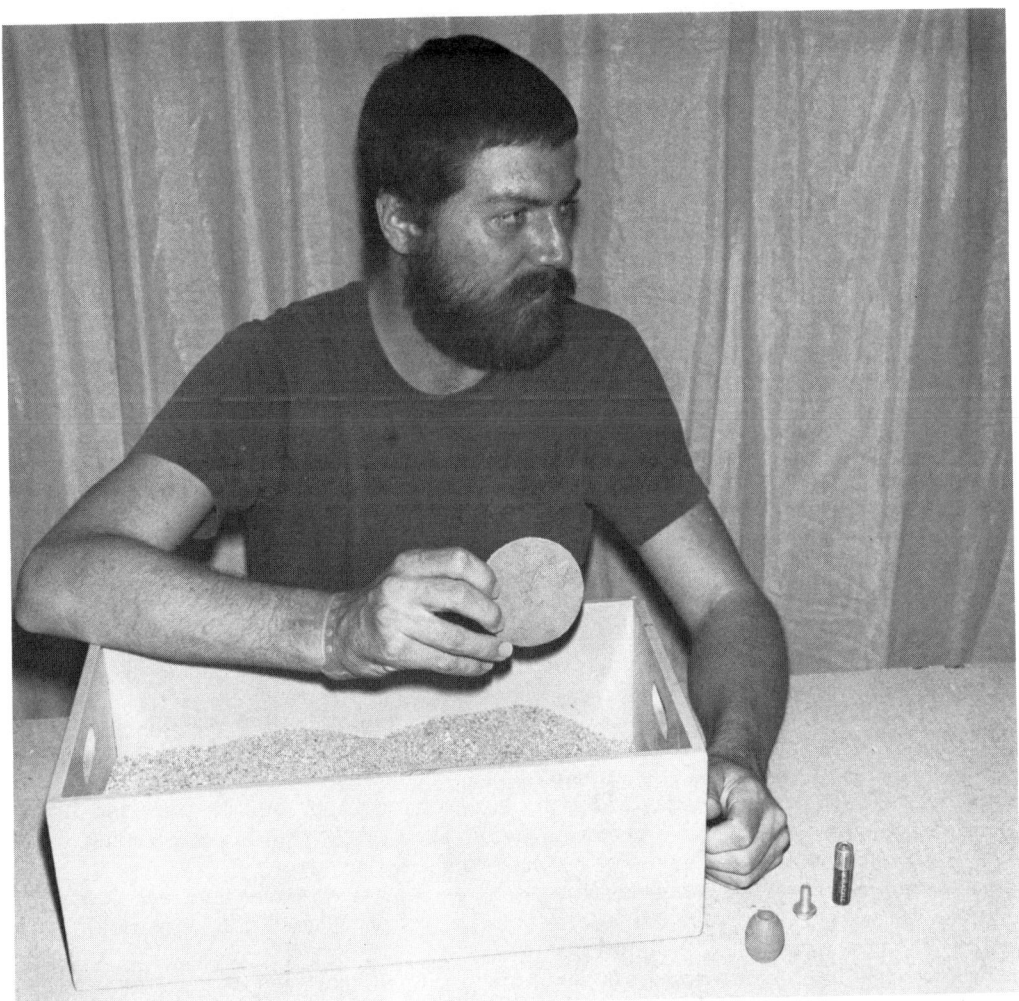

FIGURE 23-1. Developing tactile stimulation by digging small objects from a sandbox.

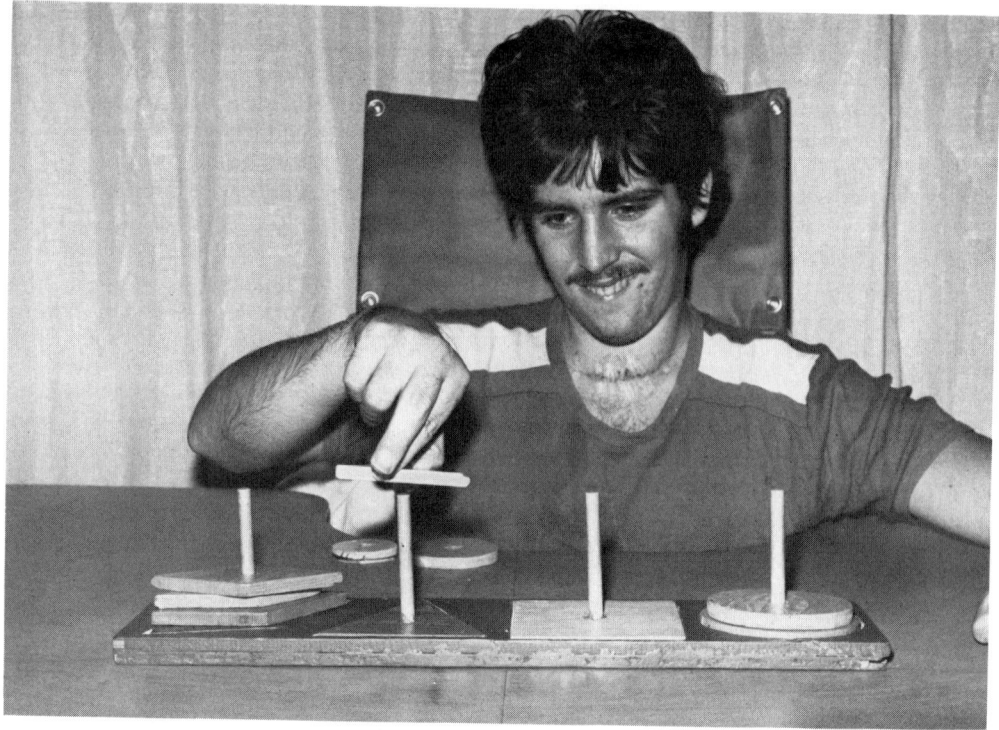

FIGURE 23-2. Learning to classify objects by shape, size, and color.

POSITIONING TECHNIQUES

Usually, the aforementioned activities are done on table top with the patient in the wheelchair. More benefit can be derived from using positioning to increase vestibular, tactile, and proprioceptive stimulation and to normalize muscle tone and inhibit reflex activity.

Increased muscle tone and reflex activity limit normal motor activity. Techniques for reflex inhibition or normalizing muscle tone as described by Bobath[4] are appropriate. Positions that incorporate the levels of development of normal motion are useful to facilitate motor control. Discussion here will be primarily concerned with those providing vestibular, proprioceptive, or tactile input, thereby providing a basis for the higher-level perceptual activities mentioned previously.

As the integration of these three "old" systems is believed to precede and enhance the processing of higher-level ("newer") perceptual skills, providing this stimulation before or during the activity should make treatment more effective.[5]

Tactile integration precedes and is the basis for the visual form in space and somatosensory systems. Tests of this function have correlated highly with motor planning ability.[6] Vestibular integration underlies motor activity and visual perception.

Proprioceptive integration aids in sensory perception of visual impulses through the extraocular muscles preceding visual form and space capabilities. It enhances motor activity by facilitating normal muscle contractions.

Typically, the overall goal of treatment with the minimally responsive patient is to increase motion. The sensory-integrative approach of positioning the patient paired with simple perceptual tasks is useful. The higher-level patient with some motor abilities may begin to

REMEDIATION OF PERCEPTUAL DYSFUNCTION

exhibit perceptual problems. These are best approached by pairing the gross positioning techniques with challenging perceptual tasks.

There are precautions to be taken when using the following techniques. Two therapists are required to safely transfer and position the patient; this also helps put the patient at ease. If occupational and physical therapists can treat the patient together, many benefits can be derived. Each one can contribute an area of expertise and be aware of changes in the patient's perceptual skills that have implications for functional activities. Having two therapists present allows one to initiate the activity and the other to observe the response.

Many patients may still have nasogastric (NG) tubes in place. If the patient is to be prone, especially with head at or below stomach level, the tube should be removed. When the NG tube is in place, the cardiac sphincter of the stomach remains open and the stomach contents can be regurgitated and possibly aspirated.[7]

Care should be taken when initiating vestibular activities to be alert to seizure possibilities. If the patient has a history of recent seizures, these activities should not be attempted.

Proprioceptive stimulation can be provided by doing joint approximation, especially to the large joints—shoulders and pelvis. The minimally responsive patient can be seated and pressure provided to the shoulders and through the trunk. A higher-level patient can be positioned on all fours and joint approximation applied to the shoulder girdle and pelvic areas. Resistance to forward and backward motions can also be given in this position (Fig. 23-3).

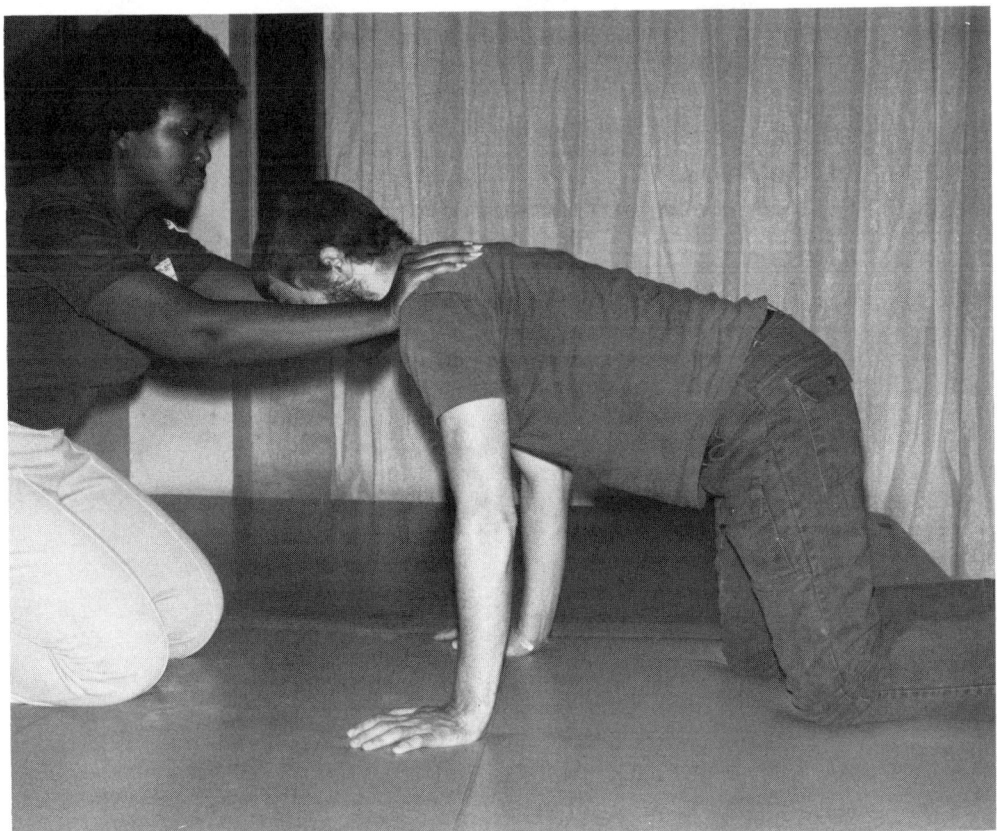

FIGURE 23-3. Providing proprioceptive feedback by doing joint approximation and testing resistance to forward and backward movements.

The patient who is ambulating but exhibiting decreased trunk rotation and fluidity of motion may benefit from the proprioceptive and vestibular stimulation of jumping on a "spring-a-ling." This is a 3-ft square board supported at the corners by heavy-gauge springs (Fig. 23-4). Initially, the patient may be permitted to hold a post or door jamb for support. Emphasis should be placed on performing smooth, evenly spaced jumps with equal weight on both lower extremities. As the patient improves, the patient can do the activity unsupported.

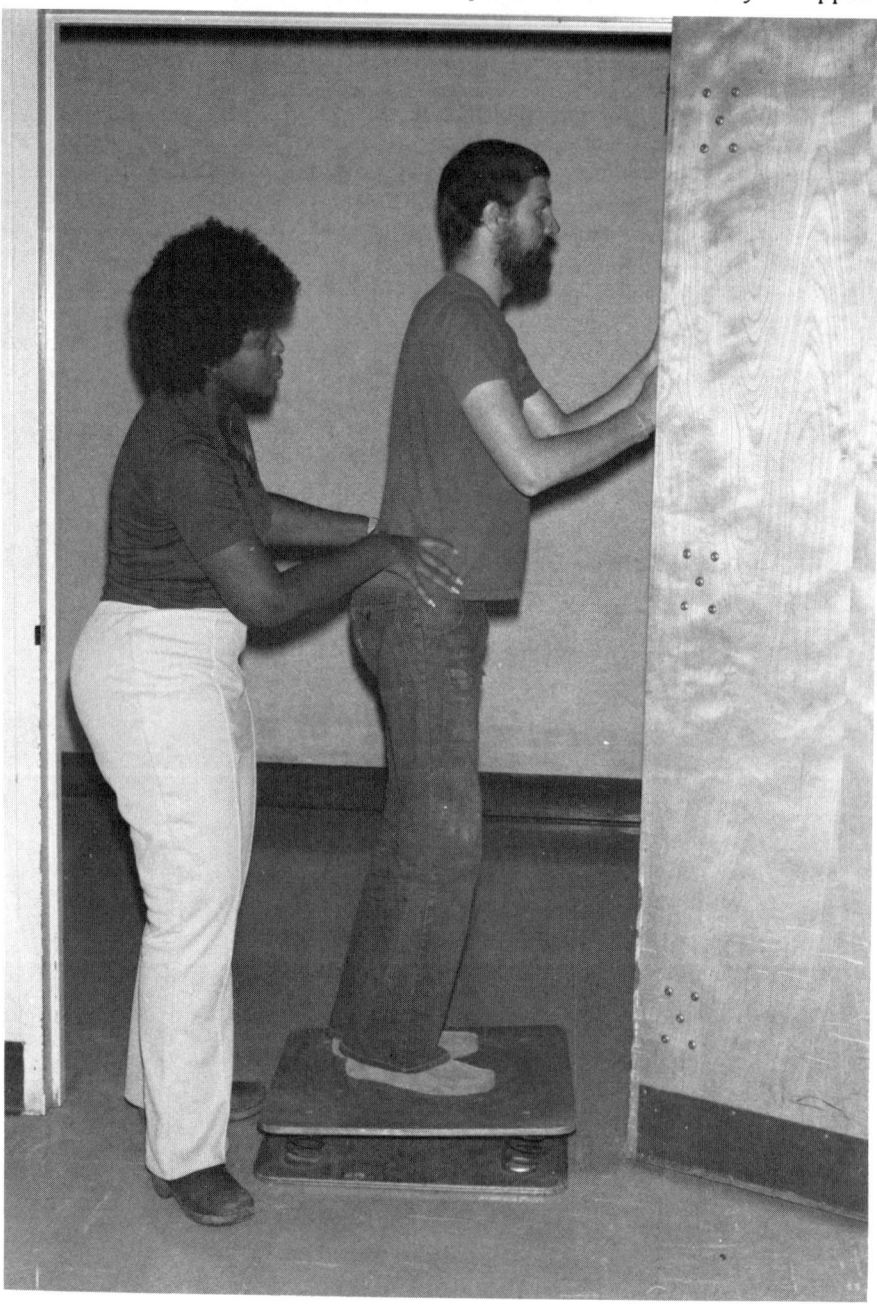

FIGURE 23-4. Using a "spring-a-ling" to provide vestibular and proprioceptive stimulation.

REMEDIATION OF PERCEPTUAL DYSFUNCTION

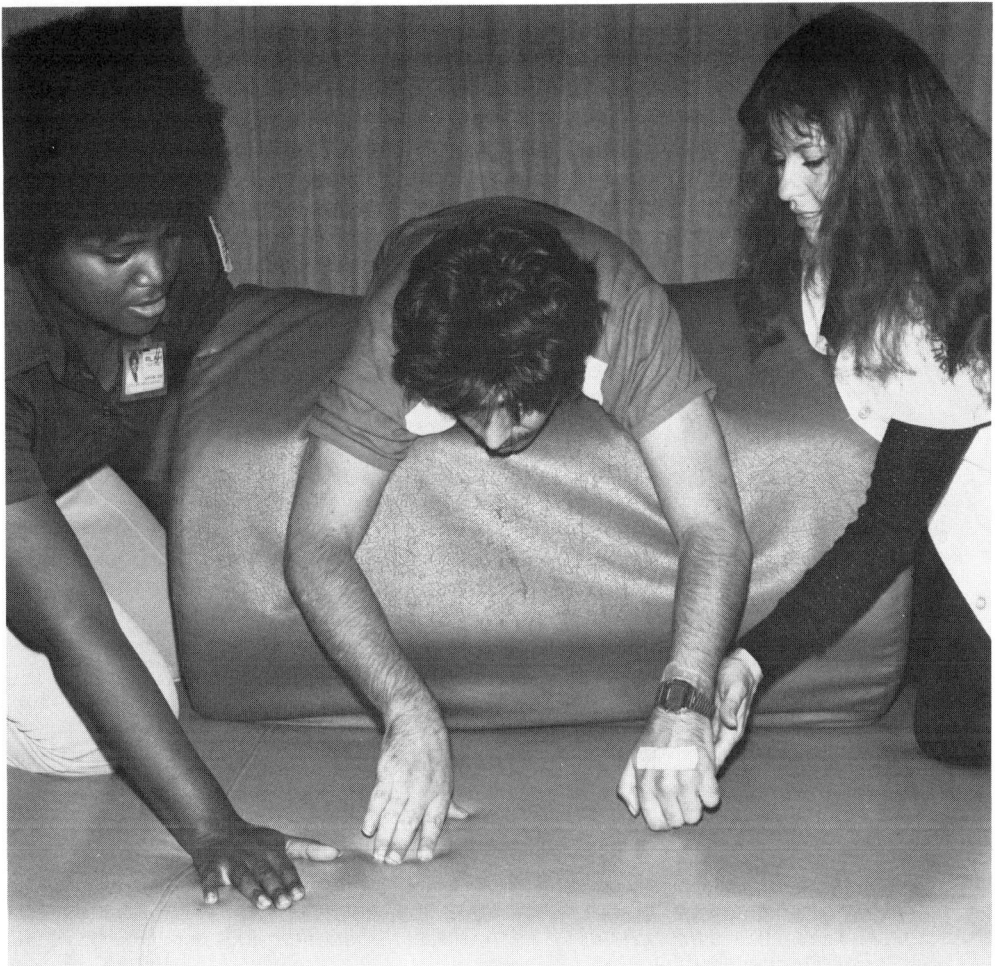

FIGURE 23-5. Placing the patient prone on an inflated cylinder, move the patient forward and ask him to extend his head upward. This activity provides vestibular stimulation.

Vestibular stimulation has the quality of being able to stimulate activity or calm overactivity. This depends on the source and rate of the stimulation. Rocking a minimally responsive patient on a rocking or balance board can be stimulating. Using this technique more gently can be calming to an agitated patient. In either case, the stage is set for higher-level activity. The patient can be placed prone over a large inflatable ball or cylinder and moved in all directions by holding the lower extremities. As the patient is moved forward, the patient can be instructed to attempt to extend the head up. This encourages prone extension and head righting (Fig. 23-5). Note the precaution regarding nasogastric tubes during this activity.

The high-level patient requiring vestibular input to increase visual perception may benefit from riding an adult-sized tricycle. This activity stimulates proprioceptive centers as well.

Tactile stimulation can be provided by means of brisk rubbing of neglected body parts with different textured materials. Agitated patients may become increasingly agitated with this. They may tolerate it better if they do it themselves. The higher-level patient may apply lotion to a neglected extremity. Follow this with a gross activity to help "channel" the stimulation. Tactile stimulation will generally increase extension tone.[4]

CASE STUDIES

As examples of the incorporation of the above information into a treatment program, three cases will be presented and a portion of their program discussed.

Case #1: D.G. was a minimally responsive patient 3 months postinjury. The patient exhibited active motion in the right arm that was dominated by increased tone in the elbow flexors and throughout the shoulder girdle. The left arm exhibited minimal active motion and postured in flexion at the elbow and wrist. His left leg was dominated by adductor tone and amputated below knee secondary to a previous accident. The right leg had selective motion with plantarflexion tone at the ankle. His head postured to the left, though he could bring it to midline with verbal cueing. When sitting, his neck flexed forward onto his chest. D.G. could be awakened with verbal or tactile stimulation and inconsistently would comply with one- or two-step commands. His attention span could be maintained for approximately 3 to 5 minutes.

The initial program consisted of stimulation to increase attention to a task, head righting, and motor control of right upper extremity. D.G. was placed prone on a wedge on a mat table with his chest and upper extremities over the high edge. He was presented with a set of colored rings to be stacked on a peg. The activity required him to choose the color ring requested from a pile of loose rings and place it on the peg, thereby challenging visual perceptual skills. In order to see the task, he had to bring his head to horizontal, encouraging head righting skills. The positioning provided some proprioceptive input to trunk and helped to decrease upper extremity flexor tone. He was able to complete the task with close supervision (verbal cueing). The task was later graded by moving the activity to the right and requiring the patient to track across the visual field.

Case #2: M.W. was a 32-year-old man 2½ months postinjury. He was confused and inappropriate, with a low frustration tolerance exhibited by combativeness. His attention span was approximately 15 to 20 minutes. M.W. was assisted with all activities of daily living secondary to cognitive deficits and decreased body mobility skills.

His physical picture included a right side that was dominated by tone. He postured in flexion at the elbow but could be ranged into full extension. There was minimal active motion in the hand and beginning motion at the elbow and shoulder. Sensation was impaired. The right leg was dominated by tone in hip extensors, knee flexors, and plantar flexors. He had slow and delayed motion in this limb. The left side had selective motion in upper and lower extremities, but both were influenced by tone. M.W. was particularly protective of his right arm; he avoided using it or allowing others to touch it.

Part of his initial program consisted of increasing motor control in the right upper limb. Before the activity was begun, tactile stimulation was given to the entire arm. M.W. was encouraged to do this himself. Proprioceptive input was provided by passively ranging the limb at each joint.

A relatively simple perceptual activity was chosen: assembling large-piece puzzles. The motor component of the task was the most challenging aspect. The patient required assistance to place the upper extremity because of shoulder weakness. The amount of motor planning and control needed to manipulate the puzzle pieces provided the right amount of challenge.

Case #3: A.B. was a 20-year-old man 4½ months postinjury. He had minimal physical findings: good to normal muscle strength in both arms and minimal sensory deficits. Both legs were intact throughout. Cognitively, he was functioning at an automatic and appropriate level, and he had a severe memory deficit. His functional skills (self-care, home, and community) were limited secondary to cognitive problems and deficits in the areas of figure-ground, body image, and spatial relations. He had difficulty finding toilet articles in drawers, putting clothes on correctly, and fastening buttons.

His perceptual problems were approached through gross motor activities. He rode the adult tricycle, which provided vestibular and proprioceptive input. Obstacle courses were set up for him to jump, crawl, and walk through. He jumped up and down on the spring-a-ling, a 3-ft square of wood supported at the corners by large springs. These activities all provided vestibular and proprioceptive stimulation. Form and space activities were interspersed. Shuffleboard, horseshoes and dart boards were some activities that were used.

After performing some of the above activities, the patient performed more fine motor tasks. One was a mosaic tile project. The tiles were placed in a predetermined pattern that A.B. had to copy to further challenge his spatial relations skills. Re-evaluation consisted of observation of changes in functional ability.

FUNCTIONAL SKILLS

There is frequently discussion concerning the transference of perceptual skills learned in the clinic to functional activities, for example, dressing or hygiene/grooming. Theoretically, if treatment for these problems is instituted at the basic low levels described, the foundation of higher-level skills is established. The patient does not learn just splinter skills, but the basis for sound functional and motor activity. The patient has a better chance for follow-through in the functional setting.

GOAL SETTING

Perceptual deficits can limit the patient's achievement in the area of functional skills. The therapist should bear this in mind when setting goals for activities of daily living.

Left-sided neglect with a field cut and body part denial make it difficult for the patient to relearn the most rudimentary self-care skills. Patients exhibiting persistent problems with neglect cannot be expected to be better than a level requiring assistance with self-care.

Problems in the area of visual perception can be subtle and interfere with high-level functional tasks when the patient approaches normal cognitive and motoric levels. Typically, such problems become apparent during a prevocational evaluation or driving evaluation. As the patient is cognitively able to cooperate with extensive therapy, these problems usually resolve or the patient can be made aware of them and how they affect performance. Patients with these problems may initially require supervision in the community but may eventually reach independence.

Severe persistent apraxia is seldom seen in this patient group. Subtle problems are frequently identified early and respond well to many of the suggestions made previously. Goal achievement may be slightly delayed, but the patient usually does well with the "old, familiar" tasks of self-care. The problem is more evident when severe arm involvement requires a change in dominance. In this case, a goal of "dominant hand or assist" for tasks requiring fine motor skills may be reasonable.

CONCLUSION

Many of the abovementioned evaluation and treatment procedures were standardized on the pediatric population. Other techniques have been borrowed from the treatment of hemiplegic patients. The adult head-injured patient exhibits characteristics of both groups, but the cognitive component makes a significant difference and must be taken into account in any evaluation or treatment procedure.

The identification and treatment of this patient population as a separate entity are relatively new; as this develops, clinicians will continue to standardize treatment procedures especially for this patient population.

REFERENCES

1. AYERS, AJ: *Sensory Integration and Learning Disorders.* Western Psychological Services, Los Angeles, 1972.
2. HAGEN, C, ET AL: *Levels of cognitive functioning.* In *Rehabilitation of the Head-Injured Adult: Comprehensive Physical Management.* Professional Staff Association of Rancho Los Amigos Hospital, Downey, Calif, 1979.
3. FROSTIG, M: *Developmental Test of Visual Perception.* Consulting Psychologists Press, Palo Alto, Calif, 1964.
4. BOBATH, B: *Adult Hemiplegia: Evaluation and Treatment.* William Heinemann, London, 1970.
5. WILSON, EB: *The application of principles of sensory motor integration to occupational therapy for the adult hemiplegic.* In *Studies in Sensory Integrative Dysfunction.* Center for the Study of Sensory Integrative Dysfunction, 1974.
6. AYERS, AJ: *Sensory Integration and Learning Disorders,* Chapter 5. Western Psychological Services, Los Angeles, 1972.
7. GUENTZ, S: *Rehabilitation nursing techniques.* In *Rehabilitation of the Head-Injured Adult: Comprehensive Physical Management.* Professional Staff Association of Rancho Los Amigos Hospital, Downey, Calif, 1979.

Chapter 24

REALITY ORIENTATION THERAPY

Jean Cerny, O.T.R.
Robin McNeny, O.T.R.

Reality orientation therapy is a technique used with head-injured adults who exhibit symptoms of confusion, disorientation, withdrawal, and difficulty interacting with the environment. Reality orientation addresses these symptoms through a process of continuous stimulation of the patient and repetition of basic orientation information. Hence, the patient is led to understand that knowledge about self and the environment is essential. It is the task of the reality orientation program to reverse these symptoms and aid the patient in the reintegration process.[1] To be effective, the reality orientation program requires a total team effort and a consistency of approach.

The Reality Orientation Program was originated by Dr. James Folsom in 1958 in Topeka, Kansas, at the Winter Veterans Administration Hospital and was further refined in 1965 while Folsom was at the Veterans Administration Hospital in Tuscaloosa, Alabama. It was designed by Folsom for use with geriatric patients to combat memory loss, confusion, and time-place-person disorientation.[2] These same symptoms are frequently seen in the individual who has sustained a traumatic head injury.

GOALS OF THE REALITY ORIENTATION PROGRAM

Reality orientation therapy with the head-injured individual has two basic goals. The first goal is to reinforce oriented behavior, which includes awareness of time, place, and person, and appropriate responses to the environment.

The newly admitted head-injured adult experiences increased disorientation owing to results of the injury itself compounded by the effects of the strange new environment of the rehabilitation unit. A further complication of the patient's rehabilitation program is the duration of post-traumatic amnesia, which seems linked to disorientation and confusion.[3] Involvement in reality orientation therapy helps diminish the patient's level of confusion.

The second goal of reality orientation therapy is to extinguish negative behaviors that are frequent outgrowths of the disoriented state. These behaviors include withdrawal from the environment and social interaction, decreased awareness of the surroundings, and bizarre behavior. The rehabilitation staff and family may notice increased agitation, hostility, withdrawal, or an unwillingness to communicate with others. Impaired memory and a failure to carry over information and instructions may be present. There may be increased motor behavior, such as pacing the halls, reckless wheelchair management, or combativeness. Interaction with staff, patients, and family members may be inappropriate; however, these behaviors tend to improve as overall orientation improves.

COMPONENTS OF REALITY ORIENTATION PROGRAM: ENVIRONMENTAL PROGRAM

A complete, well-designed reality orientation program on the rehabilitation unit includes two components, the environmental program, which is an individualized approach used by the staff during all contacts with the patient; and a series of structured reality orientation group sessions.[2]

The environmental program operates on a 24-hour basis and has been observed to be a critical factor in the total program's success. The chief modality in this phase is the role played by all persons in contact with the disoriented person. There should be continual stimulation with basic orientation information on an informal basis. As soon as the patient's degree of disorientation is established, the environmental program should be initiated.

The reality orientation program should begin immediately after the patient arouses from coma, while still in the acute phase of recovery. At this point, the environmental program is crucial. The acute-care staff focuses on techniques meant to stimulate the semicomatose, combative, or lethargic individual. The aim of their efforts is re-orientation to the self and the environment. Hopefully, this early intervention lessens the effects of disorientation and will allow for earlier transfer to the rehabilitation unit.

Once the patient is transferred to the rehabilitation unit, a more structured reality orientation program is possible. This program is composed of three basic components: (1) a positive staff attitude, (2) a consistent approach to the patient by staff and visitors, and (3) environmental stimulation.

POSITIVE STAFF ATTITUDE

The attitude of the staff and family is critical in helping the patient to establish appropriate feelings of self-worth. Friendly, warm encounters with others offer support and encouragement to the head-injured adult. When possible, the staff should help the patient learn to recognize inappropriate behavior and, hopefully, assist the patient in controlling it. Structured and supervised encounters between the patient and others on the unit allow the patient to practice social skills. Phillips[4] notes that social interaction with peers helps the head-injured adult regain contact with reality and thus self-esteem and dignity.

CONSISTENT APPROACH

The staff should be consistent in their approach to the patient. Good communication regarding the patient's level of disorientation, program components and goals, and the therapeutic strategy being used to improve orientation help staff establish the type of approach required for each patient. There should be an awareness of the patient's performance among staff members; depending on the facility, this might be best accomplished through the medical record, physician's rounds, and/or patient conferences.

ENVIRONMENTAL STIMULATION

Even before the head-injured adult awakens from coma, environmental stimulation is thought to be beneficial. This aspect of the program optimally involves family and friends.

Several techniques have been used to provide stimulation at the bedside. Tape-recorded messages from family and friends to the patient may be played for the comatose or semi-comatose patient. Familiar voices seem to be more attractive to the patient. Some families record favorite poems or songs. Radios tuned to a favorite station are also recommended for a confused individual. Of particular importance is a blend of music and news-weather reports. However, it is just as important to turn off the radio for intervals so there is not an accommodation to the sound or overstimulation.

As the patient progresses, families are asked to provide snapshots of the patient prior to this injury as well as pictures of relatives, pets, and home. If the pictures are mounted on a portable surface, such as poster board, and are identified with labels, all of the staff are able to use them during informal discussion periods with the patient. Favorite possessions, such as wall posters, clothing, or plants, can provide additional stimulation. Personalization of the patient's environment tends to make it more familiar and comfortable. Clocks and calendars are needed in every patient room, lounge area, and treatment area. They are necessary for cueing the patient about schedule and time orientation.

For the patient confined to bed, a mobile hung from the overhead trapeze is an excellent source of visual and/or auditory stimulation. Constructed from dowels or rigid plastic tubing, the mobile is designed to convey basic orientation information to the patient, such as the patient's name, where the patient is, and family members' names. Decorations for the mobile include colorful sponge balls (useful for stimulating, reaching, and grasping), unbreakable wind chimes (for auditory input, if needed), photographs, and mirrors. One professional on the team should assume responsibility for the construction of the mobile; however, all staff, once they understand its purpose and use, should employ it to orient the patient.

Regardless of the patient's level of function, the staff should strive to create the best environment to foster oriented behavior. Phillips[4] states that a good reality orientation program encompasses "a calm environment, a set routine and . . . consistency."

There are other techniques that appear to be more useful on the rehabilitation unit. These approaches include a personal notebook, environmental cueing, daily schedule cards, family visits, and home reality orientation programs.

The patient notebook is used in many centers as both a record book and resource manual for confused, disorganized patients. It accompanies the patient to all appointments; the therapists record daily activities and any assignments they wish the patient to complete for "homework." On the unit, nursing personnel periodically record information regarding the patient's activities and note changes in functional abilities. Families are requested to record complete reports of the patient's performance while on pass. The maintenance of the daily activity records assists with the re-orientation process. Staff and family use the log to help the patient recall therapy activities and assignments. As orientation improves, the patient learns to refer to the log whenever necessary.

In some instances, the physical environment may require alteration to enhance the reality orientation program. Failure to remember room numbers or the route to a therapy area is frequently seen in head-injured adults. Among the techniques recommended to help confused patients locate their rooms are to hang a name sign outside the door or put a familiar poster or wall decoration on the door itself. Some facilities paint lines on walls and floors in a variety of colors indicating pathways to therapies, the recreational area, bathrooms, and dining areas.

A well-organized, consistent daily schedule is important for the disoriented head-injured patient who has difficulty productively managing time and is unable to monitor behavior. As part of the reality orientation program, each patient is provided a daily schedule card outlining therapy appointments, meals, recreational programs, rest periods, and evening activities. Initially, the staff needs to help the patient follow the schedule. However, as the program continues, the staff is able to offer fewer reminders and encourage the patient to take greater initiative in attending therapy independently.

As the head-injured adult becomes more mobile and begins to relate more to others, disorientation and inappropriate behavior often distress the family and staff. Their support of and participation in the program help them cope with the patient's altered personality in a more constructive manner. Family instruction is needed to increase their understanding of the goals of the program and specific techniques used to attain them. Individual instruction, conferences with staff, and family education classes are all satisfactory means of teaching (see Chapter 28).

It is unfortunate that disorientation sometimes persists to the end of the rehabilitation program and thus must be a consideration during discharge planning. In this case, the family is provided a written reality orientation program to follow after discharge. It contains the same basic elements as the hospital program and is intended for use on a 24-hour basis. The individual's level of orientation is then re-evaluated by staff during follow-up visits, and necessary changes in the program are made.

COMPONENTS OF REALITY ORIENTATION PROGRAM: STRUCTURED GROUP SESSIONS

The second part of the reality orientation program is the structured group sessions. These sessions are held one to three times daily and are led by a trained staff member, usually a member of the nursing or occupational therapy staff.

Six factors should be considered when planning and organizing the group sessions for the head-injured patient.

1. *Structure, content, meeting time, and frequency.* The group's structure and content must be predetermined, as should the time for each session and the frequency of the sessions. Early morning sessions seem to orient the patients at the beginning of the day, and this appears to carry over into a large part of the day. In some settings, a second session is scheduled for the afternoon. Owing to space or personnel restrictions, the number of patients per group often is limited; various authors differ on the optimal number for each group.[4-6] The presence of agitated patients should be a factor to consider, as they require more management by the group leader. One solution to the problem of too many patients at varied levels for one session is to divide them according to age and/or functional level.
2. *Evaluation.* Prior to inclusion in a Reality Orientation Program, the head-injured patient's level of disorientation is determined through evaluation. The Reality Orientation Questionnaire[5] provides a systematic approach to evaluation (Fig. 24-1). Administered immediately following admission, the questionnaire identifies the patient's basic level of orientation and general awareness of the environment. Informal assessment of the patient's behavior on the unit and in therapy augments findings of the questionnaire and should not be underestimated. Barnes[6] has discovered that behavioral measures are actually more reliable indicators of improvement than are the results of the questionnaire.
3. *Treatment media.* The principal treatment modality is the Reality Orientation Board.[7] This board contains basic information and is displayed in a prominent location on the unit. In some facilities, several boards are placed in key areas, that is, in the dining room, at the nurses' station, and in the recreational room. The board is an essential part of the group session. (The use of the board is described later.) Other treatment media can be collected from many sources. Colorful, clear pictures depicting one large object or scene are found in magazines, posters, or calendars. Pictures are conveniently stored in a file. Sensory stimulation materials also are a

REALITY ORIENTATION THERAPY

NAME: _____ AGE: _____ BIRTH DATE: _____

ADDRESS: _____

DIAGNOSIS: _____ ONSET: _____

ADMISSION DATE TO REHAB. SERVICE: _____ PHYSICIAN: _____

INITIAL EVALUATION DATE: _____ WAS R. O. THERAPY RECOMMENDED? ____

R. O. THERAPY INITIATED (DATE): _____ DISCONTINUED (DATE): _____

EXAMINER: _____

	DATE:	INITIAL	TWO WEEKS
1. What is your name?			
2. What hospital is this?			
3. Why are you in the hospital?			
4. In what city is this hospital?			
5. In what city is your home?			
6. Are you married?			
7. What year is it?			
8. What month is it?			
9. What day of the week is it?			
10. What season is it?			
11. What is the weather today?			
12. What is our next holiday?			
13. What is our next meal?			
14. On what floor of this building is your room?			
15. What is your doctor's name?			
Scores:			

FIGURE 24-1. Reality orientation questionnaire. (Designed by Robin McNeny, O.T.R., 1979.)

valuable medium for the group sessions. A variety of scents, such as extracts, alcohol, and coffee, challenge the olfactory sense. A box of assorted textures and basic shapes is used for tactile sensation. Tape recordings of familiar sounds are used for auditory discrimination and are commercially available from educational supply firms.

The treatment repertoire also should include a collection of objects representative of the world around us—nature, holiday items, flags from different countries, maps, household tools, and toileting articles. Simple games such as Bingo, bean bag toss, and dominoes; rhythm instruments; large pads and markers; and craft and cooking supplies allow for a variety of activities. Disoriented patients need the structure of games and crafts; the need to work cooperatively with others and to follow rules and instructions can generalize to on-ward and therapy situations.[4]

4. *Staff education.* Staff education in the principles and techniques of a reality orientation program is needed prior to initiation of the program. This is best accomplished through in-service training sessions. A thorough knowledge of the basic program principles enables the staff to provide consistency. The entire staff need to feel their importance in the program's success. Consistency is indeed the key to the success of the program, and it is best developed through close communication with other team members.
5. *Designation of a group leader.* The leader is typically drawn from the nursing or occupational therapy staff. It is the responsibility of this individual to plan group sessions, maintain the treatment library, and report on patients' performance regularly.[2] In view of the amount of work required of the group leader, the leadership position often rotates among different staff professionals.
6. *Group meeting location.* A place for group meetings should be found early in the planning phase. A specific location for the group contributes to the overall effectiveness of the program; changing locations is confusing to patients and staff. The room chosen should be bright and large enough to accommodate members comfortably. A semicircular seating arrangement is ideal as it best facilitates eye contact and socialization. There should be a clear understanding among all personnel that the room is reserved daily for the reality orientation group to minimize interruptions and distractions. In some large centers, it may be necessary to post a sign on the door to remind people that the group is in progress.

Barns[2] outlined a format for a group that has been adapted for use with head-injured adults. This format includes four stages that promote interaction among participants.

Stage 1. The Climate of Acceptance. During the first 5 minutes of the session, the leader introduces himself or herself and extends a welcome to members by name. The leader interacts individually with each patient. Attempts are made to create a warm, comfortable atmosphere.

Stage 2. A Bridge to Reality. Reorientation to reality is the goal of this stage. The reality orientation board is used to stimulate recall of information and to guide the discussion. Those unable to spontaneously recall the information are encouraged to read from the board, if possible. An inability to respond to the leader's questions is best handled by providing the correct answer.[4] The leader fosters attentiveness and appropriate behavior. Negative behavior and inappropriate responses are discouraged; otherwise, the leader provides praise and positive reinforcement.

Stage 3. Sharing the World We Live in. The next 15 minutes of the session involve a discussion of a selected topic or participation in a craft, homemaking, or hygiene task. In choosing the activity, the leader should be sensitive to the interests and needs of the participants. This is particularly applicable for head-injured adults, who are often young men who respond best to relevant issues and may regard the entire group as "silly." Subjects of little interest may lead to disruptive behavior.

Audiovisual aids enliven the discussion and direct the participants' attention to the task at hand. The dialogue among patients is further stimulated as the leader asks questions regarding the topic.

Stage 4. Climate of Appreciation. During the last 5 minutes, the leader recognizes the patients' various contributions to the group that day. Feelings of pleasure and enjoyment are described by the leader and may be expressed by participants as well. Before the session ends, the next meeting is discussed, and social events, such as holidays, parties, and so forth, are brought to the participants' attention. The session closes as the group members share a handshake around the circle.

THE OCCUPATIONAL HISTORY

The end-goals of a comprehensive reality orientation program are increased environmental awareness, increased appropriate social behavior and socialization skills, and increased feelings of self-worth. In order to adequately structure the means to this end-goal of greater orientation and socialization, the occupational therapist must have adequate background information to effectively plan each patient's treatment program. Only by completing a thorough occupational history of the patient in addition to an assessment of the patient's present status can a therapist gain the necessary insight into what is *meaningful* to the patient, and thus know what stimuli must be included in treatment.

Information regarding the occupational history may be obtained from any one or more of the following: the patient (if reliable), family members, medical records, and the social history. Most critical to note from the occupational history is information about past interests, choices, habits, and preferences; the patient's past needs for rewards; past jobs or training/education; work behaviors; the patient's capacity for acceptance of failure; interpersonal competence; performance under stress; and the patient's capacity to handle conflicting role expectations.[8]

THE TREATMENT PROGRAM

The skill of the reality orientation therapist lies in the ability to abstract relevant information from the patient's history, combine it with current cognitive abilities, and design a meaningful treatment regimen for reality orientation. More simply, the therapist integrates the patient's *past* into the *present* when planning and implementing a treatment program. Realizing that "reality" for the patient is more than mere recitation of the day, date, time, and place, the therapist understands a patient's need for purposeful involvement in the world around him or her. In spite of cognitive deficits such as defective short-term memory or visual-motor impairments, patients appear capable of responding with interest and attention when given meaningful opportunities to participate.

The elements of novelty and complexity must also be considered when selecting opportunities for inclusion in a reality orientation program. Given that these elements affect one's level of interest and involvement, the therapist is conscious of grading the level of novelty and complexity of the experiences presented.[9] Overstimulation or greater disorientation may result in the absence of this awareness, but sufficient stimulation is necessary to maintain a level of adequate patient interest.

Two concepts that are basic to a reality orientation program are *repetition* and *consistency*. Day-to-day recognition of people and events may be impeded by memory deficits. In order to facilitate extension of memory, daily reiteration of the schedules of routine events (meals, dressing times, therapies) and the repeated announcement of impending events should be a matter of course.[10] Basic orientation information can be repeated when the patient is greeted by various persons throughout the day. A notebook should be set up that contains basic information (such as present day, date, name of hospital, names of family members, etc.). This notebook can serve as a reference for the patient and staff when discussing names and events in the patient's life. Some facilities use this log as a means of conveying information about a patient's performance in one therapy area to the other disciplines. It can serve as the patient's own source of information when attempting to remember the events of a given day.

If the staff members are consistent in their approach, structure is provided and undesirable behavior may be lessened. While still preserving the patient's dignity through kindness and an uncritical attitude, criticism or rechanneling of the unacceptable behavior must be handled firmly. For example, a male patient who wanders into the women's restroom should have firm redirection but should be approached in a nonjudgmental manner (e.g., "John, this is the women's restroom; the men's restroom is down the hall. If you need to use the men's room, let's turn around and go there.")

Consistency in staff contact is basic but is probably the most useful means of providing orientation early in a patient's program. If possible, a core group of professionals should work with a particular patient initially, to avoid unnecessary confusion for the patient and to provide needed structure. Primary-care nursing and one-to-one treatments by consistent therapists limit the numbers of new persons the patient must get to know in the initial days of a rehabilitation program.

Because the head-injured patient has been isolated from many normal sensory experiences during hospitalization, the occupational therapist can use these experiences as an effective starting point in a reality orientation program. Keeping each experience within its context should aid in the orientation process, by providing structure and importance for each activity. For example, if a patient's past daily routine involved the following sequence each morning: shaving, showering, eating, brushing teeth, and dressing, then every effort should be made by the staff to replicate that routine in the hospital setting. The therapist is able to assess the patient's ability to follow through with a part of or each step of the sequence, and can provide information, caring, or assistance when needed. Thus, basic daily routines can provide useful treatment settings for sensory experiences. Attention to the tastes and smells of various foods can be the focus of sensory experiences during meal times. The attention reinforces what is *real*, while providing an indelible experience within its context. Sensory stimulation for the head-injured adult should not be reduced to the passive reception of stimuli by the patient.

Prolonged hospitalization, isolation from family and friends, confusion and disorientation, and altered personality traits may all contribute to a decrease in socialization skills after head injury. Thus, the loss of social skills can be one of the most devastating sequelae of head trauma. In the early stages of marked disorientation, treatment sessions focus on one-to-one encounters in an effort to decrease confusion. As the patient progresses, resocialization can begin in small group sessions that facilitate interaction with others and reinforce appropriate social behaviors. In the structured group sessions described previously, patients and the group leader begin the session with a greeting and end it with a good-bye. Using the culturally acceptable means of introductions when new members join the group and encouraging discussion among group members are basic and necessary methods of encouraging social interaction. Discussion of culturally acceptable topics provides stimulation for the group members and should facilitate verbal interaction. Group activities, rather than discussion-only sessions, can provide excellent opportunities for practice of basic social skills such as sharing and cooperation, turn-taking, and impulse control. Since social isolation can contribute to low self-esteem, patients may be particularly helped through group sessions that foster participation, acceptance by others, and success through use of available skills. Every human being has basic needs for food and shelter, but "belonging" to a social group is also a principal human need.

The head-injured adult in the United States is typically in the young-adult age group. With prolonged disorientation and residual cognitive deficits, these individuals present with problems in the areas of vocational/avocational disruption, isolation from the community, and legal issues regarding competency. Since this population of "rehabilitated" survivors has an expected life span of many years, health-care professionals must be alerted to the impact that these residual problems have on the individual faced with a long life expectancy. Research is needed to identify the most effective means of addressing prolonged disorientation in this population and its overall impact on the individual and the society in which the individual must live.

CONCLUSION

What effects can be expected from a comprehensive reality orientation program? The efficacy of a reality orientation program may be assessed by examining elements such as loss of confusion and disorientation and by the reduction of undesirable behaviors. Therapeutic gains may be inferred from such outcomes as increased environmental awareness, modification of unsociable behavior, increased socialization skills, and greater feelings of self-worth. Patients' responses regarding the value of the aforementioned outcomes can be a valid indicator of success, as well as justification for the program. Research is needed regarding consumer attitudes about quality-of-life issues following traumatic head injury and participation in a reality orientation program. Although this research is lacking at present, the efforts of health-care professionals should continue to provide patients with the opportunities for reconstructing reality when life is interrupted by traumatic head injury.

REFERENCES

1. STEPHENS, LP (ED): *Reality Orientation.* American Psychiatric Association Hospital and Community Psychiatry Service, Washington, DC, 1970, p 1.
2. BARNS, K, SACK, A, AND SHORE, H: *Guidelines to treatment approaches: Modalities and methods for use with the aged.* Gerontologist Winter 1973: 513.
3. EVANS, CD, ET AL: *Rehabilitation of the brain-damaged survivor.* Injury. 8:80, 1974.
4. PHILLIPS, DF: *Reality orientation.* Hospitals. 47:46, 1973.
5. CORNBLETH, T AND CORNBLETH, C: *Reality Orientation for the Elderly.* Document 1593, American Psychological Association, Washington, DC, 1977.
6. BARNES, J: *Effects of reality orientation classroom on memory loss, confusion, and disorientation in geriatric patients.* Gerontologist 1974:138.
7. BOWLES, L: *Reality orientation board.* Gerontologist 1973:516.
8. MOORHEAD, L: *The occupational history.* American Journal of Occupational Therapy 23:329, 1969.
9. BERLYNE, D: *Conflict, Arousal and Curiosity.* McGraw-Hill, New York, 1960, Chapter 2.
10. HOPKINS, H AND SMITH H: *Willard & Spackman's Occupational Therapy.* JB Lippincott, Philadelphia, 1978, p 361.

Chapter 25

TREATMENT OF COMMUNICATION DISORDERS

Robert M. Smith, M.Ed.

Rehabilitative speech pathology treatment should be based on a comprehensive diagnostic and prognostic evaluation. As in any therapeutic program, the prognosis for improvement is mainly based on the premise that skills performed inconsistently have the potential to be performed consistently when an opportunity is provided for learning and practice.[1] Therefore, a major task of the diagnostician is to determine which skills the patient has in his or her behavioral repertoire and which of these skills can potentially be performed consistently. Treatment procedures for communication disorders are based on such prognostic information.

The traditional role of the speech and language pathologist is to diagnose and treat patients with communication disorders. In the treatment of head-injured patients, this role should be expanded so that the professional becomes a member of the interdisciplinary team that provides a comprehensive treatment program.

ROLE OF THE SPEECH AND LANGUAGE PATHOLOGIST

The speech and language pathologist should be an integral member of the interdisciplinary rehabilitation team working with head-injured patients.[2] The team's overall goal is physical and cognitive rehabilitation of such patients. A close working relationship is needed for the team to help each patient meet these goals effectively. During the course of rehabilitation, the team will focus its attention on various subgoals as the needs change. A task force can be organized to accomplish specific subgoals during the patient's long period of recovery.

As part of an interdisciplinary team, the speech and language pathologist should be involved in many aspects of the rehabilitation program. These include being a member of the evaluation team, a member of the coma-arousal task force, a member of the cognitive retraining task force, a member of the dysphagia task force, and the team leader in providing remedial speech and language training for specific communication problems.

EVALUATION TEAM

The speech and language pathologist takes a lead role in evaluating, diagnosing, and prognosing the speech and language of the head-injured patient. The speech pathologist may also be involved in other evaluations, such as academic and cognitive evaluations. This involvement will depend on the composition of the interdisciplinary team working with a specific patient.

COMA-AROUSAL TASK FORCE

A coma-arousal task force may be formed in an effort to awaken the comatose patient. Such a therapeutic procedure may be provided for patients who exhibit good potential for recovery. This task force should be made up of a number of professionals including the attending physician, staff nurse, psychologist, occupational therapist, and speech pathologist. Family members may also be included. The coma-arousal task force may be involved in working with the patient as soon after injury as the patient is medically stable.[3]

The task force provides stimulation in an effort to arouse the patient from the state of unconsciousness. The goal is to have the patient react to various stimulation and thereby awaken. Auditory, tactile, olfactory, and motor stimulation can be provided.

Auditory stimulation by music, environmental sounds, and voice should be provided in a structured and organized program. Talking to the patient about family, friends, and current events is sometimes helpful. Care should be taken not to overstimulate the patient with extremely loud recordings or radio. The patient's likes and dislikes of music should be considered.

Tactile stimulation of temperature, moisture, and pressure can be provided to different parts of the body. It is important that the patient be told what stimulation is being provided. Response of any kind is sought from the patient.

Aromas of perfume, flowers, onion, chocolate, and even noxious aromas such as ammonia or sulfur can be used for olfactory stimulation. Such stimulation may be helpful to patients who do not respond to auditory and tactile stimulation. Talking to the patient about what agent is being presented will help integrate the various receptive modalities.

Motor stimulation can be provided through passive range-of-motion exercises. A motorized rocking-bed may also be used to provide position stimulation and help maintain muscle tone. Motor stimulation is often necessary to prevent atrophy of muscles and spastic contractions. Some patients will be in coma for many months. If atrophy takes place during coma, later developing physical abilities will be limited.

When the patient is alert and responsive to the environment, the coma-arousal task force can be disbanded as the next stage of rehabilitation takes precedence.

TASK FORCE FOR SWALLOWING DYSFUNCTION

Swallowing problems frequently occur when head trauma results in brain stem injury. The swallowing dysfunction task force should be composed of the speech pathologist, dietitian, nurse, physician, and possibly the patient's family. The speech and language pathologist should evaluate the patient and determine what type of swallowing program will be most beneficial. Techniques to retrain swallowing usually begin with motor and sensory stimulation to the mouth and progress to instructions in specific swallowing patterns.[4]

Dysphagia programs are designed to help the patient develop conscious control of swallowing. Such a program can be started as soon as the patient is alert, demonstrates ability to follow directions, and exhibits some reflexive swallowing.[5] Swallowing programs include (1) exercises for increasing oral muscular strength, (2) exercises for improving coordination and range of motion of oral-peripheral musculature, (3) instruction in swallowing physiology, (4) exercises for improving control of laryngeal excursion, (5) instruction for correcting feeding position, and (6) practice for improving swallowing pattern.

COGNITIVE RETRAINING TASK FORCE

Remediation of cognitive problems poses the greatest challenge to the head-trauma team.[6] Such problems invariably contribute to impaired communication. Severely injured patients often require a long period of formal training in a variety of memory and cognitive tasks before they can function adequately. The speech and language pathologist, with unique skills in communication processing, can contribute much to the retraining of cognitive abilities of head-injured patients.

PROVIDER OF SPEECH PATHOLOGY THERAPEUTIC SERVICE

The speech and language pathologist will be the team leader in providing therapy for speech and language disorders. The head-injured patient may have only a transient communication problem owing to cognitive dysfunction or a permanent disorder owing to a cerebral lesion. The following is a discussion of specific treatment approaches.

TREATMENT APPROACHES FOR COMMUNICATION DISORDERS

Communication disorders exhibited by head-injured patients include confused language, aphasia, dysarthria, and apraxia of speech. These problems may be due to specific neurologic lesions or generalized cerebral dysfunction. If the cause is generalized cerebral dysfunction, then the therapy should be directed toward cognitive retraining rather than language or speech improvement.

When a head-injured patient is still in a confused cognitive state, the patient will not be able to consistently exhibit high-level mental skills and therefore may exhibit aphasia-like symptoms of dysnomia, paraphasia, neologisms, and/or unintelligible jargon. The ability to process language and express oneself linguistically necessitates high-level cognitive ability.[7] As the confusion abates and cognitive abilities improve, the functional language skills of the patient should improve. The exception is when there is a focal lesion in the language centers of the brain. Speech and language therapeutic procedures for the confused patient should aim at improving attention, orientation, and memory rather than the aphasia-like symptoms. It may be better not to label such a patient "aphasic" as this may take the therapeutic focus away from the cognitive problems. The "aphasia" in such cases is transient and will likely dissipate as cognitive abilities improve.[8]

COMMUNICATION PROBLEMS OWING TO COGNITIVE DYSFUNCTION

Many speech and language impairments exhibited by head-injured patients are secondary manifestations of cognitive disorganization and, therefore, cannot be adequately diagnosed and treated like communication disorders caused by other etiology.[9] Such patients are unable to use their memory skills consistently, to formulate language adequately, and to control thought processes. Owing to the fluctuating nature of many brain-injured patients' cognitive ability, standardized test instruments will not provide accurate prognostic information but can provide useful baseline data.

Remedial cognitive activities that deal with auditory reception, speaking, reading, and writing skills should begin as soon as the patient can interact with the speech pathologist. The goal of these activities is to improve cognitive abilities that are prerequisites to therapy for speech or language difficulty. The program should include activities that focus on improving visual and auditory attention, visual and auditory discrimination, visual and auditory memory, sequencing of information, association and integration of information, and, when possible, the analysis and synthesis of information. The therapeutic program should be directed toward the reorganization of these cognitive abilities rather than the linguistic consequences of the cognitive disorganization.[10]

TABLE 25-1 Aphasia Therapy Program

A. Understanding what is spoken
   1. Attempt to communicate with mouth movements.
   2. Respond to conversation by moving head up and down.
   3. Point to object named.
   4. Match picture of object to object—group of five.
   5. Point to object by usage.
   6. Point to picture named—group of 10.
   7. Understand question by giving appropriate yes/no response.
   8. Point to body parts.
   9. Understand verbing.
   10. Understand prepositional phrase.
   11. Follow simple two-sequence direction.
   12. Point to three consecutive items in a picture.
   13. Comprehend sentence by doing appropriate pantomime.
   14. Point to pictures rapidly.
   15. Understand oral paragraph.
   16. Place pictures in sequence following an orally read story.
   17. Understand complex directions
   18. Point to 5 consecutive pictures out of 10.
   19. Point to series of seven digits.
   20. Understand complex conversation in a group.
B. Speaking
   1. Repeat numbers 1 through 10.
   2. Repeat oral movements.
   3. Sing in unison.
   4. Repeat word with picture clue.
   5. Complete a sentence.
   6. Say a related word.
   7. Repeat structured phrase.
   8. Name picture spontaneously.
   9. Recite beginning of common poem.
   10. Answer question orally with one word.
   11. Repeat sentence of six to eight words in length.
   12. Use verb phrase.
   13. Use prepositional phrase.
   14. Brief answer to question.
   15. Describe activity with several phrases.
   16. Answer question with short sentence.
   17. Describe item in detail using sentences.
   18. Talk about use of item using sentences.
   19. Monologue.
   20. Complex conversation in a group.
C. Reading
   1. Match simple word to picture.
   2. Put days of week into sequence.
   3. Point to word named in list of five.
   4. Point to phrase in list of five.
   5. Read word orally.
   6. Pick out word in sentence of up to 10 words.
   7. Match word to associated sentence.
   8. Pick out words in list as to category.
   9. Read phrase orally.
   10. Pick out word in list of similar words.
   11. Read sentence—check yes/no answer.
   12. Answer interrogative sentence.
   13. Unscramble words into sentence.
   14. Read sentence orally—8 to 12 words long.
   15. Comprehend sentence by pantomime.
   16. Read short paragraph.
   17. Follow sequence of printed directions.

TABLE 25-1 Aphasia Therapy Program (*Continued*)

   18. Read paragraph and answer questions.
   19. Read paragraph on grade level.
   20. Read adult literature.
D. Writing
   1. Copy letters.
   2. Copy name.
   3. Print name spontaneously.
   4. Print name of common object.
   5. Print word pronounced orally.
   6. Add missing word to sentence.
   7. Write phrase dictated.
   8. Write name of item pictured.
   9. Write verb phrase to picture.
   10. Write short answer to question.
   11. Write long dictated sentence.
   12. Write declarative sentence about a picture.
   13. Write description of object.
   14. Complete a long aggregating sentence.
   15. Write definition of word.
   16. Write long answer to question.
   17. Write paragraph.
   18. Write comprehensive directions.
   19. Write a story using three to six paragraphs.
   20. Complex writing with good syntax and spelling.

A cognitive retraining program should provide language stimulation to the patient in such a manner that the relationship between stimulus input and the patient's ability to process the linguistic information is balanced. The difficulty of the materials can be manipulated by controlling the rate, amount, duration, and complexity of the stimulation. Success rate of 90 percent accuracy should be a general therapeutic goal. If the input is too difficult, the patient cannot process the material, and this may cause greater confusion and agitation. On the other hand, too little stimulation will not be therapeutic. The cognitive retraining program should help the patient learn to process information in an orderly, sequential manner.

When a particular aspect of language is consistently found to be impaired over a period of time, it is likely that this problem is due to a focal neurologic lesion. Traditional therapeutic approaches for that problem may be instituted and will be helpful when the patient is functioning at an appropriate cognitive level (*confused but appropriate* or higher on the Rancho Los Amigos Scale).[11]

APHASIA THERAPEUTIC PROGRAM

The therapeutic program for an aphasic patient, regardless of the etiology, begins with a diagnostic evaluation. The type of aphasia and the patient's linguistic level of function are determined. The program then progresses to the prognostic evaluation, at which time determination of linguistic potential is made by systematically evaluating language skills. Such evaluations take considerable time and should include the use of some sophisticated evaluative tools such as the Minnesota Test of Differential Diagnosis of Aphasia,[12] Degree of Language Impairment Scale,[13] or the Porch Index of Communicative Ability.[14] Comprehensive evaluative tools such as these will provide the examiner with diagnostic, prognostic, and prescriptive therapeutic data. There should be a direct relationship between the diagnostic and prognostic evaluation and the therapeutic program. The aphasia evaluation should determine which linguistic skills the patient can perform (diagnostic level of function), which skills the patient performs inconsistently (therapeutic levels), and which skills the patient cannot perform (prognostically unable to acquire these linguistic skills).

Treatment procedures for the aphasias should be based on psycholinguistic theory. They should deal with the four linguistic modalities of understanding spoken language, speaking, reading, and writing. The therapeutic program should provide a hierarchy of activities in each modality. As the patient improves, more difficult linguistic therapeutic activities should be available to the patient in a systematic manner.

Table 25-1 depicts a systematic therapeutic program for aphasic patients based on a hierarchy of linguistic skills in each of the modalities of language.[15] Linguistic activities are listed in each modality from very basic to normal adult function, thereby permitting this program to be used with patients who exhibit aphasia of any degree. An individual patient can be prescribed therapeutic linguistic activities from this outline. Performance level of 30 to 90 percent accuracy on any activity indicates that it should be included in the therapeutic program. Activities that can be performed only at a 20 percent level or lower are not therapeutic. With practice, using cueing techniques and reinforcement, the patient should improve in the ability to perform these therapeutic activities.

Therapeutic Facilitators

There are three basic types of speech and language therapeutic facilitators: auditory and visual cues, melodic stimulation, and gestural expressive actions.[15] All three types can be used to facilitate oral language with most aphasic patients. The more limited the patient's oral language, the greater the need for such facilitation.

Auditory and visual cueing is an integral part of most therapeutic programs for aphasic patients. Cueing is a technique that involves modifying the stimulus in such a way as to aid the patient in performing linguistic tasks in a more normal manner.[16] Cueing includes such devices as slowing the speed of presentation, giving more information about the item, providing a phonetic starter, giving a semantic starter, providing a more concrete context, repeating the stimulus, printing the word as it is spoken, and so forth. Some patients may be taught "finger writing" or a phonetic starter as a way of self-cueing.[17] By providing such appropriate linguistic cues, a patient's success rate in therapy can be kept at a high level. As the patient improves, the cues are reduced.

A second type of therapeutic language facilitator, used with aphasic patients, is melodic stimulation. The most familiar structured program of this type is Melodic Intonation Therapy (MIT).[18] The MIT program is a facilitation system whereby phrases are spoken in a melodic chant. The patient repeats the chant until the patient is able to say the phrase in a normal vocal style. Theoretically, the melodic tone helps to activate right hemisphere processing, which in turn helps to process the linguistic information from the left cerebral area. The MIT program is most helpful to patients who exhibit apraxia of speech or Broca-type aphasia. The patient's auditory processing skills must be relatively intact if melodic facilitation is to be beneficial.

A third type of speech facilitation is gestural cueing such as the Amer-Ind gestural communication system.[19] This manual communication system can often be taught to nonverbal or nonfluent patients who have adequate comprehension skills. As the patient learns to communicate manually, the patient frequently begins to speak simultaneously.

Counseling

Parallel in time and professional effort to the linguistic therapeutic program should be a counseling program for the aphasic patient and family. Counseling is necessary to help the patient adjust to altered communication skills and to help motivate the patient to work for improvement. Individual, group, and family sessions should be provided when possible.

Some aphasic patients do not have potential for improvement of communication skills. In such cases, speech and language therapy will not be provided, but help in adjusting to the language deficit will be needed. Other aphasic patients will spontaneously improve. These patients and their families should also be provided counseling to help them deal with the frustrations of the transient aphasia.

Alternate Communication

When an aphasic patient cannot functionally communicate orally, some alternative form of communication may be used. Alternate forms of communications for an aphasic patient include gestural communication and communication boards. Unfortunately, most aphasic patients do no better with a communication board than they do orally. Some patients with Broca-type aphasia can learn to use a gestural communication system.

Maximum Improvement

When maximum return of speech and language skills has been achieved and the patient and family have adjusted to the obtained level of function, dismissal from the active therapeutic program should take place. Ongoing support may be needed in the form of counseling, group therapy, or a social "stroke club." Ongoing individual speech therapy in the vain hope that "maybe something will happen" and the patient will somehow improve is not economically feasible. Speech pathology research is sophisticated enough to reliably determine when a patient has reached maximum potential.[15,20-23]

Figure 25-1 summarizes the above discussion on the aphasia therapeutic process.

TREATMENT OF DYSARTHRIA

Many head-injured patients exhibit some type of dysarthria. Dysarthria refers to a group of motor speech disorders caused by a neurologic lesion.[24] The lesion may be in the central pyramidal and extrapyramidal system or in the peripheral nerves involved in motor speech production. It may affect any one or all motor aspects of speaking, including respiration, phonation, resonance, and articulation. Typically, it affects loudness, quality, prosody, and clarity of speech. Dysarthric speech in a head-injured patient may be transient, owing to generalized cerebral dysfunction, or the disorder may be because of a permanent focal neurologic lesion. In head injury the dysarthria is usually of mixed etiology: neurologic and cognitive.

The most common communication problem that results from head injury is a mixed flaccid and spastic dysarthria. This results in soft, breathy voice with reduced prosody. Poor coordination of the muscles of respiration and reduced cognitive skills are the major contributing factors. The patient is unable to coordinate respiratory and speech muscles and is not cognitively aware of the abnormal speech quality.

A program designed to help the dysarthric patient learn control of respiration for speech has been developed at the Boulder, Colorado, Medical Center by Johnson.[25] She begins by placing the patient prone on an exercise mat. Abdominal exercises are provided passively, and this progresses to teaching the patient to move the abdominal muscles voluntarily. The exercises are provided to increase muscle strength and volitional control. Once abdominal muscle control is achieved, breathing control is practiced. The therapeutic program progresses to include control of respiration with vocalization of words and phrases. The patient slowly learns to compensate for muscular weakness by exerting greater muscle movement with a high level of conscious control. Therapy continues until the patient is able to control exhalation for adequate oral production of sentences. Once this is achieved, work on speech quality and prosody is instituted.

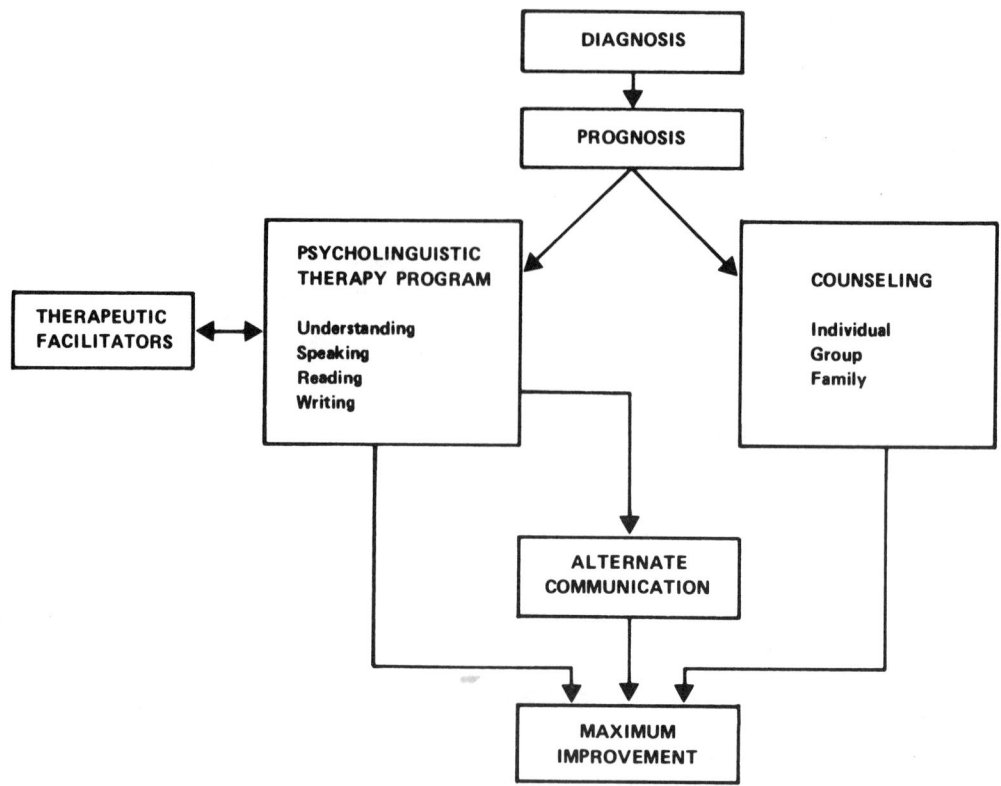

FIGURE 25-1. Schematic overview of a typical therapeutic program for aphasic patients.

Treatment of dysarthria includes procedures that help the patient improve respiratory control, phonation, resonance, and articulation of speech. The following is a brief outline of therapeutic activities involved.

Therapeutic Considerations for Improving Respiration

Respiratory control is necessary for mediation of loudness, inflection, rate, and overall prosody of speech. Improved respiration is achieved by teaching diaphragmatic breathing with proper inhalation and exhalation patterns. Blowing and sucking-type exercises can help increase muscle strength and lung capacity. Loudness control can be achieved through practice in proper breath control before and during speech. Mechanical respiratory exercises are helpful in increasing muscle strength, lung capacity, and breathing coordination. Abdominal muscle and chest muscle exercises, both dynamic and passive, are also included in a comprehensive therapeutic program.

Therapeutic Considerations for Improving Phonation

For flaccid vocal muscles, pushing exercises may help to approximate the vocal folds. Turning the neck and applying pressure on extrinsic neck muscles may help tighten the intrinsic laryngeal musculature.[26] Spastic voice difficulty, however, may require relaxation of these muscles. Mute patients can sometimes be taught to produce a vowel sound or voiced continuent consonant phoneme. Manipulation of the mouth is sometimes necessary. These sounds

TREATMENT OF COMMUNICATION DISORDERS

should be produced until they can be shaped into words. Work on proper pitch range may be indicated in some cases of dysarthria. Associated with pitch difficulty are problems of poor inflection and monotone that require practice on phrasing and inflectional patterns.

Therapeutic Considerations for Improving Resonance

A resonance problem exhibited by some head-injured patients is hypernasality. Therapy to help establish better orality can be stressed along with exercises to strengthen the soft palate and adjacent musculature. These include uvula bouncing and various soft palate movement drills. In cases where there is paralysis of the soft palate, a palatal prosthesis may be needed.[27]

Therapeutic Considerations for Improving Articulation

Many of the cranial nerves contribute to the control of the oral musculature. Therefore, articulation of speech is invariably impaired in dysarthria. Exercises for the tongue, mouth, and facial muscles can be helpful. These exercises not only help strengthen the speech muscles but, often more importantly, help the patient concentrate on the various muscles and thereby gain better control of them. The use of appropriate phrasing and pauses also helps slow speech production and thereby allows time for more precise articulation of words. When this is achieved, work on prosody will complete the dysarthria therapeutic program.

The most important aspect of dysarthria therapy is to help the patient slow the rate of speech so that the patient has time to plan and execute each speech movement.[28] The use of tape-recorder-delayed auditory feedback or a pacing board may be indicated to help the patient learn to speak slowly. Speech can then become a conscious, controlled experience rather than an unconscious but poorly executed happening.[29]

ALTERNATE FORMS OF COMMUNICATION

Patients who have sustained severe insult to motor speech centers of the brain may not be able to regain oral communication skills. Many of these patients possess normal intellectual skills. Such patients are candidates for some nonoral mode of communication. Alternatives to speech include writing, manual communication, and use of some type of communication aid. Although writing is an obvious alternative to speech, seldom is a mute head-injured patient able to write adequately.[30]

The cognitive functioning level as well as the physical function of a patient must be considered in the recommendation for an alternative form of communication. Patients exhibiting low-level cognitive skill may not be able to use any alternative forms of communication. A cognitive level of *automatic and appropriate* (on the Rancho Los Amigos Scale) or above should be obtained before adequate use of manual communication or a communication aid can be expected.

MANUAL COMMUNICATION

There are three general types of nongraphic manual communication systems. The first is finger spelling, often used by deaf individuals. The second, also associated with communication of the deaf, is sign language. The third is hand talk, or gestural communication code.

Finger spelling requires high-level linguistic skill on the part of the user. Good spelling ability and good manual dexterity of one hand are prerequisites. This system requires the user as well as persons communicating with the user to learn the finger alphabet. These prerequisites make finger spelling of limited value to many speechless head-injured patients who have reduced ability to learn a new linguistic-based system and/or have limited motor control of their hands. Sign language of the deaf has some of the same limitations. Sign language is an abstract linguistic system that must be formally learned and can be understood only by persons who have been trained in its use.

Hand talk, or gestural communication, is not a language. The signals do not represent discrete words but rather concepts. It has no grammatical structure; therefore, it can be presented in a rapid telegraphic style. The Amer-Ind Code is a popular means of hand talk. Shelly[19] has shown that this modern form of the ancient American Indian pantomime system is an excellent tool for nonverbal patients. The Amer-Ind system is relatively easy to learn and can be interpreted with no formal training. It is especially useful for patients with apraxia of speech.

COMMUNICATION AIDS

Nonverbal patients can often use some type of communication aid, such as a communication chart, picture board, word lists, or electromechanical device, to communicate with others. There are three basic communication aid systems. They are direct selection (pointing to object), scanning a list of responses, and visual-graphic encoding.[31] Any one or a combination of these approaches can be used to help the patient communicate. Good visual acuity, visual memory, and visual tracking skills are needed for patients using these approaches.

Direct Selection Communication Aids

Direct selection requires the patient to point to specific items in the environment or point to a message element on a chart or list. The message element may be a picture, a word, or a sentence. All message elements must be prepared in advance for the patient. The vocabulary and structure of the material are often custom-made to meet the needs of the individual. Pointing may be accomplished with a finger, a movement of the head, a foot, or a pointer attached to the head.

Scanning-Type Communication Aids

The scanning technique requires a minimum amount of physical control. The patient signals when the desired element appears in a series of pictures, words, or letters that are presented. Scanning systems are usually slower but more involved than direct selection. Since very little physical control is needed, they can be used with persons who have severe physical limitations. Any consistent response can be used as an indicator of the correct item: blink of the eye, raise of an eyebrow, or nod of the head.

A common scanning system uses an alphabet that is scanned with the aid of an observer. The observer sequentially points to each letter. When the appropriate letter is found, the patient responds by giving the prearranged signal. More complex systems may use a series of words, phrases, or pictures to convey particular needs. For some patients, the scanning technique is often too slow. In this case, a unit combining direct selection and scanning can be used.

Encoding Communication Aids

An encoding communication aid uses a pattern or code of signals to indicate a message. The code is usually displayed on a chart for both the message sender and message receiver to use as reference during conversation. This system requires fairly high cognitive ability. Typically, a finger motion is sufficient to indicate the message elements. A numerical code, which is a list of letters or words placed on a chart, is usually used. As the sender points to the numbers, the receiver is directed to the appropriate letter or word on the chart and "reads" the message. Some electromechanical communication aids use such an encoding system.

Electromechanical Communication Aids

During the past 10 years many electromechanical devices have been developed to aid the speechless patient.[32] Some include LED readout panels or strip printers. Some can be attached to video displays or controlled by typewriters. Electric scanning units can be activated with microswitches attached to an eyebrow or mouth-activated switch that the patient can control by a sucking or blowing action. Other units require adequate manual ability to push keys or levers that print out messages. Unfortunately, most electromechanical communication devices are very expensive.

SUMMARY

The speech and language pathologist should be an integral member of the interdisciplinary head-trauma team. This role includes providing periodic speech and language evaluation, coma-arousal therapy, cognitive retraining, dysphagia training, and counseling, as well as providing systematic speech therapy service.

Communication disorders exhibited by head-injured patients include confused language, aphasia, dysarthria, and apraxia of speech. These problems may be due to specific neurologic lesion, general cerebral dysfunction, or a combination of both. If the cause is generalized cerebral dysfunction, then the therapy should be directed toward cognitive retraining rather than speech and language improvement.

When traditional speech and language treatment approaches do not result in adequate oral speech, alternative methods of communication may be developed. These may include the use of a gestural communication system or a nonoral communication device.

REFERENCES

1. GOLDEN, CJ: *Diagnosis and Rehabilitation in Clinical Neuropsychology.* Charles C Thomas, Springfield, Ill, 1978.
2. MELVIN, JL: *Interdisciplinary and multidisciplinary activities.* Arch Phys Med Rehabil 61:379, 1980.
3. LEWINN, EB: *The coma arousal team.* R Soc Health J 10:19, 1980.
4. ROAD, M: *The use of sensory receptors to activate, facilitate and inhibit motor response.* In SATTELY, C (ED): *Approaches to the Treatment of Patients with Neuromuscular Dysfunction.* William C Brown, Dubuque, Iowa, 1962, p 26.
5. GRIFFIN, KM: *Swallowing training for dysphagic patients.* Arch Phys Med Rehabil 55:467, 1974.
6. BEN-YISHAY, Y, ET AL: *Working approach to remediation of cognitive defects in brain damage.* Monograph Supplement, Sixth Annual Workshop for Rehabilitation, New York University, New York, 1978.
7. LEZAK, MD: *Neuropsychological Assessment.* Oxford University Press, New York, 1976.
8. GROHER, M: *Language and memory disorders following closed head trauma.* J Speech Hear Res 20:212, 1977.
9. HANSON, WR AND METTER, ES: *DAF as instrumental treatment for dysarthria in progressive supranuclear palsy.* J Speech Hear Disord 45:268, 1980.
10. LURIA, AR: *Traumatic Aphasia: Its Syndromes, Psychology and Treatment.* Mouton, The Hague, 1970.

11. HAGEN, C, MALKMUS, D, AND BURDITT, G: *Intervention strategies for language disorders secondary to head trauma.* Presentation at American Speech-Language-Hearing Association, Atlanta, Ga, 1979.
12. SCHUELL, M: *Minnesota Test for Differential Diagnosis of Aphasia.* University of Minnesota Press, Minneapolis, 1965.
13. SMITH, RM: Unpublished material, 1977.
14. PORCH, BE: *Porch Index of Communicative Ability.* Consulting Psychologists Press, Palo Alto, Calif, 1967.
15. SMITH, RM: *Prognosis of aphasia: Etiology, time and linguistic factors.* Proceedings of International Association of Logopedics, Washington, DC, 1981.
16. DILLER, L: *A model for cognitive retraining in rehabilitation.* Clinical Psychologist 6:13, 1976.
17. BREURAN, M AND PEELE, L: *Self-generated cues.* J Speech Hear Disord 32:372, 1967.
18. SPARKES, RW AND HOLLAND, AL: *Method: Melodic intonation therapy for aphasia.* J Speech Hear Disord 41:287, 1976.
19. SKELLY, M: *Amer-Ind Gestural Code.* Elsevier, New York, 1979.
20. LAPOINTE, LL: *Base-10 programmed stimulation.* J Speech Hear Disord 42:490, 1977.
21. WERTZ, R: *Neuropathologies of speech and language.* In JOHNS, DF (ED): *Clinical Management of Neurogenic Communication Disorders.* Little, Brown & Co, Boston, 1978.
22. SCHUELL, M, JENKINS, J, AND JIMENEZ-PABON, E: *Aphasia in Adults: Diagnosis, Prognosis and Treatment.* Harper & Row, New York, 1967.
23. SMITH, RM: *Prognosis after severe head trauma.* Fourth Annual Post-Graduate Course on the Rehabilitation of the Traumatic Brain-Injured Adult, Williamsburg, Va, 1980.
24. DARLEY, FL, ARONSON, AE, AND BROWN, JR: *Motor Speech Disorders.* WB Saunders, Philadelphia, 1975.
25. JOHNSON, GA: *Swallowing and oral facilitation.* Fourth Annual Post-Graduate Course on the Rehabilitation of the Traumatic Brain-Injured Adult, Williamsburg, Va, 1980.
26. ARONSON, A: *Clinical Voice Disorders.* Stratton, New York, 1980.
27. KERMAN, P, ET AL: *Palatal lift and speech therapy for velopharyngeal incompetence.* Arch Phys Med Rehabil 54:271, 1973.
28. ROSENBECK, JC AND LAPOINTE, LL: *The dysarthrias: Description, diagnosis and treatment.* In JOHNS, DF (ED): *Clinical Management of Neurogenic Communicative Disorders.* Little, Brown & Co, Boston, 1978.
29. HAGEN, C, MALKMUS, D, AND DURHAM, P: *Levels of cognitive functioning.* Head Trauma Rehabilitation Seminar, Rancho Los Amigos Hospital, Los Angeles, 1977.
30. RAO, P: *Alternate forms of communication.* Fourth Annual Post-Graduate Course on Rehabilitation of the Traumatic Brain-Injured Adult, Williamsburg, Va, 1980.
31. HARRIS, D AND VANDERHEIDEN, GC: *Augmentative communication techniques.* In SCHIEFELBUSCH, RL (ED): *Nonspeech and Language Communication.* University Park Press, Baltimore, 1980.
32. VANDERHEIDEN, GC (ED): *Non-Vocal Communication Resource Book.* University Park Press, Baltimore, 1978.

Chapter 26

COGNITIVE REMEDIATION

Yehuda Ben-Yishay, Ph.D.
Leonard Diller, Ph.D.

In the past, there has been a widespread belief that the behavioral effects of brain lesions remain "fixed" after the acute phase of recovery is over. This belief was based in part on the facts that neurons do not replicate and that the acquisition of skills is difficult and painfully slow to be of great practical usefulness.[1] Although there were exceptions,[2-4] cognitive remedial retraining as a systematic rationally based endeavor was not part of the conventional armamentarium in rehabilitation programs for head-injured patients because it was implicitly assumed that there was little justification for it.

In recent years, however, there has been a dramatic shift away from the traditionally passive view of recovery of cognitive functions after head injury. Several widely differing theories have been advanced. Comprehensive reviews of the major psychologic theories of recovery may be found in two recent books by Cotman[5] and Finger.[6] These theories have in common the emphasis they place on the analysis of synaptic processes as the key to understanding the remarkable plasticity and modifiability of brain behavior that is exhibited in normal development as well as during recovery after head injuries.

Rosner[7] provides a comprehensive review of four theories of recovery that emphasize the interactions of physiologic processes with environmental influences and that underscore the capacity of head-injured organisms to find alternate means of achieving functional goals when, owing to head injuries, their previously acquired strategies for problem solving or skill repertoires have been impaired.

The first of these is Jackson's compensatory principle,[8] which is based on his hierarchic model of central nervous system (CNS) organization. According to Jackson, a function that is presently controlled and organized by higher-level cortical processes was originally (in the ontogenesis of the function) controlled and organized by lower-level cortical centers in a hierarchic order. Hence, damage to higher-level cortical centers releases the lower levels from inhibition. The lower levels can then reassume control and carry out, to some extent, the function that, until the head injury, was assumed by the higher-level organizing centers. There have been some attempts to validate the notion that brain damage causes a regression in skills[9] and to develop instruments for diagnosis[10] and therapeutics in cognitive skills[11] along these lines.

The second theory of recovery may be termed the "substitutionist" or "replacement" theory. A modern interpretation of the substitutionist view has been presented by Gazzaniga,[12,13] who maintains that behavioral recovery after head injury is possible because existing, intact behavioral strategies can replace the functions destroyed by the brain damage. "The idea here is that one can 'shunt' around a brain lesion by setting up environmental contingencies differently and thereby requiring a different part of the brain to be used in the solution of a problem."[12] A line of current research in neuropsychology that indicates that brain-damaged people respond more effectively to cues involving intact rather than impaired abilities fits in with the idea that substitute habits can replace previously acquired habits in solving a problem.[14,15]

The third explanation was first proposed by von Monakow,[16] who argued that damage to a specific region of the brain causes a shock or diaschisis in other regions. According to this view, because the focal lesion deprives the remaining intact regions of their normal amount of afferent stimulation, the resultant shock or diaschisis leads to a general "shut-down" of other systems, with its concomitant impairment of the functions that are assumed by the areas now in a state of shock and inhibition. As the diaschisis gradually dissipates over time, the intact regions resume their normal state, hence the return of those functions that are normally subsumed by these regions. Any residual symptoms following the organism's recovery from the diaschisis would therefore be the direct result of the focal lesion.

The fourth and most recent explanation is Luria's "retraining" theory, which incorporates some of the previous theories of recovery of function. Luria[17,18] postulates that areas of the brain spared by the injury reorganize dynamically in such a way that they can carry out affected functions in new ways. His is the most directly relevant explanatory system for rehabilitation professionals because (1) it is based on extensive and very rich clinical experiences with head-injured people; (2) it explicitly states that the recovery of higher cortical functions after head injuries will not occur in the absence of "active exercises" embedded in a "re-education" program wherein specific "rehabilitation training" must be given to the patient in order to help compensate for specific deficiences in functioning; and (3) Luria's work, particularly in the diagnostic area of neuropsychology, is well known and can therefore serve as a springboard for systematic work toward the development of remedial interventions.

Luria[18] has outlined some basic principles of retraining. Stated succinctly and in a simplified manner, these are as follow: (1) The formulation of a plan of "restorative training" must be based on a detailed neuropsychologic investigation. (2) In order to enable a patient to carry out a function that has become impaired because of the head injury, it is often necessary to teach the patient compensatory strategies to achieve the same function by other means. (3) During the initial phases of the restorative training, it is necessary to fully "extend" and "program" the restorative activity. This means that the training task should be broken down into a series of highly articulated routines and subroutines capable of rendering the underlying processes of the activity fully explicit for the patient. Implicit in this principle is also the idea that the retraining should follow the logical course of the ontogenesis of the disturbed function and that the initial "extended programming" stage of retraining should be followed by a gradual withdrawal (in Luria's term, "condensation") of the cues, until the patient can carry out the specific action in the usual manner.

DEFINING THE OBJECTIVES OF COGNITIVE REMEDIATION

CONSIDERATIONS OF CONTEXT

Cognitive remediation after head injuries is inseparable from the context within which it is supposed to take place and the objectives that it aims to achieve. The context includes the level of analysis of cognitive deficits and the extent to which the relationships between the generic cognitive skill structures and functional behaviors are elucidated. The objectives depend on the way in which the desired outcomes, that is, the criterion behaviors, that are the targets of the remedial intervention are defined. In rehabilitation, people are generally referred for remediation of cognitive problems because a more direct attack on deficits in functional behaviors of daily living has proven unsuccessful and the patient still has major residual dysfunctions. However, if one chooses cognitive remediation, where does one begin?

In a rehabilitation setting for head-injured patients, the targets of cognitive remedial intervention should be those areas of functioning that have been shown by means of various correlational studies[19-21] to have the greatest relevance, that is, predictive value, to outcome competencies in (1) daily life functions and self-care, (2) skill complexes that have a direct bearing on the person's subsequent work abilities, and (3) interpersonal skills and social (re)adaptability. This is, in short, a rehabilitation-relevant approach to the delimitation of the area of concern with cognitive remediation in head injury.[22,23]

Over the past 15 years, there has been an increasing number of reports on the results of rehabilitation interventions with head-injured people.[24-30] For the most part, these studies do not report on the impact of the interventions on the cognitive deficits and on the outcomes, nor are they specific enough about the precise nature of those interventions. There are clinical studies reporting marked improvements in cognitive functions after some intervention or other, and many clinicians can provide anecdotal accounts of improvements. However, it is clear that success in cognitive remediation and rehabilitation is still spotty and there is a great need for a more systematic and detailed work in this area as well as for more evidence for the credibility of the effects of cognitive remediation on functional behaviors. During the past decade, we have reported on a series of successful remedial interventions to ameliorate various types of cognitive deficits in stroke patients, and we have attempted to outline some of the conceptual and the methodologic issues in this type of work.[31-34] More recent attempts to develop the building blocks for cognitive remediation in head-injured people are documented in a series of monographs developed by Ben-Yishay and associates.[23,35-37]

CONSIDERATIONS OF SCOPE

In a rehabilitation context, the remedial enterprise with the head injured patient is often a process that must unfold over a period of many months, sometimes years. This process consists of a series of multilayered, time-sequenced, prioritized, and carefully orchestrated program elements whose ultimate purpose is the overcoming of three principal barriers[23] that stand in the way of realization of the patient's functional potential. These three barriers are:

1. Problems in persistent goal-directed behavior owing to suboptimal levels of basic arousal, fluctuating attention, poor concentration, poorly modulated behavior, and psychomotor impersistence
2. Problems in the acquisition of new information, owing to the interactions among aspects of anterograde amnesia, the attentional disorders, and the disorders in higher-level thinking that affect the assimilation, retention, and generalization of newly acquired information
3. Problems in the integration of multiple remedial inputs (which are given both simultaneously and in a sequential manner during the course of the rehabilitation process) and their application toward effective action in context-appropriate, real-life situations.

In Search of an Answer

Can there be an adequate answer to the challenges posed by the three "barriers" to the rehabilitation of the severely head-injured person? Our tentative answer is in the affirmative and is based (1) on compelling outcome and follow-up data that are being gathered on more than 60 cases to date; and (2) on two parallel, long-term clinical studies on neurologically plateaued head-injured patients who proved intractable to conventional rehabilitation methods and who, prior to their participation in these programs, remained cognitively, vocationally, and socially unrehabilitated. These studies—one in Israel and one at New York University Medical Center, Institute of Rehabilitation Medicine—have been in existence since 1975. These programs have been specifically designed to test whether head-injured patients who exhibit the type of problems characterized by the three barriers can be helped in becoming functional. Both employ essentially the same treatment techniques; the staffs of both received, before beginning to implement the treatment plans, in-depth orientation and specific training; and both are conducted under the same leadership.[35-40]

Distilled to the essentials, these programs were designed to possess three mutually reinforcing properties:

(1) The programs represent a structure of multilayered interventions that are prioritized and "programmed" in a manner conducive to optimal integration of the various remedial and "therapeutic" interventions. Figure 26-1 illustrates schematically how the programs are organized to maintain that integrative function both on a daily and long-term basis.

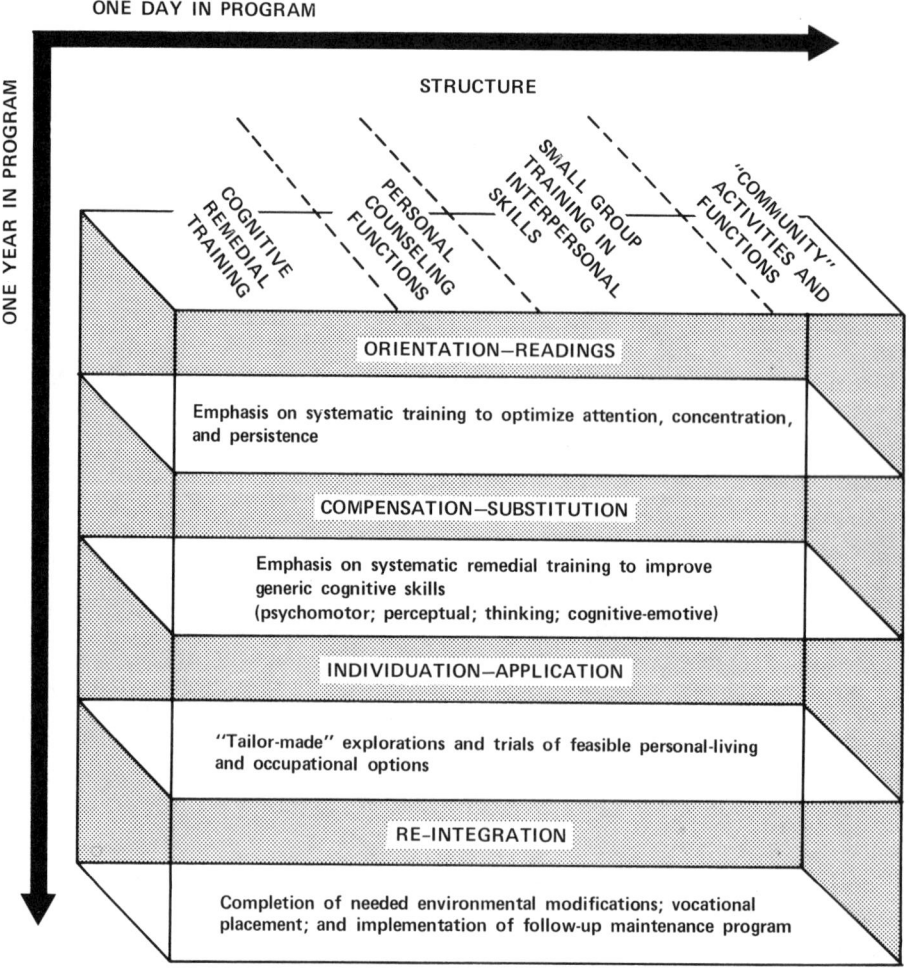

FIGURE 26-1. A cross-sectional and longitudinal overview of the multi-layered cognitive remediation program.

The programs administer a comprehensive and systematic method of cognitive remedial training "modules" according to a "master plan of treatment," to improve generic deficits across the entire range of cognitive skill domains in which are nested psychomotor skills, perceptual cognitive integrational skills, verbal ideational (logical reasoning) and cognitive-emotive integrational skills, and cognitive-interpersonal skills. Each of these domains has within it a range of difficulty of tasks that are arranged in a hierarchic fashion.

(2) The programs operate as modified, miniature "therapeutic communities" wherein the individual patient is provided with a supportive "reference group" of peers and with a variety of healthy "models"—the staff members and various "surrogates"—who combined provide (a) a natural milieu in which to "practice" improved cognitive, personal, and social skills and (b) the therapeutic leverages that are necesary to induce modification of maladaptive behaviors in the desired direction.

These programs provide a framework within which an initially disorganized, demoralized, and maladapted individual is aided in coming to terms with the existential situation (i.e., drastically altered, deflected, or reduced zone of potential for future development) and in accepting, at the end of the program, the realistic alternatives for a future life-style and occupational opportunities that are personally "meaningful" and "satisfactory" substitute outlets for deflected drives toward "self-actualization."[23]

(3) The programs also provide the framework and the means for making an orderly transition from the remedial intervention phase to the application phase, which, in the case of severely head-injured patient, must be done in a systematic and carefully graduated fashion. The principal guidelines for this process are (a) the matching of the patient's present skill band with existing and feasible "job descriptions"; (b) considering the questions of the efficiency (quality), productivity, and persistence (stability) aspects of the patient's performance; (c) considering the question of the patient's "work-relations" adequacy (i.e., the adequacy of interpersonal skills repertoire) for the specifically chosen occupational activities; (d) obtaining the patient's and significant others' endorsement of the plan; (e) considering and effecting the needed "environmental engineering" interventions (e.g., orienting and briefing, sometimes even "treating" the patient's human environment; setting up the required "logistics" and environmental modifications) that will enable and ensure the patient's stability of functioning in the "natural milieu; and (f) establishing the liaison system, the clinical procedures, and the required network of supportive systems to ensure the uninterrupted and immediate response to arising needs for crisis intervention.

An Integrated System of Cognitive Remedial Modules

Within the abovementioned rehabilitation-relevant settings, the cognitive retraining functions of the programs are confined to a certain portion of the time of a larger day program, via a series of training "modules" that are administered in a specified order. Further, the transition from module to module is based on the individual patient's rate of progress within each of the specific cognitive skill training domains that are applied after the patient has either reached criterion levels of performance or plateaued at some level below criterion. The contents of these task hierarchies (the cognitive modules), the logic of their construction, and the theoretical underpinnings have been described elsewhere.[19-21,23,33-37,41,42] In the present context, a brief restatement of the underlying logic of the construction of these task hierarchies is in order.

Figure 26-2 illustrates the multidimensional thinking that went into forming the rationale for the construction of the various remedial intervention modules. As can be seen, our rationale is the result of a synthesis of neuropsychologic theory, didactic notions, and the consideration of clinical management issues such as strategy and timing of specific interventions. Briefly summarized, we considered five dimensions of the problem:

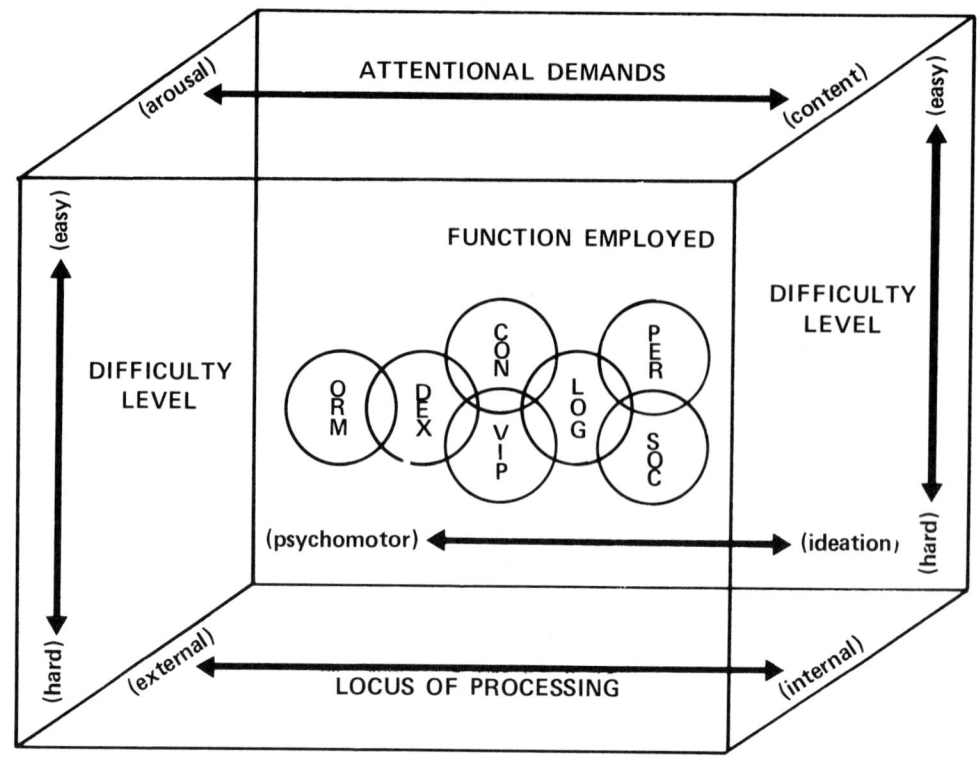

FIGURE 26-2. Factors inherent in the construction of the remedial modules.

(1) *The attentional demands of the task hierarchies.* From the standpoint of attentional demand, the task hierarchies were so constructed that they range from those that principally involve the basic arousal aspects of the consciousness continuum[43] to those that place the emphasis on the other end, the "content" aspects of the consciousness continuum. Basic arousal refers to the neurophysiologic and neuropsychologic substrata of consciousness, the underlying processes that are responsible for normal arousal level. This system originates in the brain stem reticular formation and extends to the cortex via the diffuse or nonspecific thalmic projection system.[44,45] Content refers to the higher cortical functions, the mental operations that guide the subject matter of consciousness at any given moment in time.

(2) *Choice of the materials and the way the task hierarchies were constructed.* Accordingly, by ensuring that the first tasks involve primarily simple psychomotor functions and the last ones involve predominantly higher-level ideation or verbal reasoning types of functions, it became possible to gradually increase the attentional demands on the patients via the task selections.

(3) *Locus of processing.* The third dimension considered was the locus of processing of the stimulus and the response components of the various tasks. In this connection, special attention was paid to ensure that the primary locus of the processing in the first of the series of tasks be "external" (e.g., watch for onset of signal light, press button), whereas the locus of processing in the last of the task series be predominantly "internal" (i.e., comprehend the oral instructions, translate them into a series of internal complementary self-commands, reason out a plan for solving the problem, and respond according to the plan).

(4) *Difficulty level of tasks within modules.* The fourth dimension has already been mentioned earlier. It concerns scaling each of the given modules in such a way that they

represent a graduated series of subtasks that are administered in order from the easiest to the hardest.

(5) *Order of priorities in intervening.* The last, the fifth, dimension needs little elaboration. It is implicit in the former considerations. In dealing with the severely head-injured patient, it is desirable to administer first those remedial interventions that place the least attentional demands on the patient and to administer last those that require higher levels of demand in attention and concentration; to commence with tasks involving the simpler, psychomotor functions and to end with those involving the more complex ideational functions; and, finally, to proceed from tasks whose processing is predominantly external to those whose processing is primarily internal. This order conforms both to the general notion of the neuropsychologic ontogenesis of cognitive functions and to empirically proven clinical and didactic principles.

Considerations of the Structural Aspects of Cognitive Remediation

What makes a given activity cognitive remedial and not some other kind of activity?

In a recent paper, Ben-Yishay[37] examined (1) the essential structural characteristics of all cognitive remedial tasks and (2) the necessary and sufficient conditions for the optimal unfolding of the cognitive remedial endeavor. The following section summarizes the highlights of that analysis.

(1) *Defining the overall characteristic of cognitive remedial tasks.* Procedures qualifying as cognitive remedial training were defined to be those routines or exercises that, through systematic engagement, permit the head-injured patient to correct, or at least significantly ameliorate, some generic deficit that hampers problem-solving abilities.

(2) *Problem solving based on Luria's model.* This was defined according to a modified version of Luria's working model[17] of (the verbal and nonverbal) problem-solving process in normal life. Figure 26-3 depicts the eight stages of the problem-solving cycle.

As depicted in the figure, the problem-solving process can be said to consist of a chain of overlapping and interdigited cognitive routines and subroutines. Some of the links in this chain of mental events are "convergent" in nature (i.e., their end-product is the emergence of some crystallized, core ideas); other links in the continuum are "divergent" in nature (i.e., the sought-after by-products of the thinking process are the generation of multiple, "exploratory," alternative ideas, and following that, the choosing from among those alternatives the particular ideational "strand" that seems most relevant in the specific situation at hand); whereas other links in the chain of the mental processes can be termed "executive" in nature (i.e., they involve the instrumental behaviors and responses that are necessary for rendering thoughts and plans into action sequences).

Against the above background, Ben-Yishay[37] classified the various existing (and as yet to be developed) remedial interventions that would qualify as cognitive remedial routines into three subtypes.

TYPE ONE. Type one routines include tasks designed to improve the head-injured person's higher-level analytic-synthetic (a) "convergent" thinking abilities; (b) general capacity and "flexibility" of thought required for "divergent" reasoning processes; (c) "executive" skills—planning, prioritizing, sequencing, coordinating, and self-monitoring activities; and (d) evaluative-integrative abilities.

TYPE TWO. Type two routines include remedial tasks designed to correct or ameliorate deficits in various generic, "compound" mental functions like (a) basic arousal and level of orientation—basic attention, concentration, and persistence; (b) psychomotor skills—integrating eye-hand motion cycles with finger dexterity; (c) cognitive perceptual integrative skills—constructional praxis abilities; (d) visual information processing abilities; (e) various memory

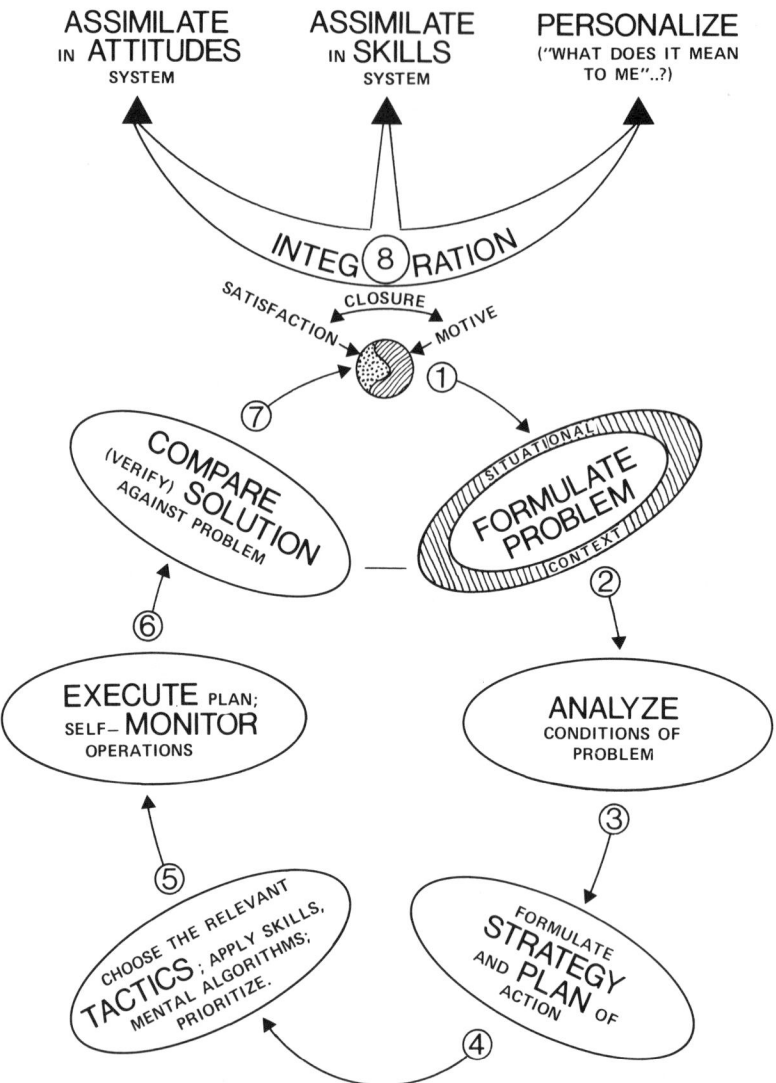

FIGURE 26-3. Stages of the problem-solving process.

functions—tasks designed to enhance the processing, acquisition, and retention of new information; and (f) communications skills—general and interpersonal communications functions.

TYPE THREE. Type three routines include two special variants of remedial training: (a) The first variant of remedial tasks includes special exercises designed to "bypass" or "neutralize" interferences or localized defects in some perceptual or motor subskills, or components of such subskills, that are employed by the patient in the course of attempts at problem solving. The aim of these special exercises is to help the patient compensate or substitute for some isolated subskill that is employed in the process of problem solving; but the subskill itself is not part of the mental process, proper, of problem solving. (b) The second variant of the type three tasks are those remedial routines that are designed to strengthen "weakened" or "slowed-down" associations among the patient's ontogenetically acquired "schemata," "kinetic melodies," "mental algorithms," "sets," "habits"—in short, the repertoire of semiautomatic (and automatic) action or thought dispositions, which are the "building blocks" or the "tools" with which problem solving is accomplished.

Systematic remedial retraining techniques of the first type have been described by Ben-Yishay and associates.[23,35] Remedial techniques of the second type have been successfully employed by Ben-Yishay and others.[23,35,36,46,47] And remedial techniques of the third type were employed by Diller and associates[33,42,43] in stroke patients and more recently by Piasetsky[48,49] with various types of head-injured patients.

Mode and Order of Presentation and Meaningfulness of the Stimuli

The cognitive remedial endeavor with severely head-injured patients requires that particular attention be paid to two interrelated dimensions of task performance. The first dimension concerns the requirements for articulating the field—the stimulus and the performance properties of the task—in a manner to fit the particular constraints of the given patient's syndrome. The second, a corollary of the first, is the "pedagogic" dimension of the remedial process. Although from a practical point of view it is difficult to separate the concern with the field properties of tasks from didactic considerations (since the dividing line between the two is not clear-cut), these are nevertheless clearly distinguishable facets of the problem and merit separate consideration.

STIMULUS AND PERFORMANCE PROPERTIES OF THE TASK. If head-injured patients have difficulties in creating their own "order" when confronted with a field of stimuli (task to perform; materials to handle), the stimulus and the performance conditions must be so ordered and presented as to enable patients to adequately cope with the task. Too complex stimuli, too many "pieces" of information to absorb, and too few cues as to the order in which to proceed or where to begin will become part of the problem, instead of helping to solve problems. Several points must be kept in mind in this connection:

(1) The precise nature of the assignment (including the "operationalized" formulation of the problem to be solved and the sought-after solution) must be conveyed to the patient, right at the outset of the remedial process. This must be accomplished by means of display and by modes of presentation that are "tailor-designed" to fit the particular constraints imposed by the patient's deficits, and they must be kept in focus to ensure that the patient remains oriented toward the final solution.

(2) The remedial task must be broken down into (phenomenologically meaningful and syndrome-appropriate) units of performance, meaning that major routines should be further broken down into subroutines, all of which should then be properly sequenced and organized to comprise a continuous process. These units and subunits of performance must conform with the salient "points of intersection and interaction" among the important cognitive component functions in this task.

(3) Following the task analysis, a system of cueing, graded for levels of difficulty, must then be developed. The training must follow the principle of "saturation cueing," which is the gradual and orderly "fading" of cues, one at a time, from the most explicit to the least explicit cueing step.

In connection with the second—the pedagogic—dimension of the remedial enterprise, several points need to be considered:

(1) Different types of head-injured patients require different, syndrome-specific, "induction." Induction refers to the preparatory phase, prior to the specific instructions, during which the patient is made "ready" to engage in the specific task. The following example illustrates one particular variant of a syndrome-appropriate induction. Consider a patient with a severe impairment of basic arousal mechanisms, which manifests itself by suboptimal vigilance, fluc-

tuating attention, insufficient concentration powers, and psychomotor impersistence. The patient is about to commence remedial training on a special instrument designed to ameliorate the attentional deficit.

Clinically, the patient appears to be insufficiently oriented to the surroundings, the patient's gaze is not focused on the examiner or the instrument in front of the patient, and the patient appears passive, remote, and uninvolved. The therapist who wishes to engage the patient in the specific activity must first prepare and "warm up" the patient by means of the induction task.

Typically, the induction in a case like this would consist of several steps:

(a) *Focusing the patient's gaze and attention on the training instrument.* The examiner would exclaim: "Look at this!" and activate the instrument, turning on all the colored lights on the display panel.

(b) *Activating the patient.* Then the examiner would say, "Now you put your finger on this button and see what happens." (Often the examiner would actually place the patient's finger on the button and press, thereby together they would activate the instrument again.)

(c) *Engaging the patient's interest in the activity.* At this point, the examiner, seeking to arouse the patient's interest and will to engage in the activity at hand, would typically deliver a short, rousing, and evocative "speech."

As shown by repeated clinical experiences with severely head-injured patients, the induction "speech" is most effective when it combines—in its content, style of delivery, and tone—elements of a sports coach's rallying pep talk with the exhoratory style of a commercial advertisement and the inspirational technique of the revivalist spiritual leader. One variant of such an induction speech would go something like this: "Now! The sharper your reflexes, the more ready you will be to respond when this signal light goes on. And the more agile your response, the faster you will be able to push this button. When you push the button real fast, you turn on all these colored lights. Go ahead! Show me your stuff! Let me see how fast you can push this button; how many lights can you turn on? Watch out for this little signal light. When it comes on you "jump" as fast as you can and push this button! Imagine that you are a champion sprinter in the Olympics, ready to sprint when the gun goes off . . . Here we go! On your mark! Get set! . . ." For continuation, see the following section.

(d) *The "countdown."* The examiner then continues: "Get set! We begin the countdown (alluding to the "blast off" phase of a space shot): Five, four, three, two, one, Push! . . ." With the induction over, the examiner then instructs patients into the specifics of the task, and the training proper is commenced.

(2) Different types of syndromes require different methods of instruction, feedback, and behavior monitoring during the remedial exercise. The rate of presentation of material, the "rhythm" in which the material is presented, the extent to which repetitions and recapitulations should be made, the means employed by the instructor to "bridge" between auditorily presented information and visually presented information, running commentaries concerning "housekeeping" aspects of the patient's behavior (e.g., "do not crowd the pieces together . . ."), and the means employed by the instructor to maintain continuity from minute to minute within a single session and between sessions all require special attention, "tailor-made" for the individual patient at hand.

(3) No cognitive remediation with the severely head-injured patient can take place without proper clinical management of what Goldstein[50] termed the minor and major "catastrophic reaction" phenomena. The term refers to a variety of "shock" reactions, to impending or actually experienced failure, manifestations of anxiety, and "refractory" periods (wherein the patients may become temporarily incapable of coping with even simple routines, well within the patient's ken of competence under "calmer" circumstances). Catastrophic reactions are the inevitable by-products of problem-solving behavior in head-injured persons and must be successfully dealt with so that the remedial process can go on unimpeded.

Problems Inherent in the Nature and Conditions of the Remedial Tasks

It would be highly desirable in cognitive remediation to train the head-injured person to perform those types of tasks that are most directly related to the solving of specific problems in daily life functions. The more readily a patient can identify an activity as being concretely related (i.e., "relevant") to personal problems, the more meaningful it becomes to the patient, hence the easier the task of inducing the patient to engage in and persist at the activity. The fact that in normal development and education no real learning takes place without a minimum degree of involvement of the learner in the act of learning (which includes both active participation and motivation) is well known and needs little emphasis. There are, however, several aspects to this issue that are specific to the way severely head-injured people learn and assimilate new information, which need be touched upon in this context.

Carrying out the remedial intervention directly within, or very near, the "real-life" events is usually impractical from the standpoint of sustained and systematic intervention. Since most of the more complex, higher-level, functional activities are of a compound nature (i.e., consisting of various mixtures of generic cognitive and interpersonal skills), they are multidetermined (i.e., usually stemming from multiple intentional-motivational sources), and they usually occur within specific contexts and are part of extended processes. Hence, such activities do not lend themselves to the kinds of treatments (e.g., didactic interruptions, analyses, amplifications, articulations, simplified restatements, repetitions, and so on) that characterize all systemic teaching or remedial endeavors. Moreover, the interruption of spontaneous activities, of a "real-life" nature, in the severely head-injured person, frequently results in the loss of the patient's sense of continuity or, worse yet, in temporary disorientation plus frustration. In addition, the patient's already significantly lowered tolerance for error and "failure" tends to become further exacerbated when failure occurs during the performance of "naturalistic," personally meaningful acts.

Thus, for the reasons mentioned above, the tasks that are employed during cognitive remedial training are usually specially designed and carefully delineated (somewhat contrived) action sequences whose principal characteristics are that they lend themselves to precisely "calibrated" and controlled activities. These tasks, of course, rarely resemble "real-life" behaviors. Hence, the therapist who engages in cognitive remediation must face a seemingly paradoxic situation: The therapist must relate the remedial task, which is not a part of the patient's "naturalistic" repertoire of behaviors, to the patient's own perceived life goals and "priorities" of rehabilitation. Only thus can head-injured patients be optimally engaged in and motivated to perform the remedial exercises and to view these as being personally relevant, meaningful, and important exercises.

Although the precise nature of the underlying mechanism needs to be further studied and elucidated, the accumulated evidence from clinical experiences over the past few years is most persuasive. It has been repeatedly shown that in order to actively and dynamically engage severely head-injured patients and to induce them to persist at various cognitive remedial exercises, several techniques proved to be particularly effective motivating tools: (1) the use of exhortatory techniques (e.g., "Come on, give it all you have got!" ... "Show me/us your stuff/determination" ... "Come on, don't be 'stingy,' don't hold back; get cracking!"); (2) the use of powerfully evocative metaphors (e.g., "like a champion sprinter, ready to jump at the sound of the gun" ... "like a rocket, ready to lift off" ... "concentrate, focus your mind/eyes like a powerful laser beam, right on the target" ... "steady, and cool at the controls, like a test pilot; ready for everything" ... "your mind/will is the master, the mouth/hand/foot is the servant; make the ... obey!" ... "here we go! coming in for the last sprint; one last surge of effort and we cross the 'finish' line ..."); (3) the use of inspirational techniques (e.g., "What a pleasure and privilege to watch a *mind* in action ..." "Yes, sir, this is something to behold, this should be videotaped; this is what life is all about, *mind* over muscle, *will* over weakness...."); (4) the use of "psychodrama" with role reversals; the patient is coaxed into accepting the challenge of role reversal (and is provided "modeling" how to do it), whereupon the patient in effect ends up explaining to a "mirror image"—the therapist—the rationale for the particular exercise at hand and exhorts the self to greater and more sustained mental efforts; and (5) requesting that the patient make repeated assertions regarding intent to comply with the task demands and to explicitly verbalize the importance of the exercises for rehabilitation. Then after some preliminary "rehearsals," these assertions are videotaped or audiorecorded "so that little doubt should be left in anyone's mind that you know exactly *what* you are going to do and *why*...."

Traditionally, engaging the individual via exhortatory techniques has been commonly associated with the worlds of commercial advertisements and sports, and the use of inspirational techniques with religious revivalism or with politics; the "extraction" or "public" assertions of intent and compliance, plus the request that these be delivered "with feeling" and in a "convincing" manner, conjure up in one's mind the methods employed by (the Chinese version of) "thought reformers." The use of such techniques for the purpose of motivating individuals and to induce attitudinal and behavioral changes has been frowned upon by traditionalists in educational psychology and psychotherapy. However, such methods have been found to be most effective, even indispensable, in the remedial retraining of severely head-injured patients and, when judiciously applied as part of a well-thought-out clinical-remedial strategy, they should be employed to enhance the potential effects of the remedial enterprise.

In this we clearly subscribe to the notions that were so aptly articulated by Frank.[51] In his now classic work on persuasion and healing, Frank pointed out that the worlds of religion, religious healing, and thought reform contain some important lessons for the modern psychotherapist that should be heeded. In a similar vein, McClelland[52] noted that in an attempt to develop a program to induce changes in the "achievement drive" in a village in India, it was necessary, among other things, to resort to exhortatory and inspirational techniques in order to effect the desired changes in behavior.

SUMMARY

This chapter briefly summarized the neuropsychologic rationale for cognitive remediation after a head injury; defined the objectives of cognitive remediation; briefly outlined the main considerations concerning the setting, scope, and organizational aspects of a remedial program; outlined the structural-cognitive features of remedial training tasks and identified the three main subtypes of cognitive remedial training tasks; pointed out some of the most important considerations concerning the order of presentation, meaningfulness of the stimuli, and the pedagogic and clinical aspects of the application of remedial training exercises; and, finally, called to attention the importance of optimizing the patient's involvement in the remedial activity and maintaining the patient's motivation to persist at the remedial task, in order to enhance learning and assimilation.

REFERENCES

1. KOTTKE, FS: *From reflex to skill: The training of coordination.* Arch Phys Med Rehabil 61:551, 1980.
2. GOLDSTEIN, K: *Human Nature in the Light of Psychopathology.* Harvard University Press, Cambridge, Mass, 1951, pp 56–57, 85–119.
3. LURIA, AR: *Restoration of Function After Brain Injury.* Macmillan, New York, 1963.

4. ZANGWILL, OL: *Psychological Aspects of Rehabilitation in Cases of Brain Injury.* Annual Extended Meeting, British Psychological Society, Durham, April 12, 1946.
5. COTMAN, CW: *Neuronal Plasticity.* Raven Press, New York, 1978.
6. FINGER, S: *Recovery from Brain Damage.* Plenum Press, New York, 1978.
7. ROSNER, BS: *Recovery of function and localization of function in historical perspective.* In STEIN, DG, ROSEN, JJ, AND BUTTERS, N (EDS): *Plasticity and Recovery of Function in the Central Nervous System.* Academic Press, New York, 1974.
8. JACKSON, JH: *Selected Writings,* Vol 2. Basic Books, New York, 1969.
9. BORTNER, M AND BIRCH, HG: *Perception and perceptual motor disassociation in cerebral palsied children.* J Nerv Ment Dis 130:49, 1960.
10. ESON, ME, YEN, JK, AND BOURKE, RS: *Assessment of recovery from serious head injury.* J Neurol Neurosurg Psychiatry 41:1036, 1978.
11. BUSSE, TV AND LIGHTHALL, FF: *Conceptual retraining of brain damaged adults.* Percept Mot Skills 22:899, 1966.
12. GAZZANIGA, MS: *Determinants of cerebral recovery.* In STEIN, DG, ROSEN, JJ, AND BUTTERS, N (EDS): *Plasticity and Recovery of Function in the Central Nervous System.* Academic Press, New York, 1974.
13. GAZZANIGA, MS: *Is seeing believing: Notes on clinical recovery.* In FINGER, S (ED): *Recovery from Brain Damage.* Plenum Press, New York, 1978.
14. FORDYCE, WE AND JONES, RH: *The efficacy of oral and pantomime instructions for hemiplegic patients.* Arch Phys Med Rehabil 47:676, 1966.
15. BINDER, IM AND SCHREIBER, J: *Visual imagery and verbal mediation as memory aids in recovering alcoholics.* Journal of Clinical Neuropsychology 2:71, 1980.
16. MONAKOW, C VON: *Die lokalisation in grosshirnrinde und der abbau der funktion durch korticale herde.* JF Bergmann, Wiesbaden, 1914.
17. LURIA, AR: *The Working Brain.* Penguin Press, London, 1973.
18. LURIA, AR, ET AL: *Restoration of higher cortical function following local brain damage.* In YINKEN, RJ AND BRUYN, GW (EDS): *Handbook of Clinical Neurology,* Vol 3. North-Holland, Amsterdam, 1969.
19. BEN-YISHAY, Y, ET AL: *Prediction of rehabilitation outcomes from psychometric parameters in left hemiplegics.* J Consult Clin Psychol 34:436, 1970.
20. BEN-YISHAY, Y, ET AL: *Relationships between initial competence and ability to profit from cues in brain damaged individuals.* J Abnorm Psychol 75:248, 1970.
21. BEN-YISHAY, Y, DILLER, L, AND MANDLEBERG, I: *The ability to profit from cues as a function of initial competence in normal and brain injured adults: A replication of previous findings.* J Abnorm Psychol 76:378, 1970.
22. DILLER, L: *A model for cognitive retraining in rehabilitation.* The Clinical Psychologist 29(2):13, 1976.
23. BEN-YISHAY, Y (ED): *Working Approaches to Remediation of Cognitive Deficits in Brain Damaged.* New York University, IRM Behavioral Science, Rehabilitation Monograph No. 61, New York, 1980.
24. WALKER, AF, CAVENESS, WF, AND CRITCHLEY, M: *The Late Effects of Brain Injury.* Charles C Thomas, Springfield, Ill, 1969.
25. NAJENSON, TL, ET AL: *Rehabilitation after severe head injury.* Scand J Rehabil Med 5:1, 1973.
26. NAJENSON, TL, ET AL: *Rehabilitation after severe head injury.* Scand J Rehabil Med 6:5, 1974.
27. NAJENSON, TL, ET AL: *Prognostic factors in rehabilitation after severe head injury.* Scand J Rehabil Med 6:101, 1975.
28. GRONWALL, DA: *Paired auditory serial addition task as a measure of recovery from concussion.* Percept Mot Skills 44:367, 1977.
29. REYES, RL, BHATTACHARYYA, AK, AND HELLER, D: *Traumatic head injury: Restlessness and agitation as prognosticators of physical and psychologic improvement in patients.* Arch Phys Med Rehabil 62:20, 1961.

30. TOBIS, JS: *Physical medicine and brain rehabilitation in brain injury.* Arch Phys Med Rehabil 55:56, 1974.
31. BEN-YISHAY, Y, ET AL: *Similarities and differences in Block Design performances between older normal and brain-injured persons: A task analysis.* J Abnorm Psychol 78:17, 1971.
32. BEN-YISHAY, Y, ET AL: *Differences in matching persistence behavior during Block Design performance between older normal and brain-damaged persons: A process analysis.* Cortex 10:121, 1974.
33. DILLER, L, ET AL: *Studies in Cognition and Rehabilitation in Hemiplegia.* New York University Medical Center, IRM, Behavioral Science, Rehabilitation Monograph No. 50, New York, 1974.
34. DILLER, L, ET AL: *Methods for Evaluation and Treatment of Visual Perceptual Difficulties of Right Brain Damaged Individuals.* New York University Medical Center, IRM, Behavioral Science, Rehabilitation Monograph, New York, 1980 (Supplement to 1980 Eighth Annual Workshop).
35. BEN-YISHAY, Y (ED): *Working Approaches to Remediation of Cognitive Deficits in Brain Damaged.* New York University, IRM Behavioral Science, Rehabilitation Monograph No. 59, New York, 1978.
36. BEN-YISHAY, Y (ED): *Working Approaches to Remediation of Cognitive Deficits in Brain Damaged.* New York University, IRM Behavioral Science, Rehabilitation Monograph No. 60, New York, 1979.
37. BEN-YISHAY, Y (ED): *Working Approaches to Remediation of Cognitive Deficits in Brain Damaged Persons.* New York University Medical Center, IRM Rehabilitation Monograph No. 62, New York, 1981.
38. BEN-YISHAY, Y: *An outline of a comprehensive theoretical framework for the rehabilitation of persons with severe head traumas.* Keynote address, Sixth Annual Rehabilitation Day Symposium, Chaim Sheba Medical Center, Tel Hashomer, Israel, November 1975.
39. BEN-YISHAY, Y: *Setting up a therapeutic community for comprehensive rehabilitation of Israeli outpatient war casualties with severe head injuries: Structure and remedial systems.* Invited panelist, The 13th World Congress of Rehabilitation, Israel, June 1976.
40. BEN-YISHAY, Y AND DILLER, L: *A multi-impact clinical experiment in rehabilitation of problematic outpatient brain injured veterans.* Post Congress Workshop, The Brain Injured: Rehabilitation and Bio-Engineering, The 13th World Congress of Rehabilitation, Israel, June 1976.
41. WEINBERG, J, ET AL: *Visual scanning training on reading related tasks in acquired right brain damage.* Arch Phys Med Rehabil 58:479, 1977.
42. WEINBERG, J, ET AL: *Training sensory awareness and spatial organization in people with right brain damage.* Arch Phys Med Rehabil 60:491, 1979.
43. PLUM, F AND POSNER, J: *Diagnosis of Stupor and Coma.* FA Davis, Philadelphia, 1972.
44. STRUB, RL AND BLACK, FW: *The Mental Status Examination in Neurology.* FA Davis, Philadelphia, 1977.
45. MAGOUN, H: *The Waking Brain.* Charles C Thomas, Springfield, Ill, 1963.
46. GIANUTSOS, R: *What is cognitive rehabilitation?* J Rehabil 5:36, 1980.
47. MILLER, E: *The training characteristics of severely head injured patients: A preliminary study.* J Neurol Neurosurg Psychiatry 43:525, 1980.
48. PIASETSKY, G: *Implications of brain behavior relationships for rehabilitation.* Presented at Symposium on Models and Techniques of Cognitive Rehabilitation, Community Hospital of Indianapolis, Indianapolis, Ind, January 1981.
49. PIASETSKY, G: *Process oriented training: A case study depicting treatment of verbal-cognitive deficits in a chronic aphasic.* Presented at the Ninth Annual Workshop on Remediation and Management of Cognitive and Perceptual Problems in Brain Damaged Adults, New York University Medical Center, IRM, New York, May 1981.
50. GOLDSTEIN, K: *Aftereffects of Brain Injuries in War.* Grune, New York, 1948.
51. FRANK, JD: *Persuasion and Healing.* Shocken Books, New York, 1963.
52. MCCLELLAND, D: *The Achieving Society.* Van Nostrand, New York, 1968.

Chapter 27

TREATMENT OF BEHAVIORAL DEFICITS

Craig A. Muir, Ph.D.
William J. Haffey, Ph.D.
Kathryn J. Ott, B.S.N.
Diane Karaica, A.A.
Jane H. Muir, R.P.T.
Margaret Sutko, Ph.D.

The purpose of this chapter is to present a behavioral perspective that can be helpful to clinicians treating head-injured patients. The chapter begins with a discussion of the behavioral nature of rehabilitation. This is followed by definitions of some behavior modification principles. The next section reviews published applications of these principles to rehabilitation, with emphasis on head-injured patients. It includes reports of chemotherapeutic approaches to behavioral problems. The final section describes several kinds of settings in which behavioral approaches are currently being used for the rehabilitation of head-injured individuals.

REHABILITATION AS A BEHAVIORAL PROCESS

The problems addressed by rehabilitation specialists involve observable, quantifiable events. Range of motion in an extremity, the amount of assistance needed for a transfer, continence or incontinence of bladder, and so on are events that can be seen by trained observers (therapists). In the sense that these actions occur in the observable, public domain, they are behaviors. This is not to say that events that occur within the patient are unimportant. Understanding the patient's emotional and cognitive processes is vital to successful rehabilitation.[1] However, the understanding of those inner processes is based on observable phenomena. The patient demonstrates the ability or inability to do a task, expresses fears, or exhibits depression through overt behavior. These external events and our interpretation of them constitute the behavioral basis of rehabilitation.

Patient progress is also measured behaviorally. If a person needed assistance from two people to walk when admitted to a rehabilitation program and walks independently upon discharge, that is a behavioral change. These changes in behaviors are defined as rehabilitation progress. Rehabilitation, then, can be conceptualized as a process in which some persons (treators) try to change the behaviors of other persons (patients) in particular directions.

An enormous amount of research has been done to establish the most effective ways of helping people change their behavior. Unfortunately, the knowledge gained through that research is not usually applied systematically in rehabilitation. Behavior modification methods are not easily transferred from the laboratory to clinical settings. The level of consistency that is the sine qua non of an experimental laboratory is difficult to achieve in clinical situations. Without a high level of consistency, behavior modification often loses its effectiveness. Behavior modification also requires that treators respond to patients in ways that may seem contrary to "common sense" or to one's usual ways of thinking about and dealing with patients. In essence, then, a basically behavioral process is usually carried on without the benefit of a large body of scientific work that directly addresses how to most effectively produce changes in behavior.

The need for systematic application of behavior modification procedures is especially critical in the rehabilitation of head-injured patients. Given their cognitive deficits, these individuals often cannot comprehend the connection between a therapeutic exercise regimen and long-term goals. For example, a patient may be able to indicate a desire to walk again without being able to understand that certain strengthening exercises are a prerequisite for ambulation. If the purpose of the regimen is not understood, why should a patient be "motivated" to participate in therapy? Furthermore, treatment of many head-injured patients begins when they are responding at a very primitive level, unable to establish or even to understand long-term goals.

In the acute recovery phase, cognitive disorders can include impaired attention and concentration, elementary and higher-order sensory and perceptual deficits, central language processing and production deficits, memory dysfunction, inability to use information for effective problem-solving, and inability to appreciate conceptual and symbolic relationships (e.g., cause and effect).[2-4] Behavioral and personality problems can involve emotional lability, low frustration tolerance, hyperactivity and impulsiveness, inappropriate social behavior, aggessiveness, assaultiveness, and disconnected thinking.[3-7] The interaction of these cognitive and behavioral deficits can seriously impede rehabilitation.[8,9]

After discharge from the acute setting, persistent cognitive and behavioral disorders contribute to the continued disability of head-trauma victims, despite improvements in physical functioning.[6,8-15] Failure to reintegrate adequately into the family, school, work, and the community often leads to further psychologic deterioration. Prolonged denial of disability, withdrawal, severe anxiety and depressive reactions, suicidal ideation and behavior, uncontrollable outbursts of anger and aggression, and frank psychotic episodes are frequent symptoms of this psychologic deterioration. Post-traumatic cognitive and behavioral deficits appear to be the most significant factors in the long-term disability of head-trauma victims.

Rehabilitation specialists seek to teach coping behaviors that maximize functional capabilities and minimize dependence on others. The methods and goals of rehabilitation efforts must be attuned to the patient's needs. For head-injured patients, the initial needs are typically in the areas of physical and medical restoration. Cognitive, psychosocial, and vocational difficulties emerge as the primary foci in the more chronic stage of recovery.[16-18] In both stages, cognitive and behavioral disorders often thwart the efforts of treatment staff.

DEFINITIONS OF BEHAVIORAL PRINCIPLES

Target behaviors are the foci of behavioral programs. Of all the behaviors that a patient displays, it is necessary to choose a few on which to concentrate at any one time. These target behaviors may be specific to a given activity (such as walking, reading, and maintaining bowel and bladder control) or may traverse all areas of patient response (initiation, attention, agitation, or physical assaultiveness). They may be large, functional goals or very small increments of change that eventually make up a functional behavior.

The identification and analysis of target behaviors are crucial to the effectiveness of any program. Choosing target behaviors requires input from all members of the interdisciplinary team, both to identify the behaviors that should be the initial and subsequent foci of treatment and to ensure cooperation in carrying out the behavioral programs. Once a behavior such as chair-to-chair transfers is identified as the target behavior, it is critical to analyze why the performance is not adequate. If the patient is unable to learn the sequence of steps needed to perform the transfer, no amount of reinforcement for hard work will improve performance. If the patient can learn but is disinclined to participate in therapy, then reinforcement for sustained effort would be appropriate.

Once a target behavior is identified and analyzed, its *baseline* must be established. For our purposes, a baseline may be defined as the level of performance demonstrated by the patient before a behavioral program is instituted. This level is the basis for measuring all future performance. It is therefore also the standard against which the effectiveness of the behavioral program is evaluated.

Target behaviors are usually observed by many staff members in different settings. Any behavior will vary across situations. These differences must be taken into account when establishing baselines. Inadequate sampling of behaviors across time and conditions makes it impossible to know if real changes are taking place or if natural variations in performance are leading to spurious observations by different staff members.

Contingencies are the events that follow a specific behavior. Contingencies may be random in the absence of behavioral programs or may be based on what staff or family members feel is the right thing to do. For example, a transfer may be followed by verbal encouragement, comments about the adequacy of performance, and so on. Contingencies vary in a nonsystematic way across a variety of situations unless they are part of a consistent program.

A *positive reinforcer* may be defined as any contingency that increases the probability that a target behavior will be produced. That is, if a particular contingency increases the frequency of the behavior it follows, it is a positive reinforcer. Sometimes obvious "rewards" such as food or social attention increase a response, but other times obvious "rewards" do not increase the frequency of a behavior—they may even decrease it. The patient's performance identifies positive reinforcers. This is in contrast to selecting contingencies that staff and family members feel "ought" to be positively reinforcing.

Positive reinforcement is the systematic application of positive reinforcers to attain a specified behavior. A program is most effective when the reinforcement is immediate. This requirement may be met by providing contingencies that are intrinsically reinforcing, such as food or praise. Another strategy is to give the patient something immediately after a target response that can be exchanged later for a reinforcer (for example, points or tokens to be used to purchase things the patient wants). The latter approach is often the basis for a "token economy" system in which patients earn points toward reinforcers much as they would earn money to be spent if they were employed.

Behavior shaping relies on the notion of successive approximations.[19,20] When a target behavior is selected, the patient is reinforced for any movement in the direction of the target behavior. As performance approaches the level designated as the target behavior, each successive approximation is reinforced until the goal is reached.

Fading is the gradual reduction of external reinforcement as behavior becomes self-reinforcing. As the patient masters each level of target performance, a higher level of response is required in order to obtain reinforcement. Fading of reinforcement is a systematic way of moving from a target behavior that takes place only in the presence of multiple cues to that same target behavior without external cueing.

Extinction is the elimination of a target behavior by withholding positive reinforcement. Head-injured patients often display problems ranging from verbal aggression to agitation and even physical assaultiveness. Typically, these problems produce a great deal of social interaction with staff (e.g., trying to persuade the patient to calm down, verbally castigating the patient, and so on). Unfortunately, social interaction is usually a positive reinforcer, even when the tone and content of the interaction are "negative." In other words, even the most well-intentioned social interaction during and after a patient's outburst will probably increase the incidence of those outbursts. Consequently, many behavioral programs simply remove the patient from the sources of interaction. This is often called a *"time-out"* procedure, meaning time away from positive reinforcement. Patients may be taken to their rooms, to a quiet corner, or to a designated "time-out room," or they may be ignored. The best procedure to use with a given patient is determined by assessing the effectiveness of various contingencies in eliminating, or extinguishing, a problem behavior. After all, one person's "time out" may be another person's positive reinforcement.

The use of behavioral principles does not automatically ensure complete control over patients' participation in their therapeutic programs. Nor do extinction procedures eliminate all agitation and assaultiveness. But the behavioral approach does provide a systematic, proven way of increasing or decreasing the overall incidence of target behaviors. The approach can be applied to large, functional behaviors or to very small increments of change. The next section of the chapter reviews the published reports of behavioral management procedures used in the rehabilitation of brain-damaged individuals. The final section describes the behavioral components of several types of programs currently treating traumatically head-injured persons.

PUBLISHED APPLICATIONS

Reports of the application of behavior modification principles to the problems of physically disabled persons have appeared frequently since the early 1960s.[9,21-25] These applications are, of course, based on the notion that many of the dysfunctions displayed by brain-damaged individuals can be altered by behavior modification.[26] However, it has also become clear that each patient's cognitive deficits and capacities must be taken into account when structuring a program.[27] This can be achieved by integrating neuropsychologic assessment data into the behavioral planning process.[1]

In the acute phase of recovery from head trauma, traditional psychotherapeutic approaches are rarely successful in altering behavior patterns that are interfering with therapy. This is primarily due to patients' cognitive deficits. Similarly, therapists' attempts to reason with a patient regarding the importance of therapeutic exercises usually prove fruitless and frustrating. Traditional rehabilitation practice relies on the intrinsic reinforcement that comes from the patient sensing improvement in therapy and taking satisfaction in functional gains. However, intrinsic reinforcement is often insufficient to evoke sustained participation in therapy.[9]

The systematic application of behavior modification techniques using tangible, extrinsic reinforcement has proven successful in improving head-injured patients' participation in therapy sessions. Hollon[28] reported the extinction of disruptive, assaultive behaviors in a 22-year-old trauma patient. Initially, verbal and social reinforcement were given for any alert, appropriate responses. Later, reinforcement was contingent on appropriate responses within the context of specific therapy tasks.

Kusher and Knox[29] demonstrated the effectiveness of an apparently paradoxic conditioning paradigm. A 25-year-old man with diffuse brain trauma resisted participation in therapy by throwing his head back and staring at the ceiling. The paradoxic directive to stare at the ceiling was given as therapy materials were placed in front of him. The patient reported that he didn't like being told what to do and wouldn't look at the ceiling because he couldn't see the therapy materials. Repetition of the paradoxic conditioning approach extinguished the negative behavior and allowed therapy to proceed.

Ince[23] applied the Premack principle to increase performance in speech and occupational therapy in two cerebrovascular accident patients who participated faithfully in physical therapy. The Premack principle uses the more frequent response (in this case, participation in physical therapy) as a reinforcement for performing the less frequent response (participation in speech and occupational therapy). Each patient's attendance reached 100 percent in all therapies. Head-injured patients also respond to such a treatment paradigm.

Behavior modification has also proven successful in the more chronic stage of recovery from head trauma. Sand and colleagues[30] extinguished the temper tantrums (kicking, spitting, and so on) of a 7-year-old who had been injured 2½ years previously in a fall from a horse. They used a variety of techniques, including social reinforcement for appropriate behavior, a token economy system, and "time-out" procedures. In treating a 28-year-old trauma victim, Hurwitz[31] made permission to wear his own clothes instead of hospital clothing contingent on the cessation of assaultiveness, abuse of alcohol, and escaping from the hospital grounds. A token economy system was also used. Rosenbaum and associates[32] treated 13 severely head-injured veterans in a therapeutic workshop. The veterans spent 30 hours a week in the therapeutic community. A token economy technique was used in vocational training to reinforce production and appropriate behaviors, with excellent results.

CHEMOTHERAPEUTIC APPROACHES

Cognitive and behavioral deficits after head injury have also been treated chemotherapeutically. Luria's group[33] reported the successful use of the anticholinesterase agents *neostigmine* and *galanthamine* to improve motor, sensory, and higher cognitive functions. They believed that the improvement in cognitive capacity was a function of "de-inhibition" in accord with von Monakow's "diaschisis" hypothesis. Brailowsky[34] notes that these experiments have not been replicated but merit continued research. Stern[35] successfully altered the severe behavioral disinhibition, apathy, and indifference to environmental events in 8 of 11 prefrontal trauma patients. *Dextroamphetamine* (10 to 15 mg, administered in the morning) resulted in increased alertness and responsiveness to therapeutic training without negative side effects such as seizures or acute psychotic manifestations.

In both the acute and chronic stages, brain-damaged patients' responses to tranquilizers and sedatives are often equivocal, but some good results have been reported. Kirschbichler[5] treated two patients with acute traumatic bilateral temporal lesions with *chlorpromazine* (Thorazine). Delusional behavior, excessive religiosity, and mood swings were controlled with *thioridazine* during acute recovery phase. Rosenbaum and Barry[36] described the case of a 57-year-old man with a basilar artery aneurysm and trauma to the right temporal lobe from retraction. Initial combative behavior was treated with chlorpromazine. Owing to persistent episodes of euphoria, excessive talkativeness and religiosity, delusions, and mood swings, he was placed on a regimen of 2 mg haloperidol (Haldol) four times daily. When he did not respond to the haloperidol, lithium carbonate therapy was instituted. As long as the patient remained on lithium, the symptoms were diminished.

Research regarding the relationship between the neuroleptics (phenothiazines, butyrophenones) and the neurotransmitters (e.g., norepinephrine, acetylcholine, dopamine, epinephrine, and serotonin) may have bearing on the use of the neuroleptics in the management of behavioral disturbances in head-injured patients.[37-40] The relationship between the inhibition of neurotransmitters and recovery from head trauma is as yet unclear. As Brailowsky points out, the precise action of pharmacologic agents in the presence of brain damage is uncertain, but it is known that the effects of these agents ". . . can change both quantitatively and qualitatively when administered to a lesioned organism."[34] Najenson and associates[6] express the belief that the reliance on chemotherapeutic management of behavior disorders can be reduced if the staff is trained in behavior modification. The systematic manipulation of the patient's environment often provides an alternative to chemotherapeutic management.

CURRENT TREATMENT APPLICATIONS

The remainder of the chapter describes the behavior modification aspects of several different types of programs that currently treat head-injured patients. We begin with examples of inpatient rehabilitation and proceed toward more community-based treatment.

INPATIENT SETTINGS

Casa Colina Hospital for Rehabilitative Medicine has taken a programmatic approach to treatment. That is, one interdisciplinary team is dedicated solely to the treatment of head-injured patients. This programmatic approach has enabled team members to focus on treatment methods particularly suited to this patient group. Annual census is 90 to 100 new inpatients per year.

Behavioral programming is viewed as one of the necessary components of treatment.[4] It is an integral part of therapy, not adjunctive to it. In practical terms, this has meant that behavioral programs are not optional. Once the team has decided on a particular approach, treators are required to apply the structured contingencies just as they are required to practice aseptic techniques or to be aware of a patient's neuromuscular capacities and deficits. The emphasis given to behavior modification by program management has provided continued positive reinforcement to those who have wanted to develop behavioral approaches but realized that doing so required consistent application by all staff.

Several mechanisms have been found to be extremely helpful in structuring and maintaining the behavioral component of the brain injury program. Training in behavioral techniques is an ongoing activity necessary to orient new staff and to help others who are continuing to develop their skills. Initial patient evaluations by the various disciplines include the behavioral parameters of the patient's responses. A specific behavioral assessment is done by the team psychologist. Since these are brain-damaged patients, a neuropsychologic evaluation is considered essential to establish the cognitive parameters within which the patient can be expected to perform.[42]

A multidisciplinary behavior committee meets twice weekly to devise particular programs; all staff whose patient is being discussed on a given day take part in the behavior committee's deliberations. Team meetings of all members are also held frequently to discuss behavior programs. Specialized training in physical management techniques has been provided to help staff handle combative patients effectively. All of these assessments and meetings, plus the informal discussions that proceed daily, coalesce into a behavioral approach to treatment. This approach includes attempts to conceptualize behavior in the terms defined earlier, as well as specific behavior programs for specific patients.

Many potential positive reinforcers for a given patient are identified by the analysis of the patient's cognitive status, premorbid likes and dislikes, and current evidence of preferences (e.g., types of food, attention of a particular sort, and specific activities). The analysis produces a list of responses that are tested with the patient in a systematic way.

Once the positive reinforcers are identified, it is necessary to observe what contingencies actually follow the target behaviors. Frequently, it turns out that well-meaning staff and family members are not positively reinforcing the desired behaviors at all and may even be doing the opposite. For example, in the case of a recent inpatient, social attention was found to be a positive reinforcer. He seemed either depressed or lethargic, so his father and mother, as well as some staff members, were offering him verbal encouragement regardless of his level of performance in therapy. Since attention was a positive reinforcer, whenever encouragement followed a poor performance the patient was actually receiving positive reinforcement for doing badly. This is true despite the good intentions of the person doing the encouraging. Once the interactions between the patient and others were analyzed behaviorally, staff and family members could see that their encouragement was actually not in the patient's best interests. A program was designed that gave him social reinforcement following target-level responses and no interaction following poor performance. After an initial period of 1 week during which the patient increased his demands for attention, performance was consistently above baseline. Although this is an elementary program, it could not have worked without a consistent adherence to behavioral principles by all staff and family members.

A slightly more complex program was devised for another inpatient, Ronald H.:

> This premorbidly active 22-year-old had suffered bilateral frontal lobe lesions in a car accident. He demonstrated many of the classic signs of mild frontal lobe syndrome: his ability to initiate complex actions was severely deficient; he often lost track of what he was doing; his affect was flat.
>
> Ronald was physically capable of doing many things but rarely did them. He was, for instance, able to transfer from one chair to another with moderate assistance and to walk in the parallel bars with two therapists helping him. When asked directly, he was able to indicate bowel and bladder needs. Despite these abilities, and the predictions by experienced therapists that he could reach supervised or independent levels in many areas, Ronald was making no progress.
>
> When urged to practice transfers, he pushed the transfer chair away and took his shoes off. Placed in front of the parallel bars, he sat in apparent indifference. When asked why he urinated and defecated in his pants and in bed rather than alerting staff to his needs, he simply replied "I don't know."
>
> The inability of staff to specify long-term goals added to their frustration. Despite all the work and stress involved in trying to treat Ronald, what goals could be foreseen after discharge besides lifelong placement in a nursing home?
>
> Team members devised the following program, based on identification and analysis of target behaviors, reinforcers, and of Ron's specific cognitive abilities and deficits. Ron was given his three basic meals a day, but no snacks in between. Several target behaviors were chosen, including grooming and transfers. Each of these functional categories was divided into small, well-defined steps. Chair to commode transfers, for example, were broken down into 14 sequential movements. This enabled treators to record and reinforce very small increments of change. Movements were shaped in therapeutic directions by spoonfuls of yogurt. As soon as one level of a target behavior was reached, reinforcement was faded and applied to higher levels. Progress became rapid, and continence was added to the target behaviors. A timed voiding program was begun. Ron received social reinforcement each time he spent 5 minutes on the commode during an hour, and yogurt for any production of urine or feces near the commode.
>
> As Ron's behavior came under greater control, he was re-evaluated by the neuropsychologist. Ron's mechanical abilities were found to be fairly intact for repetitive tasks. Upon discharge, the behavior program was continued in a transitional sheltered workshop. He has made substantial progress despite occasional episodes of incontinence. His willingness to do repetitive tasks makes him a good candidate for eventual placement in a light industrial setting. He is unlikely to be able to live independently, but at least has the possibility of earning a living in a job that he finds satisfying.

This case demonstrates the value of behavior modification techniques in an acute rehabilitation setting. Without this approach, Ron's "lack of motivation" would have led to an early discharge owing to poor functional progress. The behavioral program produced changes that otherwise would not have occurred. Consistency of approach by the whole treatment team was necessary to make the program effective.

The Kemsley Unit of St. Andrew's Hospital in Northampton, England, was developed for those head-injured individuals who could not benefit from rehabilitation programs owing to behavioral problems. It is an example of a structured behavioral program based on a token economy system.[43]

Physical rehabilitation services are provided in the context of this structured behavioral setting. All privileges—such as receiving visitors, visiting home, or even participating in meals—

are purchased with tokens earned for periods of "appropriate" behavior. Each patient's period of earning tokens varies, but the rate of four tokens per hour is constant for all patients. Additionally, each patient has individual goals that are reinforced behaviorally. Social reinforcement is withdrawn only when a patient acts inappropriately. "Time-out" periods within the therapy setting consist of temporarily withdrawing reinforcement. For more disruptive behaviors (such as acts of physical aggression), the patient is removed to a small, barren room for a set period of isolation ranging from 5 to 10 minutes.

The unit manages 12 to 15 patients at a time; they range from 3 to 5 years postonset. They have significant residual cognitive impairments, especially in the areas of attention and memory. A neuropsychologically based retraining program is an integral part of treatment. Nonetheless, these persistent cognitive deficits place constraints on learning, even within the context of the behavioral approach.[44]

The current projected length of stay on the Kemsley Unit is 6 to 18 months. The staff are beginning to foresee the necessity of planning resettlement for some patients in the community surrounding the hospital. This would allow the Kemsley Unit staff to actively assist patients to reintegrate into community life.

The Brain Injury Project of Woodrow Wilson Rehabilitation Center in Fishersville, Virginia, incorporates inpatient behavioral treatment and self-structured intermediate facility (or dormitory) living by using a system of four levels.[45]

Most patients are at least 1 year postinjury and have been discharged from other rehabilitation facilities. Each patient is admitted to the hospital unit for a 2-week multidisciplinary evaluation. The culmination of the assessment period is a set of individualized goals and an initial program. The patient may begin in an intermediate facility or in the first level of the adjacent dormitory, depending on coping skills. The dormitory is divided into four levels, beginning with a highly structured program (Level 1) and graduating to virtual independence (Level 4). For example, at Level 1, a patient would have the entire day structured for him or her, with frequent monitoring to ensure compliance. When less structure is required, the patient moves to Level 2, where an entire day of assignments is given at one time. Level 3 patients work on a weekly assignment basis. Level 4 patients develop their own schedules.

Reinforcement is built into the program by structuring the social environment to emphasize the value of moving up the levels system. Additional privileges are also contingent upon showing greater responsibility. For example, each level has a weekly outing, but Level 4 patients are also allowed to plan and initiate their own separate outside activity without staff involvement.

Those patients who need additional help are given individualized behavioral contracts with specified contingencies. This approach frequently uses intermediate reinforcement such as tokens, points, rating sheets, and so on. Patients who have difficulty controlling their agitation are taught deep relaxation techniques and learn to look for the antecedents of their own agitation.

Preliminary indications are that this combination of a levels-of-structure system and behavioral contracting may prove very helpful to chronic head-injured patients who have behavioral problems.

TRANSITIONAL LIVING PROGRAMS

The difficulties encountered by the Kemsley Unit staff are shared by treators of head-injured patients in the United States and Canada. Even when patients achieve inpatient physical and medical restorative goals, their persistent cognitive, behavioral, and psychosocial deficits can so severely impede reintegration into the community that long-term, 24-hour behavioral programming is required.

The original transitional living program specifically designed to meet the needs of these head-injured patients was pioneered in 1974 by Ashby. Ashby House, located in Toronto,

Canada, provides an invaluable model for others who care to venture into this difficult arena. Staff and residents of the facility have shared their experiences in several forums, and the program is described in detail elsewhere.[46] The specific behavioral components are based primarily in social learning theory. Residents participate in role-playing twice daily. Many of the interactions, including the group counseling sessions, are videotaped. Residents can then observe their own and each other's behavior and critique it on the basis of the goals of each individual's program. Levels of independent living are also used as positive reinforcement. Level 1 is a residence for five head-injured patients, with house parents and a highly planned program. Level 2 consists of nearby apartments where former residents live together and are visited regularly by residence staff.

The Transitional Living Center at Casa Colina Hospital for Rehabilitative Medicine was established in 1980.[47] It was designed for long-term head-injury patients who were physically capable of relatively independent living but whose behavioral and cognitive problems had resulted in psychiatric placements or total attendant care. Prior to its opening, house staff were trained to observe and document responses of head-injured patients and to apply the behavioral principles outlined earlier in this chapter. Three psychologists experienced in the treatment of head-injured patients design behavioral programs for each of the residents. The psychologists, project director, therapists, and house staff meet weekly to review behavioral charting, reinforcement strategies, and the goals of each individual program. Although each resident has his or her own specific program and goals, the overall thrust is to help the patient develop the skills needed for community living.

A daily group meeting of the residents focuses on developing problem-solving strategies. Role playing and modeling are employed to increase residents' awareness of how their actions affect others. The individual behavioral programs include social reinforcement, token economies, and successive approximations of independent living skills. One resident, for example, was fearful of crossing streets because he walks very slowly. He began by walking across sparsely traveled streets with a staff member, then by himself with a staff person observing. Praise for speed of crossing was employed as a positive reinforcer. He then graduated to busy streets that had median dividers and finally to busy streets without a midway stopping point. When he achieved the final target behavior, focus was shifted to functional use of his new skill, reinforced by points that he could exchange for money and home visits.

Increasing the frequency of adaptive behaviors is a major focus of each resident's program. There appears to be a lowered level of activity in general, and of adaptive behaviors in particular, that accompanies long-term adjustment after head injury. The reluctance to engage in an activity may be due to prior negative experiences (as with a dysarthric patient who had had people hang up on him when he tried to make phone calls), emotional adjustment issues (such as the resident who wanted to postpone activities until that magic day when he could walk again), or other internal events. Although the emotional aspects are treated psychotherapeutically, behavioral programs have been found to be necessary to decrease the amount of learned passivity in this group of chronic patients.

Preliminary results after 8 months indicate improvements in some areas for each of the residents. One man has been able to move into his own apartment and return to work. Another has decreased the frequency of his temper outbursts to the point where he will soon be able to live with a member of his family. A third has made major gains in initiation and self-care, and a fourth has progressed to independent living. As with the Kemsley Unit patients, the length of stay ranges from 6 to 18 months.

DAY TREATMENT PROGRAMS

Some head-injured patients who achieve inpatient rehabilitation goals experience cognitive and behavioral residuals of a less severe nature than the previously described individuals.

Many of them receive cognitive retraining for part of the day to develop strategies essential for return to work and/or school.

> Sam is a 19-year-old who remained bladder incontinent; his craniotomy scar was still healing. He became somnolent easily. If given a structured task, he performed it well despite intermittent periods of diminished arousal. Otherwise, he initiated little. He did not interact with others and rarely attended to events in his surrounding environment.

In the Day Hospital Restorative Program of Casa Colina's Adult Day Treatment Center, Sam's bladder incontinence was the target of a timed voiding program. Once his arousal problems were resolved, whenever his behavior approximated the timed voiding schedule he was reinforced positively. After 2 months of training, Sam now remains continent using a self-guided schedule and is responsible for his own medication regimen. Social reinforcement and modeling have been the main behavioral means of increasing his interaction with others. Both the frequency of interactions and the length of his responses in interactions have increased. Moreover, he is now demonstrating greater interest in his environment as measured by behaviors such as watching the televised news and reading the daily paper.

The Adult Development Center at Santa Clara Valley Medical Center in San Jose, California, was established in 1975 to provide head-injured patients with a structured learning center for social and cognitive problems.[48] It is an educational setting for 15 to 20 young adults who are too cognitively or physically disabled to qualify for sheltered workshops, community college programs, and so on. Each individual's program focuses on the behaviors or deficits that are preventing the use of other community resources. A primarily volunteer staff is trained in role-modeling and in giving immediate verbal feedback to patients about their behavior. Other special reinforcements include rounds of applause by patients and staff for target behaviors achieved, charting of behavioral progress, and a therapeutic group for discussion and role-playing of effective and ineffective behaviors in social and vocational settings. Patients who initially need controlled visual and auditory input are provided with room partitions or ear muffs. A "time-out" room is also available for extinction of problem behaviors or for brief limitation of stimulation. The program has been successful in helping 45 percent of its enrollees move on to other, more traditional community resources.

SUMMARY

Traumatically head-injured patients present challenges at all stages of rehabilitation. Behavioral and cognitive deficiencies and the high degree of variation in recovery patterns often thwart rehabilitation efforts. The difficulties encountered with these patients, plus the uncertainty of long-term outcomes, have caused some clinicians to be reluctant to treat them at all.

The systematic application of behavior modification principles to the treatment of head-injured patients, although certainly no panacea, has resulted in demonstrably better outcomes. Inpatient rehabilitation staff have discovered that behavior modification enables patients to reach higher functional goals. Problems with "motivation," initiation, and disruptive behaviors have been managed more successfully. Performance in functional tasks has been improved based on careful analysis of target behaviors and reinforcement contingencies. Patients who would previously have been discharged owing to aggressive behavior have more often been treated successfully. Those head-injured patients whose persistent behavioral and cognitive deficits produce failure in more traditional outpatient and community-based programs have been placed in highly structured, intensive behavioral programs. Preliminary results are promising. Head-injured patients with less severe behavioral and cognitive deficits have responded well when behavior modification is applied in less intensive settings, such as day treatment centers.

Despite these promising beginnings, behavior modification remains an underutilized resource. The systematic application of behavioral principles to the rehabilitation of head-injured patients is still rare. In settings such as those described above, additional research is needed. Formal clinical studies need to be conducted to evaluate the effectiveness of specific behavioral techniques.

REFERENCES

1. MUIR, C AND HAFFEY, W: *Psychological and neuropsychological interventions in the mobile mourning process.* In EDELSTEIN, B AND COUTURE, G (EDS): *Behavioral Assessment and Rehabilitation of the Traumatically Brain Damaged.* Plenum, New York, in press.
2. LEISCHNER, A: *The pathological brain syndrome in the brain-injured.* In WALKER, AE, CAVENESS, WF, AND CRITCHLEY, MACD (EDS): *The Late Effects of Head Injury.* Charles C Thomas, Springfield, Ill, 1969, p 364.
3. LEVIN, HS AND GROSSMAN, RG: *Behavioral sequelae of closed head injury: A quantitative study.* Arch Neurol 35:720, 1978.
4. BENTON, A: *Behavioral consequences of closed head injury.* In ODOM, GL (ED): *Central Nervous System Trauma Research Status Report.* National Institutes of Health, Public Health Services–National Institute of Neurological and Communicative Disorders and Stroke, Washington, DC, 1979, p 220.
5. KIRSCHBICHLER, T: *Mental disorders in the early stage of brain injury.* Scand J Rehabil Med 4:106, 1972.
6. NAJENSON, T, ET AL: *Rehabilitation after severe head injury.* Scand J Rehabil Med 6:5, 1974.
7. FORD, B: *Head injuries: What happens to survivors.* Med J Aust 1:603, 1976.
8. NAJENSON, T, ET AL: *Prognostic factors in rehabilitation after severe head injury.* Scand J Rehabil Med 6:5, 1975.
9. INCE, L: *Behavior Modification in Rehabilitation Medicine.* Charles C Thomas, Springfield, Ill, 1976.
10. LISHMAN, WA: *Brain damage in relation to psychiatric disability after head injury.* Br J Psychiatry 114:373, 1968.
11. MILNER, B: *Residual intellectual and memory deficits after head injury.* In WALKER, AE, CAVENESS, WF, AND CRITCHLEY, MACD (EDS): *The Late Effects of Head Injury.* Charles C Thomas, Springfield, Ill, 1969, p 84.
12. TEUBER, H-L: *Neglected aspects of the posttraumatic syndrome.* In WALKER, AE, CAVENESS, WF, AND CRITCHLEY, MACD (EDS): *The Late Effects of Head Injury.* Charles C Thomas, Springfield, Ill, 1969, p 13.
13. JENNETT, B: *Predictors of recovery in evaluation of patients in coma.* In THOMPSON, RA AND GREEN, JR (EDS): *Advances in Neurology,* Vol 22. Raven Press, New York, 1979, p 129.
14. GOGSTAD, AC AND KJELLMAN, AM: *Rehabilitation prognosis related to clinical and social factors in brain injured of different etiology.* Soc Sci Med 10:283, 1976.
15. ROSENBAUM, M AND NAJENSON, T: *Changes in life patterns and symptoms of low mood as reported by wives of severely brain-injured soldiers.* J Consult Clin Psychol 44:881, 1976.
16. DIKMEN, S AND REITAN, RM: *Emotional sequelae of head injury.* Annals of Neurology 2:492, 1977.
17. LEZAK, M: *Living with the characterologically altered brain injured patient.* Journal of Clinical Psychiatry 39:592, 1978.
18. WEDDELL, R, ODDY, M, AND JENKINS, D: *Social adjustment after rehabilitation: A two year follow-up of patients with severe head injury.* Psychol Med 10:257, 1980.

19. BACON, F: *Instauratio Magna,* 3 pts in 1 v. Apud Bonhamum Nortonium et Joannem Billium, London, 1620. (Translated in BACON, F: *Advancement in Learning and Novum Organum.* Wiley Books, New York, 1944.)
20. WHALEY, DL AND MALOTT, RW: *Elementary Principles of Behavior.* Prentice-Hall, Englewood Cliffs, NJ, 1971.
21. GOODKIN, R: *Case studies in behavioral research in rehabilitation.* Percept Mot Skills 23:171, 1966.
22. MEYERSON, L, KERR, N, AND MICHAEL, J: *Behavior modification in rehabilitation.* In BIJOU, SW AND BAER, DM (EDS): *Child Development: Readings in Experimental Analysis.* Appleton-Century-Crofts, New York, 1967, p 214.
23. INCE, LP: *A behavioral approach to motivation in rehabilitation.* Psychological Record 19:105, 1969.
24. FORDYCE, WE, ET AL: *Behavioral systems analyzed.* J Rehabil 37:29, 1971.
25. GOODKIN, R, DUEER, L, AND SHAH, N: *Training spouses to improve the functional speech of aphasic patients.* In LAHEY, B (ED): *The Modification of Language Behavior.* Charles C Thomas, Springfield, Ill, 1973, p 218.
26. MINKE, KA: *Behavioral engineering.* In INCE, LP (ED): *Behavioral Psychology in Rehabilitation Medicine: Clinical Applications.* Williams & Wilkins, Baltimore, 1980, p 3.
27. FORDYCE, WE: *Psychology and rehabilitation.* In LICHT, S (ED): *Rehabilitation and Medicine.* Licht, New Haven, Conn, 1968, p 129.
28. HOLLON, TH: *Behavior modification in a community hospital rehabilitation unit.* Arch Phys Med Rehabil 54:65, 1973.
29. KUSHNER, H AND KNOX, AW: *Application of the utilization technique to the behavior of a brain-injured patient.* J Commun Disord 6:151, September 1973.
30. SAND, PL, ET AL: *Behavior modification in the medical rehabilitation setting: Rationale and some applications.* Rehabilitation Research and Practice Review 1:11, 1970.
31. HURWITZ, R: Unpublished material, 1976.
32. ROSENBAUM, M, ET AL: *A description of an intensive treatment project for the rehabilitation of severely brain-injured soldiers.* Scand J Rehabil Med 10:1, 1978.
33. LURIA, AR, ET AL: *Restoration of higher cortical function following local brain damage.* In VINKEN, PJ AND BRUYN, GW (EDS): *Handbook of Clinical Neurology, Vol 3: Disorders of Higher Nervous Activity.* North-Holland, Amsterdam, 1969, p 368.
34. BRAILOWSKY, S: *Neuropharmacological aspects of brain plasticity.* In BACH-Y-RITA, P (ED): *Recovery of Function: Theoretical Considerations for Brain Injury Rehabilitation.* University Park Press, Baltimore, 1980, p 187.
35. STERN, JM: *Cranio-cerebral injured patients.* Scand J Rehabil Med 10:7, 1978.
36. ROSENBAUM, AH AND BARRY, MJ, JR: *Positive therapeutic response to lithium in hypomania secondary to organic brain syndrome.* Am J Psychiatry 132(10):1072, 1975.
37. AXELROD, J: *Central catecholamine neurotransmitters and psychoactive drugs.* In VAN PRAAG, HM AND BRUINVELS, J (EDS): *Neurotransmission and Disturbed Behavior.* Bohn, Scheltema & Holkema, Utrecht, 1977, p 6.
38. COOLS, AR: *The influence of neuroleptics on central dopaminergic systems.* In VAN PRAAG, HM AND BRUINVELS, J (EDS): *Neurotransmission and Disturbed Behavior.* Bohn, Scheltema & Holkema, Utrecht, 1977, p 73.
39. BARTHOLINI, G: *Interaction of dopaminergic and other transmitter systems in the brain: Relation to the action mechanism of neuroleptic drugs.* In VAN PRAAG, HM AND BRUINVELS, J (EDS): *Neurotransmission and Disturbed Behavior.* Bohn, Scheltema & Holkema, Utrecht, 1977, p 103.
40. IVERSEN, LL: *The Chemistry of the Brain.* In *The Brain.* WH Freeman & Co, San Francisco, 1979, p 70.
41. HAFFEY, WJ: *Behavior deficits in head injured adults: Implications for management.* Presented at the Third Annual Conference, "Head Trauma Rehabilitation: Coma to Community," San Jose, Calif, March 1980.

42. MUIR, CA: *Qualitative neuropsychological assessment: Implications in rehabilitation strategy.* Presented at the Fourth Annual Post-Graduate Course on the Rehabilitation of the Traumatic Brain-Injured Adult, Williamsburg, Va, June 1980.
43. EAMES, P: *Establishing and maintaining a transitional living facility: The Kemsely Unit experience.* Presented at the Third Annual Conference, "Head Trauma Rehabilitation: Coma to Community," San Jose, Calif, March 1980.
44. EAMES, P: *Applications of behavior modification to brain-injury.* Presented at the Third Annual Conference, "Head Trauma Rehabilitation: Coma to Community," San Jose, Calif, March 1980.
45. BOLGER, J AND FRANCIS, B: Personal communication, 1980.
46. ASHBY, M: *It Is Not the End: Take One Step at a Time.* Canada Printers, Toronto, 1980.
47. JOYCE, D: *The development of transitional living facilities for brain injured adults.* Presented at American Congress of Rehabilitation Medicine, Washington, DC, October 1980.
48. CERVELLI, L: Personal communication, 1980.

Chapter 28

PATIENT-FAMILY EDUCATION

Linda Nielson Diehl, R.N., M.S.

The primary goal of the rehabilitation effort is to assist the head-injured person and the family in making the transition back into the community and society as a participating member and as a functioning unit. For this move to be successful, learning must occur—learning new skills and how to apply these skills to, perhaps, very different life situations than those prior to the injury, and learning skills that contribute to the attainment of a healthy state. Educational programs within the rehabilitation setting assist the patient and family to acquire new information, develop skills, achieve competence, assume behaviors that aid in the coping process, and adapt to future situations.

For learning to be effective, the patient and family need to be partners in the rehabilitation process, working with other members of the health-care team. This is particularly true with the head-injured person and family. Often, the most complex problems addressed in a rehabilitation setting are those associated with traumatic head injury, thus necessitating a unified, comprehensive approach to learning.

The problems encountered by the head-injured person and the family are numerous and varied. Although sophisticated measurements for prediction of outcome have been developed and serve as a valuable guide in evaluating the severity of injury and its ramifications, few systematic educational programs have been developed in the field of head injury for the person who has sustained the injury and for those individuals who are significant to the patient. The manifestation of problems associated with head injury mandates an integration of approaches to help these individuals successfully return to community life.

Whether the head injury be diagnosed as mild, moderate, or severe, the consequences can have a devastating effect on the individual's life. Problems can include changes in motor and sensory functioning, perceptual difficulties, behavior, cognitive processes, social skills, and communication skills. An individual may be exhibiting denial, impulsive behavior, emotional lability, decreased attention span or tolerance to stimuli, confusion, combative or disoriented behavior, frustration, fright, and depression. The patient may be threatened with decreased opportunities for socialization, changes in financial status, vocational disruption, altered roles within the family and community, and difficulties in pursuing avocational activities.

As indicated by Bond[1] in addressing the needs of the head-injured person, the emphasis has been on the improvement of physical impairments, with a lesser priority on emotional changes, which may be the most relevant in affecting the individual's ability to return to community life. Although the interrelationship of the consequences of brain injury has not been substantially researched, it is imperative that the entire scope of deficits be addressed early in the rehabilitation program. The element of time is further emphasized in considering the faster recovery rate during the 6 months postinjury as compared with the slower recovery rate following this time span.

Inherent with head injury, regardless of its degree of severity, is uncertainty for the individual, family, and health professionals involved in the rehabilitation program. Traumatic head injury brings about a sudden unexpected change in the individual's life as well as in the lives of those who are close to him or her. The consequences of the injury, the deficits incurred, and the adaptive responses by the individual and family have a profound effect on the rehabilitation process.

In setting the environment, no other condition requires as careful environmental control as head injury. Early in the therapeutic program, activities need to be carried out in an area of minimal stimuli with a consistent approach used by both staff and family members. This is imperative during the evaluation process as well as during the activities of the various treatment modalities.

As a restorative process, rehabilitation encourages a continuous interchange with the total environment—adapting to appropriate demands and stresses. The patient, as the control figure, functions within the context of family, friends, and community members. When the patient enters the health-care system, there are an exchange and flow of support systems, including the influences of health professionals as well as the patient's own resources, values, and priorities as they relate to the patient's total environment. This process is exemplified in an adaptation of a model developed by Hazzard[2] (Fig. 28-1).

When designing a learning program for the head-injured person and family, several essential components need to be addressed. The nature of head injury requires the program to be flexible and varied, considering the relevancy of content and learning potential of the patient and family. Consideration must be given to the complexity and interrelationship of the problems or deficits, in order to gain a better understanding of the patient's and family's needs, reinforce the efforts of team members, and jointly assess progress and redirect the

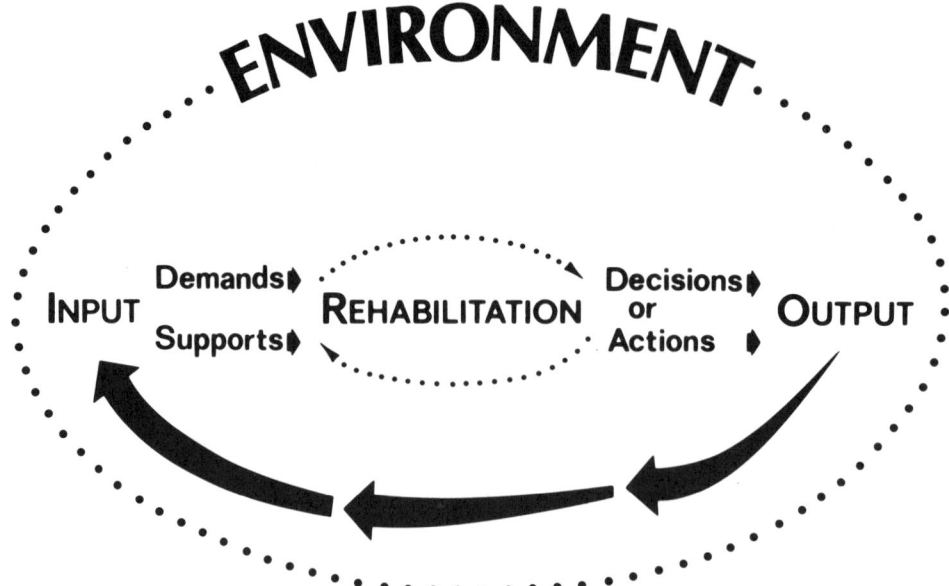

FIGURE 28-1. Comprehensive client learning. (From Hazzard, ME: *An overview of systems theory.* Nurs Clin North Am 6:385, 1971, with permission.)

program as necessary. A team effort needs to be directed toward meeting both individual and family needs. Although each discipline emphasizes its unique focus within the rehabilitation process, the nature of head injury requires that each team member be prepared to address a broad range of problems.

FACTORS IN PLANNING AN EDUCATIONAL INTERVENTION

In determining learning readiness, the team needs to take into account the kinds of questions asked by either the patient or family, their primary concerns, and their emotional readiness to learn. Factors that impinge on the learning process include (1) information given, (2) skills already mastered, (3) participation, (4) attitudes perceived, (5) observations made, (6) questions asked, and (7) bodily responses. All these factors interrelate and need to be considered when developing specific learning activities or the overall program. It is then imperative that the rationale for the program be defined on a collaborative basis with other team members and that the content be designed in terms of what learning environment is most appropriate for the individual.

Although educational programs may be of a conceptual, affective, or cognitive nature, a broad range of approaches should be used in order to address all levels of comprehension. These approaches, including individual, one-to-one, and group situations, can include such activities as direct purposeful or simulated experiences, behavior modification, demonstration, use of instructional media, role playing, recreation, and environmental stimuli.

TYPES OF INTERVENTIONS

REALITY ORIENTATION

Reality orientation is a vital component of the learning program. It serves to improve perception, alertness, awareness of the environment, communication, and overall functional abilities and socialization skills. It can also serve to alter and improve patterns of behavior as well as restore a feeling of self-worth. The approaches to reality orientation are innumerable, ranging from purposeful activities related to orientation of time and place to self-care.

Reality orientation aids in helping the individual to strengthen associations with basic everyday situations and the environment. Primary candidates are those patients demonstrating confusion, disorientation, withdrawal, and more generally an inability to interact with the environment. Although contact with the individual is established on a one-to-one basis, the program should be designed both on a one-to-one and group basis. Every person with whom the individual has contact can serve as a therapeutic agent in a reality orientation program—not only clinicians, family, and friends, but also other patients and support staff who are in daily contact with the head-injured person.

Key points to consider when designing a reality orientation program include (1) focus the program on specific behavior the individual is exhibiting; (2) incorporate the program into all aspects of treatment: one-to-one contacts, activities of daily living, learning events, recreational activities, and so forth; and (3) emphasize in each aspect of the program who the patient is, where the patient is, and what the appropriate activity or response should be. (See Chapter 24 for additional details about reality orientation.)

HOME VISITS

Home visits serve as a learning tool by promoting reality orientation, bringing the family together in its own environment, and providing a realistic setting to try out recently acquired skills, improve socialization, and evaluate the home in terms of architectural barriers. To help the family view the visit as a therapeutic one, a home visit evaluation form (see Appendix at end of chapter) can assist the patient, family, and rehabilitation staff to make appropriate revisions in the patient's program and also modify the home environment. Topics to be included in evaluating the visit include (1) transportation, (2) outside architectural barriers, (3) inside architectural barriers, (4) self-care and activities of daily living, (5) relationship with family members and/or friends; (6) summary of average day's activities, (7) success of the visit, and (8) recommendations.[4]

Since the broad goal of a rehabilitative program is to assist the client in making a smooth transition from the hospital or rehabilitation center to community, home visits should be incorporated early in the program. Often, dramatic improvements are seen after an early visit to the home.

EDUCATIONAL GROUP APPROACHES

As the person's orientation improves and the patient can cope with more diversified stimuli, group learning can be initiated. Group learning activities can be used to provide specific information, promote socialization, and reinforce that which the individual and/or family is learning in the various therapeutic programs. As adults have traditionally been exposed to educational activities in a group setting, the rehabilitation program is also viewed as a learning, participatory activity rather than the usual hospital environment in which the client's expectations are those of being "cared for." The Department of Rehabilitation Medicine at the Medical College of Virginia has developed a series of 12 classes designed to meet the specific learning needs of the client who has experienced a stroke or traumatic head injury.

The rationale for this program is based on the philosophy that patient and family education is the process of assisting individuals in acquiring knowledge, skills, competencies, or desirable qualities of behavior. This can be accomplished, in part, through the patient and family attending educational activities together. In addition, it is desirable that they be exposed to a broad spectrum of educational experiences. The program is also designed to improve quality of care, strengthen the facility as a therapeutic environment, encourage patients and families to be more involved in the rehabilitation process, and provide them with an opportunity to increase their knowledge of disability, its implications, and its management. Benefits to the rehabilitation staff include further awareness of patient and family needs, increased standardization and formalization of health-care procedures, increased documentation, and team participation. Criteria for participation in the series include the following:

1. Classes will be available to patients who have a diagnosis of stroke or traumatic head injury.
2. Individuals must have reached the level of comprehension and have the ability to participate in a group learning situation.
3. Classes will be open to family members and/or friends who are serving as a support system to the patient.
4. Aphasic patients with altered ability to understand and comprehend will be evaluated on an individual basis.
5. A referral must be made by a rehabilitation team member.
6. Efforts will be made to have a mix of patients and families that will facilitate learning.

Topics of the classes include the following:

1. What is stroke and traumatic head injury?
2. What is rehabilitation?
3. Coping with change
4. Communication

5. Bowel and bladder management
6. Range of motion and positioning
7. Self-care training
8. The role of sexuality in rehabilitation
9. Wheelchair maintenance
10. Medications
11. Community resources
12. Safety, prevention, and risk factors
13. Leisure time utilization
14. Vocational rehabilitation

Classes are held twice a week for 45 minutes. Since the classes include a broad range of topics, patients and families can join them at any point within the series. This provides flexibility in using learning readiness as a criterion for participation.[4] Within the past several years, many head-injury units in the United States have developed educational groups for head-injured persons as an integral part of the rehabilitation program.

As discussed by Romano,[5] patients often have a clearer perspective of their limitations than those perceived by their families. This may be due, in part, to the family's fears, uncertainties, and denial of the problems at hand or potential problems in the future. However, the family may have difficulty in recognizing progress the head-injured person has made or in recognizing its own abilities to assist the person.

FAMILY CONFERENCES

Family conferences, either as a multidisciplinary meeting or on a one-to-one basis, facilitate information sharing among patient, family, and rehabilitative professionals. Conferences are a valuable source for jointly defining and modifying goals. By demonstrating the team's availability, concern, and interest in mutual planning, families can not only participate in the rehabilitation program but also evaluate the program as consumers. As indicated by Kreger,[6] mutual goal setting aids families in becoming more informed and in being better able to cope with situations outside the hospital environment. It helps the multidisciplinary team see the priorities of the patient and family in the context of their life-style and environment.

Family conferences need to be an ongoing part of the rehabilitation program, not solely a discharge planning session. They can be used initially to orient the patient and family to the program, to help them recognize themselves as students within the program, to give them support throughout the program, to provide them with specific information (such as prognosis), and to answer their questions and concerns.

SELF-HELP GROUPS

Self-help groups provide an effective means for individuals, their families, and friends to receive information, solve specific problems, or share mutual concerns. They can also serve as a form of patient care through the association with and support from those who have successfully coped with the multifaceted problems consequent to head injury. Other benefits of self-help groups are self-evaluation of progress, increased motivation, identification with the group, attainment of new referral systems, and increased social skills.[7] It is advantageous to the patient and family that they be introduced to this type of experience early in the recovery and rehabilitation process; all too often this referral is made on discharge or only when a specific problem arises. These groups offer such supportive relationships. (See Chapter 29 for further discussion.)

METHODOLOGIC CONSIDERATIONS

Supplemental to participatory educational activities is the use of printed material to (1) introduce patients and families to the activities they will be involved in during the rehabilitation program, (2) provide them with specific information, and (3) reinforce material covered in the various therapeutic activities. Examples of material that may be included are a description of the nature of head injury; an introduction focusing on the rehabilitation unit as a learning center; and information on communication, diet, seizure precautions, mobility, and use of community resources. Through use of a looseleaf manual, material included can be individually tailored to each client's situation.

As emphasized earlier in this chapter, literature discussing educational programs for head-injured individuals is minimal. Consequently, little is written on evaluating learning programs for these individuals. Jennett and Teasdale[8] indicate that recovery curves may be used as an indicator of the results of spontaneous recovery and the results of treatment modalities. These indicators could be of greater value than using the site of the lesion as a determinant, since the head-injured person frequently sustains diffuse damage, making it difficult to correlate therapeutic activities with the site of the lesion. Clinicians need also to develop tools to evaluate learning effectiveness that correlate with prognosis and outcome.

Evaluation of educational systems aids in determining strengths and weaknesses, identifying effects of specific strategies, supporting accountability and how resources are expended, and measuring effectiveness. Methods for evaluation may include pretests and post-tests using a control group; random assignment and/or representative samples; or a follow-up survey using admission and discharge records, observations, checklists, and interviews. Redman[9] emphasizes in her standards for evaluation that multiple evaluation measures should be used—a method particularly true when working with individuals who have sustained diffuse injuries.

Another aspect of evaluation that can assist rehabilitation professionals in measuring effectiveness is consumer satisfaction with and evaluation of our efforts throughout the rehabilitation program. This can be incorporated in the clinical setting or after discharge from the clinical setting. Individuals and families can be one of our greatest resources in determining the effectiveness of our programs.

Socialization is the process by which one learns to relate with others and assume roles within the family, community, and society. The head-injured person is frequently a young adult who is just beginning to develop his or her own place within society, still dependent on family but also developing independence. As the person is recovering from the head injury and relearning skills or developing new ones, we often need to assist the individual in learning again to relate to others. An individual can develop these skills through activities such as community dining, group support sessions, leisure skills development classes, recreational activities, a buddy system to help orient the person to the environment, group coffee breaks, and community meetings.

These events not only enhance social development and the improvement of communication skills but can also have a profound effect on judgment, memory, agitation, short attention span, and altered cognitive processes. The head-injured person's ability to participate and gain from activities that promote socialization should not be underestimated; it is through these programs that the person often is able to move on to more specific tasks.

CONCLUSION

Early in the recovery phase and throughout the rehabilitation process, the head-injured person needs exposure to a broad range of learning experiences. The consequences of head injury are often of such a fundamental nature that the entire scope of the individual's life may be drastically altered. In turn, the family and others significant to the patient will also be affected by the abrupt, unexpected change that has also altered their lives. To reach a successful outcome, all concerned must be knowledgeable and skilled in the therapeutic aspect of the rehabilitation program—through active participation rather than only as recipients. The educational program must be a collective team effort in which accomplishments are made through collaborative efforts. This is imperative when addressing the interrelated problems associated with head injury.

Although we are only at the threshold of developing educational programs directed toward the unique situations of the head-injured person and family, valuable resources are available to further develop educational programs for these individuals. If collaborative efforts are developed with fellow rehabilitation professionals and consumers, we will have an even greater potential in reaching the goal of providing more comprehensive programs to assist the head-injured person and family in resuming a life that is integrated within society.

REFERENCES

1. BOND, MR: *Assessment of the psychosocial outcome of severe head injury.* Acta Neurochir (Wien) 34:57, 1976.
2. HAZZARD, M: *An overview of systems theory.* Nurs Clin North Am 6:385, 1971.
3. DIEHL, L, RIANI, R, AND GRIFFITH, E: *The home visit: A self-evaluation tool.* Poster Presentation, American Congress of Rehabilitation Medicine Annual Session, Washington, DC, November 1980.
4. DIEHL, L: *Educational systems as an integrating factor in the rehabilitation setting.* Poster Presentation, American Congress of Rehabilitation Medicine Annual Session, Honolulu, Hawaii, November 1979.
5. ROMANO, MD: *Family response to traumatic head injury.* Scand J Rehabil Med 6:1, 1974.
6. KREGER, SM AND WHELON, RC: *A procedure for goal setting: A method for formulating goals and treatment plans.* Rehabilitation Nursing 2: March-April 1981.
7. JAQUES, M AND PATTERSON, K: *The Self-Help Group Model: A Review.* In MARINELLI, R AND DELL ORTO, A (EDS): *The Psychological and Social Impact of Physical Disability.* Springer Publishing, New York, 1977.
8. JENNETT, B AND TEASDALE, G: *Management of Head Injuries.* FA Davis, Philadelphia, 1981.
9. REDMAN, BK: *The Process of Patient Teaching in Nursing.* CV Mosby, St Louis, 1980.

Appendix

Home Visit Evaluation Form

DEPARTMENT OF REHABILITATION MEDICINE
MEDICAL COLLEGE OF VIRGINIA,
  VIRGINIA COMMONWEALTH UNIVERSITY
RICHMOND, VIRGINIA

NAME _____
CHART # __
DATE _____

HOME VISIT EVALUATION FORM

Your visits home are an important part of the rehabilitation program. They give you the chance to practice new skills you have learned. While at home you and your family should identify the activities you are able to carry out successfully as well as those which are still difficult for you. The information will be helpful as we continue to set goals and modify your program to make the transition from the rehabilitation unit to home a smooth one.

Please fill out this form as completely as you can, adding any additional information you think will be helpful. When you return from your visit home, please give the completed form to your nurse.

TRANSPORTATION	Yes	No	Comments
1. Did you have trouble getting into and out of the car?			
2. Did you receive help from others? Who helped you?			
3. Did you wear a seat belt in the car?			
4. Did you have any trouble with your balance in the car?			
5. Did the motion of the car bother you in any way?			
6. Did you have trouble getting any equipment into or out of the car?			
7. What would make transportation home easier for you?			

OUTSIDE ARCHITECTURAL BARRIERS			
1. Was it difficult getting from the car to the entrance of your home?			

	Yes	No	Comments
a. Rough driveway?			
b. Curbs?			
c. Hills?			
d. Grass?			
e. Stairs?			
f. Other?			

INSIDE ARCHITECTURAL BARRIERS

When moving about in your home did you have trouble with any of the following?

	Yes	No	Comments
1. Doorways too narrow.			
2. Door sills too high.			
3. Room layout.			
4. Furniture in the way.			

INSIDE ARCHITECTURAL BARRIERS

Describe any difficulties you encountered in any of the following rooms:

	Yes	No	Comments
1. Kitchen.			
2. Bathroom.			
3. Living room.			
4. Bedroom.			
5. Porch.			
6. Other.			

SELF-AID AND ACTIVITIES OF DAILY LIVING

Did you need help with any of the following activities:

	Yes	No	Comments
1. Mobility			
a. Moving around in bed.			

PATIENT-FAMILY EDUCATION

	Yes	No	Comments
b. Getting into or out of bed.			
c. Getting on or off the toilet.			
d. Getting into or out of the bathtub.			
2. Activities of Daily Living			
a. Bowel or bladder care.			
b. Eating.			
c. Preparing meals.			
d. Taking medicine.			
e. Combing your hair.			
f. Brushing your teeth.			
g. Shaving.			
h. Bathing.			
i. Dressing.			
3. Leisure Time and Fun Activities			
a. Visiting.			
b. Sports.			
c. Games.			
d. Reading.			
e. Hobbies.			
f. Other.			
g. Was there anything you needed or wanted to do at home that you have not yet learned or were unable to do?			

RELATING TO FAMILY MEMBERS

1. Did your family let you do as much for yourself as possible?

2. How many people at home helped?

3. Did one particular person help more than others?

4. Did you have any problems communicating your needs or desires to your family?

5. Were there any problems concerning your sexuality?

SUMMARY OF AVERAGE DAY'S ACTIVITIES

1. What was your average day like?

2. What did you enjoy doing the most?

3. What did you enjoy doing the least?

4. When and how often did you take rest periods?

5. Were there any unusual problems at home (sickness, falls, drinking, or others)?

SUCCESS OF VISIT

1. Was your home visit a success?

2. Do you plan to go home next weekend?

3. How can we be of most help to you and your family?

COMMENTS: Please use this section for any additional information you think will be helpful.

Chapter 29

METHODS OF FAMILY INTERVENTION

Mitchell Rosenthal, Ph.D.
Craig A. Muir, Ph.D.

In planning the comprehensive rehabilitation of the head-injured adult, it is essential to consider the close relatives of the patient as important partners in the treatment program. Because of the numerous physical, cognitive, and behavioral sequelae of head injury, the rehabilitation effort cannot be conducted solely within the confines of the rehabilitation facility. The treatment program must be extended to the home environment and community to which the patient inevitably returns. Within the community, often the family of the head-injured patient bears the burden of executing the physical and psychologic rehabilitation program prescribed by the rehabilitation team.

Because the improved neurosurgical management of head-injured patients has appeared to increase the numbers of survivors of head injury, a greater percentage of patients return to the home environment after discharge, rather than to another institution for long-term care. Recent epidemiologic studies[1,2] have indicated that the significant proportion of this population is between ages 15 and 35. Unlike other young, severely disabled adults (e.g., spinal-cord-injured), these victims of head injury lack the cognitive and behavioral capabilities to manage for themselves. The prolonged, unpredictable duration of the recovery process often results in a state of dependence on family. It is often the case that this state of dependence, rather than the pure mental or physical impairments, can become an obstacle to successful social and vocational rehabilitation.

In the recent past, research efforts have been more concerned with the description of the natural recovery process and determining specific physical and psychosocial outcomes[3-6] rather than examining how head injury as a disability uniquely alters the family system and interaction within it. Very few investigations have addressed the manner in which the family can be used as an effective resource in helping to remediate the multifaceted deficits of their relatives. It should be clear, however, that the most dramatic and effective neurosurgical intervention may be of little consequence if the patient is unable to resume a useful role within the family and home environment.

Research conducted by Bond,[7] who studied the families of 52 patients with severe head injury, revealed that mental rather than physical deficits were most closely associated with lack of family cohesion after head injury. This is easily confirmed in clinical experience, where so often the family quite readily accepts and learns the approaches to managing physical care, but is perplexed and confused as to the appropriate ways of handling the psychosocial sequelae. One of the earliest studies on family reaction to head injury was performed by Romano,[8] who found that the relatives of 13 head-injured adults tended to deny both the presence and permanence of disability after injury. Mental disability is especially conducive to denial, as its manifestations may be more subtle and less apparent than the physical deficits. It may be argued, however, that denial as a coping mechanism is quite adaptive in the early phases of recovery from head injury. Yet if this pattern of denial continues for many months or years after the onset of injury, the family may be unwittingly preventing their loved one from accepting the disability and resuming a productive role within society.

Several studies have described the degree to which families experience stress and burden after head injury. Panting and Merry[9] reported that 61 percent of families interviewed after head injury indicated that they were under considerable stress as a direct result of the injury and its consequences. Oddy and coworkers[10] studied 54 head-injured patients and their families and found that the level of stress did not appear to diminish over time (e.g., 1 year postinjury). In the examination of reactions of wives of Israeli head-injured soldiers, Rosenbaum and Najenson[11] found that these spouses had a more restricted social life than either the wives of spinal-cord-injured men or control subjects. Thus, as suggested by Bond and Brooks,[12] stresses caused by head injury may vary in intensity and duration but certainly create a heavy burden on all members of the family system.

The foregoing review provides enough data to suggest that the family needs to be considered as an additional member of the total rehabilitation effort. In this chapter, a theoretical framework for understanding family adaptation to head injury will be described and methods for intervention will be proposed. (For a more detailed review of the effects of head injury on the family system, see Chapter 15.)

THEORETICAL FRAMEWORK FOR FAMILY INTERVENTION

Traumatic head injury produces losses of a particular kind. To be effective, interventions must be based on a theoretical model that approximates the reality experienced by the victim of head injury and the family.

> His nickname was "Mule" but I only call him Dan now because that was the tender, sensitive, thoughtful part of him. "Mule" was the wild-haired, bike-riding, hard-drinking, woman-chasing part. "Mule" is dead; but Dan is still alive because he is still sensitive, like to pain, and he squeezes my hand when I come to sit by him.

This lament is from the sister of a minimally responsive head-injured patient. There are several applicable concepts illustrated in this excerpt. These include *personal system*, *partial death*, and *mobile mourning*.[13]

Every person who suffers a head injury is part of a unique personal system of pretraumatic experiences, abilities, aspirations, fears, family members, friends, and lovers. This combination of persons and emotions that surrounds the patient is a system. All the "parts" of this system interact with each other. A change in one area of the system requires change in all the other areas. Second, the interactions within each system follow patterns that are logical once the system is understood. The dynamics of a given personal system must be understood to understand the interactions between patient and family after traumatic head injury.

The losses suffered by a head-injured patient can be conceptualized as a *partial death*.[14] Partial deaths can consist of those small changes everyone experiences as we move from what we once were to what we are at present. Change itself produces loss, regardless of the positive or negative nature of the change. Major losses are partial deaths of a more serious, even devastating, nature.

The partial death that results from head injury likewise varies from minor sequelae to virtually complete characterologic metamorphoses. In the abovementioned case, the patient's sister clearly felt that a part of her brother's personality—the "mulish" part—was dead. The patient's mother and father experienced the "death" of their hope that he would grow up out of his rebelliousness and become financially independent. Since the recovery process is an uncertain one, filled with reasons for hope and despair, feelings of partial death may continue unabated for months and years. This uncertainty and concomitant disorganization of the grieving process has led to the coining of the term "mobile mourning."

Unlike the finality that accompanies an actual death, partial death leaves the members of the personal system in a state of extended turmoil. In effect, they are uncertain as to what to mourn because they are unclear as to the permanence of the losses in physical and mental function. In contrast to the classic mourning process—that is, progression through stages of denial, euphoric hope, despair, and resignation[15,16]—the uncertainties about the nature of the losses from head injury produce long-term disorganization of the mourning process. The wild fluctuations from euphoria to despair may continue indefinitely because the patient continues to change from time to time. Denial can continue for many months or years and can, on occasion, be an adaptive mechanism in preventing complete disruption of the family system.[17] However, the longer the denial exists, the greater the likelihood that it will create a pathologic condition. In the third year after injury, Dan's tendency to use denial resulted in an exaggeration of a premorbid tendency toward grandiosity and a psychotic state. The problem with head injury is that there are often enough indications of improvement to allow such grandiose thinking to persist unchecked for a very long time.

The mobile mourning process after head injury is intense and disorganized and often requires professional intervention to facilitate the grieving process. Since the rehabilitation of the head-injured patient requires a multidisciplinary effort over a prolonged period of time, it is likely that several members of the rehabilitation team may have frequent contact with the patient and family. Thus, there is a need for all of the treatment team to be aware of this conceptual framework and be prepared to participate in this process of adaptation.

EFFECTS OF PSYCHOSOCIAL DEFICITS ON THE FAMILY SYSTEM

Though each head-injured victim and family are unique entities, owing to the nature of the injury and personal system, it is possible to categorize those common psychosocial deficits that exert the most profound effects upon the family system.[17] Certainly, behavioral excesses and deficiencies are most troublesome sequelae of head injury. Newly head-injured patients often display behavior patterns reminiscent of childhood or early adolescence, manifested by an inability to delay gratification, excessive dependency, and a craving for constant attention. This *"emotional regression"* was well characterized by Symonds,[18] who noted that the head-injured adult is often observed to be "less of a man and more of a child." Closely related to these deficits are the variety of *inappropriate social behaviors* that are frequently seen. This generic category would include antisocial behavior, overt sexual displays, and a general lack of regard for social norms.

Perhaps the most severe behavioral problems exhibited after head injury are those that accompany injury to the frontal lobes. This *frontal lobe syndrome,* as it has been termed, usually consists of a variety of maladaptive behaviors, including aspontaneity, lethargy, irritability, reduced drive, dull or flat affect, and a lack of goal-directed behavior.[19] The following case vignette illustrates the magnitude of the problem:

> W.B. was a 17-year-old boy who sustained bifrontal injury in a football game. The patient had a left frontal subdural hematoma removed and was in coma for approximately 1 week. He spent 6 weeks in a rehabilitation program and was then discharged to the home setting. The family reported that the patient seemed to lack any desire to initiate conversation, would sit in front of the television 16 hours a day, and would rarely show any sign of emotion. When asked to perform a household task, he would reluctantly comply, but usually became tired after 10 to 15 minutes.

He seemed to lack any interest in being around his friends and showed no motivation to return to school or seek employment.

Such a patient tends to require constant stimulation and supervision and is unlikely to achieve independence should these deficits persist. Family members are often confused and perplexed by these behaviors and need considerable assistance in understanding and managing these problems.

Alterations in premorbid cognitive function tend to be the rule, rather than the exception, after head injury. Though cognitive deficits may be quite diverse (e.g., impaired learning, slower rate of information processing, inability to problem-solve), perhaps the most common and debilitating deficit involves the impairment of *immediate and recent memory*. When severe, this problem can persist for years after injury and pose almost insurmountable obstacles to successful educational and vocational rehabilitation. Families often experience frustration and despair in their attempts to develop or find programs that can successfully remediate problems in the retention of information.

It is unfortunate that the natural peer support system of the young head-injured person frequently vanishes within several months after the patient is returned to the community. Head-injured persons often begin to acknowledge their deficits shortly after discharge from the hospital. This realization often results in decreased self-esteem and feelings of depression. Head-injured persons perceive themselves as different, unattractive, and handicapped. This perception is often reinforced by the loss of peer contacts and social relationships. With the loss of these relationships that are so vital in adolescence and young adulthood, the family is compelled to fill the void and assume the responsibility of trying to provide a rewarding social life for their relative.

The alterations in cognitive and behavioral functioning of the head-injured person necessitate changes in patterns of *role relationships* and interactions within the family. The "big brother" may now be functioning as the "youngest child"; the "breadwinner" may now be financially dependent on spouse or other resources; the dominant, strong, aggressive marital partner may now be the weak, passive, dependent spouse. It should also be noted that siblings are often adversely affected by head injury. Cunning[20] noted the frequent observation that siblings of head-injured persons often did poorly in school in the year following the injury. Depending on the circumstances of the injury, a sibling may experience guilt feelings about the injury itself or about not experiencing the pain that the brother or sister feels. Each of the aforementioned problems can create undue strain, tension, and stress in family relationships.

This analysis of psychosocial deficits and their effects on the family system provides a sampling of the manner in which families can be adversely affected by head injury. The clinician involved with families of head-injured persons should recognize that the full impact of these deficits is rarely experienced until the patient has been living with the family for several months after discharge from the rehabilitation hospital. In most rehabilitation centers, outpatient follow-up programs are less well organized than inpatient programs. Thus, it becomes more likely that the emergence of family dysfunction will be unrecognized by the health-care team.

ESTABLISHING THE NEED FOR INTERVENTION

Early identification of the need for intervention and the type of intervention required is essential. The "diagnosis" of the family and "prescription" for treatment will aid in preventing secondary disability produced by maladaptive interactions between the patient and family. The assessment process may be conceptualized as consisting of at least three major components: (1) carefully analyzing the premorbid history of the patient and family; (2) establishing accurate estimates of the likely severity and duration of the physical and mental sequelae; and (3) attending to "signals" from the family that might reflect a need for instruction.

ANALYSIS OF PREMORBID HISTORY

As stated earlier, each patient and family bring a unique set of experiences, attitudes, and behaviors (described as the personal system) to the situation. As is the case with spinal cord injury, head-injured persons often have a premorbid history of impulse-control problems, antisocial behavior, and/or excessive alcohol intake. The therapist should obtain a detailed and comprehensive history from the patient (when possible) and the family. This may be accomplished through interviews and/or by questionnaire. In either case, the information obtained should provide data regarding peer, marital, and family relationships; educational and vocational history; avocational activities; description of premorbid behavior patterns; and a description of the circumstances of the injury itself. The importance of the premorbid history cannot be overstated, as it is often the best predictor of the degree to which the patient and family will make a satisfactory postinjury adaptation.

Earlier in this chapter, the concept of stress was discussed as an important factor in family adaptation. It would be useful to understand how the patient and family members handled stress. Was stress a stimulus for aggression, denial, or avoidance behavior? Could the stresses of certain situations (e.g., work) be tolerated better than other stresses (e.g., family)? Management of stress can be viewed as a critical concept in adaptation since disability often imposes a series of stresses that greatly tax the adaptive resources of the patient and family.

IDENTIFYING THE NATURE, SEVERITY, AND DURATION OF DEFICITS

Though the prediction of global outcome of head injury has achieved a measure of reliability and validity, it is still difficult to accurately predict the nature, severity, and duration of the many individual psychosocial deficits that accompany the injury. This is a truly unfortunate state of affairs in that the prediction of deficits is often the most burning question in the minds of the patient and family. The unpredictable nature of recovery often leads to the process of incomplete or *mobile mourning,* as noted earlier.

In the physical domain, it is often the case that one can assess, with a reasonable degree of probability, the likelihood that physical deficits existing at 6 months postinjury will become permanent residuals of the injury. This is especially true for functional deficits such as impaired mobility or self-care skills. In the case of more subtle deficits—as in vision, hearing, seizure activity, balance problems, and so forth—the rehabilitation professional should consult with those specialists who can best provide an accurate prediction as to the duration of the deficits. Such information becomes critical in planning the future educational and vocational programs that will best serve the patient's needs.

The prediction of residual mental deficits is less precise because of a variety of factors, including a slow and less consistent pattern of recovery, problems in accurately measuring deficits (especially behavioral deficits), and the unknown environmental factors that may aid or adversely affect the rehabilitation process. Within the early inpatient rehabilitation phase, family members are often told that *some* degree of mental deficit may persist indefinitely. This level of information is rarely helpful for families concerned with the long-term adjustment of their loved one. In the course of extended family intervention, it is important that the therapist provide a milieu wherein the family can ask questions and gain an understanding about the nature, severity, and duration of mental deficits. The therapist should be ready to give the family an honest appraisal and an analysis of deficits, especially within the areas of memory, learning ability, and behavioral function. Of course, the manner in which this information is conveyed to both patient and family depends on their willingness to listen and their ability to emotionally accept the answer provided to them.

UNDERSTANDING "SIGNALS" FROM THE FAMILY

Since family members rarely request counseling or psychosocial support, the therapist should be attuned to subtle indications from the family that might symbolize a request for help. The expression of severe anxiety and/or fears about prognosis is often symbolized by statements like, "How will I manage if he can't ever return to work?" Confusion and helplessness about observed behavioral problems may also indicate a need for intervention. A wife may express despair about her husband's strong degree of emotional and physical dependence. She may have serious misgivings about their ability to ever have a normal marital relationship. Another problem that may indicate a need for intervention is conflict between the head-injured adolescent and the siblings. This may be due to the patient's childlike behavior or perhaps the inability of the siblings to understand and accept the fact that the brother or sister is a changed person and may never be the same.

All these "signals" are indications that the family is in need of some education, guidance, emotional support, or psychotherapy. If the therapist is alert to these concerns, appropriate intervention may be initiated at the proper time to minimize family dysfunction.

HIGH-RISK FAMILIES

Not all families experience problems after head injury that require intervention. Yet there are several categories of high-risk families that would be most likely to experience the greatest degree of dysfunction.

From the comprehensive analysis of the premorbid history, one can identify those families with a history of *maladaptive behavior patterns.* For example, a family with a history of marital discord, alcoholism, antisocial behavior, or financial problems may become totally overwhelmed by the advent of traumatic head injury. Once the initial period of rehabilitation has been completed, it has often been observed that maladaptive behavior patterns become intensified as a consequence of the sequelae of the injury.

The *prolonged use of denial* by either patient or family is likely to result in an inability to effectively plan for the future. For example, the family continues to maintain the belief that total recovery will occur and therefore fails to take the necessary steps to enroll the patient in the appropriate educational, vocational, or community programs that would facilitate the recovery process. In this case, the eventual outcome is a feeling of despair and intense disappointment with resultant tension and bitterness among family members.

Finally, a high-risk family may be one in which *severe chronic physical and/or mental deficits* persist. A case in point would be the young head-injured person who displays a frontal lobe syndrome, marked by dull affect, decreased initiative, apathy, and lethargy. For the family, it is as if they were living with an entirely different family member. Such a patient requires continual care, emotional support, and supervision, resulting in an intense burden for all concerned.

FACTORS TO CONSIDER BEFORE INITIATING AN INTERVENTION

As in any clinical situation, one must be aware of a variety of factors before starting a treatment procedure. One important factor is the *timing of the intervention.* Since each person's recovery pattern is unique, as is the ability of family members to understand and accept the disability, it is vital that a given intervention not be initiated before a patient or family is ready. For example, in the case of prolonged denial, early intervention (i.e., in the initial 6 weeks postinjury) may create more harm than good. So, even after determining a need for intervention, the question of readiness must be addressed.

Another important question concerns the *assignment of staff members* to family intervention. In other words, which staff members should be involved in family intervention? Rehabilitation is perhaps unique in its emphasis on a diverse multidisciplinary team approach with areas of overlapping expertise. Though the family is often considered the sole province of the social worker, it is our view that this is no more the case than the treatment of motor dysfunction is the exclusive domain of the physical therapist. Because of the complexity of head injury, all members of the rehabilitation team are involved and may have frequent contact with the family. The degree to which a certain professional should be involved in family intervention depends on that person's degree of expertise in head injury, ongoing involvement with the individual patient and family, previous background in family intervention, and the level of intervention required.

TYPES OF FAMILY INTERVENTION TECHNIQUES

Family intervention techniques may be discussed in two broad categories, that is, those initiated and conducted by the rehabilitation professional, and those initiated and conducted by nonprofessionals (e.g., peers, family).

Three categories of professionally initiated techniques can be considered: (1) patient-family education; (2) family counseling; and (3) family therapy.

PATIENT-FAMILY EDUCATION

Oddy and colleagues[10] reported that families often are dissatisfied with the amount and type of information received regarding nature and extent of the injury and prediction of outcome from head injury. Within the past few years, patient-family education programs have become a popular technique in rehabilitation centers throughout the United States. In some centers, educational programs about sexuality and disability, spinal cord injury, rheumatoid arthritis, and strokes have become a formalized and routine component in the rehabilitation program. A prototype for educating patients and families about head injury was developed by Diehl and colleagues[21] at the Medical College of Virginia. In this program, patients with head injury (e.g., stroke and trauma) attend a series of 10 to 12 sessions that cover a wide range of topics, including communication, cognitive deficits, mobility, and community resources. The group consists of six to eight patients and their families and is held twice weekly for 5 weeks. The response to this educational group format has been extremely positive. It appears to fulfill the families' need for education and results in peer support as a by-product (for further details see Chapter 28). Other rehabilitation programs are using this technique in a variety of modified formats and are attempting to assess their effectiveness. At the Good Samaritan Hospital in Phoenix, Blackwood[22] and colleagues are attempting to objectively determine the effectiveness of family education by comparing the knowledge base of families who participate in such a program and those who do not receive the formal educational approach.

Patient-family education appears to be an intervention that can be of great benefit for the majority of families who experience head injury. It is especially useful in the early stages of recovery, when there are many uncertainties and unanswered questions. In the aforemen-

FAMILY COUNSELING

Another level of intervention often practiced by rehabilitation professionals is family counseling. This type of intervention often is directed toward the family of the head-injured patient. A major goal of family counseling is to assist the family in the mourning process that accompanies adaptation to head injury. Another goal of family counseling is to assist the family in understanding and accepting the disability and its potential consequences—for example, increased dependence, impaired cognitive and behavioral functioning, and decreased physical abilities. Often, this intervention is initiated by the psychosocial member of the rehabilitation team. It is useful to commence family counseling sessions while the patient is in the acute rehabilitation phase. Though a family may be initially resistant to psychosocial intervention, once initiated, family counseling usually provides a vehicle for emotional support that is often critical during the first few months after injury.

Case Illustration—Bobby F.

Bobby F. was a 23-year-old unmarried man who was driving home from a New Year's Eve party while intoxicated and sustained a severe head injury resulting in 2 weeks of unconsciousness and diffuse head injury. After 2 months of hospitalization, the patient was independent in activities of daily living (ADL) and mobility skills but had mild residual deficits in memory and speech, dull affect, impaired coordination, decreased motor speed, periodic violent outbursts, and inappropriate social behavior. During the hospitalization, the family met weekly with a psychologist in family counseling sessions. The family vented their anger about the circumstances surrounding the injury. The family expressed their grief and feelings of loss because "Bobby will never be the same again." Prior to the injury, Bobby was in the second year of law school and was engaged to be married. The family voiced their fears that their son would never be able to return to law school, get married, and live independently. Mr. and Mrs. F. asked many questions about whether the patient would regain his memory, the effects of the seizure medication, and his ultimate capability to have relationships with his peers. In addition to providing emotional support in working through the grieving process, specific suggestions were made as to the management of inappropriate behaviors in the home environment.

The foregoing case illustrates the variety of needs for ongoing family counseling and emotional support during the hospitalization and after discharge into the community. In these sessions, family members (often parents or spouse of victim) are given the opportunity to express their feelings of guilt, anguish, anger, sadness, and loss. The family is given the opportunity to ask questions about the nature of the disability, prognosis, and anticipated level of care that may be required. Families that experience head injury and subsequent prolonged periods of hospitalization are often taxed to the limit of their adaptive resources. Frequent visits to the hospital may necessitate changes in family work schedules, impose strain on marital and parent-child relationships, and create physical stresses that may lead to psychosomatic illnesses. Often, perceived progress is painstakingly slow, and the ultimate goal of restoration of premorbid function appears to be an "impossible dream." As discharge approaches, families become apprehensive since they have been given an implicit or explicit message that a "plateau" has been reached.

During the transition from hospital to community, the counselor can play a key role in assisting the family to anticipate future problems and be more psychologically and physically prepared to assume the burden of care. Frequently, the patient and family may maintain unrealistic expectations that restoration of function will magically occur once the patient can return home. To prevent an experience of overwhelming disappointment and frustration, the counselor can gently prepare the family for the realities of life with a head-injured relative and maintain close communication to provide support during this most difficult transition period. It is important to schedule periodic follow-up sessions with the family to provide additional support so often needed, but rarely requested.

Ideally, family counseling should be initiated prior to discharge from the rehabilitation hospital and should continue during the transition from hospital to home and beyond. Since many families have not reached the point of accepting the reality of the injury during the hospitalization, it is likely that family counseling will be initiated after discharge in many cases. Families often verbalize, "I didn't really understand about the behavioral problems while he was in the hospital; but now that I am with him 24 hours a day, I understand why the staff was so concerned." Family counseling is usually performed by a member of the psychosocial team (e.g., psychologist, social worker, psychiatrist, rehabilitation counselor), but other team members may play an important role in identifying the need for family counseling on follow-up visits and making the appropriate referrals.

FAMILY THERAPY

Family therapy can be defined ". . . as a professionally organized attempt to produce behavioral changes in a disturbed marital or family unit by essentially interacting non-physical methods."[23] With families who experience dislocation after head injury and have a premorbid history of dysfunction, family therapy can be an invaluable treatment. The primary goal of this procedure is to alter maladaptive communication and interaction patterns within the family system. In contrast to family education and family counseling, the focus in family therapy is on the family system as a unit. To be successful, the entire family should be included in the sessions, including the identified patient. Because of the various cognitive and behavioral deficits accompanying head injury, the therapist should be wary about instituting family therapy sessions unless the patient can emotionally tolerate and meaningfully participate in the sessions.

Glick and Kessler[23] describe several specific goals for family therapy, which we have modified slightly:

1. To provide a supportive environment where all family members can freely verbalize feelings about the trauma and its effects upon the family;
2. To educate the family about the nature of the deficit in communication and interaction and develop methods for resolving conflicts within the relationship patterns of the family system;
3. To examine and clarify role relationships and restructure roles and responsibilities within the family system.

Ideally, family therapy is initiated prior to discharge, as the need for this type of intervention should have been clearly defined. However, in reality, it is difficult for the family to express readiness to participate in this process until the patient has returned home and specific problems become manifest. Rosenthal[24] has suggested some specific techniques that can be employed in family therapy, including:

1. Emphasizing the mutuality of responsibility for the maladaptive communication and interaction within the family—shifting the burden of guilt and blame from the identified patient to the family system.
2. Analyzing and emphasizing the positive aspects of the family system—reinforcing evidence of appropriate and healthy interaction which occurs within the sessions.
3. Exploring dysfunctional patterns of interaction by re-enacting family conflicts and assisting family members in problem-solving to alleviate conflicts.

4. Prescribing "homework assignments" for the family to practice outside the sessions to foster generalization of behavior change. Homework assignments may be defined as specific tasks that family members are asked to perform between sessions to create desirable behavior change. These tasks may involve altering methods of communication between parent and child, specific problem-solving techniques to employ when conflicts arise, or perhaps engaging in alternative, and more adaptive, ways of expressing feelings and frustrations.

Case Example—Patty R.

Patty R. was a 16-year-old girl who was in junior high school when she sustained a closed head injury in an automobile accident. The head injury resulted in diffuse brain disease, with mild bilateral motor impairment and cognitive deficits in memory, learning, and abstract reasoning. Because of a neurosurgical procedure, her head was shaven and her beautiful, long blonde hair was gone. The patient's family consisted of her parents (on the verge of divorce prior to the injury), a 14-year-old brother who was heavily involved in drugs, and an 11-year-old adopted sister who was in psychotherapy because she was failing in school and running away from home. Though the "identified" patient and family would accept the disability, the premorbid maladaptive communication and interaction within the family created a variety of problems. Maladaptive communications within parent-child and sibling relationships were explored. Patty, who had always been the "big sister" who helped her brother and sister, was now the dependent little sister. This role reversal was difficult for all the family members to accept. Because of her physical appearance (i.e., loss of hair), Patty refused to leave the house for many months after the injury. She became withdrawn and alienated from her peer group. Mr. and Mrs. R. were frustrated because their son encouraged Patty to use drugs to "escape from her problems." Family therapy sessions were held once weekly for 9 months following discharge from the hospital.

Family therapy enabled a more open dialogue for communication and problem-solving to exist. Family members were each given "assignments" to alter their communication and interaction, based on role-playing during the sessions. In addition, family members expressed and clarified their own feelings about the trauma and were able to achieve greater comfort in relating to each other.

NONPROFESSIONAL INTERVENTION

For a variety of reasons, families do not always find rehabilitation professionals the optimal resource for providing emotional support and helping to solve the everyday problems imposed by the head injury and its consequences. The consumer involvement movement within rehabilitation has recently reached the families of head-injured patients and has resulted in various self-help organizations.

Within the United States, one of the first parent-initiated programs was the High Hopes Recovery Group in Costa Mesa, California. This program was designed by the parents of a young head-injured victim with the aid of local professionals. A major accomplishment of this program has been a free-standing prevocational workshop program. The goal of this program is to retrain cognitive and vocational skills, provide peer group support, and improve social skills. In addition, parents are involved in an active support group. (See Chapter 30 for additional details.)

In 1980, parents of head-injured persons coalesced to form an organization known as the National Head Injury Foundation (NHIF). At this point, chapters are being developed in 15 states and will likely become the major advocacy group for head-injured persons in this country. The NHIF is developing a wide variety of services to aid the families of head-injured persons. Some of the current activities include the following[25]:

METHODS OF FAMILY INTERVENTION 417

1. To provide a centralized resource and clearinghouse for the gathering and dissemination of information related to head injury for parents and others responsible for the care of head-injured persons.
2. To provide emotional support to families and others responsible for the care of their head-injured loved ones.
3. To encourage the formation of family groups throughout the United States as chapters of the organization.
4. To develop parent support groups and "hot-line" counseling services.

At present, regional support groups conducted by parents of head-injured patients have been developed throughout Massachusetts. The purpose of a family support group is to provide peer support, exchange of information, and practical problem-solving, and to assist each other in coping with the unsettling realities and frustrations that are associated with the burden of care for the head-injured person. Similar support groups run by consumers have been established in other parts of the country and have been found to be a much-needed resource for families. In addition, a "hot-line" crisis intervention service is planned to provide immediate emotional support for those in need of such a service.

The proliferation of consumer organizations dedicated to providing emotional support and other services to head-injured persons and their families is an important, exciting new development. The perspective provided by families is a unique one, having experienced the anguish, frustrations, and uncertainties associated with recovery from head injury. Professionals concerned with the rehabilitation of the head-injured adult should provide guidance and assistance in fostering the growth of these organizations.

CONCLUSION

This chapter has provided a theoretical rationale for family intervention, proposed a method for the assessment of family dysfunction, and suggested several methods of professional and nonprofessional inventions. The significance of the family in the rehabilitation process has become greater as we have come to understand the nature of the recovery process and the likelihood of permanent mental sequelae of head injury. The lack of adequate community-based educational, vocational, and socialization programs has forced the family to assume a primary role in the long-term rehabilitation of their loved one.

The process of family adaptation parallels the grieving process that exists after the loss of a loved one. Some important differences exist, however; the composition of the individual's unique personal system may be an important factor in determining the family's ability to successfully adapt to the trauma of head injury. Owing to the multifaceted losses in function experienced by head-injured persons, the injury creates a feeling of "partial death." Finally, the uncertainty of the recovery process results in an extended period of grieving, known as mobile mourning.

The need for intervention should be established through a careful analysis of the premorbid history of the family; an understanding of the nature, severity, and duration of the psychosocial deficits; and an ability to understand "signals" from the family. Prior to initiating an intervention, one must consider the timing of the intervention as to the readiness of the patient and family members to participate. One must also determine which member or members of the treatment team should be involved in any intervention.

A variety of options may be considered in family intervention. Patient-family education, especially in the early phases of inpatient rehabilitation, is a treatment of choice for most families. The brief, focused educational group format allows families to gain an understanding of head injury and receive support but not necessarily to confront the rather overwhelming problems that lie ahead.

As the patient approaches the end of inpatient rehabilitation, many families can benefit from periodic family counseling sessions. These sessions are useful in identifying potential problems that will be encountered when the patient returns home. The counselor can aid the family in developing a realistic assessment of the patient's abilities and limitations. In addition, the counselor can help family members "work through" their grief and feelings of loss that accompany a growing recognition of the significant and perhaps permanent changes in cognitive and behavioral functioning manifested by their loved one.

A select number of families are in need of family therapy, which involves a psychotherapeutic process whereby communication and interaction patterns within the family are explored and, hopefully, altered. This type of intervention is usually effective only when the entire family unit, including the patient, can participate in the sessions. It is recommended for "high-risk" families, in which there is a significant premorbid history of family dysfunction or in which a persistent tendency to deny the disability and its consequences is observed. The goal of family therapy is to develop specific techniques to alter maladaptive patterns of interaction and communication within the family.

A newer form of family intervention has been developed by the consumer community, that is, families of head-injured persons. Organizations such as the National Head Injury Foundation have been developed by parents and spouses of head-injured persons to provide education, advocacy, referral information, and peer support. Family support groups have been developed wherein emotional support is provided in an environment that may be less threatening and provide greater reassurance than the traditional health-care setting. This method of treatment will certainly be expanded in the future and is as important as professionally initiated interventions.

To date, some research performed has documented the need for family intervention, but none has demonstrated that successful family intervention differentially affects outcome. Despite this lack of scientific evidence, clinicians are reporting that the inclusion of family intervention into the broad spectrum of rehabilitative treatment for head-injured persons is essential. The tasks that are yet to be accomplished involve more controlled research into the effects of head injury on the family system and determining the most effective and reliable methods of intervening to maximize patient and family adaptation.

REFERENCES

1. RIMEL, R: *An assessment of recovery following head trauma.* Presented at the Third Annual Conference on the Rehabilitation of the Traumatic Brain Injured Adult, Williamsburg, Va, June 1979.
2. JENNETT, B AND MACMILLAN, R: *Epidemiology of head injury.* Br Med J 282:101, 1981.
3. BOND, MR: *Assessment of psychosocial outcome of severe head injury.* Acta Neurochir (Wien) 34:57, 1976.
4. EVANS, CD, ET AL: *Rehabilitation of the brain damaged survivor.* Injury 8:80, 1976.
5. JENNETT, B AND BOND, MR: *Assessment of outcome after severe brain damage.* Lancet 1:480, 1975.
6. NAJENSON, T, ET AL: *Rehabilitation after severe head injury.* Scand J Rehabil Med 6:5, 1974.
7. BOND, MR: *The psychosocial consequences of head injury.* Presented at the Fourth Annual Conference on the Rehabilitation of the Traumatic Brain Injured Adult, Williamsburg, Va, June 1980.
8. ROMANO, MD: *Family response to traumatic head injury.* Scand J Rehabil Med 6:1, 1974.

9. PANTING, A AND MERRY, PH: *The long term rehabilitation of severe head injuries with particular reference to the need for social and medical support for the patient's family.* Rehabilitation 38:33, 1972.
10. ODDY, M, HUMPHREY, H, AND UTTLEY, D: *Stresses upon the relatives of head injured patients.* Br J Psychol 133:507, 1978.
11. ROSENBAUM, M AND NAJENSON, T: *Changes in life patterns and symptoms of low mood as reported by wives of severely brain injured soldiers.* J Consult Clin Psychol 44:881, 1976.
12. BOND, MR AND BROOKS, DN: *Understanding the process of recovery as a basis for the investigation of rehabilitation for the brain-injured.* Scand J Rehabil Med 8:127, 1976.
13. MUIR, CA: *Mobile mourning: Psychodynamics of family and patient in brain trauma.* Presented at the Western Psychologists Association Annual Meeting, San Francisco, Calif, April 1978.
14. SCHNEIDMAN, ES: *Deaths of Man.* Penguin Books, Baltimore, 1974.
15. BOWLBY, J: *Attachment theory, separation anxiety, and mourning.* In ARIETI, S (ED): *American Handbook of Psychiatry,* Vol 6. Basic Books, New York, 1975, p 292.
16. SYALITA, AB: *Grief and bereavement.* In ARIETI, S (ED): *American Handbook of Psychiatry,* Vol 6. Basic Books, New York, 1975, p 673.
17. MOOS, RH: *Coping with Physical Illness.* Plenum Press, New York, 1977.
18. SYMONDS, CP: *Mental disorders following head injury.* Proc R Soc Med 30:1081, 1937.
19. FREEDMAN, AM, KAPLAN, HI, AND SADDOCK, BJ: *Comprehensive Textbook of Psychiatry,* Vol 1. Williams & Wilkins, Baltimore, 1975, p 218.
20. CUNNING, JE: *Emotional aspects of head trauma in children.* Rehabil Lit 37:335, 1976.
21. DIEHL, L: *Patient-family education.* Presented at the Second Annual Conference on the Rehabilitation of the Traumatic Brain Injured Adult, Williamsburg, Va, June 1978.
22. BLACKWOOD, D: Personal communication, 1981.
23. GLICK, ID AND KESSLER, DR: *Marital and Family Therapy.* Grune & Stratton, New York, 1974, p 1.
24. ROSENTHAL, M: *Family intervention strategies.* Presented at the Second Annual Conference on the Rehabilitation of the Traumatic Brain Injured Adult, Williamsburg, Va, June 1978.
25. National Head Injury Foundation, Framingham, Mass, 1980.

Chapter 30

REINTEGRATION INTO THE COMMUNITY

Emily Hackler, R.N., M.A.
Jerome S. Tobis, M.D.

BACKGROUND OF THE PROBLEM

The incidence of traumatic head injuries has reached epidemic proportions in the United States and is creating an alarming mortality and morbidity among the youthful population of this nation. Particularly tragic is the fact that this type of trauma occurs most frequently to young people who are in the prime of their lives. Trauma is the leading cause of death in people under age 45, and craniocerebral trauma accounts for the majority of deaths. This indicates the extreme results of head trauma but does little to demonstrate the alarming morbidity associated with such accidents.[1] All too often the survivors are consigned to lives of frustration, disorganization, and despair. Brain damage seriously impairs the quality of life for the patients and their entire social constellation. To the family, it means an enormous financial burden, as well as emotional stress that may lead to disruption of family relationships. To the communities, it means the loss of potential human productivity of its youth, which incurs additional responsibilities to provide costly lifelong supervision for those who do not recover sufficiently. Essentially, head trauma turns the potential taxpayer into a lifelong tax burden.

However significant the mortality associated with traumatic head injuries, the problems related to remediating the disabilities associated with the survivors are staggering. Persistent disability that usually occurs after traumatic brain damage includes both mental and physical handicaps. The mental component is often the more important in contributing to the overall disability. The combination of mental and physical handicaps not only complicates the assessment but also tends to make the total disability seem greater than the sum of all its parts. This may be due to the interactions between the two components; either the mental or physical symptoms might well be compensated for, but when they occur together the result is devastating.[2] Clinicians are apt to underestimate the sequelae in head-injured persons because the patients often are euphoric and unaware of their difficulties. Although nearly one third of people with head injuries also have associated problems such as spasticity, hemiplegia, traumatic epilepsy, or language disorders, those rarely contribute significantly to the persisting mental disability.[2]

Advancements in emergency medical care, computerized diagnostic equipment, and space-age medical and neurosurgical techniques literally have created this handicapped population, which is growing in alarming numbers each year. Unfortunately, little is being done in the community to parallel the outstanding achievements in acute care. There are few adequate resources for this population that is particularly vulnerable to discrimination and denial of rights for special services. Many of them appear to be within normal limits of physical and intellectual function because they lack obvious disfigurements and often maintain a high level of verbal skills; yet in reality they lack adequate memory skills, have impaired judgment, are socially inappropriate and disinhibited, and lack insight into their own disabilities.[3] They lack skills that are necessary to process and give order to their surroundings, and as a result, they encounter difficulty in interacting with their environment. For these reasons they have few friends in the years that follow the trauma and often fail in school or employment when they try to re-enter the competitive worlds of education and employment.

Basically, head injury requires three levels of care that contribute to the optimal physical, social, and vocational survival of the total person. First, there is the acute phase where life-saving techniques are the primary goals of care, and both the hospital staff and family members focus attention on preserving the lives of the injured individuals. The second phase of care, physical rehabilitation, generally concentrates on assisting patients to regain motor and language skills as well as independence in activities of daily living. Again, most activities during this phase of care take place in a hospital setting. Thus, staff and family focus their rehabilitation efforts within the walls of a medical model. The final phase, community rehabilitation, focuses on reintegrating injured individuals to the mainstream of life. It requires the provision of appropriate social, vocational, educational, and independent living services that are located within the community.

Most people with head injuries return to their homes after discharge from the hospital, but in many cases the families are not physically, financially, or emotionally prepared for the responsibilities that ensue. Fatigue, despair, and depression of the patients and families are symptoms that appear in the months following hospital discharge. Fears of long-term disability insidiously grow into terrible reality for families who frequently did not comprehend the problems related to home and community care.

ABOUT LONG-TERM SURVIVORS

The self-help group that was organized in southern California in 1975, High Hopes Neurological Recovery Group, Inc., began its activities with a hopeful attitude of helping head-injured persons. Originally, the goal of the new organization was to provide opportunities for social and recreational activities for the patients who complained of being lonely, depressed, and confused. However, it also offered supportive rap sessions for parents and siblings who are experiencing similar heartbreaking problems of coping with shattered hopes and dreams about the injured family member and their own futures.

At the outset, the program was managed entirely by the parents because there were no funds to hire staff. The meetings were held in private homes or in community recreational facilities. It was not until professional help was offered to the program that planned and structured activities began. Inadequate state and federal financing for these types of programs presents barriers because the participants are considered to be chronically disabled and reimbursement for services is difficult to obtain. Fortunately for this program, the community college in the area later agreed to provide staff, facility space, and equipment, and it has been the primary support system in the community that has enabled the program to move forward.

Although the agency began its service primarily by offering resocialization, information, and referral help to families who requested assistance, an additional component of prevocational training was initiated in 1977. The daily classes that now are offered through the local community college district have attracted more than 50 students in 3 years of existence. The population represented in the first 2 years of service from 1977 to 1979 appears to typify the people who have entered the program since that time. Thirty-four students ranged in age from 17 to 36 years, with a mean of 23.7 years for males and 24.8 years for females. They averaged 3.8 years post-trauma. There were 26 males and 8 females, and all but 2 were from white middle class or upper middle class families. Fourteen were injured in automobile accidents, 13 in motorcycle accidents, and the remainder by a variety of causes ranging from attempted suicide by hanging to football injuries, to encephalopathy from brain tumors and encephalitis (Table 30-1).

The majority of students lived within a 20- to 40-mile radius of the school. With the exception of two men who were confined to wheelchairs, all participants were ambulatory and able to learn to use public transportation to attend classes. This particular population displayed severe memory loss and a variety of motor problems ranging from contractures and hemiplegia to varying degrees of motor apraxia. Poor balance, endurance, and coordination and limited vital capacity were common physical problems among the students. Four of them displayed overt speech problems. However, all were able to communicate their basic needs, usually by pantomime. All the students displayed socially limiting behaviors, such as lability, restlessness, short attention span, and verbal and/or physical aggression.[4]

Basically, most of the people enrolled in the program were in the fourth category of outcome, moderate disability, as described by Jennett. These patients can travel by public transportation, can participate in a sheltered environment, and are independent in activities of daily living. The disabilities found in this group usually include varying degrees of dysphasia, hemiparesis, or ataxia, as well as intellectual and memory deficits and personality change.[2]

Following their injuries, 20 of the 34 students returned to complete high school or attend junior college. Most students who returned to regular classes demonstrated marked learning disabilities and required extensive tutoring to meet minimum requirements to complete their courses. Although some of the people were awarded high school diplomas, few actually completed the required courses for the credential. All of the people who entered the community college system were placed in special education programs and took a variety of remedial learning and adaptive physical education classes. Only one person was able to complete all the basic requirements for an associate of arts degree, although most of them had attended college for several years (Table 30-2).

Several people had participated in sheltered workshops as part of vocational training programs planned by the state Department of Rehabilitation. All the participants in this group left the setting of their own volition because they reported that work assignments were insulting and menial and their coworkers were unacceptable. Four people had been employed prior

TABLE 30-1. Etiology of Trauma and Age at Time of Injury for Students in High Hopes Program

Cause	Incidence	Average Age at Time of Accident
Automobile	14	19
Motorcycle	13	20.7
Sports accident		
Football	1	16.9
Diving	1	16.2
Hanging	1	17.4
Gunshot wound	1	16.1
Nontraumatic injury		
Brain tumor	1	15.4
Encephalitis	1	15.7
AVM	1	37.6

TABLE 30-2. Premorbid Vocational Status for Students in High Hopes Program

Status	No.
High school student	20
College student	3
Housewife	1
Employed	10
Unemployed	0

to admission to the program but were discharged for a variety of reasons. Poor attendance, failure to complete assignments, and inability to accept supervision were the most common causes of dismissal.

The head-injured individuals who participated in the daily prevocational training program appeared to be "people of the moment," responding to the dominant external stimuli in their immediate environment. At first, most of them demonstrated little evidence of planning for future events or learning from past experiences. They seemed to lack the cognitive skills to process or give order to their environment and, as a result, responded to it moment by moment. In that sense, their behaviors were predictable. For example, if the room was noisy, specific work assignments were lacking, and work materials were not distributed, one could expect students to move about randomly or even elope from the classroom, and to talk with each other; or if the frustration level became high for any reason, they might become physically or verbally abusive to each other. On the other hand, if assignments had been verbally established by the instructor and later posted in writing on a designated bulletin board, most participants were quietly cooperative and productive. Clearly, they were more functional when the environment was enriched with visual and verbal cues that informed them about expected behaviors. Often, it seemed that they had a latent awareness of their expectations, but they could not initiate activity that would enable them to achieve their goals unless they received some sort of a cue. A cueing system needed only to provide minimal clues to stimulate an appropriate behavioral response in the classroom setting. The main obstacle in establishing a cueing system for this head-injured population was that a lengthy and intensive indoctrination period was required because of their memory losses, and little deviation in the procedure could be tolerated. However, at the end of a 16-week semester, most students were capable of absorbing the concept and using the technique, which enabled them to become substantially more dependable and productive in a controlled vocational training environment.

ANOSOGNOSIA

One of the most perplexing and bewildering disabilities observed in this population of young adults suffering from long-term effects of traumatic head injuries was anosognosia: a real or pretended ignorance of disease or disability.[5] Because of the consistent appearance of this symptom in the group, it seems unlikely that the disability was collectively fabricated. In several cases where moderate to severe physical deficits had been present for more than 5 years, it was baffling to observe people refuse to use various forms of assistive devices such as walkers, canes, braces, or special shoes because they felt they did not need them. Many of the participants in the program suffered from poor balance, spasticity, and lack of coordination that caused them to fall and hurt themselves frequently. Yet when confronted with the reality of contusions and bruises on their bodies, many would appear to be totally puzzled by their presence.

Most of the people with this problem reported that they could not remember how they hurt themselves and denied any physical discomfort associated with the injury. In a few cases where the accident had not been observed and serious injury had been incurred, the patients did not seek medical intervention until staff or a family member observed unusual symptoms in the affected extremities. If the head-injured youths were questioned specifically about falls that occurred in the presence of staff members, they would report that they fell but did not know why; however, in most cases they indicated that they did not feel they had a serious balance problem that could imperil their safety in community-based activities. In reality, most of these people were observed to fall repeatedly when crossing streets, descending stairs, or boarding buses. Maintaining safe environments for this particular group required extreme consideration of staff and family members because the head-injured persons did not seem to recognize their physical limitations or the potential hazards that were imposed by their deficits.

Problems associated with anosognosia and memory loss had ramifications on almost every aspect of the patients' social and vocational lives. They could not recognize the significance of their physical problems. Moreover, they demonstrated lack of awareness of their cognitive deficits. For example, most of the entrants to the program reported they did not have memory deficits and seemed indifferent to the need for followthrough on assignments for classroom work or completion of job tasks in the work skills laboratory. Furthermore, they could not identify the impact that their rage or other socially inappropriate behaviors created on people in their environment because they could not evaluate that they were behaving adversely. Problems with inability to interpret their own behavior or remember what they had done were reported by families to be the most common causes of social isolation in the long years that follow trauma. Participants demonstrated heightened awareness of some of these problems after participating in the program for several months. However, families and friends reported that the problems remained significant outside the classroom. Apparently, the students were unable to apply a system of self-control without an environment that consistently offered them the clues for appropriate behaviors. This suggests that learning is possible but that the head-injured person has difficulty in generalizing from the experience.

Case Example

An example of lack of self-awareness was demonstrated in the case of a 23-year-old man who sustained brain stem injuries in a motorcycle accident at age 16. He was unconscious for 2 months. His findings included spasticity of all extremities, poor balance, lack of coordination, memory loss, dysphasia, and learning disabilities. He fell frequently. However, he appeared oblivious to the problem and was totally unconcerned when it was brought to his attention. He lived at home with his middle-aged parents and was totally independent in all aspects of self-care. He attended the local community college where he took a variety of courses, mostly related to a vocational interest or adaptive physical education. His unrealistic vocational goal was to become a business manager or teacher. This young man was independent in his ability to travel by bus about the country without becoming lost. Upon completing a year in the prevocational training program, he demonstrated marked improvement in his perception of time and money management. Therefore, his educational program was expanded to phase the young man back into the regular community college system where he would be placed in a special job assignment. This plan required that he take several more buses each day, which required precise time management to coordinate the transportation between the two schools. The young man, who usually was articulate, pleasant, and cooperative, became agitated by the amount of time he was spending in transportation and decided to buy himself a moped. He proceeded with the purchase before his family or the staff became aware of his clandestine efforts. When the purchase was discovered and he finally was confronted with the dangers of driving a vehicle that required balance and coordination, the young man denied that he had any problems that would prohibit him from riding the bike. When he was confronted with the numerous scars, cuts, and bruises on his body that he had sustained during the 7 years following his accident, he was unconvinced and reported that his family and staff members were only trying to prevent him from becoming independent.

Supervising the safety of the long-term survivors of severe traumatic head injury both in their homes and in the community was a significant concern among staff and family members. The clients lacked global comprehension of things outside their bodies as much as they did about themselves. For example, several students were found huddled around a stove where the griddle inadvertently had been turned on in the kitchen classroom by a student who thought he had heated the oven. The top of the stove was blistering hot, and the students collectively decided that the first priority in safety was to cool the top of the range. They soaked paper towels in cold water and spread them over the hot plate, using the logic that water puts out fire. Curiously, even when the water-soaked papers shriveled and charred and the stove remained red hot, most of the students were unable to solve the problem. The cooking mitt of another student caught fire as he impassively watched it without attempting to remove the glove. He appeared to lack the awareness that he could have been burned even though he reported that his mitt was on fire.

Although the students were reasonably safe in the classroom setting because they were so closely supervised, parents stated that these problems also were common at home. Because the head-injured people did not appear to comprehend the dangers of fire, unlit gas jets, or hot water or food, many families were unwilling to place them in responsible roles in the household out of fear that they would jeopardize the safety of other family members. For this particular population, the provision of a safe environment is a top priority in planning long-term care programs.

FACT OR FICTION

It often was difficult to determine the world of reality when working with head-injured persons because of their collective skills in confabulation. Individuals in the program responded to questions about themselves and their recent activities with self-assuredness and determination. Others in the room often provided affirmation with such group unity that it was difficult to dismiss the responses, unless a staff member or volunteer could provide an accurate account of what actually had taken place. For example, a 21-year-old man who had been injured 5 years earlier in an automobile accident insisted that his freshly lacerated lip and bruised cheek were results of a fist fight he had with another member of the class. His response could have been truthful because he was incorrigibly abusive, both physically and verbally. He provided a colorful description of the altercation with the fellow, who was much taller and stronger than he. The alleged opponent did not exhibit any signs of being in battle, but he collaborated with his classmate and, in fact, apologized for his inappropriate behavior. However, the teaching assistant who was in the classroom at the time of the accident reported that the injured student had wandered out of the classroom and attempted to ride a two-wheeled bicycle that had been left near the classroom door. The young man, who was afflicted with severe left hemiplegia, fell off the bike when he tried to ride away and struck his face on the pavement. There had been no fist fight that day.

These types of incidents occurred often, and family members and inexperienced staff had difficulty handling them because it appeared that the head-injured people were deliberately lying or trying to conceal physical disabilities that they denied or ignored most of the time. At other times, their responses were blatantly absurd, but it appeared that they were trying to make some sort of response to a situation that they neither comprehended nor remembered in totality. It was as if they tried to latch onto any fragment of past reality that was immediately accessible and seemed to fit plausibly into the context of the present event.[6] Perhaps the confabulation represented an effort to achieve some sense of coherence and orientation that otherwise was unattainable, given their gross memory deficits. But perhaps it merely was a reflexive response that represented little or no effort to bring sense to the moment because, in many cases, it appeared that something they saw or heard in their immediate environment triggered their unreliable responses.

Case Example

A 26-year-old man who had sustained brain stem injuries in a motorcycle accident 8 years prior to entering the training program had a serious problem with confabulation. It interfered with his social and vocational life, eventually causing him to be fired from a variety of jobs and be virtually friendless except for social relationships with people in the program. His past employers listed insubordination, lack of motivation, and unreliability as causes for dismissal. To them it appeared that the glib young man deliberately fabricated situations to avoid doing his assigned work and being on time. He was a handsome young man who demonstrated minimal physical disabilities, so it was not difficult to understand why the average lay person did not comprehend the nature of his problems. He frequently talked about his goal to be a physician and carried medical textbooks with him most of the time. He often spent his break periods in school hunched over the large tomes, with his chin cupped studiously in one hand while he followed each line with the index finger of his other hand as he appeared to be reading, frequently knitting his brows and nodding in apparent affirmation or confirmation of the material. One day he was asked where he got the book, and he immediately responded that he bought it at the book store near the university. When he was confronted with the stamp of a local public library on the front page, he immediately corrected himself. "Oh yes," he said, "I bought it at a used book sale at the library." Neither response was correct because he had borrowed it from a library where the class had been taken on a classroom assignment to learn to use public resources. The head librarian had called the office to request help in getting the expensive book returned. When the circumstances of the situation were explained to him, he shrugged his shoulders and said, "Well, you must know because you're the boss." With that remark, he closed the book and threw it at the instructor.

This young man demonstrated a high level of receptivity to the High Hopes training program and within 15 months went to work in a kitchen of a large department store. He has remained employed for more than a year but required some staff help in interpreting the nature of his problems to the employer. At present it appears that he has managed to control himself well enough to handle supervision and perform adequately in competitive employment. Unless problems of confabulation are identified, head-injured young adults such as this man will remain socially and vocationally paralyzed because they appear to be unreliable and insincere in their efforts to participate in mainstream activities.

It is curious that the verbal abilities of many head-injured persons appear more effective than they actually are. Studies have indicated that significant linguistic defects are common in patients with closed head injury.[6] Perhaps it is an indication of the limited verbal skills that are required to establish "superficial" communications between people.

THE POLICE AND HEAD-INJURED INDIVIDUALS

The head-injured people in the prevocational training program had frequent encounters with the local police for various reasons during the first 2 years of the operation. The program was located in a resort community that bordered the beach cities, an area frequented by a large population of healthy young adults. Use of drugs, alcohol, and marijuana was common among the beachgoers. The police were sensitive to these issues, and they scouted the streets for individuals who demonstrated suspicious behaviors. The participants in the program were stopped on several occasions because of their unsteady gaits, slow and slurred language, and expressionless faces. Most of them were unable to defend themselves when confronted by questions from the police, but owing to their physical disabilities, they were seldom retained because it was obvious that something other than alcohol or drugs was the cause of their unsteady appearances.

However, on a few occasions, students with minimal physical deficits were taken to police headquarters for further questioning. Occasionally, the head-injured person became physically and verbally aggressive with the police, who misinterpreted the behaviors as being deliberately resistive. Parents reacted with frustration and anger at the occurrence of these problems because they felt inadequate in handling these recurring situations. Orientation to the police department in the local vicinity easily alleviated this problem in the area of the educational program; unfortunately, it continued in other sites more remote from the program.

Not all encounters were initiated by the police. Often they were requested to help locate head-injured people who became lost after wandering away from home or school, or who became lost on the bus lines. Most of the assistance offered by the law enforcers was polite and helpful; however, head-injured individuals often became resistant to assistance when officers attempted to return them to their homes.

Another problem that caused police investigation was inappropriate sexual behavior in public by men in the program. Primarily, the difficulties centered around young men making suggestive advances to women at restaurants, recreational facilities, or other public places. They were accused of touching, feeling, and trying to kiss strangers. One 23-year-old man was accused of indecent exposure to girls under age 6 and masturbation in public. These men also occasionally had temper outbursts over seemingly insignificant incidents, such as a passing pedestrian bumping into them or someone telling them to improve their behavior or clean up their language, which in some cases was extremely profane. Their outbursts often were misunderstood and mishandled by the family, the public, and the police. It seemed that the more people tried to reason with head-injured persons or subdue their acting-out behavior, the more violent they became. Again, the head-injured individuals appeared to care little about the consequences of their behavior when they responded to whatever stimuli dominated the moment. Several of the older men in the program gave accounts of being placed in the "cooler" because of their aggressive behavior but related the experience without emotion or concern.

LOCKED IN GRIEF SYNDROME

Family members related memories of the numb shock they felt when first observing the care given to their unconscious relatives in the early hours and weeks following the accident.

They were observers in strange care units dominated by electronic sounds, unempathetic equipment, and staff members preoccupied with their lifesaving missions. During this time, most family and friends maintained life-and-death vigils close to the bedside of the loved one. Their entire thoughts and efforts were directed toward the patient surviving the crisis, and little consideration was given to the long-term impact of severe brain damage.

During the phase of physical rehabilitation, the families became more involved in the physical care of the patient, but they remained buffered from the long-term realities of home care because most services continued to be rendered in the hospital. Families and friends rejoiced in the physical progress once it began, and they identified each sign of increasing strength as an indication of the beginning of total recovery. One father explained that he thought that the injured brain was like a broken bone in that it required time to heal, but once the process was established it would continue to complete a total recovery loop. During the early days and months following the accident, the father was confident that his 16-year-old son's preaccident personality and physical abilities would resurface despite the presence of obvious physical disabilities and cognitive deficits. He related that health professionals had predicted the postaccident status but he did not believe the prognosis. It seemed obvious to him that the boy had made miraculous strides considering his moribund state for more than 2 months, and the father had no reason to doubt that total recovery was possible, despite what he was told by the doctors and nurses. He and his wife were not prepared for the next 5 years, which were filled with tribulations of providing care to a severely disabled teenager who lacked memory, had learning disabilities, and was prone to violent outbursts of rage. He physically abused family members if they were within his reach.

This parent and others like him developed symptoms of "locked in grief." Shock, grief, guilt, and depression were common problems reported by the parents that continued to last over the years that followed the trauma. Divorce and alcoholism were common among the group. At first, parents had difficulty in articulating negative feelings about their head-injured children, but as time progressed they began to ventilate their feelings in parent group meetings. They felt that the "potential" of the injured child had been killed in the accident. However, they were unable to resolve their grief over the loss of hope and anticipation of a bright future. The handicapped, forgetful, and uncooperative stranger inhabiting the body was alien and unwanted in many cases. Resentment of caring for these difficult people, who appeared not to recognize or appreciate the help the parents offered, was staggering; unfortunately, it merely served to fan the flames of guilt to higher levels. Thus the parents remained trapped in a vacuum of grief, unable to bury the dead child because the body and fragments of the old self still walked in their midst. Many parents in the group appeared to handle care of their children much more realistically when they were assisted to complete the grieving process and accept the injured child as a person with different needs and potentials.

Sibling rivalry was a serious problem in families, especially if younger sisters and brothers were left with minimal attention and supervision during the long months that the parents were maintaining their vigilant watch at the hospitals. The young people expressed confusion, anger, and jealousy toward the injured member who was the center of attention. Siblings were reported to be extremely cooperative and contrite immediately after the accidents. However, they became confused by the personality changes and confabulation, which they often misunderstood as deliberate lying. Often, they retaliated with equally abusive behavior to the patient who was prone to rage and temper tantrums. The siblings were caught in a dilemma of being unable to attract attention except when they too developed their own techniques of surviving head injury in the family. Depression, withdrawal, drug abuse, and leaving home were reported to occur most often. Parents reacted with guilt and anger at themselves for not being able to handle the situation more adequately and at the injured person because he or she was the source of the problems.

The entire family reels under the impact of head injury, but experience with this population indicated that the parents are most heavily hit by the tragedy. Not only have their hopes and dreams about the futures of their young ones been abruptly and mercilessly dashed, but the future of the entire family seems imperiled. Financial concerns remain an underlying problem that insidiously contributes to the erosion of hope for freedom from this burden, which they eventually realize will be their lifelong responsibility.

THE COMMUNITY

Group meetings with the parents, friends and spouses of head-injured persons identified many notable gaps in the community resources once the patient was discharged from the hospital. These problems ranged from finding long-term placement facilities for the unconscious patient who no longer could remain in an acute-care hospital to locating adequate independent-living care programs for those who were ambulatory but in need of minimal supervision.

The first 25 patients and families who applied for admission to the community-based prevocational training program listed the following problems in order of priority: (1) lack of socialization opportunities, (2) inadequate physical fitness programs to prevent continued physical deterioration, (3) lack of vocational training programs specifically for the head-injured population, (4) lack of adequate educational programs to correct the learning disabilities that had occurred as a result of the head injury, and (5) lack of counseling services for the patients and their families.

Long-term survivors of traumatic head injuries shared many common problems, of which memory deficits, anosognosia, and indifference to the environment appeared to be most dominant. Lack of memory caused them to be unreliable, difficult to train, and incapable of supervising themselves. Inabilities to recognize their physical deficits created problems in maintaining a safe environment because they tended to overestimate their capabilities and ignore dangers. Therefore, it seems reasonable that care plans for head-injured persons should include a variety of services that provide an environmental feedback system that clues the patients into some sort of functional coherence.

IMMEDIATE ENVIRONMENT

Clocks, large calendars, time schedules, mirrors, and pictures of family members, friends, or pets should be placed in close proximity to patients early in their hospitalization, preferably as soon as they give indications of heightened consciousness. They should be encouraged to explore their environments for information they ask about. Staff and family should develop a sensitivity to these questions and refer the patient to the objects that are posted within easy reach and with good visibility. The purpose of this system is to prevent patients from becoming dependent on others to do their internal data search.

Experience with long-term survivors revealed that many of them were completely dependent on others for verbal cues in order to initiate or complete basic tasks in self-care and independent living. They literally required an interpreter to be with them all the time. In some cases, parents accepted the roles of being the visual and conceptual extensions of their children and accompanied them everywhere because there were no other alternatives. Family members had not been taught to be facilitators who encouraged the head-injured persons to search for answers; rather, they provided the cognitive assessments and verbal instructions for appropriate responses. As a result, the head-injured persons became lost when they were alone because they did not recognize the value of street signs; they took the wrong bus because they did not attend to the bus numbers; they used the wrong restrooms because they did not pay attention to signs on the doors; they bought the wrong grocery supplies because they did not use their shopping lists. Interestingly, most people in the program responded well in learning to scan their environments when they were students; unfortunately, years of dependence on the family made the process more complicated because the family members also had to change their behaviors. Sometimes, the parents were more resistant to the change than the head-injured persons because it threatened the roles they had accepted in coping with a precarious situation.

It seems imperative in planning care for head-injured persons to teach them to scan their surroundings for information as early as possible in the rehabilitation program. Families must be introduced to the cueing system while the patient still is in the hospital so that a smooth transition can be facilitated from the institution to the community. For those unfortunate people who suffer long-term memory deficits, an individually designed system might well be a lifetime need. Without it, they are certain to remain dependent on others to provide motivation and direction for functional living. For example, teaching them to use pocket-sized engagement calendars was one method of helping them remember their daily schedules. Use of large engagement calendars at home that contained lists of chores and appointments also helped them become functional family members. Although this may sound simplistic, it is not because head-injured persons required months of repetitive work before they finally remembered to use these tools regularly.

BEHAVIORAL CONTROLS

In many cases, the cognitive and emotional functions are the most powerful predictors of an individual's social and vocational adjustment potential. Motor difficulties may confine a person to a wheelchair, but the person may be able to lead a normal life if the cognitive capacities are reasonably intact and the emotional status is satisfactory. On the other hand, even a moderate cognitive impairment can make the person vocationally unfit and a heavy burden to self and others.[10] Dealing with the cognitive problems clearly requires more research in the long-term management of head-injured persons because they appear to be the primary cause of social and vocational disabilities.

Experience with the people in the community program indicated that they improved in many areas of social and vocational aptitudes when taught to assess themselves and their own behaviors. The assessment was handled in much the same manner as the environmental cueing system. Every time something unusual happened—good or bad—the students were asked to identify what they had done and, in the event of desirable behavior, it was immediately reinforced. Conversely, they were required to identify their inappropriate responses and immediately correct them. Use of mirrors and videotapes appeared to be extremely helpful in this approach, but this was not conclusively substantiated because lack of finances and adequate staff made further explorations of these techniques impossible. Family and friends reported that student behaviors improved considerably at home during the time that this program was being administered.

An additional problem was the management of the enormous degree of confabulation in the classroom setting. Staff and family alike fell into traps of responding to students who obviously were confabulating and being verbally negative. Often students refused to participate in classroom activities. These answers simply were not accepted and the students again were instructed to participate in the activity. An explanation that the purpose of the task was to help them get better so that they could return to a more normal and productive life was offered with the command. Few students refused to cooperate with this approach. Group feedback was encouraged when negative or confabulating behaviors were observed in fellow classmates, and in some students, these problems were remediated in a short time.

It appeared that clearly defined assignments for head-injured persons reduced the amount of confabulation and socially inappropriate behaviors, but this required a consistent and coordinated effort between the classroom and the home environment. Helping head-injured persons to relearn accountability is an awesome task, but from empirical experiences, people with long-term problems associated with head trauma appeared to make progress in a daily program that was enriched with both verbal and visual cues.

OTHER CONSIDERATIONS

Families and patients need to be educated about other rehabilitation needs that are significant in the recovery process. One of them is adequate rest. Impairment of attention and concentration, emotional instability, and lowered tolerance to frustration and noise remained significant problems in the course of recovery for head-injured persons.[9] Hence, it is recommended that frequent rest periods be provided in a quiet setting. As care progresses to a daily therapy regimen, the patient should be given adequate rest time between sessions to avoid sensory overload and cerebral fatigue, which often manifest themselves in verbal and physical aggressiveness. The routine of daily rest periods should continue when the patient returns to home life and gradually be phased out as physical strength and cognitive coherence return.

Most of the participants have been socially isolated and were virtually nonparticipative in any type of sports activity. In fact, most of them spent the majority of time watching television and smoking cigarettes. Many of them exhibited weakness, increased spasticity, and limited vital capacities, which the families reported had become progressively worse as the years passed. This supports the findings of Becker and others,[7] who reported that both circulatory and ventilatory responses of patients with craniocerebral injury were less efficient, probably owing to deconditioning because of their passive way of life, overprotection, and lack of self-confidence. Families and patients need to be educated that adequate nutrition and continued physical conditioning are essential in the years that follow discharge from the hospital. Health-team members should help design a physical activity schedule that will incorporate sports and games to replace the exercises that were given in the therapeutic settings. Referrals to the local YMCA or other health clubs are sources that families can be encouraged to use in their communities. Also, adult education classes and community colleges offer special adaptive education classes to all handicapped people in their districts.

Discharge of a head-injured patient should be accompanied by a referral to a home-care agency to provide follow-up that will ease the stressful transition from hospital to home. Families usually require counseling and support in the months that follow discharge because that is when the bottom-line realities of brain damage begin to materialize. Referral to local community-based family social service agencies might be indicated to assist needy families in coping with the long-term emotional and financial burdens of caring for a head-injured young adult. In all instances, health professionals should provide the families with realistic hope for attainable goals, being careful not to be too optimistic or too bleak about expectations for the future.

OPTIMAL CARE FOR HEAD-INJURED PERSONS

Success in care of head-injured persons should not be measured by the survival rate alone. It should include the quality and productivity that the survivors achieve when they are returned to family and community life. This will depend largely upon communities mobilizing to provide essential rehabilitation outreach services.

Specifically, optimal care for head-injured persons begins with high-quality emergency medical care and acute-care services; however, it is essential that families receive early education about the nature of brain damage and the sequelae of mental, cognitive, and physical disabilities. This process should continue throughout the three levels of patient care. Families should be educated that an unconscious brain is not a sleeping brain. Many people are under this misapprehension, and it is one of the reasons that they often anticipate better recovery than is expected by health-team members. Levels of consciousness should be stressed at the outset when working with the patients and their families.

Physicians, nurses, and therapists should guard against making prognostications about the recovery of head-injured persons in the early days and weeks following the accident. Although considerable information is known about the sensory functions and motor control, we possess fragmentary knowledge about the processes that govern thinking, reasoning, motivation, and other cognitive aspects of the brain's function. These problems present the primary obstacles in long-term recovery from head injuries. Peer counseling with both patients and families who successfully have handled the problems of living with disabilities associated with brain damage should be considered in facilities where the program could be closely monitored by a professional member of the health team.

Efforts to include family members and friends in the care of injured individuals should be stressed during the second level of care. They also should be included in staff conferences where short- and long-term care plans are being established. Basically, families should be informed and educated as much as possible during the patient's hospital stay so that home and community care will be less threatening to the families.

Restructuring of social, vocational, and educational programs for head-injured persons is essential if they are to be assisted to achieve their highest social and vocational potentials. Most of the students in the community-based rehabilitation program in southern California had been misdiagnosed and misplaced in various rehabilitation services. Many of them had been placed in classes with mentally ill or developmentally disabled clients because staff of those programs did not comprehend the problems unique to this population. Emphasis must be placed on obtaining adequate state and federal funds to support services for this new population of survivors, who are growing in numbers each year.

Clearly, the plight of survivors of head injury is a health concern in the United States. They are a new population of disabled people with very limited advocacy at this time. Their special needs for long-term community-based services are urgent in the total scope of rehabilitation services.

CONCLUSION

The observations presented in this chapter reflect more than 3 years' experiences with head-injured young adults in a community-based prevocational training program, High Hopes Neurological Recovery Group, Inc., Costa Mesa, California. Initially, it was organized and managed by a group of committed parents of head-injured young adults and later was made operational by volunteered professional help at the outset of its prevocational training service. However, other similar organizations with equally innovative programs are beginning to spring up across the nation to accommodate the burgeoning needs for special social, educational, and vocational services for head-injured persons. These agencies represent the collective efforts of family members—mostly parents—friends, and interested others who are unwilling to compromise the futures of young people who survive acute head trauma.

The pool of survivors of traumatic head injuries has grown steadily over the years, slowly at first because few people lived through the acute episodes of trauma. However, advancements in diagnostic techniques and medical care dramatically reduced the mortality over the past decade, thus enabling severely injured individuals to survive. The issue at hand is that long-term services have not kept pace with medical advancements for a wide variety of reasons, the most significant being that there is limited reimbursement for services related to long-term care. This particular population of disabled people apparently has reached a critical mass, and suddenly the incidence of people being returned to communities after head injuries seems overwhelming. Social change is needed to provide the kinds of services that these individuals require; like most other movements that developed at a grassroots level to improve the quality of life for the disabled and other minorities, families and friends have rallied their efforts to overcome lack of adequate resources for head-injured persons. They are creating the services themselves.

Most of these organizations are established as nonprofit services since state and federal dollars generally are limited for these types of community-based services. Some parents at High Hopes volunteered countless hours beyond their normal working schedules to work on boards of directors, organize tedious and time-consuming fundraising projects, give evening talks to local philanthropic service groups to educate the community about the needs of head-injured persons, and staff programs within their own agency to keep it operational until staff could be found. For these parents, the work was considered to be a vital part of their lives because it was their only alternative to a desperate situation. They preferred working at that strenuous pace rather than giving up hope for a better future for their injured young family members.

High Hopes is but one of the many agencies being formed by parent support groups. The Neurological Learning Center in Pasadena, California, and the National Head Injury Foundation in Framingham, Massachusetts, are examples of two such groups that focus on a variety of problems, ranging from the provision of educational programs to advocating and educating the public about the problems related to head injuries. It is important that a communication network be formed to link the efforts of support groups from rural United States to the great metropolitan areas.

Health professionals and medical facilities also are beginning to address the problems of long-term care needs of head-injured persons. Most large communities and rehabilitation centers now are developing specialized programs for head-injured persons. Facilities such as Casa Colina Rehabilitation Hospital in Pomona, California, are providing highly specialized treatment programs for head-injured adults who are placed in transitional living experiences for periods of 6 to 9 months. Santa Clara Valley Medical Center in San Jose, California, offers day treatment for head-injured people after they are discharged from inpatient care. The Ashby House in Toronto, Canada, has been providing group living services under the direction of Mrs. Mira Ashby, a social worker, since 1978 and has served as a model for that kind of program in the United States. The Center for Comprehensive Services also is offering unique community-based services in Illinois. There are many other fine programs in the country that are providing worthwhile assistance to head-injured persons; the key of this national thrust is to work collectively and cooperatively in sharing information and providing consultation to each other as the needs arise. We have much to learn from each other.

REFERENCES

1. RIMEL, R: *Epidemiology and recovery patterns in adult head trauma.* Presented at the Third Annual Conference on Current Trends in Later Rehabilitation Treatment, Community Care and Research, San Jose, Calif, March 1980.
2. JENNETT, B AND BOND, M: *Assessment of outcome after severe brain injury.* Lancet 1:480, 1975.
3. HACKLER, E: *Accountability: A moral issue in care for the head injured.* Rehabilitation Nursing (submitted for publication).
4. CUE, M: *An adapted physical education program for the traumatically head injured young adult: Movement patterns.* Graduate thesis, Department of Physical Education, California State University of Long Beach, Long Beach, Calif, June 1979.
5. *Dorland's Illustrated Medical Dictionary,* ed 24. WB Saunders, Philadelphia, 1965, p 100.
6. BENTON, A: *Behavioral consequences of closed head injury.* In ODOM, GL (ED): *CNS Trauma Research Statistic Report,* National Institute of Health-National Institute of Neurological, Communicative Disorders and Stroke, Washington, DC, 1979, Chapter 15, p 220.
7. BECKER, E, ET AL: *Pulmonary functions and responses to exercise of patients following craniocerebral injury.* Scand J Rehabil Med 10:47, 1978.

CONCLUSION

Mitchell Rosenthal, Ph.D.

As rehabilitation of the head-injured adult proceeds from the first few hours, which are devoted to lifesaving intervention, to the later attempts to remediate the deficits created by the neurologic insult, management techniques become less based on controlled scientific research and more determined by clinical experience and intuition. Yet the treatment techniques described in this section are, in large part, innovative procedures derived from accumulating data comprised of clinical observation and empirical testing of theoretical models.

A fundamental principle underlying head-injury rehabilitation is the notion that the significant cognitive deficits resulting from head trauma can be ameliorated through procedures known as "cognitive remediation techniques." Ben-Yishay and Diller, pioneers in the application of rehabilitation principles to the remediation of cognitive deficits in stroke and head-trauma patients, describe a complex but systematic model for effective remediation. Their treatment protocol has already yielded promising results and has stimulated researchers and clinicians throughout the international rehabilitation community to develop similar methods.

The presence of behavioral dysfunction is often characterized as the most difficult of all the problems confronting therapists involved in the rehabilitation of head-injured persons. Muir, Haffey, and their colleagues describe the application of behavior modification procedures to reduce and eliminate negative behaviors, as well as to foster more appropriate social behaviors. The incorporation of the procedures in a controlled residential treatment setting, as described in their chapter, would appear to be an ideal environment to test the effectiveness of their treatment techniques. The use of behavior shaping, token economies, and contingency contracting is not an entirely new idea—in fact, these procedures have been used effectively with other neurologically impaired individuals, for example, mentally retarded, cerebral palsied, autistic, and learning disabled persons. It remains to be determined whether behavioral treatment will prove to be as effective with traumatically head-injured persons.

The traditional therapeutic disciplines in rehabilitation—physical therapy, occupational therapy, and speech-language pathology—base their treatment interventions largely but not exclusively on procedures used for other disabilities, for example, stroke. Many researchers and clinicians have noted the similarities in residual deficits of the stroke patient and head-injured patient; however, there are important differences. Owing to the differential age of the brain in the typical head-injured patient and the usual stroke victim, the prognosis for recovery of function is usually better in the case of head injury. Second, the typical neuroanatomic pattern is one of diffuse injury in the case of head trauma, whereas cerebrovascular accident most often results in unilateral or focal damage to the brain. Nelson, in describing a set of procedures that have resulted in objective improvements in ambulation in head-injured persons, notes the similarities between the treatment of this population and the stroke population. The traditional methods of perceptual retraining, as described by Wahlstrom, are akin to those used with the stroke victim but incorporate treatment techniques based on an understanding of the unique cognitive deficits that accompany traumatic head injury. The therapeutic procedures described by Smith in speech-language rehabilitation and Cerny and McNeny, in discussing reality orientation, depend on the successful use of attention and orientation training. These procedures are necessary precursors to the development of higher-level skills training, designed to improve abstract thinking, conceptual thought, and an insightful understanding of the complex environment surrounding the patient. In each of the therapeutic areas just described, the treatment procedures borrow from established protocols of treatment with stroke patients but build on the newly developed understanding of the pattern of cognitive deficits that accompany head injury.

Only recently has the role of the family been addressed as a significant variable in the total rehabilitation process. As Bond described in an earlier chapter, the presence of head injury often exerts an overwhelming stress on the adaptive resources of the family. In spite of the emotional trauma experienced by family members, they are required to assume major responsibility for the case of their loved one. Therefore, the needs of the family must be addressed. Diehl describes a multifaceted approach to patient-family education, which recognizes the importance of the patient and family as partners in the rehabilitation process. Rosenthal and Muir present a theoretical model for understanding the methods that families use to cope with head injury. In addition, a variety of intervention techniques are described, which may be of considerable value in mobilizing the family system in aiding in the rehabilitation process. The emergence of family-initiated self-help groups, such as the National Head Injury Foundation, can only assist in meeting the unmet needs of the family.

Finally, the role of the community and home environment has been addressed by Hackler and Tobis. Their description of the difficulties inherent in re-entry into the community underscores the notion that rehabilitation does not cease upon discharge from the rehabilitation hospital. In fact, one can infer that the most difficult part of the rehabilitation process occurs after the patient returns home and attempts to re-establish a sense of identity and a meaningful role within the community. At present, there are more barriers to successful reintegration than there are adequate programs in the community that effectively meet the social, psychologic, and vocational needs of this population. But this unfortunate set of circumstances is slowly changing as more community-based programs are developing.

In reviewing the last major text on the rehabilitation of head-injured persons—*The Late Effects of Head Injury* by Walker, Caveness, and Critchley, published in 1969—it is apparent, that the state of the art has improved significantly but is far from an exact science. One can be encouraged by the new developments in early diagnosis and neurosurgical management; prediction of outcome; specification of the deficits imposed by head injury; more sophisticated rehabilitation assessment procedures; and exciting new techniques of cognitive remediation, behavioral management, transitional living programs, and family intervention techniques. But the work of the rehabilitationist is still in a primitive stage; we have many "miles to go" before the riddle of head-injury rehabilitation has been solved.

INDEX

A "t" following a page number indicates a table. A page number in *italics* indicates a figure.

ACCIDENTS, traffic, as cause of head injuries, 13–14
Activities
    form and space, for perceptual dysfunction, 337, *338*
    group learning, patient-family education and, 398–399
    motor, for perceptual dysfunction, 337
    somatosensory, for perceptual dysfunction, 336, *337*
    visual, for perceptual dysfunction, 336
Activities of daily living, 26t, 276
    advanced
        communication skills, 148–149
        driving, 151–152
        family relationships, 149–150
        financial management, 151
        home living skills, 149
            case history of, 149
        other issues affecting, 152
            case history relating to, 153
        social roles, 151
        time management, 150–151
    basic
        dressing, 146–147
        feeding, 143
            behavioral and cognitive problems and, 145
            case history of, 145–146
            oral dysfunction and, 144
            physical limitations and, 144–145
        hygiene skills, 147
            case history of, 147–148
    community skills, 277
    home skills, 276
    self-care skills, 276
Adjustment, social, outcome and, 111–112

Age
    of head-injured patients, 11–12, *11*
    outcome from head injury and, 55
Aids, communication, 364
    direct selection, 364
    electromechanical, 365
    encoding, 364–365
    scanning-type, 364
Airway, obstruction of, 237
Alcohol use as contributing factor to head injuries, 14
Ambulation training, 324–325
Amnesia
    post-traumatic, 4–5, 5t, 41, 185–186, 188–191, 233
        assessment of, 100–101
        outcome and, 109–110, 109t, 110t
Anemia, 42
Anosognosia, 424–426
Anticonvulsants, prophylactic, 123
Antispasticity drugs, 136–137
Aphasia
    traumatic and vascular, 158–159
    treatment of, 358–359t, 359–361, *362*
Approach, consistent, in reality orientation therapy, 346
Apraxia, 24
    of speech, 283
Arm, motor control of, 326–328
Arm-dropping test, 249
Arousal, 60
Arterial hypotension, 42
Arterial hypoxemia, 41–42
Articulation, 284
    therapeutic considerations for improving, 363
Assaults as cause of head injuries, 14

Assessment. *See also* Evaluation; Examination; Diagnosis
  medical, 231
    criteria for rehabilitation and
      airway obstruction as, 237
      cranial nerve deficits as, 233–234
      cranioplasty as, 236
      effects of facial bone fractures, 234
      epilepsy as, 235
      medical stability as, 232
      neurologic improvement as, 232
      oral-feeding status as, 236
      heterotopic ossification as, 236–237
      hypothalamic functions as, 237–238
      infections as, 235
      post-traumatic amnesia as, 233
      post-traumatic hydrocephalus as, 235–236
      skeletal trauma as, 237
  motor, 241
    arm-dropping test and, 249
    dynamometry and, 255–259, *256, 257, 258*
      validity and reliability of, 259
    equilibrium reaction and, 249
    Functional Ambulation Score and, 253, *254*
    hand function and, 253, 255
    head-dropping test and, 245
    locomotion and, 253
    motor behavior inventory and, 261, *262–265*
    motor examination and, 242–244
    motor problems of head-injured patient and, 242
    movement from sitting to standing and, 251, *251*
    muscle tonus and myotatic reflexes and, 244–245
    pronation and supination of forearms and, 249–250
    recording of motor behavior and, 255
    righting reflex and, 248–249
    shoulder-shaking test and, 249
    sitting balance and, *250,* 250–251
    standing position and, 252–253, *252*
    tonic reflexes, 248
  neurologic
    case history of, 303, 304t, 305, 305t, 306t
  neuropsychologic
    definition and background of, 291–292
    Halstead-Reitan battery and, 292–293, 294–295t
    in rehabilitation settings, 299
      baseline determinations and, 299
      data organization and presentation, 302, *303*
      identification of strengths and weaknesses, 299, *299,* 300t
      prediction and determination of outcome, 300–301, 302t
      prescriptions for treatment, 300
    language functions and, 297–298
    Luria-Nebraska Neuropsychological Battery and, 293, 296, 297t
    Luria's Neuropsychological Investigation and, 293, 296t
    memory functions and, 298
  of cognitive deficits, 176–181, *176, 178, 179*
  of sensory responsiveness, 245–246
    bilateral simultaneous stimulation and, 246–247
    body schema and, 247–248, *247*
    sensory inventory and, 266, *267–269*
    stereognosis and, 246
    two-point discrimination and, 246
    visual function and, 248
  speech and language, 279
    cognitive evaluation and, 279–280
    language evaluation and, 281–282
    natural recovery from head injury and, 285–287, 285t, 287t
    neuromuscular speech system and, 283
      apraxia of speech and, 283
      articulation and, 284
      dysarthria and, 283
      phonation and, 284
      prosody and, 285
      resonance and, 284
      respiration and, 284
Asymmetric tonic neck reflex, 243
Ataxia, 24
Attitude, staff, positive, 346
Awareness, 60
  visual, 274–275
Axial rotation of trunk, improvement of motor control and, 316–317

Baclofen, 136
Balance
  movement from sitting to standing and, 251, *251*
  sitting, *250,* 250–251
  standing, 252–253, *252*
  weight shift and, 320, *321*
Bed positioning, 315–316
Behavior
  assessment of, outcome and, 107–108
  disturbances of, feeding and, 145
  effects of head injury on, 211t
  motor
    inventory of, 261, *262–265*
    recording of, 255
  target, 382–383
Behavior shaping, 383

Behavioral Competence Index, 180
Behavioral controls, patient reintegration into community and, 431
Behavioral deficits. *See also* Behavioral dysfunction
  behavioral principles and, 382–384
  chemotherapy for, 385
  rehabilitation as a behavioral process and, 381–382
  treatment of, 386
    day programs for, 389–390
    inpatient, 386–388
    transitional living programs, 388–389
Behavioral dysfunction. *See also* Behavioral deficits
  contributing factors to, 197
    environmental factors as, 200–201
    premorbid factors as, 198
    site of lesion as, 198–200
  minor head injury and, 205–206
  outcome of, 202–203
  recovery from, 201–202
  secondary, 203
    denial as, 203–204
    dependence as, 205
    depression as, 204–205
Behavioral principles, 382–384
  published applications of, 384–385
Behavioral substitution, 314
Benton Visual Retention Test, Revised, 298
Bilateral reciprocal isokinetic exercise, effectiveness of, 325–326, *326*, 327t
Bilateral reciprocal training program, 322, *323*, 324
Bilateral simultaneous stimulation, 246–247
Blood chemistries, management of coma and, 63–64
Blood pressure
  coma and, 64
  low, 42
Body schema, 247–248, *247*
Boston Diagnostic Aphasia Examination, 298
Boston Test for Aphasia, 159
Bradykinesia, 24
Brain
  focal damage to, memory deficits and, 189–190
  premorbid status of, 37–38
  primary impact damage to, 38
    diffuse, 39
    local, 38
    polar, 38–39
  secondary damage to
    brain distortion, shift, and herniation, 45–46
    hypoxic/ischemic brain damage, 46
  secondary insults to, 41
    anemia and, 42
    arterial hypotension and, 42
    arterial hypoxemia and, 41–42
    brain swelling and, 43
    hydrocephalus and, 44–45
    hyponatremia and, 42
    intracranial hematoma and, 43
    intracranial infection and, 44
    post-traumatic epilepsy and, 45
    raised intracranial pressure and, 43–44
Brain stem, dysfunction of, evoked potentials to detect, 82, *83*, *84*, 84–87, *85*, *86*

CARE, patient
  optimal, for patient reintegration into community, 432–433
  pre-hospital, severity of head injury and, 14–15
Case history
  anosognosia, 425–426
  confabulation, 427
  family counseling, 414
  family therapy, 416
  feeding difficulties, 145–146
  home living skills, difficulty with, 149
  hygiene difficulties, 147–148
  inadequate skills in advanced activities of daily living, 153
  neuropsychologic assessment, 303, 304t, 305, 305t, 306t
  remediation of perceptual dysfunction, 342–343
Casting
  for spasticity, 134
  total contact, motor control and, 330–331
Cause of head injury, 13–14
Cerebral shock, 313
Chemistries, blood, management of coma and, 63–64
Chemotherapy for behavioral deficits, 385
Chlorpromazine, 137, 385
Clinical course of head injury, 16–18
Clinical features of spasticity, 129–130
Clonazepam, 137
Cognitive deficits, 167–168. *See also* Cognitive dysfunction; Cognitive disorders
  assessment of, 176
    barriers to functional normalcy and, 176–177, *176*
    baseline measures and, 178–181
    core deficits and behavior dysfunctions, 177, *178*
    IRM system of, 178, *179*
    process and outcome measures and, 181
  clinical neurologic approach to, 168–169
  functional limitations and, 172–173, 174–175t
  learning theory approach to, 169
  long-term, problems in establishing, 171–172

Cognitive deficits—*continued*
  psychometric tradition and, 168
  rehabilitation approach to, 170
  use of norms to define, 170–171
Cognitive disorders
  remediation of, 367–368
    considerations of context and, 368–369
    considerations of scope and, 369–378, *370, 372, 374*
Cognitive disturbances, feeding and, 145
Cognitive dysfunction
  treatment of communication problems owing to, 357, 359
Cognitive evaluation, 279–280
Cognitive functions, assessment of, outcome and, 105–107, *106*
Cognitive remediation, 367–368
  considerations of context and, 368–369
  considerations of scope and, 369–378, *370, 372, 374*
Cognitive retraining task force, 356–357
Cold, application of, for spasticity, 132
Collateral sprouting, 315
Coma
  definition of, 102
  duration of, 101–103, 102t, 103t
  evaluation of patient in, 48–49, 48t, *50*
  management of, 63t
    blood chemistries and, 63–64
    blood pressure and, 64
    dextrose administration and, 63–64
    fever and, 65
    hypothermia and, 64
    maintenance of respiration and, 63
    nasogastric intubation and, 64
    neurologic evaluation and, 65–68, 65t
    pulse and, 64
    traumatic injuries and, 64
  multimodality evoked potentials in, 77–78
  outcome of, assessment of, 70–71
  pathophysiology of
    central downward transtentorial herniation and, 61–62
    herniation of temporal lobe uncus, 62
    subtentorial lesions and, 62
    supratentorial lesions and, 61
    toxic-metabolic encephalopathy and, 61
    unconsciousness due to head trauma and, 62
  prediction of outcome of, 68–69
    head injury and, 69
    medical coma and, 69–70
  regulation of consciousness and, 60–61
Coma-arousal task force, 356
Communication
  disorders of, 155–156
    aphasia, traumatic and vascular, 158–159
    duration of unconsciousness and, 157
    dysarthria, 160–161
    focal versus diffuse damage and, 157–158
    open versus closed injury and, 156–157
    specific speech and language deficits, 159–160
  manual, 363–364
  recovery of, 161–163
Communication aids, 364
  direct selection, 364
  electromechanical, 365
  encoding, 364–365
  scanning-type, 364
Communication disabilities, 27, 28t
Communication disorders
  alternate forms of communication and, 363
    communication aids, 364
      direct selection, 364
      electromechanical, 365
      encoding, 364–365
      scanning-type, 364
    manual communication, 363–364
  role of speech and language pathologist in, 355
    cognitive retraining task force and, 356–357
    coma-arousal task force and, 356
    evaluation team and, 355
    provision of speech and language pathology therapy, 357
    task force for swallowing dysfunction and, 356
  treatment of, 357
    aphasia and, 358–359t, 359–361, *362*
    dysarthria and, 361–363
    problems owing to cognitive dysfunction and, 357, 359
Communication skills, 148–149
Communicative Activities of Daily Living technique, 298
Community, patient reintegration into
  background of problem of, 421–422
  behavioral controls and, 431
  community resources for, 429–430
  family grief and, 428–429
  immediate environment and, 430
  long-term survivors and, 422–424, 423t, 424t
    anosognosia in, 424–426
    confabulation in, 426–427
    police encounters of, 427–428
  optimal patient care and, 432–433
  other considerations for, 431–432
Community skills, 277
Complications
  neurologic, 27t
  neurologic and systemic, multimodality evoked potentials and, 91, 92t
Computed tomography, 49, *50*, 67–68
  outcome from head injury and, 56

INDEX

Concussion, 40–41
Confabulation, 426–427
Conferences, family, patient-family education and, 399
Consciousness
  lack of
    due to head trauma, pathophysiology of, 62
    duration of, communication disorders and, 157
  level of
    disturbance of, prediction of memory deficits and, 188–189
    neurologic evaluation and, 65
    outcome from head injury and, 55
  regulation of, 60–61
Consistency, reality orientation therapy and, 351–352
Context of cognitive remediation, 368–369
Contingencies, as behavioral principle, 383
Controls, behavioral, patient reintegration into community and, 431
Counseling, family, as family intervention technique, 414–415
Cranial nerve deficits, 233–234
Cranioplasty, 236
Cryotherapy, 330, *331*
Cushing reflex, 64

DAILY living, activities of. *See* Activities of daily living
Damage
  brain
    diffuse, 39
    hypoxic/ischemic, 46
    local, 38
    polar, 38–39
  to scalp, skull, dura, and other structures, 39–40
Dantrium. *See* Dantrolene sodium
Dantrolene sodium, 136–137
Data, neuropsychologic, organization and presentation of, 302, *303*
Day treatment programs for behavioral deficits, 389–390
Death, partial, 408–409
Deficits
  behavioral
    behavioral principles and, 382–384
    chemotherapy for, 385
    rehabilitation as a behavioral process and, 381–382
    treatment of, 386
      day programs for, 389–390
      inpatient, 386–388
      transitional living programs, 388–389
  cognitive, 167–168
    assessment of, 176
      barriers to functional normalcy and, 176–177, *176*
      core deficits and behavior dysfunctions, 177, *178*
      IRM system of, 178, *179*
      process and outcome measures and, 181
    baseline measures and, 178–181
    clinical neurologic approach to, 168–169
    functional limitations and, 172–173, 174–175t
    learning theory approach to, 169
    long-term, problems in establishing, 171–172
    psychometric tradition and, 168
    rehabilitation approach to, 170
    use of norms to define, 170–171
  cranial nerve, 233–234
  educational and vocational, 219
    brain function and, 219–220
    pre-injury status and, 220
    remediation of, 222–223
    specific, effects of, 221–222
    universal, effects of, 220–221
  identification of, family intervention and, 411–412
  language, specific, 159–160
  memory
    delayed, 186
    early after injury, 185–186
    methods for improvement of, 192–194
    prediction of, 188
      disturbance of consciousness level and, 188–189
      signs of focal brain damage, and, 189–190
    reason for, 186–187
      long- and short-term memory and, 187
      memory sensitivity and, 187
      storage or retrieval and, 187
    recovery from, 190–191
    test performance and, 192
  psychosocial
    effects of, on family system, 409–410
  speech, specific, 159–160
Definition(s)
  behavior shaping, 383
  coma, 102
  contingencies, 383
  disability, 23
  extinction, 383–384
  fading, 383
  handicap, 23
  impairment, 23
  neuropsychologic assessment, 291–292
  positive reinforcer, 383
  spasticity, 125–126
  target behaviors, 382–383
Degree of Language Impairment scale, 359
Denervation, supersensitivity of, 314–315

Denial, 202–204
Dependence, 205
Depression, 204–205
Dextroamphetamine, 385
Dextrose, administration of, management of coma and, 63–64
Diabetes insipidus, 237–238
Diagnosis of head injury
  determinants of head injury and, 46–47
  triage and, 47–48
Diaschisis, 313
Diazepam, 136
Dilantin. *See* Phenytoin
Direct selection communication aids, 364
Disability. *See also* Disorders; Dysfunction
  communication, 27, 28t
  definition of, 23
  due to brain damage, classification of, 109t
  educational and vocational, 30–31
  from head injury, nature of, 5–6
  minor brain trauma, 31
  physical
    functional physical disabilities, 25–26
    motor impairments, 24, 24t
    pre-existing, 26
    resulting from associated injuries, 26
    resulting from medical complications, 26–27, 27t, 28t
    sensory impairments and aberrations, 24
  psychologic, 27, 29t
  social, 30, 30t
Disability Rating Scale, 301, 302t
Discrimination, two-point, 246
Disorders. *See also* Disability; Dysfunction
  cognitive
    remediation of, 367–368
      considerations of context and, 368–369
      consideration of scope and, 369–378, 370, 372, 374
  communication, 155–156
    alternate forms of communication and, 363
    communication aids, 364
      direct selection, 364
      electromechanical, 365
      encoding, 364–365
      scanning-type, 364
    manual communication, 363–364
    aphasia, traumatic and vascular, 158–159
    duration of unconsciousness and, 157
    dysarthria, 160–161
    focal versus diffuse damage and, 157–158
    open versus closed injury and, 156–157
    role of speech and language pathologist in, 355
    cognitive retraining task force and, 356–357
    coma-arousal task force and, 356
    evaluation team and, 355
    provision of speech and language pathology therapy and, 357
    task force for swallowing dysfunction and, 356
    specific speech and language deficits, 159–160
    treatment of, 357
      aphasia and, 358–359t, 359–361, 362
      dysarthria and, 361–363
      problems owing to cognitive dysfunction and, 357, 359
Distortion, brain, 45–46
Disturbances
  behavioral, feeding and, 145
  cognitive, feeding and, 145
Doll's eye reflex, 49, 67
Dressing, 146–147
Driving, 151–152
  epilepsy and, 123–124
Dura, primary impact damage to, 39–40
Dynamometry, 255–259, *256, 257, 258*
  validity and reliability of, 259
Dysarthria, 160–161
Dysfunction. *See also* Disability; Disorders
  behavioral
    contributing factors to, 197
      environmental factors as, 200–201
      premorbid factors as, 198
      site of lesion as, 198–200
    denial as, 203–204
    depression as, 204–205
    minor head injury and, 205–206
    outcome of, 202–203
    recovery from, 201–202
    secondary, 203
      dependence as, 205
  brain stem, evoked potentials to detect, 82, *83, 84,* 84–87, *85, 86*
  cognitive, treatment of communication problems owing to, 357, 359
  extent of, multimodality evoked potentials and, 88, 90t
  oral, feeding and, 144
  perceptual, remediation of, 335
    case histories of, 342–343
    functional skills and, 343
    goal setting and, 343
    positioning techniques for, 388–341, *339, 340, 341*
  severity of, multimodality evoked potentials and, 87–88, 89t
  swallowing, task force for, 356
Dyskinesias, 24

EDUCATION, patient-family, 395–397, *396*
  as family intervention technique, 413–414
  factors in planning, 397
  family conferences and, 399
  group learning activities and, 398–399
  home visits and, 397–398
    evaluation form for, 402–405
  methodologic considerations of, 400
  reality orientation and, 397
  self-help groups and, 399
Educational and vocational deficits, 30–31, 219
  brain function and, 219–220
  pre-injury status and, 220
  remediation of, 222–223
  specific, effects of, 221–222
  universal, effects of, 220–221
Electric stimulation for spasticity, 135
Electroencephalogram, abnormal, frequency of after head injury, 122
Electromechanical communication aids, 365
Electronic feedback, 332
Emergency room, management of severe head injury in, 51–52
Encephalopathy, toxic-metabolic, 61
Encoding communication aids, 364–365
Environment
  behavioral dysfunction and effect of, 200–201
  reintegration of head-injured patient into community and, 430
Environmental program of reality orientation therapy, 346
  consistent approach and, 346
  environmental stimulation and, 346–348
  positive staff attitude and, 346
Environmental stimulation, reality orientation therapy and, 346–348
Epilepsy, 235
  driving and, 123–124
  post-traumatic, 45
    early, 119–120
    late
      features of, 120
      prediction of, 120–122, 121t, *122*, 122t
      prevention of, 122–123
Equilibrium reaction, 249. *See also* Balance
Equipotentiality, 313–314
Evaluation. *See also* Assessment; Diagnosis; Examination
  cognitive, 279–280
  language, 281–282
  neurologic, 53t, *54*, 65, 65t
    acute phase and, 59–62
    computed tomography in, 67–68
    in recovery stage of coma, 68
    level of consciousness and, 65
    motor responses and, 66
    neuro-ophthalmologic examination and, 66–67
  of cognitive deficits, 168–169
  of outcome, 103, *104*, 105, *105*
  occupational therapy
    activities of daily living and, 276
      community skills, 277
      home skills, 276
      self-care skills, 276
    general procedures, 272–273
    goal setting and, 277
    motor control and, 273
      muscle strength, 273–274
      muscle tone, 273
      range of motion, 273
    perceptual-motor abilities and, 274
      form and space perception, 275–276
      motor planning, 276
      somatosensory functions, 275
      visual awareness, 274–275
    review of medical history and, 271–272
    sensation and, 274
  of comatose head-injured patient, 48–49, 48t, *50*
  of home visits, 402–405
  of serial multimodality evoked potentials, recovery and, 91, *93*
  of spasticity, 130–131
Evaluation team for communication disorders, 355
Evoked potentials
  multimodality, 77
    analysis of, 78, *79*, *80*, *81*
      somatosensory brain stem response and, 79–81
      somatosensory cortical response and, 78–79
      auditory brain stem responses, and, 81–82
    in comatose patients, 77–78
    prognosis and, 87–88, 89t, 90t, 91, 92t, *93*, 93, 94t, 95
    visual cortical evoked responses and, 82
  sensory, 75–77, *76*, *77*
    detecting brain stem dysfunction with, 82, *83*, *84*, 84–87, *85*, *86*
Examination. *See also* Assessment; Diagnosis; Evaluation
  neuro-ophthalmologic
    doll's eyes, 67
    eye movements, 66–67
    ice-water caloric test, 67
    pupillary findings, 66
Exercise, bilateral reciprocal isokinetic, effectiveness of, 325–326, *326*, 327t
Exteroceptive feedback for coordination, 332

Extinction, as behavioral principle, 383–384
Extracranial injuries, 17t
Etiology of spasticity, 126–129
Eye(s)
   doll's, 67
   movements of, in coma, 66–67

FACIAL bone fractures, effects of, 234
Fading, as behavioral principle, 383
Falls as cause of head injuries, 13
Family
   effects of psychosocial deficits on, 409–410
   grief of, patient reintegration into community and, 428–429
   head-injured patient and, 209–210
   high risk for problems after head injury and, 412
   physical and mental consequences of head injury and, 210–213, 211t, 212t, 213t
   psychosocial consequences of head injury and, 213–216, 216t
   signals from, need for family intervention and, 412
Family conferences, patient-family education and, 399
Family counseling as family intervention technique, 414–415
Family education. See Patient-family education
Family intervention, 407–408
   establishing need for, 410–411
      identifying deficits for, 411–412
      premorbid history for, 411
      signals from family and, 412
   factors to consider before initiating, 412–413
   high-risk families and, 412
   nonprofessional, 416–417
   techniques of, 413
      family counseling as, 414–415
      family therapy as, 415–416
      patient-family education as, 413–414
   theoretical framework for, 408–409
      effects of psychosocial deficits on family system and, 409–410
Family relationships, 149–150
Family therapy as family intervention technique, 415–416
Feedback
   electronic, 332
   exteroceptive, for coordination, 332
Feeding, 143
   behavioral and cognitive problems and, 145
   case history relating to, 147–148
   oral dysfunction and, 144
   oral, status of, 236
   physical limitations and, 144–145
Fever, coma and, 65

Financial management, 151
Foot, motor control of, 329
Forearms, pronation and supination of, motor assessment and, 249–250
Form and space activities for perceptual dysfunction, 337, *338*
Form and space perception, 275–276
Fractures
   facial bone, effects of, 234
   skull, 17t
Function
   hand, 253, 255
   language, neuropsychologic assessment and, 297–298
   memory, neuropsychologic assessment and, 298
   respiratory, improvement of motor control and, 316
   somatosensory, 275
   vicarious, 314
Functional Ambulation Score, 253, *254*
Functional Communication Profile, 162–163
Functional reorganization, 314

GLASGOW Coma Scale, 4, 15–16, 16t, 48, 48t, 54–55, 102–103, 102t, 103t, 189, 231–232
Glasgow Outcome Scale, 19, 97, 98t, 99, 301
   at discharge, 19t
   at three months postinjury, 20t
   outcome and, 109t, *110*
Goal setting, 277
   for perceptual dysfunction, 343
Goals of reality orientation therapy, 345–346
Grief, family, patient reintegration into community and, 428–429
Group learning activities, patient-family education and, 398–399
Group sessions in reality orientation therapy, 348–351
Groups, self-help
   as nonprofessional family intervention, 416–417
   patient-family education and, 399

HALDOL. See Haloperidol
Haloperidol, 385
Halstead-Reitan Battery, 292–293, 294–295t
Hand
   activities of, motor control and, 329
   function of, 253, 255
Handicap, definition of, 23
Head injury
   cognitive deficits and, assessment of, 176–181, *176, 178, 179*
   communication disorders and
      aphasia, traumatic and vascular, 158–159

duration of unconsciousness and, 157
dysarthria, 160–161
focal versus diffuse damage and, 157–158
open versus closed injury and, 156–157
specific speech and language deficits, 159–160
diagnosis of
  determinants of injury and, 46–47
  evaluation of comatose patient and, 48–49, 48t, 50
  triage and, 47–48
epidemiology of, 3–4
factors influencing outcome from, 55–56
frequency of problems after, 20t
incidence of, 9, 10t, 11
management of
  in emergency room, 51–52
  in intensive-care unit, 52–53, 53t, 54
  operative, 52
  pre-hospital, 51
  treatment of raised intracranial pressure and, 53
mechanisms of recovery from central nervous system lesions, 313–315
nature of disability from, 5–6
outcome of, 18–19
  assessment of, 70–71
  at discharge, 19, 19t
  at three months, 19–20, 20t
pathophysiology of, 37
  concussion and, 40–41
  premorbid status of brain and, 37–38
  primary impact damage to brain and, 38–39
patient characteristics and,
  age and sex, 11, *11*, 12
  cause of injury, 13–14
  location of injury, 14
  medical history, 13
  socioeconomic status, 12–13, *12*
  time of injury, 14
physical and mental consequences of, 210–213, 211t, 212t, 213t
post-traumatic epilepsy and, 119–124, 121t, *122*, 122t
prediction of outcome from coma in, 69
recovery from, 6–7, 53–55
  speech and language assessment and, 285–287, 285t, 287t
secondary damage to brain from
  brain distortion, shift, and herniation, 45–46
  hypoxic/ischemic brain damage and, 46
secondary insults to brain, 41
  anemia and, 42
  arterial hypotension, 42
  arterial hypoxemia, 41–42
  brain swelling and, 43

hydrocephalus and, 44–45
hyponatremia and, 42
intracranial hematoma and, 43
intracranial infection and, 44
post-traumatic epilepsy, 45
raised intracranial pressure and, 43–44
sequelae of
  long-term, problems in establishing, 171–172
  mental, functional limitations and, 172–173, 174–175t
severity of, 4–5, 5t
  clinical course and, 16–18
  extracranial injuries and, 17t
  Glasgow Coma Scale and, 15–16, 16t
  length of hospital stay and, 18
  pre-hospital care and, 14–15
  skull fractures and, 17t
unemployment after, 20t
vegetative state after, 71
Head-dropping test, 245
Hearing disorders, 25
Hematoma
  computed tomograms of, *50*
  intracranial, 43
  presence of, outcome from head injury and, 55
Hemiparesis, 24
Herniation
  brain, 45–46
  central downward transtentorial, 61–62
  temporal lobe uncus, 62
Heterotopic ossification, 236–237
High Hopes Recovery Group, 416
History
  medical, of head-injured patients, 13
  occupational therapy evaluation and, 271–272
  occupational, in reality orientation therapy, 351
  premorbid, family intervention and, 411
Home living skills, 149, 276
  case history relating to, 149
Home visits
  evaluation form for, 402–405
  patient-family education and, 397–398
Hospitalization, duration of, severity of injury and, 18
Hydrocephalus, 44–45
  post-traumatric, 235–236
Hygiene skills, 147
  case history relating to, 147–148
Hypercalcemia, 237
Hypertension, intracranial, outcome from head injury and, 56
Hyponatremia, 42
Hypotension, arterial, 42
Hypothalamic functions, 237–238

Hypothermia, coma and, 64
Hypoxemia, arterial, 41–42
Hypoxic brain damage, 46

ICE-WATER caloric test, 67
Impact, primary
    damage to brain from, 38–39
    damage to scalp, skull, dura, and other structures from, 39–40
Impairment
    definition of, 23
    motor, 24, 24t
    sensory, 24–25, 25t
Infection, 235
    intracranial, 44
Injuries
    extracranial, 17t
    head. See Head injury
    traumatic, coma and, 64
Instruments. See Tests
Insults, secondary
    mass lesions, multimodality evoked potentials and, 88, 91
    other complications, multimodality evoked potentials and, 91, 92t
Intensive-care unit, management of head injury in, 52–53, 53t, 54
Intervention, family, 407–408
    establishing need for, 410–411
        identifying deficits for, 411–412
        premorbid history for, 411
        signals from family, 412
    factors to consider before initiating, 412–413
    high-risk families and, 412
    nonprofessional, 416–417
    techniques of, 413
        family counseling as, 414–415
        family therapy as, 415–416
        patient-family education as, 413–414
    theoretical framework for, 408–409
        effects of psychosocial deficits on family system and, 409–410
Intracranial hematoma, 43
Intracranial infection, 44
Intracranial pressure
    raised, 43–44
        mannitol to reduce, 51–52, 53
        treatment of, 53
Intubation, nasogastric, management of coma and, 64
Ischemic brain damage, 46

KINETRON, 322, 323, 325–326

LABYRINTHINE reflex, tonic, 248
Language evaluation, 281–282. See also Speech and language assessment
Language functions, neuropsychologic assessment and, 297–298
Learning activities, group, patient-family education and, 398–399
Learning, tests of, 99t
Learning theory, cognitive deficits and, 169
Lesion(s)
    central nervous system, mechanisms of recovery from, 313
        behavioral substitution, 314
        collateral sprouting, 315
        diaschisis, 313
        equipotentiality, 313–314
        functional reorganization, 314
        regeneration and, 315
        supersensitivity of denervation, 314–315
        vicarious function, 314
    mass, multimodality evoked potentials and, 88, 91
    site of, behavioral dysfunction and, 198–200
    subtentorial, 62
    supratentorial, 61
Limitations, physical, feeding and, 144–145
Lioresal. See Baclofen
Living, daily, activities of. See Activities of daily living
Location of injury, 14
Locomotion, forward, 253
Luria-Nebraska Neuropsychological Battery, 293, 296, 297t
Luria's Neuropsychological Investigation, 293, 296t

MANAGEMENT. See also Therapy; Treatment
    financial, 151
    of coma, 63t
        blood chemistries and, 63–64
        blood pressure and, 64
        dextrose administration and, 63–64
        fever and, 65
        hypothermia and, 64
        maintenance of respiration and, 63
        nasogastric intubation and, 64
        neurologic evaluation and, 65–68, 65t
        pulse and, 64
        traumatic injuries and, 64
    of head injury
        in emergency room, 51–52
        in intensive-care unit, 52–53, 53t, 54
        operative, 52
        pre-hospital, 51
        treatment of raised intracranial pressure and, 53

of memory disorders, 192–194
of spasticity, 132–139, 132t, 133t
time, 150–151
Mannitol, 51–52, 53
Manual communication, 363–364
Measurement of outcome
  aims of, 100
  duration of coma and, 101–103, 102t, 103t
  instruments for, 100
  need for objectivity in, 114
  need for realism in, 115
  overall, 108–111, 109t, *110*, 110t
  post-traumatic amnesia and, 100–101
  process of, 97, 98t, 99–100, 99t
  reasons for, 97
  social adjustment and, 111–112
Medical assessment, criteria for rehabilitation and, 231
  airway obstruction as, 237
  cranial nerve deficits as, 233–234
  cranioplasty as, 236
  effects of facial bone fractures as, 234
  epilepsy as, 235
  heterotopic ossification as, 236–237
  hypothalamic functions as, 237–238
  infections as, 235
  medical stability as, 232
  neurologic improvement as, 232
  oral-feeding status as, 236
  post-traumatic amnesia as, 233
  post-traumatic hydrocephalus as, 235–236
  skeletal trauma as, 237
Medical history
  occupational therapy evaluation and, 271–272
  of head-injured patients, 13
Memory
  deficits of
    delayed, 186
    early after injury, 185–186
    methods for improvement of, 192–194
    prediction of, 188
      disturbance of consciousness level and, 188–189
      signs of focal brain damage and, 189–190
    reason for, 186–187
      long- and short-term memory and, 187
      memory sensitivity and, 187
      storage or retrieval and, 187
    recovery from, 190–191
    test performance and, 192
  tests of, 99t
Memory functions, neuropsychologic assessment and, 298
Metabolic encephalopathy, 61
Minnesota Test for the Differential Diagnosis of Aphasia, 298, 359

Mobile mourning, 408–409
Modules, cognitive remedial, 371–373, *372*
Motion, range of, 273
Motor activities for perceptual dysfunction, 337
Motor behavior inventory, 261, *262–265*
Motor behavior, recording of, 255
Motor control
  muscle strength, 273–274
  muscle tone, 273
  occupational therapy evaluation and, 273
  principles of improving
    during acute phase
      axial rotation of trunk, 316–317
      bed positioning, 315–316
      respiratory function and, 316
      sensory stimulation, 316
    during subacute phase, 317–318, *318*, *319*
      ambulation training, 324–325
      bilateral reciprocal training program, 322, *323*, 324
      effectiveness of bilateral reciprocal isokinetic exercise and, 325–326, *326*, 327t
      foot control and, 329
      hand activities and, 329
      linking vestibular stimulation to voluntary movement, 318–320
      motor control of upper limb and, 326–328
      stimulation of weight bearing, 320–322
      stimulation of weight shift and standing balance, 320, *321*
    supplemental treatment and, 329–330
      cryotherapy, 330, *331*
      electronic feedback, 332
      exteroceptive feedback for coordination, 332
      total contact casting, 330–331
      vibratory stimulation, 332–333
Motor impairments, 24, 24t
Motor neurons, spasticity and, 126–129
Motor planning, 276
Motor re-education techniques for spasticity, 135–136
Motor responses, neurologic evaluation of, 66
Mourning, mobile, 408–409
Movement(s)
  assessment of, 241
    arm-dropping test and, 249
    dynamometry and, 255–259, *256*, *257*, *258*
      validity and reliability of, 259
    equilibrium reaction and, 249
    from sitting to standing, 251, *251*
    Functional Ambulation Score and, 253, *254*
    hand function and, 253, 255
    head-dropping test and, 245
    locomotion and, 253
    motor behavior inventory and, 262, *262–265*

Movement(s)—*continued*
    motor examination and, 242–244
    motor problems of head-injured patient and, 242
    muscle tonus and myotatic reflexes and, 244–245
    pronation and supination of forearms and, 249–250
    recording of motor behavior and, 255
    righting reflex and, 248–249
    shoulder-shaking test and, 249
    sitting balance and, *250*, 250–251
    standing position and, 252–253, *252*
    tonic reflexes, 248
  disorders of, 24t
  eye, in coma, 66–67
  voluntary, vestibular stimulation and, 318–320
Multimodality evoked potentials, 77
  analysis of, 78, *79*, *80*, *81*
    somatosensory brain stem response and, 79–81
    somatosensory cortical response and, 78–79
    auditory brain stem responses and, 81–82
  in comatose patients, 77–78
  prognosis and, 87–88, 89t, 90t, 91, 92t, *93*, 93, 94t, 95
  visual cortical evoked responses and, 82
Muscle(s)
  strength of, 273–274
  tone of, 273
Muscle tonus, assessment of, 244–245
Muscle vibration for spasticity, 135
Myelotomy, 139
Myotatic reflexes, assessment of, 244–245

NALOXONE, 64
Nasogastric intubation, management of coma and, 64
National Head Injury Foundation, 416–417
Neck reflex, tonic, 248
Neurologic evaluation, 65, 65t
  acute phase and, 59–62
  case history of, 303, 304t, 305, 305t, 306t
  computed tomography in, 67–68
  in recovery stage of coma, 68
  level of consciousness and, 65
  motor responses and, 66
  neuro-ophthalmologic examination and, 66–67
  of cognitive deficits, 168–169
  of head-injured patient, 53t, 54
  of outcome, 103, *104*, 105, *105*
Neurolysis
  intramuscular, 137
  peripheral nerve, 137

Neuromuscular speech system, 283
  apraxia of speech and, 283
  articulation and, 284
  dysarthria and, 283
  phonation and, 284
  prosody and, 285
  resonance and, 284
  respiration and, 284
Neurons, motor, spasticity and, 126–129
Neuro-ophthalmologic examination
  doll's eyes, 67
  eye movements, 66–67
  ice-water caloric test, 67
  pupillary findings, 66
Neuropsychologic assessment
  definition and background of, 291–292
  Halstead-Reitan Battery and, 292–293, 294–295t
  in rehabilitation settings, 299
    baseline determinations and, 299
    data organization and presentation, 302, *303*
    identification of strengths and weaknesses, 299, *299*, 300t
    prediction and determination of outcome, 300–301, 302t
    prescriptions for treatment, 300
  language functions and, 297–298
  Luria-Nebraska Neuropsychological Battery and, 293, 296, 297t
  Luria's Neuropsychological Investigation and, 293, 296t
  memory functions and, 298
Neurosensory Center Comprehensive Examination for Aphasia, 298
Neurosurgery for spasticity, 138–139
Norms, use of, to define cognitive deficits, 170–171

OBJECTIVITY, need for, in assessing outcome, 114
Obstruction, airway, 237
Occupational history in reality orientation therapy, 351
Occupational therapy evaluation
  activities of daily living and, 276
    community skills, 277
    home skills, 276
    self-care skills, 276
  general procedures, 272–273
  goal setting and, 277
  motor control and, 273
    muscle strength, 273–274
    muscle tone, 273
    range of motion, 273
  perceptual-motor abilities and, 274
    form and space perception, 275–276

INDEX

motor planning, 276
somatosensory functions, 275
visual awareness, 274–275
review of medical history and, 271–272
sensation and, 274
Oculocephalic reflex, 49
Oculovestibular response, 49
Ophthalmologic examination. *See* Neuro-ophthalmologic examination
Oral dysfunction, feeding and, 144
Oral-feeding status, 236
Orientation, reality, patient-family education and, 397
Orthoses for spasticity, 134
Ossification, heterotopic, 236–237
Outcome
  aims of measurement of, 100
  instruments for measuring, 100
  measurement of
    duration of coma and, 101–103, 102t, 103t
    need for objectivity in, 114
    need for realism in, 115
    overall, 108–111, 109t, *110,* 110t
    post-traumatic amnesia and, 100–101
    social adjustment and, 111–112
  mental, assessment of
    cognitive and perceptual functions, 105–107, *106*
    personality and behavior, 107–108, *108*
  neurologic assessment of, 103, *104,* 105, *105*
  of behavioral dysfunctions, 202–203
  of coma, 70–71
    prediction of, 68–69
      head injury and, 69
      medical coma and, 69–70
  of head injuries, 18–19, 70–71
    at discharge, 19, 19t
    at three months, 19–20, 20t
    factors influencing, 55–56
  prediction and determination of neuropsychologic, 300–301, 302t
  process of measuring, 97, 98t, 99–100, 99t
  reasons for measuring, 97

PARTIAL death, 408–409
Pathologist, speech and language, role of, in communication disorders, 355
  cognitive retraining task force and, 356–357
  coma-arousal task force and, 356
  evaluation team and, 355
  provision of speech and language pathology therapy and, 357
  task force for swallowing dysfunction and, 356
Pathology, speech and language, therapy for, 357

Pathophysiology
  of coma
    central downward transtentorial herniation and, 61–62
    herniation of temporal lobe uncus and, 62
    subtentorial lesions and, 62
    supratentorial lesions and, 61
    toxic-metabolic encephalopathy and, 61
    unconsciousness due to head trauma and, 62
  of head injury, 37
    concussion and, 40–41
    premorbid status of brain and, 37–38
    primary impact damage to brain and, 38–39
  of spasticity, 126–129, *126, 127*
Patient(s), head-injured
  age and sex of, 11–12, *11*
  cause of injury in, 13–14
  comatose, evaluation of, 48–49, 48t, *50*
  family and, 209–210
  location of injury and, 14
  medical history of, 13
  motor problems of, 242
  physical and mental consequences of injury and, 210–213, 211t, 212t, 213t
  psychosocial consequences of injury and, 213–216, 216t
  reintegration of, into community
    background of problem of, 421–422
    behavioral controls and, 431
    community resources for, 429–430
    family grief and, 428–429
    immediate environment and, 430
    long-term survivors and, 422–424, 423t, 424t
      anosognosia in, 424–426
      confabulation in, 426–427
      police encounters of, 427–428
    optimal care and, 432–433
    other considerations for, 431–432
  socioeconomic status of, 12–13, *12*
  time of injury of, 14
  triage of, 47–48
Patient-family education, 395–397, *396*
  as family intervention technique, 413–414
  factors in planning, 397
  family conferences and, 399
  group learning activities and, 398–399
  home visits and, 397–398
    evaluation form for, 402–405
  methodologic considerations of, 400
  reality orientation and, 397
  self-help groups and, 399
Perception of form and space, 275–276
Perceptual dysfunction, remediation of, 335
  case histories of, 342–343
  functional skills and, 343

Perceptual dysfunction, remediation of—*continued*
    goal setting and, 343
    positioning techniques for, 338–341, *339, 340, 341*
    treatment approaches to, 336–337, *337, 338*
Perceptual functions, assessment of, outcome and, 105–107, *106*
Perceptual-motor abilities, 274
    form and space perception, 275–276
    motor planning, 276
    somatosensory functions, 275
    visual awareness, 274–275
Personal system, 408
Personality
    assessment of, outcome and, 107–108, *108*
    effects of head injury on, 211t
Phenytoin, 123, 137
Phonation, 284
    therapeutic considerations for improving, 362–363
Physical limitations, feeding and, 144–145
Planning, motor, 276
Police, encounters of head-injured patients with, 427–428
Porch Index of Communicative Ability, 159–160, 162, 298, 359
Positioning, bed, 315–316
Positioning techniques for perceptual dysfunction, 338–341, *339, 340, 341*
Positive reinforcer, as behavioral principle, 383
Postconcussion syndrome, 5, 31, 206
Post-traumatic amnesia, 4–5, 5t, 41, 185–186, 188–191, 233
    assessment of, 100–101
    outcome and, 109–110, 109t, 110t
Post-traumatic epilepsy, 45
    early, 119–120
    late
        features of, 120
        prediction of, 120–122, 121t, *122,* 122t
        prevention of, 122–123
Post-traumatic hydrocephalus, 235–236
Posture, disorders of, 24t
Potentials, evoked
    multimodality, 77
        analysis of, 78, *79, 80, 81*
            somatosensory brain stem response and, 79–81
            somatosensory cortical response and, 78–79
        auditory brain stem responses and, 81–82
        in comatose patients, 77–78
        prognosis and, 87–88, 89t, 90t, 91, 92t, *93,* 93, 94t, 95
        visual cortical evoked responses and, 82
    sensory, 75–77, *76, 77*

detecting brain stem dysfunction with, 82, *83, 84,* 84–87, *85, 86*
Pre-hospital care of head-injured patient, 51
Premorbid history, family intervention and, 411
Pressure
    blood, coma and, 64
    intracranial, raised, 43–44
        mannitol to reduce, 51–52, 53
        treatment of, 53
Principles, behavioral, 382–384
    published applications of, 384–385
Problem solving, 373, *374*
Problems, frequency of, after head injury, 20t
Pronation, forearm, motor assessment and, 249–250
Proprioceptive stimulation for perceptual dysfunction, 339–340, *339, 340*
Prosody, 285
Psychologic disabilities, 27, 29t
Psychometric tradition and cognitive deficits, 168
Psychosocial deficits, effects of, on family system, 409–410
Pulse, coma and, 64
Pupils, findings in coma, 66
Purdue Peg Board test, 180

QUESTIONNAIRE, Reality Orientation, 348, *349*

RANGE of motion, 273
Reaction, equilibrium, 249
Realism, need for, in assessing outcome, 115
Reality orientation, patient-family education and, 397
Reality Orientation Questionnaire, 348, *349*
Reality orientation therapy, 345
    environmental program of, 346
        consistent approach and, 346
        environmental stimulation and, 346–348
        positive staff attitude and, 346
    goals of, 345–346
    group sessions in, 348–351
    occupational history and, 351
    treatment program in, 351–353
Recovery
    early multimodality evoked potentials and, 91, 93, 94t, 95
    from coma, neurologic evaluation during, 68
    from head injury, 6–7, 53–55
        speech and language assessment and, 285–287, 285t, 287t
    mechanisms of, from central nervous system lesions, 313
        behavioral substitution, 314
        collateral sprouting, 315
        diaschisis, 313

equipotentiality, 313–314
functional reorganization, 314
regeneration, 315
supersensitivity of denervation, 314–315
vicarious function, 314
of communication, 161–163
serial multimodality evoked potentials and, 91, 93
Reflex
asymmetric tonic neck, 243
Cushing, 64
doll's eye, 49
myotatic, 244–245
oculocephalic, 49
righting, 248–249
symmetric tonic neck, 244
tonic labyrinthine, 248
tonic neck, 248
tonic vibratory, 332–333
Regeneration, 315
Regulation of consciousness, 60–61
Rehabilitation
as approach to assessing cognitive deficits, 170
as behavioral process, 381–382
criteria for
airway obstruction as, 237
cranial nerve deficits as, 233–234
cranioplasty as, 236
effects of facial bone fractures as, 234
epilepsy as, 235
heterotopic ossification as, 236–237
hypothalamic functions as, 237–238
infections as, 235
medical stability as, 232
neurologic improvement as, 232
oral-feeding status as, 236
post-traumatic amnesia as, 233
post-traumatic hydrocephalus as, 235–236
skeletal trauma as, 237
of educational and vocational deficits, 222–223
Rehabilitation settings, neuropsychologic assessment in, 299
baseline determinations and, 299
data organization and presentation and, 302, 303
identification of strengths and weaknesses, 299, 299, 300t
prediction and determination of neuropsychologic outcome and, 300–301, 302t
prescriptions for treatment and, 300
Reinforcer, positive, as behavioral principle, 383
Relationships, family, 149–150
Relaxation techniques for spasticity, 135–136
Reliability of dynamometer, 259
Remediation. See also Therapy; Treatment
cognitive, 367–368

considerations of scope and, 369–378, *370, 372, 374*
considerations of context and, 368–369
of perceptual dysfunction, 335
case histories of, 343–343
functional skills and, 343
goal setting and, 343
positioning techniques for, 338–341, *339, 340, 341*
treatment approaches to, 336–337, *337, 338*
Reorganization, functional, 314
Repetition, reality orientation therapy and, 351–352
Resonance, 284
therapeutic considerations for improving, 363
Resources, community, for patient reintegration, 429–430
Respiration
maintenance of, in comatose patient, 63
speech and, 284
therapeutic considerations for improving, 362
Respiratory function, improvement of motor control and, 316
Responses
auditory brain stem, to evoked potentials, 81–82
motor, neurologic evaluation of, 66
oculovestibular, 49
somatosensory brain stem, to evoked potentials, 79–81
somatosensory cortical, to evoked potentials, 78–79
visual cortical, to evoked potentials, 82
Responsiveness, sensory, assessment of, 245–246
bilateral simultaneous stimulation and, 246–247
body schema and, 247–248, *247*
sensory inventory and, 266, *267–269*
stereognosis and, 246
two-point discrimination and, 246
visual function and, 248
Retrieval, memory, 187
Rhizotomy, 138
Righting reflex, 248–249
Rigidity states, 24
Roles, social, 151
Rotation, axial, of trunk, improvement of motor control and, 316–317

SCALP, primary impact damage to, 39–40
Scanning-type communication aids, 364
Schema, body, 247–248, *247*
Scope of cognitive remediation, 369–378, *370, 372, 374*
Secondary insults
mass lesions, multimodality evoked potentials and, 88, 91

Secondary insults—*continued*
  neurologic and systemic complications, multi-modality evoked potentials and, 91, 92t
Self-care skills, 276
Self-help groups
  as nonprofessional family intervention, 416–417
  patient-family education and, 399
Sensation, occupational therapy evaluation and, 274
Sensory evoked potentials, 75–77, *76, 77*
  detecting brain stem dysfunction with, 82, *83, 84,* 84–87, *85, 86*
Sensory impairments, 24–25, 25t
Sensory inventory, 266, *267–269*
Sensory responsiveness, assessment of, 245–246
  bilateral simultaneous stimulation and, 246–247
  body schema and, 247–248, *247*
  sensory inventory and, 266, *267–269*
  stereognosis and, 246
  two-point discrimination and, 246
  visual function and, 248
Sensory stimulation, improvement of motor control and, 316
Sequelae of head injury
  long-term, problems in establishing, 171–172
  mental, functional limitations and, 172–173, 174–175t
Severity of head injury
  clinical course and, 16–18
  extracranial injuries and, 17t
  Glasgow Coma Scale and, 15–16, 16t
  length of hospital stay and, 18
  pre-hospital care and, 14–15
  skull fractures and, 17t
Sex of head-injured patients, 11–12
Shaping, behavior, as behavioral principle, 383
Shift, brain, 45–46
Shock, cerebral, 313
Shoulder-shaking test, 249
Signal detection theory, 187
Signs of spasticity, 129–130
Sitting balance, *250,* 250–251
Skeletal trauma, 237
Skills
  communication, 148–149
  community, 277
  driving, 151–152
  family relationship, 149–150
  financial management, 151
  functional, perceptual dysfunction and, 343
  home living, 149, 276
    case history relating to, 149
  hygiene, 147
  self-care, 276
  social roles, 151

  time management, 150–151
Skull
  fractures of, 17t
  primary impact damage to, 39–40
Social adjustment, outcome and, 111–112
Social disabilities, 30, 30t
Social roles, 151
Socioeconomic status of head-injured patients, 12–13, *12*
Sodium, serum level of, 42
Somatosensory activities for perceptual dysfunction, 336, *337*
Somatosensory cortical response, 78–79
Somatosensory functions, 275
Space and form activities, for perceptual dysfunction, 337, *338*
Space and form perception, 275–276
Spasticity
  clinical features of, 129–130
  definition of, 125–126
  etiology and pathophysiology of, 126–129, *126, 127*
  evaluation of, 130–131
  management of, 132–139, 132t, 133t
Speech and language assessment, 279
  cognitive evaluation and, 279–280
  language evaluation and, 281–282
  natural recovery from head injury and, 285–287, 285t, 287t
  neuromuscular speech system and, 283
    apraxia of speech and, 283
    articulation and, 284
    dysarthria and, 283
    phonation and, 284
    prosody and, 285
    resonance and, 284
    respiration and, 284
Speech and language pathologist, role of, in communication disorders, 355
  cognitive retraining task force and, 356–357
  coma-arousal task force and, 356
  evaluation team and, 355
  provision of speech and language pathology therapy and, 357
  task force for swallowing dysfunction and, 356
Speech and language pathology, therapy for, 357
Speech system, neuromuscular, 283
  apraxia of speech and, 283
  articulation and, 284
  dysarthria and, 283
  phonation and, 284
  prosody and, 285
  resonance and, 284
  respiration and, 284
Splinting for spasticity, 133–134
Spring-a-ling, 340, *340*

Sprouting, collateral, 315
Staff attitude, positive, 346
Standing balance, motor assessment and, 252–253, *252*
  weight shift and, 320, *321*
Stereognosis, 246
Stimulation
  bilateral simultaneous, 246–247
  electric, for spasticity, 135
  environmental, reality orientation therapy and, 346–348
  proprioceptive, for perceptual dysfunction, 339–340, *339, 340*
  sensory, improvement of motor control and, 316
  tactile, for perceptual dysfunction, 341
  vestibular, for perceptual dysfunction, 341, *341*
    voluntary movement and, 318–320
  vibratory, 332–333
Storage, memory, 187
Strength, muscle, 273
Strengths and weaknesses, neuropsychologic assessment of, 299, *299*, 300t
Stress, family, head injury and, 215–216, 216t
Stretching techniques for spasticity, 133
Substitution, behavioral, 314
Subtentorial lesions, 62
Supersensitivity of denervation, 314–315
Supination, forearm, motor assessment and, 249–250
Supratentorial lesions, 61
Surgery
  indications for, in head injury, 52
  neurosurgery, for spasticity, 138–139
  orthopedic, for spasticity, 137–138
Swallowing dysfunction, task force for, 356
Swelling, brain, 43
Symmetric tonic neck reflex, 244
Symptoms of head injury, 212t, 213t
Syndrome(s)
  pain, 25, 25t
  postconcussion, 5, 31, 206
System, IRM, of assessing cognitive deficits, 176–181, *176, 178, 179*

TACTILE stimulation for perceptual dysfunction, 341
Target behaviors, 382–383
Task force
  cognitive retraining, 356–357
  coma-arousal, 356
  for swallowing dysfunction, 356
Techniques
  motor re-education, for spasticity, 135–136
  relaxation, for spasticity, 135–136
Temperature, body

  high, coma and, 65
  low, coma and, 64
Test(s)
  arm-dropping, 249
  Behavioral Competence Index, 180
  Boston Diagnostic Aphasia Examination, 298
  Boston Test for Aphasia, 159
  Communicative Activities of Daily Living technique, 298
  Degree of Language Impairment Scale, 359
  Disability Rating Scale, 301, 302t
  for measurement of outcome, 100
  Functional Ambulation Score, 253, *254*
  Glasgow Coma Scale, 4, 15–16, 16t, 48, 48t, 54–55, 102–103, 102t, 103t, 189, 231–232
  Glasgow Outcome Scale, 19, 19t, 20t, 97, 98t, 99, 109t, 110, 301
  Halstead-Reitan Battery, 292–293, 294–295t
  head-dropping, 245
  ice-water caloric, 67
  learning and memory, 99t
  Luria-Nebraska Neuropsychological Battery, 293, 296, 297t
  Luria's Neuropsychological Investigation, 293, 296t
  Minnesota Test for the Differential Diagnosis of Aphasia, 298, 359
  Neurosensory Center Comprehensive Examination for Aphasia, 298
  Porch Index of Communicative Ability, 298, 359
  Purdue Peg Board, 180
  Revised Benton Visual Retention, 298
  shoulder-shaking, 249
  Token, 298
  Wechsler Memory Scale, 298
  Western Aphasia Battery, 162–163
Theory
  learning, cognitive deficits and, 169
  signal detection, 187
Therapy. *See also* Treatment; Remediation
  family, as family intervention technique, 415–416
  reality orientation. *See* Reality orientation therapy
Thiamine, 64
Thioridazine, 385
Thorazine. *See* Chlorpromazine
Time management, 150–151
Time of injury, 14
Token Test, 298
Tomography, computed, 49, *50*, 67–68
  outcome from head injury and, 56
Tone, muscle, 273
Tonic vibratory reflex, 332–333

Tonus, muscle, assessment of, 244–245
Total contact casting, 330–331
Toxic encephalopathy, 61
Traffic accidents as cause of head injuries, 13–14
Training
    ambulation, 324–325
    bilateral reciprocal, 322, *323*, 324
Transitional living programs, behavioral deficits and, 388–389
Trauma, skeletal, 237
Traumatic injuries, coma and, 64
Treatment. *See also* Remediation; Therapy
    neuropsychologic, 300
    of behavioral deficits, 386
        transitional living programs, 388–389
        day programs for, 389–390
        inpatient, 386–388
    of communication disorders, 357
        aphasia and, 358–359t, 359–361, *362*
        dysarthria and, 361–363
        problems owing to cognitive dysfunction and, 357, 359
    of raised intracranial pressure, 53
    of spasticity, 132–139, 132t, 133t
    program of, in reality orientation therapy, 351–353
Tremors, 24
Triage, patient, 47–48
Trunk, axial rotation of, improvement of motor control and, 316–317
Two-point discrimination, 246

UNCONSCIOUSNESS
    due to head trauma, pathophysiology of, 62
    duration of, communication disorders and, 157
Uncus, temporal lobe, herniation of, 62
Unemployment after head injury, 20t
Upper limb, motor control of, 326–328

VALIDITY of dynamometer, 259
Valium. *See* Diazepam
Vegetative state, 71
Vestibular stimulation
    for perceptual dysfunction, 341, *341*
    voluntary movement and, 318–320
Vibration, muscle, for spasticity, 135
Vibratory stimulation, 332–333
Vicarious function, 314
Visits, home
    evaluation form for, 402–405
    patient-family education and, 397–398
Visual activities for perceptual dysfunction, 336
Visual awareness, 274–275
Visual function, 248
Visual impairment, types of, 25t
Vocational and educational disabilities, 30–31
Vocational deficits. *See* Educational and vocational deficits
Voluntary movement, vestibular stimulation and, 318–320

WEAKNESSES and strengths, neuropsychologic assessment of, 299, *299*, 300t
Wechsler Memory Scale, 186, 188, 298
Weight bearing, stimulation of, 320–322
Weight shifting
    from sitting to standing, 251, *251*
    in standing position, 252–253, *252*
    sitting, *250*, 250–251
    standing balance and, 320, *321*
Western Aphasia Battery, 162–163